QUANTUM LEADERSHIP

SIXTH EDITION

CREATING SUSTAINABLE VALUE IN HEALTH CARE

Nancy M. Albert PhD, CCNS, CHFN, CCRN, NE-BC, FAHA, FCCM, FHFSA, FAAN
Associate Chief Nursing Officer Research and Innovation
Cleveland Clinic Health System
Cleveland, Ohio

Clinical Nurse Specialist
Kaufman Center for Heart Failure
Heart, Vascular, and Thoracic Institute
Cleveland Clinic
Cleveland, Ohio

Sharon H. Pappas, PhD, RN, NEA-BC, FAAN
Chief Nurse Executive
Emory Healthcare
Atlanta, Georgia

Clinical Professor
Nell Hodgson Woodruff School of Nursing
Emory University
Atlanta, Georgia

Tim Porter-O'Grady, DM, EdD, ScD, APRN, FAAN
Senior Partner
Health Systems TPOG, LLC
Atlanta, Georgia

Clinical Professor
Nell Hodgson Woodruff School of Nursing
Emory University
Atlanta, Georgia

Kathy Malloch, PhD, MBA, RN, FAAN
President
Kathy Malloch Leadership Systems, LLC
Glendale, Arizona

Clinical Professor
The Ohio State University, College of Nursing
Columbus, Ohio

Case studies prepared by
Jaynelle F. Stichler, DNS, RN, NEA-BCr, FACHE, FAAN
Founding Co-Editor Emerita, HERD Journal
Consultant, Caster Institute for Nursing Excellence,
Sharp HealthCare
San Diego, California
Professor Emerita, San Diego State University
San Diego, California

World Headquarters
Jones & Bartlett Learning
5 Wall Street
Burlington, MA 01803
978-443-5000
info@jblearning.com
www.jblearning.com

Jones & Bartlett Learning books and products are available through most bookstores and online booksellers. To contact Jones & Bartlett Learning directly, call 800-832-0034, fax 978-443-8000, or visit our website, www.jblearning.com.

Substantial discounts on bulk quantities of Jones & Bartlett Learning publications are available to corporations, professional associations, and other qualified organizations. For details and specific discount information, contact the special sales department at Jones & Bartlett Learning via the above contact information or send an email to specialsales@jblearning.com.

Copyright © 2022 by Jones & Bartlett Learning, LLC, an Ascend Learning Company

All rights reserved. No part of the material protected by this copyright may be reproduced or utilized in any form, electronic or mechanical, including photocopying, recording, or by any information storage and retrieval system, without written permission from the copyright owner.

The content, statements, views, and opinions herein are the sole expression of the respective authors and not that of Jones & Bartlett Learning, LLC. Reference herein to any specific commercial product, process, or service by trade name, trademark, manufacturer, or otherwise does not constitute or imply its endorsement or recommendation by Jones & Bartlett Learning, LLC and such reference shall not be used for advertising or product endorsement purposes. All trademarks displayed are the trademarks of the parties noted herein. *Quantum Leadership: Creating Sustainable Value in Health Care, Sixth Edition* is an independent publication and has not been authorized, sponsored, or otherwise approved by the owners of the trademarks or service marks referenced in this product.

There may be images in this book that feature models; these models do not necessarily endorse, represent, or participate in the activities represented in the images. Any screenshots in this product are for educational and instructive purposes only. Any individuals and scenarios featured in the case studies throughout this product may be real or fictitious, but are used for instructional purposes only.

The authors, editor, and publisher have made every effort to provide accurate information. However, they are not responsible for errors, omissions, or for any outcomes related to the use of the contents of this book and take no responsibility for the use of the products and procedures described. Treatments and side effects described in this book may not be applicable to all people; likewise, some people may require a dose or experience a side effect that is not described herein. Drugs and medical devices are discussed that may have limited availability controlled by the Food and Drug Administration (FDA) for use only in a research study or clinical trial. Research, clinical practice, and government regulations often change the accepted standard in this field. When consideration is being given to use of any drug in the clinical setting, the health care provider or reader is responsible for determining FDA status of the drug, reading the package insert, and reviewing prescribing information for the most up-to-date recommendations on dose, precautions, and contraindications, and determining the appropriate usage for the product. This is especially important in the case of drugs that are new or seldom used.

21607-3

Production Credits
VP, Product Management: Amanda Martin
Director of Product Management: Matthew Kane
Product Manager: Tina Chen
Content Strategist: Christina Freitas
Manager, Project Management: Kristen Rogers
Project Specialist: Kelly Sylvester
Senior Digital Project Specialist: Angela Dooley
Senior Marketing Manager: Jennifer Scherzay
VP, Manufacturing and Inventory Control: Therese Connell
Product Fulfillment Manager: Wendy Kilborn
Composition: S4Carlisle Publishing Services
Cover Design: Michael O'Donnell
Senior Media Development Editor: Troy Liston
Rights & Permissions Manager: John Rusk
Cover Image (Title Page, Chapter Opener): © Pobytov/iStock/Getty Images
Printing and Binding: Sheridan Books

Library of Congress Cataloging-in-Publication Data
Names: Albert, Nancy, author. | Pappas,
  Sharon, author. | Porter-O'Grady, Timothy, author. | Malloch, Kathy, author.
Title: Quantum leadership : creating sustainable value in health care /
  Nancy Albert, Sharon Pappas, Tim Porter-O'Grady, Kathy Malloch.
Description: Sixth edition. | Burlington, Massachusetts : Jones & Bartlett
  Learning, [2022?] | Tim Porter-O'Grady's name appears first in the
  previous edition. | Includes bibliographical references and index.
Identifiers: LCCN 2020025768 | ISBN 9781284216073 (paperback)
Subjects: MESH: Leadership | Health Services Administration |
  Organizational Innovation
Classification: LCC RA971 | NLM W 84.1 | DDC 362.1068--dc23
LC record available at https://lccn.loc.gov/2020025768

6048

Printed in the United States of America
24 23 22   10 9 8 7 6 5 4 3

Chapter Three	Innovation Leadership and Professional Governance: Building the Structure for Transformation 105

Definitions and Concepts 107
Rationale for Healthcare Innovation 108
Innovation Label Versus Innovation Role 115
Conclusion 125

Chapter Four	Innovation and Opportunity: Leading Through the White Water of Change 139

Driving the Culture of Innovation 140
Equity and Partnership 142
Decisions and Structures 143
The Centrality of the Point-of-Service 147
Alignment, Not Motivation 149
Creating Stakeholder Value 154
The Contextual/Strategic Role of the Board 155
The C-Suite and the Context for Innovation 158
First-Line Leaders: The Catalyst for Innovation 159
Creating a Context That Supports the Innovator 162
Innovation and the Membership Community 164
Balancing Innovation with Value 166
Differentiating Roles in Innovation 167
Leadership and the Will to Innovate 170
Conclusion 172

Chapter Five	From Evidence to Innovation: Measuring the Foundations of Practice and Value 187

Key Drivers for Change 188
A Very Complex System 193
Emergence and Uncertainty 194
New Healthcare Valuation Model 196
Conclusion 207

Chapter Six	Diversity and Difference: Managing Conflict in a Transdisciplinary Network 217

Growth and Transformation 220
Avoiding Unnecessary Conflict 222
Team-Based Conflict Issues 227
Identity-Based Conflicts 229

CONTENTS

Preface viii
Acknowledgments xii
Case Study Instructions xiv

Chapter One   **A New Landscape for Leadership: Changing the Health Script in an Age of Value** 1

Leading in a World of Constant Movement 2
Newton and Organizational Design 4
Leading in the Postdigital Age 5
Change Is 7
Postdigital Leadership 8
Endless Change 10
The Quantum Character of Leadership 14
The Compression of Time Will Affect How Work Is Done 35
Change and Effectiveness 38
Conclusion 40

Chapter Two   **Ten Complexity Principles for Leaders Advancing Value in the Quantum Age** 53

Chaos and Complexity and the Drive for Value 56
Principle 1: Wholes Are Not Just the Sum of Their Parts 59
Principle 2: All Health Care Is Local 63
Principle 3: Value Is Now the Centerpiece of Service Delivery 66
Principle 4: Simple Systems Aggregate to Complex Systems 68
Principle 5: Diversity Is Essential to Life 71
Principle 6: Error Is Essential to Success 72
Principle 7: Systems Thrive When All of Their Functions Intersect and Interact 74
Principle 8: Equilibrium and Disequilibrium Are in Constant Tension 79
Principle 9: Change Is Generated from the Center Outward 82
Principle 10: Revolution Results from the Aggregation of Local Changes 85
Conclusion 90

Interest-Based Conflicts 245
People and Behavior 257
Conclusion 259

Chapter Seven   Leading Constant Movement: Transforming Chaos and Crisis 271

Normative and Nonnormative Crisis 272
The Leader's Perception of Crisis. 273
Understanding Crisis. 274
Complexity and Technology. 275
Complexity and Organizations 276
Adaptive Capacity and Change 277
The Human Resources Focus 279
Adaptive Capacity in Human Organizations 280
Strategic Crisis Management 282
Macro Considerations for Organizational Crisis. 285
Synthesizing External and Internal Factors 287
Strategic Core 288
Team Performance. 289
Team Outcomes 290
User Expectations. 292
The Partnership Team Process Factors 293
Impact on Outcomes 299
Internalization and Externalization. 301
Ensuring a Strong Service Core 303
Crisis and Environmental Scanning 304
Crisis Preparedness 308
Planning 308
Recovery/Salvage Stage 310
Adaptive Effectiveness. 312
Conclusion 315

Chapter Eight   The Focused Leader: Embracing Vulnerability, Risk Taking, and the Potential to Succeed 325

Leadership Fitness in the New Millennium 326
Vulnerability 327
Power 328
The Cycle of Vulnerability. 331
New Relationships 343
Complexity Communication 348
Collective Mindfulness 352

    Strategies for Cultivating Leadership Vulnerability. 353
    Is There a Choice? 357
    Conclusion 357

Chapter Nine — Transforming Error and Engaging Failure Toward a Culture of Safety 371

    Creating the Context for Safety 372
    Just Culture 373
    Learning 375
    Teamwork 376
    Evidence-Based Practice 382
    Patient-Centered Care 383
    Leadership 383
    Healthcare Leadership: Issues and Opportunities 385
    Highly Reliable Organizations and Safety Culture 404
    Conclusion 404

Chapter Ten — The Fully Engaged Leader: Demonstrating Capacity to Sustain Relationships. 417

    Underpinnings of Emotional Competence 419
    Nature of Emotional Competence 422
    Emotional Risks of Leadership 433
    Benefits of Emotional Competence in Health Care 434
    Developing Emotional Competence 439
    Emotionally Incompetent Behaviors 442
    Team Emotional Competence 443
    Connecting with Generations of Workers 446
    Conclusion 448

Chapter Eleven — Toxic Organizations and People: The Leader as Transformer 459

    Cultures Depend on Healthy Individuals to Help Patients Heal 461
    How Does Toxicity Develop? 462
    How Leaders Shape Culture 463
    Leadership Polarity Dominates 464
    Millennial Nurses Crave Connection 464
    Toxic Behaviors 466
    Ten Principles for Minimizing Toxic Behavior in Organizations 480
    Conclusion 489

Chapter Twelve   **Coaching for Unending Change: Transforming the Membership Community** **503**

From Responsibility to Accountability 504
Transforming Work and the Transforming Worker 508
Evolution and Revolution 510
The Learning Organization 511
Organizing for Transformation 516
Dealing with the Lack of Time 520
The Leader as Revolutionary 524
Innovation Coaching 527
Making Integration Work 532
Addressing Problems Head On 534
Eliminating Firefighting Altogether 537
Conclusion 540

Chapter Thirteen   **The Leader's Courage to Be Willing: Building a Context for Hope** **551**

A Context for Hope 552
Will 553
Strategies to Facilitate Willingness 561
Relighting the Lamp 574
Conclusion 576

Chapter Fourteen   **Engaging the Spirit of Leadership: Becoming a Living Leader** **587**

Chaos and the Call to Leadership 588
Self-Management and Creativity 591
Creativity and Innovation 594
Exercising the Spirit 604
Spiritual Intelligence: 10 Mindful Rules of the Road 608
Becoming Self 613
Listening for the Sounds of Change 614
Finding Spirit in the Chaos 616
The Compensations of Ignorance 617
Mystery 619
Synthesis and Synergy 620

Appendix: Quiz Answers 631
Index 633

PREFACE

When this text was first written in 2002, health care was on the verge of many shifts and transformations. After years of preparing for major transformation in health care, we are now experiencing multiple transformations that are reconfiguring our healthcare delivery systems. Political transitions are reshaping healthcare reform. Other changes that are shifting the very foundation of health care are the continual progression of information technology used in community and individual prevention, assessment, management, and evaluation and in healthcare provider and clinician work. The digital age has brought us artificial intelligence, apps, and software that allow us to predict risk, prevent untold events, and plan care in ways we could not imagine many years ago. Further, as the world changes, there is a need to explicitly share and understand new notions of how to advance the work of organizations and people, and to develop new patterns of behavior. Just like other segments of society, health care is going through the drama and trauma of reconceptualizing its work and priorities to take into account the new global reality, sustainable health reform, value-driven care, changing payment models, and the advances in therapeutics and clinical technology. Multiple advances are already bearing fruit and radically altering both quantity and quality of life. Changes yet to come will have an even greater impact than did those that have already occurred. We hope this *Sixth Edition* has kept up with recent changes and reflects the best thinking on the state of the art of contemporary leadership. For healthcare leaders, transformational changes can help us work smarter, faster, and with greater accuracy. We can monitor quality and safety more accurately, facilitate and maintain a highly reliable culture, support the well-being of our clinicians, and develop just-in-time solutions to work issues or needs.

As we update this *Sixth Edition*, we are still surprised and pleased that much of what is included in this text remains relevant and essential to both guiding and thriving in the emerging healthcare milieu. We are dedicated to ensuring that the most current and relevant information is contained in this text, and we are committed to updating its contents every 2 years. Ultimately, we strive to ensure that the most current and relevant insights related to "quantum leadership" are contained within, in a way that helps prepare and inform contemporary leaders. As an example, contemporary healthcare leaders are relying more and more on the ever-increasing digitalization and mobility of health services, the increasing availability and complexity of "big data," and the growing utility that digitalization and big data have in informing healthcare decisions and actions. Accountability for choice and proper action are coming to rest in the hands of "users" of data. Healthcare leaders have the important job of enabling providers to alter their practices to include use of connected technologies and preparing users to assume accountability that is increasingly being appropriately transferred to them. Newer therapies and technologies are making it necessary to build evidence regarding clinical work that truly makes a difference in the lives of those we serve and in the health of our communities. Leaders in all health settings must be grounded in evidence, and they have a central role in the creation and utilization of innovations in clinical therapeutics, delivery models, and supporting infrastructures. Although the themes seem to be opposed, a delicate balance exists between current evidence and novelty; these two factors are in motion together and together can lead to transformational leadership changes.

A leadership book like this one serves as a dynamic snapshot, if you will, of the leadership role at a particular moment in time. In our attempt to identify and describe the correct behaviors and strategies for the role, we focus on the issues that are most representative of the current era. One of the earmarks of our era, of course, is the accelerating rate of change in the substantive reformatting of the delivery of health care, including the obvious challenges of ensuring access, availability, and payment for health care for all Americans regardless of socioeconomic status, disabilities, and institutional healthcare disparities. Another dynamic earmark is leaders' responsibilities in responding to a pandemic or other crises. We include current and emerging issues related to the value-based drivers influencing payment to facilitate unique opportunities for more effective contemporary leadership.

The peculiarity of books on leadership is that they can never be truly finished or even "current." Leadership is essentially a never-ending work in progress—an endless journey with facets and elements that add up to a broad and complex mosaic. Embedded in the leadership role is a host of behavioral, relational, interactional, and structural considerations that give form to the activity of leading. Research in each of these areas could line the shelves of libraries for generations. We submit that no one person could comprehend all that has been said and written about leadership or all the actions that have been done in its name. Ultimately, healthcare leaders must push their organizations further into the value-driven age as well as into the fray of reformatting health delivery. They must be able to see into the darkness of the future, and also to live comfortably inside the potential—that risky, unsettled space between the present and the future. And because leaders cannot pull people into a future that only they have conceived of, they must bring everyone to the table to shape the future through collective dialogue and concerted action at all times, understanding both the value to health care and the benefit to clinicians of engaging them in the process because they know best what the changes must be.

As professionals, it is becoming increasingly important to build an evidentiary foundation that provides a clear demonstration of the relationship between the processes and the impact of our work. For too long, the focus of professional work has been on the work itself: the quality of that work, the content of the work, and how well the work was done. Increasingly, the challenges between appropriate resource use and the outcomes of clinical work have raised the specter of incongruity and our often frequent failure to advance the health status of those we serve. Value now calls for health professionals to make a strong case for practice and establish a firm foundation that demonstrates a goodness-of-fit between the action of clinical practice and the impact of advancing social health. And now, this must be done within the context of equity-based provider teams committed to advancing the health of those they serve in a cost-effective and price-sensitive environment. Evidentiary dynamics is now a fundamental subset of both leadership and clinical work. Improvement sciences and value-based practices and payment require both technological and practice frames that elicit best practices and advance the user experience. Ultimately, leaders have an obligation to ensure that there is a tight relationship between the aggregated net health status of the community and the resources used to obtain and sustain it.

In this *Sixth Edition*, we try to conceptualize the newer complexity-based realities in health care and use the emerging foundations as a template to prioritize leadership skills and behaviors—those skills and behaviors that leaders can use to ensure that their organizations are guided accurately and effectively. Our strategy is first to provide a glimpse into the future and then to present some of the implications of the maturing sciences of complexity and chaos. We delineate the context of the leadership role as we all move further into the 21st century in order to help leaders make sense of this continuously emergent sociotechnical world with all its risks and opportunities.

Anticipating change requires the ability to predict and adapt to transformation and the crisis that both stimulates it and represents the appropriate response. Leaders must now recognize the ever-constant company of the serendipitous occurrences that are reflected in a fast-paced and highly changing environment. Leaders must model and inculcate a predictive and adaptive capacity into the life of their organizations and into the skills of all staff in the organization.

There is simply no way that reforming and advancing health care can unfold without a great deal of conflict. Most people assume that conflict in the workplace is bad and should be avoided. Nothing could be further from the truth. Conflict is a normal element of all interaction. Leaders must understand this and acquire the necessary skills to manage conflict in a way that yields the benefits that it is capable of delivering. By handling conflict appropriately, leaders also are better positioned to create a healing environment for providers as well as consumers of health care and to undertake the healing of a wide variety of emotional and spiritual injuries suffered by people as they struggle with the work of transforming the healthcare system. Building a healthy environment by being fully present and demonstrating compassion and accountability is a fundamental responsibility of contemporary leaders.

Not only is it necessary to handle conflict effectively, it is necessary to see organizations as being in constant flux and subject to continuous change. Leaders now must both predict and adapt to the patterns of change that affect their people and their organizations. An adaptive and predictive capacity is a necessity for good leaders if their organizations are going to continue to thrive and change as new conditions and technology emerge. Developing these insights and the skill of predictive and adaptive capacity provides a good skill foundation to ensure that organizations of the future continue to change and sustain themselves.

Over the previous two decades, a host of authors and researchers have reminded us that leaders must possess not just intellectual ability but also mindfulness and emotional competence. After all, establishing and maintaining relationships are an essential part of leadership, and all relationships have an emotional component. To ensure that leaders' relationships exhibit emotional maturity, they need to understand themselves through mindful reflection expressed through a high level of emotional competence in a way that touches the emotional center in themselves and others. The value of personal mindfulness and emotional maturity for leadership is just beginning to be understood.

Behavior does not exist in a vacuum, and thus the context within which people interact and work together requires as much consideration as what they do. The enormous changes that are occurring, some of them very traumatic, cause people to see themselves awash in a sea of movement that does not make much sense. Staff members often fail to understand the direction in which their leaders are taking them and begin to lose hope and any sense that their work is meaningful. Leaders, in their actions, can provide the foundations for hope and meaning and value. They must first find these things for themselves and then translate them into a language that others can comprehend and own.

Why are some leaders more successful than others at leading an organization through transformational change? Why do some create an environment of hope and calm despite difficult or even desperate circumstances? The answers can be found in the notion of personal willingness. Willing leaders are the cocreators of change. They recognize that no one person or situation can take away their personal peace, joy, or sense of competence. They transmit these feelings to others in a way that encourages and enables them to embrace the new script and share in the writing of it.

In the contemporary context for health care, a capacity for innovation is no longer optional. Every leader now must operate within an innovation mental model that includes both stimulating and guiding innovations. Leaders need to demonstrate an availability to the inventive and the creative that are so much a part of our fast-paced sociotechnical existence. Innovation is more than a process. It is increasingly evident that there is a science that drives it. As we become more aware of the action of complexity and its consonance with the movement of systems, the role of the emergent and transformational substrate of existence becomes more definitive. It is the role of a leader to create both context and conditions that harness this energy and facilitate the discourse, discovery, and application of this knowledge in advancing the quality of life and our human experience. Creating the context for the dynamics of innovation is now a central role of leadership capacity and is essential to the ability to be sustained and to thrive.

Coaching people into the future they must live in requires special skills. Unlike in the past, leaders cannot simply force people into a mold or into compliance with demands that they played no part in setting. Allowing people to be investors, partners, and stakeholders in their own processes is a talent necessary in new leaders. Leading workers out of a toxic and perennially sick or stuck work environment is a part of this process. It requires leaders to understand the characteristics of neurotic and pathological organizations and those behaviors that prevent people and their organizations from embracing the changes they must adapt to in order to thrive in the new world of health care.

Finally, leaders must focus on the energy and spirit within to be innovative and grow and thereby act as models for others in their own search for meaning and value in what they do. But the ability to exhibit creativity, self-understanding, and personal growth is not obtained accidentally or without effort; it requires regular mental and spiritual exercise, including periods of reflection, to refine it. In the future, leaders, to sustain their effectiveness in the leadership role, will need to engage in reflective personal work and increase their level of creativity and well-being.

Like others of its kind, this book is always a work in progress. It is necessarily and forever incomplete. There is already a host of good books on contemporary leadership, with more arriving on the bookshelves every day. They, too, are incomplete. What individuals who want to learn about leadership must do is see the myriad available resources on the topic as making up a single dynamic and growing body of knowledge. Thus, if they want to improve their leadership skills, they should use this book as one resource along with others, understanding at the same time that the theories of leadership and their application will advance as more information becomes available.

We hope that the contents of this Sixth Edition of *Quantum Leadership* stimulate reflection and discussion. We believe that this book extrapolates newer ways of conceiving and exercising the leadership role. At this time, leaders are challenged to take the next step in the journey toward better and more relevant methods of leadership. Those whose lives leaders impact have a right to expect the best that leaders have to offer, especially as more is demanded of professionals than ever before. We hope this *Sixth Edition* plays some small role in ensuring that those who provide healthcare services get from their leaders what they have every right to expect and, as a result, the health of our nation is advanced.

—Nancy Albert, Sharon Pappas, Tim Porter-O'Grady, and Kathy Malloch

ACKNOWLEDGMENTS

We acknowledge Cathleen Krueger Wilson, PhD, RN, nurse, therapist, consultant, colleague, and friend to Tim and Kathy, who first conceived the possibility of this kind of book on leadership. Her creativity and imagination in applying leadership to all venues of health service were an inspiration and a joy to all who knew her. Cathleen was a role model as nurse, mother, spouse, and friend and brought the full weight and energy of her person to her work and relationships. In death, as in life, she still serves to stimulate and encourage the best in all whose lives she touched.

We also acknowledge and thank our leadership colleague Jaynelle Stichler, DNSc, RN, FAAN, for her excellent contribution of chapter-based case studies for each of the topical chapters in this text. Dr. Stichler serves as an exemplar of nursing leadership and leadership practice excellence, as clearly demonstrated in the quality of cases contained in this text.

My role as author of the Sixth Edition of *Quantum Leadership* is possible because of the brilliantly completed previous work by Tim Porter-O'Grady and Kathy Malloch, who envisioned the need for this leadership book and brought previous editions to life. I appreciate their trust that Sharon Pappas and I could faithfully update content to reflect current leadership expectations, and also current and upcoming challenges leaders must face head on and work through to succeed in their roles. I am grateful to my workplace and national organization colleagues, as their open communication, collaborations, and insights strengthen my own leadership capabilities, and importantly, to my wonderful family—my husband Gerard and children Samantha, Bill, Alyssa, and Stephanie—who provide a wonderful counterbalance to my work life. Their ongoing support and levity, and their ability and timing in creating memorable moments are cherished and always appreciated.

—Nancy M. Albert

Standing on the shoulders of giants is clearly how I feel as with this opportunity to continue with Nancy Albert this important leadership journey by advancing the *Sixth Edition*. I appreciate Kathy and Tim's confidence that Nancy and I can contribute to the advancement of healthcare leaders' growth in this way. My hope is that those that consume this text will benefit from its content. I learned much about leadership in my places of practice both in Colorado and Georgia, and for that I am forever grateful. What I have learned is vast, and my hope is that this book gives me a chance to give back to all of those I practiced with plus many others. I learned a lot, too, about leadership by being a parent to my amazing girls, Kristen and Ruth (who is also a nurse)—for that I am grateful. Finally, thank you to my precious husband, Greg, who always supports me and is the reason I have been able to succeed. God is good.

—Sharon Holcombe Pappas

This Sixth Edition of *Quantum Leadership* could not have been completed without the support of a good number of people. First, I thank my coauthor, Kathy Malloch, who committed full time and energy to this book and whose collaboration continually encourages me. I also acknowledge the many colleagues in nursing and health care who were both the subject source and the motivation for this book and have much to do with its content. Their encouragement kept us focused on writing a text that is both relevant and useful. Finally, I thank Mark Ponder, for his 40 years of support and partnership, and for being a sign to me that caring, loving, and nursing have nothing to do with gender.

—Tim Porter-O'Grady

The Sixth Edition of *Quantum Leadership* is the result of insights garnered from our many dedicated readers, and for this we are grateful. We acknowledge and thank our colleagues for their undying dedication to lifelong learning so they can influence and empower others to be the best they can be. Thank you, Tim, for your friendship and unquestionable support—you are one very special person: a leader, a healer, a thinker, a visionary, and a great colleague. Finally, my greatest thanks and recognition go to my husband, Bryan "Mallotchi," my very best friend and confidant, always encouraging me and tolerating my inconsistencies. Without his unconditional support, my work as a leadership advocate and healer would not be nearly as meaningful.

—Kathy Malloch

CASE STUDY INSTRUCTIONS

The use of case studies in education provides a rich opportunity for students to employ situated cognition in the application of new knowledge when analyzing the case situations in a low-stakes environment. Case study analysis as a teaching method uses abstract conceptualization with active participation and experimentation as the students reflect on each case scenario, applying experiential knowledge learned from personal experience and the new cognitive knowledge from content read in the textbook chapters (Kolb et al., 2000).

In each chapter, two case studies related to the material are provided. These can be used to facilitate classroom discussion or can be assigned for individual student learning beyond reading the chapter content. Each case study presents real-life situations, complete with complexity, structured controversy, extraneous and pertinent information, emotion, and decisions that need to be made by weighing all possible options and using the new knowledge gained from reading the chapter.

In reviewing each case, students should use critical thinking and problem-solving skills to analyze the case. They can apply principles from the chapter content to identify possible methods to resolve the case or to reflect on personal insights to enrich class discussion.

Students should be encouraged to (1) identify the stakeholders in each case, (2) describe the case situation from the perspective of each stakeholder, (3) apply the chapter's content as a framework for analyzing the case, and (4) determine a course of action to resolve the case, recognizing that there is not one correct answer or best way to resolve each case.

The case studies can be assigned as reflective essays or they can be applied as a framework that students can use to write a case from their own experience. They can present their cases to the class or demonstrate knowledge and application of the chapter's content in class discussion.

The case study analyses amplify the chapter content and engage students in applying the principles to real organizational situations.

References

Kolb, D. A., Boyatzis, R. E., & Mainemelis, C. (2000). Experiential learning theory: Previous research and new directions. In R. J. Sternberg & L. F. Zhang (Eds.), *Perspectives on cognitive, learning and thinking styles*. Erlbaum.

CHAPTER ONE

A New Landscape for Leadership: Changing the Health Script in an Age of Value

> The hardest thing is not to get people to accept new ideas; it is to get them to forget old ones.
>
> —John Maynard Keynes

Chapter Objectives

At the completion of this chapter, the reader will be able to:

- Contrast the characteristics of traditional leadership with those of complexity leadership.
- Enumerate the elements of quantum leadership and explain how quantum thinking has influenced movement through the Age of Technology and throughout processes of continuous health transformation.
- Assess the impact of quantum science and recent advances in technology on healthcare value and clinical practice outcomes.
- Describe the implications of digitally driven environments on leadership actions in a time of healthcare reform.
- Identify the different skill sets for leaders in contemporary complex organizations.

The timelessness of transformation continues to influence the trajectory of healthcare reform. Every age is ever-evolving and transformative, filled with a host of inspiring and challenging opportunities that in centuries past were the stuff of science fiction. Who would have thought that this generation would see the advent of fiber-optics, virtual universities, cloning, customized DNA-based treatment modalities, genomics, lasers, 3D organ printing, and myriad technological innovations that boggle the mind, enthrall the imagination, and dramatically change the way we work? And who could have imagined that, after an intense, decades-long political and social debate, we would still be embracing and meeting the vagaries and challenges of implementing significant national health cost and quality expectations?

CHAPTER ONE   A New Landscape for Leadership: Changing the Health Script in an Age of Value

> **Key Point**
>
> Communication technology has created a world without boundaries. We now must create our own self-limiting boundaries in a way that produces a balance among the conflicting demands of our lives.
>
> The complexities of change and the overwhelming interaction and relationship between each element is enough to overwhelm even the most energized. As soon as we have the time to consider the particulars of recent changes, new changes are upon us, insinuating themselves into our culture. We do not even have the luxury of identifying their advantages and disadvantages or of considering their potential influence on our lives.

Along with these many innovations comes the challenging adjustments we must make to live in this increasingly digital universe. Instant communication, relationships across geographic boundaries, the globalization of economics and politics, internet interactions, virtual communication, and incoming knowledge that exceeds our capacity to assimilate it—all have a dramatic impact on our ability to thrive in the 21st century. For most of us, changes have come so fast that we do not fully comprehend how they will affect us; we are hard-pressed to cope with their implementation and fully understand their implications.

Our society, for instance, is just beginning to understand the impact of social media on our beliefs, knowledge, communication, business, and politics. Elements of social media already alter how we live our lives and change the questions we ask about what is passing before our very eyes. Questions of yesterday will not be answered within that context, because tomorrow has become today sooner than we ever could have imagined.

Leading in a World of Constant Movement

Fluidity has become a characteristic of doing business and managing life in every human arena. Because of the need to quickly accommodate change initiatives, the capacity to adjust course has become a necessity. In this context, leadership cannot be the same. Just as the underpinnings of our society, including how we deliver health care, are being radically transformed, so must the leadership that helps others adapt to essential change. Old models of leadership are no longer adequate to meet the demands of today. When the world was slower paced and systems theory, complexity theory, and quantum theory were not as well conceptualized or as influential, the nature and role of leadership were different. Even the operational realities of the workplace have changed to the point that work itself requires different skills and a different ethos (**Exhibit 1-1**).

Exhibit 1-1   New Versus Old Skill Sets

Knowledge Worker	Employee (Former Type)
• Conceptual synthesis/critical thinking	• Functional analysis
• Competent care	• Manual dexterity
• Multiple "intelligences"	• Fixed skill set
• Mobile skill set	• Process value
• Outcome practice	• Process practice
• Team performance	• Unilateral performance

Most of us in practice today have emerged from a time characterized by stable institutions into an increasingly contemporary framework exemplified by a more "network" context for work. The brick-and-mortar healthcare institutions of the past are breaking up, replaced by a growing digital architecture as work moves away from institutions altogether. The infrastructure of society is becoming less institutional and more information based, and the architecture of our places of work, service, and business is changing dramatically. Information structures are primarily relational and function collaterally and in multimodal ways, whereas most of our business structures have historically functioned vertically. Leading in a complex multimodal work culture is radically different from leading in a predominantly vertical or linear work culture.

In the recent past, the Industrial Age, organizations were primarily fixed, finite, and functional. Work in the Industrial Age was based on Newtonian principles, and from the beginning of the 20th century, when Frederick Taylor laid down the foundations of scientific management, to the late 1960s, business organizations were structured mechanistically and hierarchically. Even the management theorists of the 1930s, 1940s, and 1950s did not radically alter basic organizational design. Historically, the worker was mostly considered a subset of the work. Most training was gained on the job, and the apprenticeship model used for training was essentially hierarchical as well. The organization owned the work and set the rules. Communication and decision making traveled up and down the corporate ladder: the higher up the ladder, the greater a person's authority and autonomy. At the bottom were workers who performed most of the functions—under the control of those who had moved "upward." Although attention was paid to both the work and the worker, this attention was barely reflected in the management structure and the application of leadership in organizations. Leadership focused on the individual as leader and emphasized behavioral characteristics as the driving centerpiece of leadership learning. Now, leadership is seen through a lens that focuses on factors external to the person of the leader and provides different insights with regard to the requisites of good leadership.

> **Point to Ponder**
>
> The worker is increasingly in control. Knowledge necessary to get work done is now mostly in the hands of those who do the work. Because the workplace is becoming more dependent on knowledgeable workers, a major shift in power and control has occurred, and old structures are now in conflict with this new type of worker.

Much has changed in the life of the organization and the role of the leader. In the current world of work, it is not the organization but the worker who owns the work. Over the last 2 decades, the character of work has changed—it has become increasingly technical and complex, and often relies on knowledge work. Today, individuals usually need to be trained for jobs before they become eligible for them—they are expected to arrive "on the run" and start contributing from the outset. Further, organizations' increased dependence on knowledge workers has created a new power equation, shifting the locus of control from the organization to the worker and the work.

In the Industrial Age, leadership meant being a good manager, guiding one's subordinates like a good parent, and directing their activities in the interests of the organization; essentially, a bureaucratic framework (Uhl-Bien et al., 2007). The critical skills were those required for planning, organizing, leading, implementing, controlling, and evaluating (note the acronym constructed from these six words: POLICE). The ability to function well and undertake

Exhibit 1-2 Work Life Reality Shift

Old Reality	New Reality
• Scripted lives	• Own your script
• Unlimited resources	• Finite resources
• Fixed functions	• Tightness of fit
• Employee	• Stakeholder/member
• Fixed jobs	• Fluid roles
• Promotion	• Work–life balance
• Constancy of employer	• Mobility/short-term tenure

well-defined processes has traditionally been the basis of every role. Good performance and a sense of responsibility were highly valued, strongly encouraged, and heavily rewarded.

It was also expected that workers' behaviors would demonstrate compliance with the expectations of the workplace. Organizational leaders used vertical communication and command strategies exclusively to ensure that the workplace stayed focused and orderly and that the work was performed efficiently. They also refined hierarchical mechanisms and fostered congruence of workplace behavior in whatever way they could.

In this industrial context, the first contemporary notions of leadership developed. A whole host of approaches to understanding leadership in complex systems and acting as a leader in these settings emerged during the past century, and each one reflected prevailing notions of work and workplace organization (**Exhibit 1-2**). These various approaches helped to create the current framework for leadership, in the realms of both action and decision making.

Newton and Organizational Design

Newtonian mechanics had a tremendous influence on 20th-century science and business. In particular, Newton's model of the physical universe influenced social theorists to view social relationships, roles, and work as highly mechanistic. The reason that this mechanistic framework was so pervasive was its clarity and simplicity, linear structure, and coherence, and its generalized agreement with people's notions of common sense. Especially appealing was its dependence on reductionism—the tenet that any complex phenomenon could be understood simply by reducing it to its smallest components and analyzing it compartmentally. This linear simplicity was especially appealing to business and organizational leaders and was embraced by them with great veracity in ways that would define the structure of work to this very day. As a result, entrepreneurs and organizational gurus constructed models of work in which work activities were highly compartmentalized, and they succeeded in spreading the use of these models throughout the world. Subsequently, work was generally designed with efficiency and effectiveness in mind, and special attention was paid to individual performance as a means of ensuring that the work was done as planned.

> **Key Point**
>
> In the Industrial Age model, the focus of work was on performing the right processes. In the postdigital model, the focus is on aligning good process with the right outcomes.

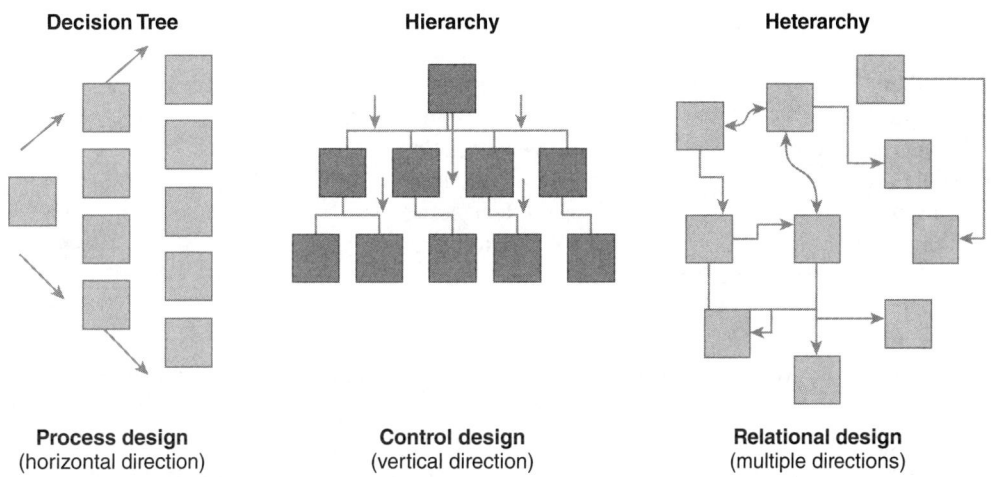

Figure 1-1 Changing Organizational Models.

Also, 20th-century organizations focused on the assumption that by constructing work processes properly, they would produce products and services of consistently good quality. Here again, the organizational literature of the time reflected a reductionist model. The organizational gurus viewed organizations as being essentially the same as always, although differing in structure in minor ways and characterized by an increased degree of control over employees. As Peter Drucker pointed out, the cornerstone of most 20th-century organizations was control, as indicated by the "line-and-box" approach to configuring the workplace (Edersheim & Drucker, 2007) (see **Figure 1-1**).

> ## Group Discussion
> We are living on the cusp of the transition between two health systems, and life in this contemporary age of health reform differs substantially from life in the traditional tertiary care system. Current changes include those involving clinical work and leadership. Brainstorm at least 10 changes that will occur in refining health reform and advancing health transformation over this next decade and discuss their implications for leaders.

Leading in the Postdigital Age

For the past 35 years or so, standard models of work and the underpinnings of society have been shifting radically. The impact of our burgeoning technology has brought about a new construct for social structures and relationships across the whole human landscape. Quantum theory, refined and applied since the middle of the 20th century, has helped to create newer technologies that affect life from the molecular to the global levels (Bilal et al., 2018).

Exhibit 1-3 Conceptual Foundations

Newtonian	**Quantum**
• Mass production	• Envision the whole
• Compartmentalism	• Integration
• Reductionism	• Synthesis
• Analysis	• Relatedness
• Discrete action	• Interdisciplinary team action

For example, consider the computer chip, which has single-handedly altered the human experience forever. Among other things, its continuing refinement generates a whole new understanding of quantum principles and has changed the very foundations of social life by connecting people in new ways. We now live with the knowledge that everything is linked, and that events in one part of the universe have an impact on events in other parts. Our understanding of the linkages among all experiences is the basis for complexity science and has led to changes in the conceptual foundations of the sciences and their social application (**Exhibit 1-3**).

Just as the understanding of convergence, relationships, and leading life at the interface or intersections of networks and systems is important, our understanding of networks as a structural framework for behavior requires leaders to conceptualize their role in the relationships between structure, process, and people, and to redefine the functional elements of leadership and of work. Newer understanding of the operation of complex adaptive systems and the resultant complex responsive processes serve to recalibrate the roles of leader and worker and reconfigure the very foundations of organization, relationships, and impact.

Along with a new understanding of changes that are congruent with complex adaptive systems, the level of conflict surrounding basic issues may be heightened, ranging from the existence and nature of God to ethical and social norms. Claims that once seemed beyond question are now open to investigation, continuous challenge, and new insights. New scientific discoveries have substantial religious, philosophical, scientific, and ethical implications and have caused social discomfort among those holding more rigid or linear beliefs (Volti, 2017).

It is into this equation that organizational leaders are now thrust. The problem is that they, too, are experiencing the conflict endemic to the times. Most leaders have spent the majority of their lives leading in Industrial Age models, just as everyone else has. They, too, are confronting newer realities with beliefs and practices acquired in the past. They, too,

Group Discussion

Healthcare providers in this time of significant health transformation must be willing to give up antiquated practices (because they will cease to have value) and to take on new practices. List some of the practices, habits, rituals, or routines that need to be left behind, and discuss symbolic acts or events that could be used to help let go of these formally. What replaces some of these "old" practices?

are struggling to make sense of the significant changes occurring globally. As an additional challenge to adapting to global changes, they must also lead others to adapt successfully to a whole new approach to understanding human organization, relationship, and behavior. Furthermore, related discoveries and innovations are occurring faster than the rate of adaptation. Dynamic changes require new or different responses; continual learning needs to become a cultural norm. To achieve transformational success and sustain change, leaders may use the science of learning health systems to operationalize change and meet goals (Meissner, 2018).

Change Is

Quantum theory continues to teach us that change is not a thing or an event but rather a dynamic that is constitutive of the universe. Change cannot be avoided because it is constant and ever present, but we can influence its circumstances and consequences. In short, although we cannot control it, we can give it direction. This notion of constant motion or change reflects foundations in quantum mechanics that suggest that matter is constantly moving in the universe and can even exist in more than one place at one time while taking different forms. Quantumness is almost counterintuitive, and reflects characteristics and dynamics of matter and energy that do not fit any logical, ordered, structured understanding of them.

Schrödinger, a mid-20th-century physicist, used his famous Schrödinger's box thought experiment to show two prevailing realities operating at any given time. He identified them as "actual reality" and "potential reality." Actual reality is that which currently occupies our immediate attention. Potential reality, however, although still current and present, is not yet experienced. Being still "potential," reality is waiting for the right moment to become expressed and visible, thus becoming "actual."

Potential reality is the realm in which leadership takes form. The leader's role is to engage with the unfolding reality; perceive it, even predict it; note its demands and implications; translate it for others; and, finally, guide others into actions to meet the demands of a reality not yet quite present. The leader must be comfortable with the ambiguity of the "in between"; that is, living in two realities, in the space between that which is ending and that which is emerging. Demonstrating this comfort with the journey provides a frame for leading others through the chaos and uncertainty of constant change.

In this transformational time between two paradigms, the leader's primary role is to live fully in the realm of potential reality. The leader is not only an operational expert and problem solver, but the leader is a good "signpost reader." To be effective, the leader must anticipate the path of change and then spell it out for those who are moving their own activities, knowingly or unknowingly, in the same direction as real change is taking form.

> **Point to Ponder**
>
> A stop sign can be used to illustrate potential reality. When first seen, it notifies a driver to stop—but not immediately. The sign is a real object, a reality, and it does require a real response. The driver's preparation to stop is the first in the chain of actions; however, it is only when the driver arrives at the stop sign that the act of actually stopping becomes real. Seeing the sign and preparing to stop is acting in consonance with "potential reality." Actually stopping at the stop sign represents "actual reality."

CHAPTER ONE   A New Landscape for Leadership: Changing the Health Script in an Age of Value

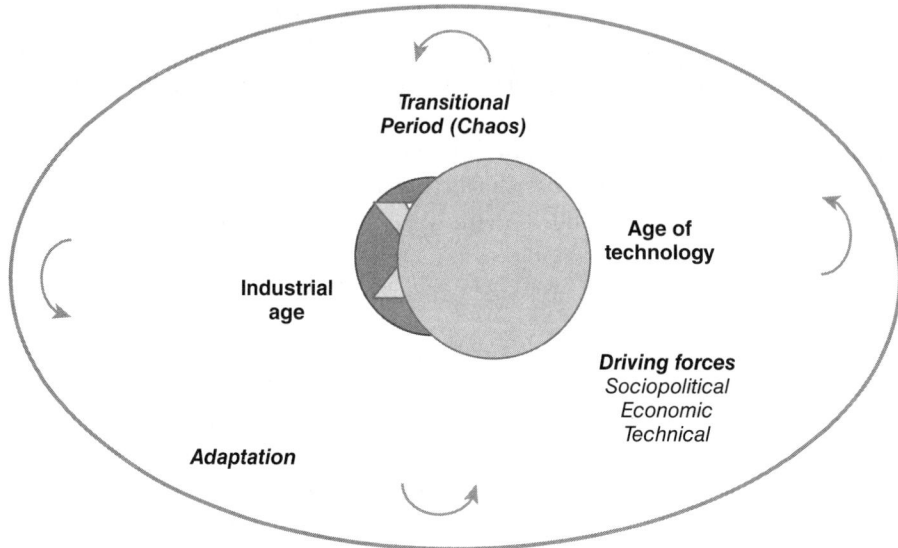

Figure 1-2 The Universal Cycle of Transformation.

Postdigital Leadership

Age changes do not occur quickly. Such massive changes generally occur over 2 or 3 decades. The challenge is not to become "stuck" in the no man's land between an extinguishing life script and an emerging one. This has occurred several times in human history. From the Middle Ages through the Age of Enlightenment and the Industrial Age and up to the current era, which we might dub the Digital Information Age, historic indicators have foreshadowed major shifts in the human experience (**Figure 1-2**).

However, an important difference exists between previous shifts and the one that is presently occurring. In hindsight, the significance of previous shifts quickly became clear, even if it was rarely apparent during the critical transition points. Today, the period between predicting future changes and confronting their unfolding is very brief—too brief to allow plans to be made to accommodate them. Indeed, today's network leaders act as agents of change, but, like everyone else, they must also undergo changes virtually at the same time as they perceive them. Wholly new leadership skills are required to manage in this kind of a world.

Think for a moment about some of the ways in which the script of life is being rewritten for all of us:

- Social media is now a primary communication and business tool, and it is fundamentally altering how business is done (Flury, 2017).
- Fiber-optics, in conjunction with satellite technology, has wirelessly connected the world into a seamless communications network in which information can be transmitted instantly from any place on the globe to any other place.

- Genetics, genomics, organ printing, and micromanipulation are demonstrating that the micronization of life processes can alter their trajectory and influence how life is experienced.
- Information has become highly portable, and, given the developments in shipping and delivery, everyone has access to almost anything they want or need from anywhere in the world. From decades of collecting and storing massive amounts of digital information, the current challenge is to be able to utilize and manage data in a way that advances the utility of it and its impact on human decision making and action.
- Technology, including voice technology and robotics, has enabled communication and interaction to become increasingly more available and portable as chips have become smaller and digital devices have become packed with technology and applications in lighter, smaller, multifunctional hardware.
- Each person has control over personal or business relationships and can personalize any interaction within any context at any time and in any way desired.
- Miniaturization has made it possible for people to be mobile and still remain connected to everything and everyone. Furthermore, miniaturization has prompted innovations in service, communication, information, wearable technology, and health care to be faster, easier, and less expensive to implement than ever before.
- Globalization has created a world community and removed traditional boundaries between people, be they political, social, or physical. The recognition of the mobility of human experience and of work has created a new virtual and global landscape for human action and relationships.

These are just a very small sample of the transformations that are occurring. These and other transformations are only the beginning of much more emergent substantive changes. Even so, they have a major impact on our understanding, on the way we live and relate, and, of course, on the way we work.

Imagine the lives of our great-grandparents, or even our grandparents, and how different our lives are from theirs as a result of technologies (keep in mind, for example, that digital cameras were not prototyped until 1984 and there were no cell phones before 1986). Then, consider the possibility that the children of current teenagers might never write or read as we have, interact and play as we have, relate to each other or travel in the same way we have. And remember, this generation is currently ushering in a new way of living and working as the baby boom generation continues to retire.

In short, our current age is a transitional generation—the last generation of the Industrial Age and the generation moving quickly and further into the Digital Age. Current generations

Group Discussion

List dramatic discoveries and inventions that occurred during the past century and compare the way life changed as a consequence with the way life changed during the preceding millennium. Then, discuss the technological changes occurring in the first decades of the 21st century that affect the future of health reform and care delivery.

are in essence the bridge between two ways of experiencing the world (i.e., compare digital immigrants to digital natives). What we do now lays the groundwork for a future that will look nothing like the world most of us have known.

Endless Change

It is important that leaders be aware of the transformative work that continually redefines their role. The Digital Age now calls for leaders to perceive their role differently, and to express it in ways that best fit the characteristics of an emerging sociopolitical, economic, technical culture (**Figure 1-3**).

The role of today's leaders is to encourage transformation. Indeed, they must make a commitment to the journey and work hard to incorporate changes in their lives in a very personal way. In other words, rather than simply suggesting that everyone and everything must change, they must lead by example. They must serve as witnesses to changes and show others how to adapt to changes by demonstrating their adaptation. Essentially, leaders must model the way and enable others to act.

> **Point to Ponder**
>
> The behavior of leaders must exemplify their commitment to sustain their own journey and to coordinate and facilitate the efforts of others to build a desired future.

In the initial stage of transformation, leaders must be able to show that the unfolding changes represent a critical shift and must, through their passion for movement, inspire responses from others. This is not the time for complacency but for truth-telling and transparent conversations. In short, it is a time to inform people how changes

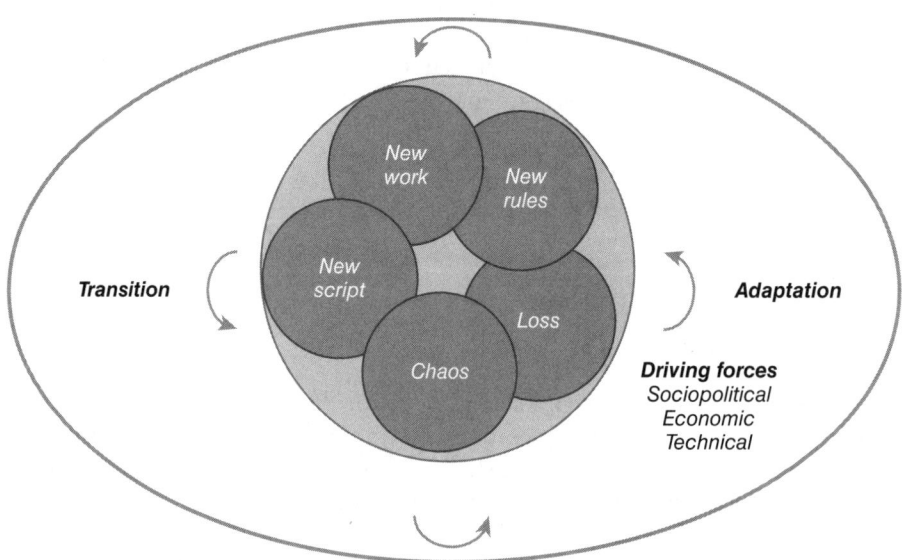

Figure 1-3 Universal Dynamics of Transformation.

will make a substantial difference in their lives and in their work. Advancing people's awareness of transformational change requires a level of honesty and directness once thought to be confrontational.

In the case of health care, the major reforms under way will lead to the end of the hospital-based sickness-oriented model of service delivery (tertiary-driven care). Our technologies and emerging clinical dynamics enable us to treat illnesses at an earlier stage (often via telemedicine) and reduce the need for costly surgical interventions or hospital stays. As a consequence, physicians, nurses, and other health professionals must make substantial changes in the way they practice their professions and provide services. The refinement of value-driven approaches and healthcare financing changes that focus on early engagement, attaining the highest level of personal health, prevention rather than treatment, and designing the system to provide a continuum of health services represents an effective model of health service (Ash et al., 2017; Birk, 2013).

Leaders in health care must help people sever their attachment to the kind of healthcare system with which they have become comfortable (Costich et al., 2015; Kane et al., 2019). Health reform requires all caregivers and leaders to focus on accountability, early engagement, prevention, cost-effectiveness, and a higher level of aggregate health for all citizens. Consumers and health professionals may mourn the loss of what is passing away or has passed away. A sense of loss is understandable, but most of what is mourned for *should not* be retained or brought back. That was then; this is now. Some factors that attracted many of us to health care have vanished for good. The question is not whether they will return, but how to adapt to new circumstances and new models of health service (Souba & Tsai, 2019).

Contemporary healthcare leaders must try to engage others in the process of making their own changes. They must take whatever action is necessary to impress upon health professionals that this is a time of great mobility and of shifting foundations. In particular, they must call all stakeholders to the table to work out what must be altered and what must be introduced to refine a new healthcare delivery system. A great tragedy will occur if healthcare leaders are unsuccessful in this task and allow stakeholders simply to react to what is perceived as established elements of healthcare delivery. Complacency guarantees failure.

Leaders may sometimes be victims of their own insights and past successes, which can cause them to use an outdated recipe for success as well as misleading measures of success. They must see the approaching challenges within the context of their becoming, not through the eyes of past triumphs. Indeed, past metrics may provide an impediment to measuring the unfolding of contemporary changes that represent an entirely different dynamic (Souba & Souba, 2018).

Not only must leaders close the door on the old models of health delivery and clinical work, but, after closing it, they must turn completely around to face the future, viewing the entire landscape to develop a workable vision. Often, healthcare leaders are too shortsighted, and their vision too tenuous. The conditions that determine the future of health care are vastly different from anything that we have experienced to date, and thus leaders must construct a radical vision of how services will be provided in the new healthcare landscape. The impact of micronization, genomics, biotherapeutics, chemotherapeutics, and new economic and service delivery models is constantly altering Western medicine (**Exhibit 1-4**), and so the structures that support the provision of Western medicine also need to change. The brick-and-mortar infrastructure and the current administrative and operational frameworks are no longer entirely relevant, and they must be adjusted in response to financial, political, and technological

Exhibit 1-4 Changing Medical Management

Old Therapies/Models	New Therapies/Models
• Surgery	• Lasers
• Salves, creams, and drugs	• Microsurgery
• Accommodation	• Genomics
• Nothing can be done	• Pharmaceuticals
• Treatments	• Chemotherapy
• Enemas	• Radiotherapy
• Bloodletting	• Synthetic products
• General supplements	• Specified supplements
• In-person treatment	• Telemedicine
• Objective provider assessment	• Patient-centered assessment
• Provider-led decisions	• Shared (participatory) decision making

pressures of a changing healthcare system. Imagine how painful that message is for the serious and talented men and women who have devoted their lives to building their image of the healthcare system. The requirement to tear it apart and begin anew is overwhelming to them, but they are called to this task by the changes that have already occurred and those anticipated as we refine and unfold health reform over the next 2 decades.

Contemporary health leaders must be able to communicate to others their vision of the future and bring as much energy and commitment to reforming the healthcare system as possible. They need to capture the hearts and minds of all health professionals and other stakeholders in the healthcare system by being relentless communicators and persistent challengers of current ways of thinking and doing. They must push against the walls of thought and work to ensure that stakeholders are fully engaged in critiquing what they do, building sustainable service partnerships, assessing the product of their work, and questioning whether what they are doing is congruent with the changing demands placed on them (Bennis et al., 2015). Every stakeholder must continually examine the appropriateness of current work rituals and routines and determine what should be retained and what should be left behind as no longer relevant. The job of leaders is to raise questions about the efficacy and effectiveness of current work processes and whether they are meeting new and emerging expectations for value-driven health care.

The most important task of healthcare leaders is to communicate their vision via inspiring stories and, importantly, by their behavior. If leaders cannot respond appropriately to the demand for change, others will not be able to either.

Their next most important task is to anticipate the blocks in the way of substantive change. Implementing any planned modification requires the integration of numerous activities and people, as well as overcoming embedded obstacles. The most notable obstacles are elements of the organizational structure, which themselves act as insulation against the demand for reform. One of the first jobs of a leader acting as a change agent is to diffuse the power of these elements, and thus remove a large barrier to concerted and dramatic action on the part of stakeholders.

Leaders must be aware that people have spent much of their lives avoiding the prospect of change. One person dedicated to blocking change can bring the entire change process to a grinding halt. Change avoiders or resisters must be identified, challenged, worked with, empowered, and placed in the midst of the change process so that they do not impede the ability of the organization to thrive. The entrenchment of behaviors and structures that reward these behaviors provides the greatest barrier to meaningful change in health care and contributes to decline in the system. Nothing is more tragic for society than the desperate stranglehold on a system in need of great change by leaders who benefit by delaying or avoiding the necessary shifts. Leaders who are change avoiders or resisters cease to be relevant or viable, and actively contribute to the overwhelming onset of great decline and ultimate failure (Aarons et al., 2015).

Because the transition from one age to another is a long-term process, leaders must continually set short-term goals to give stakeholders a sense of movement and accomplishment. The attainment of short-term goals enables stakeholders to mark their journey forward and visualize and celebrate the process of change. It also gives them a moment of respite and reflection and helps them gather the energy necessary for the next stage.

Leaders must look at change not as an event but as a journey—a never-ending journey. Every point of arrival, in other words, is also a point of departure. Therefore, leaders must carefully balance periods of effort and action with periods of rest and celebration so that stakeholders will be regularly refreshed and reenergized to meet future challenges.

Finally, change is experienced on a personal level and on a cultural level. And of the two, culture always rules. This truism must be solidly rooted in the mind of every leader engaged in transforming an organization. The task is to prove to workers that the modifications will improve their work or the workplace. Today's workers are faithful not to the workplace, but to their work. They know they can take their skills elsewhere and be welcomed. Thus, leaders must

> **Key Point**
> Moving into a transformed health system does not mean leaving everything behind. It does mean thinking about what needs to be left behind and reflecting on what should go with us as we move into an age with a different set of parameters.

> **Key Point**
> The greatest impediment to future success is past success. A capacity for change implementation is an important factor in change and transformation.

> **Key Point**
> The leader is an agent of change, responsible for providing others with a vision of change and ensuring that their response aligns with the demand for change.

> ## Group Discussion
> Along with the nature of work, the characteristics of workers are changing. Discuss how the broad contemporary social realities have an impact on the culture of the workplace. Then, discuss how the characteristics of workers (especially knowledge workers) compare with the characteristics of younger and older workers. What types of issues arise when both types of workers must perform together?

be aware of the demands regarding work that exist within the prevailing culture. Incorporating symbolic and cultural norms in the language and process of change helps cast it into a form that workers can understand and value. Every wise leader knows the political realities pertaining to a change process and adapts the process in light of them so that the needs of key stakeholders are met and stakeholders can devote their efforts to implementing and sustaining the process.

The Quantum Character of Leadership

Quantum realities are characterized by many new patterns and processes, such as those described in this section.

Linear Thinking Is Now Replaced by Relational and Whole-Systems Thinking

Perhaps the most radical shift to occur is the move away from mechanistic (Newtonian) and reductionist models of thought and research. In the 20th century, most research was based on vertical, reductionist (or linear) processes. Quantum science, in contrast, has an affinity for multidirectional complexity and uncertainty. The use of complex relational algorithms has lessened the former devotion to vertical and reductionist processing, and relational and whole-systems models now constitute a new foundation for scientific and business research. Because researchers can rapidly process and relate complex arrays of data, they can use different processes for making decisions and creating new products and technologies, such as computer chips, synthetics, bioceuticals and pharmaceuticals, and DNA-moderated clinical therapeutics.

Structure Is About Wholes, Not Parts

Our newly acquired capacity for discovering and understanding the critical vitality of linkages and intersections has made it clear to us that at some level everything is interdependent. Further, our knowledge of the interconnectedness of everything causes us to look differently not just at the physical components of the universe but also at organizations and human interactions (**Exhibit 1-5**). This is not to say, of course, that we always fully comprehend the nature of the interdependence among any particular elements, but we do recognize its significance.

Exhibit 1-5   The Language of Complexity and Chaos

Emerging language from the science of complex systems describes a world different from that which we have grown familiar. New terms and phrases express a whole set of dynamics that operate just outside our field of vision, yet they have a defining impact on our experience of life and the human journey in which we each play an important, but not always known, role. Some of the more unusual words include these:

- *Autopoiesis*: The process by which living systems continually seek to renew and reinvent themselves, yet maintain their core integrity.
- *Autocatalysis*: A process in which information enters into a system in small fluctuations that continually grow in strength, interacting with the system and feeding back upon itself.
- *Dissipative structures*: Structures in which disorder is the source of order, and vice versa. In this "dance" between order and disorder, an old form ends and a new form begins.
- *Strange attractor*: The activity of a collective chaotic system composed of interactive feedback between and among its various parts and evidencing attraction to its pattern of behavior.

Our understanding of the design of fractals (complex geometric patterns demonstrating precise similarity in that all the details of the structure viewed at any scale continuously repeat elements of the overall pattern), for example, is critical for comprehending the order that exists in chaos and for appreciating the impact of complexity on organizations and human behavior. The smallest level of a single organization and the most complex array of a large, aggregated system containing the organization are connected inexorably in a pattern, as demonstrated through the power of fractals.

If you have ever looked at a hologram, which is a three-dimensional photograph of an image, you may have noticed that no matter what size section you focus on, the entire image is present in the smaller piece. Holography thus can be used to explain the nature of fractals because in a fractal the complete pattern is present in any component regardless of the level of detail or complexity. A tree is a good example from the so-called natural world because its overall structure, including the trunk and branches, is similar to the branching pattern of each leaf (the fractal effect).

Fractals have tremendous implications for organizations. From the smallest structural elements to the very complex patterns of behavior that exist throughout an organization, the same patterns appear and are played out in precise detail. This fact implies that at every level of the organization there exists a self-organizing capacity, and that this capacity maintains a balance and harmony even in the midst of the most apparently chaotic processes. To the extent that the balance and harmony are sustained, the organization's life is advanced. To the extent that they are upset or cannot be well articulated, visualized, and acted on at every level of leadership, the organization's actions tend to impede its inherent integrity and effectiveness. It is important, therefore, that organization leaders are aware of the continuous and dynamic action, the fractal effect, in all organizational behavior and structure so that they can advance the consonance and value of the organization members' activities and enhance the organization's ability to fulfill its mission.

Perhaps it is even more important for leaders to recognize that, within the context of the dynamic action of fractals, their own actions have cascading and rippling implications throughout the organization. In fact, they should understand that no decision, action, or undertaking can occur in the organization without ultimately having an impact on every other action, decision, and undertaking. This happens because of the interdependent web of interaction and connectivity that links all of the pieces together in a reciprocal and intersecting dynamic of action that requires the action of each linked to the action of all to sustain the life of the system. In addition, once people are cognizant of the web of interaction and interdependence that exists in the organization, leaders will approach deliberation and decision making only with extreme care, caution, and thoroughness. Here, inclusiveness and engagement are not optional in providing for the sustainability of the system.

Issues of relationship, interaction, empowerment, and ownership have become increasingly pertinent in our understanding of the nature of work. We now view individuals rather than organizations as owning the work processes, and this change in our understanding has altered the relationship between workplace and worker. Further, by focusing on different descriptors in portraying how human dynamic systems work and how processes become sustained, we have created a new framework for considering design and function

> **Key Point**
> Competence is not about having skills, but about using skills to achieve desired outcomes.

within the workplace and within the entire human community. The new framework also enables us to consider what is and is not effective in the workplace and in relationships among people and to emphasize issues of accountability, productivity, and value.

For example, it is not enough for leaders to assess the functional proficiency of individual workers as a way of determining whether a work process is fully effective and sustainable. Instead, they must also examine whether each worker's competence and efforts fit with the competence and efforts of other workers. "Goodness of fit," not the individual proficiency of any single participant, leads to effectiveness and sustainability. Imagine the impact of this understanding on viable and sustainable measures of productivity and performance.

The Value of Work Is a Function of the Outcome, Not Just the Process

In the last 30 to 40 years, our understanding of the value of work has shifted. In the past, the focus of clinical work was on the excellence of process, and the existence of a good work process was taken to indicate the provision of good service. We now recognize that process is not the only determinant of good service. Indeed, a work process derives its value from the purpose toward which it is directed (the desired outcome), and if the purpose does not inform and discipline the process, the process can lose its value (we must learn to create goodness-of-fit between process and outcome).

Work is not inherently valuable, despite the historically associated Judeo-Christian ethic. Consider how many people say that their work provides meaning in their life, and that they find their life to be pointless when the function and content of the work shift. What they forgot is that work is not meaningful in itself but becomes meaningful when it fulfills the purpose to which it is directed. People sometimes feel burned out when they seek the meaning that should drive the work inside the work activity itself. When the work changes, they cannot cope because they experience the end of a way of working as well as an end of meaning. The problem is that their "how" has become their "why," and their means have become their ends.

> **Point to Ponder**
>
> Work is not inherently valuable. Instead, it is valuable to the extent that it fulfills a purpose. Therefore, the main focus should be on the good fit between work and real value, not just on the work itself.

Process is not always connected to outcome, and hence to value. Nurses and physicians, particularly, have a hard time understanding this. Sometimes their commitment to treating patients is not disciplined by the recognition that the value of any treatment activity lies in the good fit between process and final outcome or impact. Indeed, they often provide health services in cases where there is little evidence that the services dependably result in a right outcome. Medical practice variance accounts for billions of dollars a year in healthcare expenditures. Today, there is high demand for a connection between process and product—between particular treatments and their outcomes; this will play a more significant role in the management of healthcare resources and the valuing of health services.

Technology Changes What People Do, How They Live, and Who They Are

When we view the technological advances of our time objectively, it is difficult not to marvel. Many inventions that first appeared in science fiction have been realized in the past few decades; obviously, many innovations are yet to come, including some that will alter the very

---

Exhibit 1-6   New Age Imperatives

1. Value-driven health service models
2. Medicine/nursing based on cellular manipulation
3. Mass-customized diagnosis and treatment
4. User-specific insurance programs
5. Integration of allopathic and alternative therapies
6. Payment incentives (bundles) tied to outcomes (quality)
7. Focused service settings for specific populations

---

structure of life. Frightening as it may be, for the first time in human history we can manipulate our own evolution, and that of every other species on the earth.

Healthcare leaders need to realize that the medical internet and technology are driving the transformation of health care in ways that have not been seen since the development of germ theory. Genomics, micronization, 3D printing, big data, smartphones, digital health advisors, and related sciences are shifting the therapeutic framework for health care, probably for the rest of the century (Brill et al., 2019). How many of us can provide leadership in a postgenomic healthcare system? How many of us really know what that will look like?

Certainly, health care will depend less on the use of highly mechanical interventions, especially surgical interventions. The advances in bio-, chemo-, techno-, and pharmacotherapeutics enable many conditions that required traditional surgery to be handled more easily and less invasively through modern therapies. Even Alzheimer's disease will become a more treatable illness within the next 20 years. The question is, what are the implications of the switch to new therapeutic modalities, especially for the treatment of older persons and when the new modalities replace traditional institutional models of treatment (**Exhibit 1-6**)?

Leaders will have to grapple with these emerging realities and incorporate them into their own lives. Most people find it difficult, if not impossible, to imagine what new technologies will mean for life in the second and third decades and beyond in the 21st century, despite wanting to embrace them. They need help in grasping how technologies will affect them and what adjustments they must make now to thrive in the continually emerging digital reality (Ricciardi et al., 2019).

New Rules Will Apply in the New Age

Imagine not just learning to live within the context of a whole new set of emergent conditions but also leading others to embrace these shifts in their own lives and work. This is the fundamental leadership task—dealing with the same changes as everyone else while helping others thrive in a new reality. What makes this even more challenging is that people are inclined to reject the implications of the changes that are occurring.

Several late-20th-century innovations are still having a powerful impact on people's lives and on their relationship with health professionals and other service providers. These innovations include the internet, wireless communication, fiber-optics and lasers, the cloud (which helps manage large and dense information repositories), and technologies that enable these groups to converge around new clinical technologies, therapeutics, and drugs. The internet, for example, not only has influenced global communications but has altered the very way business is conducted. For a couple of decades now, people shop without leaving home, and even without any human contact. Using social media, they can access a wide variety of people and information, including information they once needed to visit a library or a professional expert to get. When people meet with their doctors (often digitally), they might already have accessed health information from other sources, have questions and concerns they want to discuss, and can share the digital media they accessed virtually in real time. The internet, in other words, is helping to shift the locus of control from providers of health services to users. This change is affecting the patient–provider relationship in the following ways:

- Patients now determine the parameters of the patient–provider relationship, setting the stage for a different kind of interaction than has historically occurred.
- Many patients develop partnerships with providers to sort through available choices and pick the best. They need providers to act as navigators and educators who are willing to assist them in making healthcare decisions.
- Patients need providers' help in verifying the accuracy of data they have gathered independently from a host of sources and in interpreting data.
- Patients are interested in options, not orders to undergo particular treatments. They want to be able to consider a range of options within the context of their personal values and priorities and to choose the one option that fits best (shared decision making).
- Providers need to be concerned with what patients know and can do in regard to controlling their own health decisions in a "user-driven" world. More of the responsibility for health care will be placed on patients and their loved ones. Providers must transfer skills to others and share the ownership of care with others.
- Providers need to focus more predominantly on the relationship between patients and the service network along the patients' continuum of care, connecting and integrating other providers and resources in a seamless link between them and with patients in a way that best advances personal and community health.

Although the locus of control has shifted to patients (users), essentially, patients are undereducated about health care. Still, ready or not, they now must take command of their own care and acquire whatever skills they need to manage it. The current role of providers in a reforming health system is to ensure that patients/users not only have the proper tools and skills, but that they actually succeed at managing their own care. Consequently, providers need to alter their priorities. Rather than intervening medically and providing care themselves, providers frequently help their patients to make proper health-related decisions and to learn how to perform necessary self-care tasks. To a certain extent, providers are becoming health service agents/navigators, using patient-centered communication to assist their patients in obtaining the knowledge, equipment, and services they and their patients have determined are needed or desired (Newell & Jordan, 2015).

Early Engagement Health Care

Over this next century, bio-, chemo-, and pharmacotherapeutics will come to dominate the health services landscape. Because technology will enable healthcare providers to assess a person's DNA and physiology in ever-greater detail, diseases will be identified sooner than they are now. Diagnostics that include genetic profiling now make it possible to predict with high levels of accuracy a person's degree of risk for particular diseases and conditions. Preventive treatment will soon be supplied before symptoms manifest, and detailed, highly customized clinical services will be configured specifically to fit individual DNA characteristics.

Health professionals must ask, how will improvements in diagnostics and therapeutics alter the practice of medicine? In the past, medical and nursing interventions often required patients to be hospitalized/institutionalized. Therapies of the future will require much less hospitalization and will hardly impede patients' normal routines. The main goals of health professionals will be to provide the right therapy at the right time and at the right dose and to educate people about their life processes, their health, their choices (including medical and lifestyle choices), and the risks associated with each choice. As these become prevalent realities for service and economies of scale are reached, cost-effectiveness and value can be more adequately assessed, and appropriate financial choices can be made.

The largest two groups of health professionals, nurses and physicians, have much to accomplish in the next 2 decades if they are to successfully make the transition to a digitally driven, value-grounded, reformed health system. Their clinical roles will change substantially during this period, and getting these groups to converge around a new way of addressing prevention, education, and service delivery will be challenging and a tumultuous experience for healthcare leaders. Leaders will require extreme diligence as well as a skill set that stretches their resources to the limit. To design the future, leaders must understand the current landscape and how it differs from the familiar territory of past experience.

Group Discussion

Consumers' expectations regarding their role in healthcare decisions and processes are changing. Discuss these changes and describe the role of health professionals in helping consumers develop the insights and skills they need to manage their own health effectively, especially in this age of value. Also discuss the dangers of consumers making their own decisions, as well as the actions that healthcare leaders can take now and in the future to mitigate the dangers and ensure that consumers become accountable decision makers.

The Context for Leadership Is Shifting

From deconstructing infrastructure to confronting "new age" workers, leaders have a new set of tasks before them—tasks they are not fully prepared to address. For many leaders, most of the foundations of their understanding and expression of the nature of leadership were formed in the early and middle 20th century and reflect outmoded models. During the last third of the 20th century and the first decade of the 21st century, newer models of leadership and its application have emerged. These models are based on new ideas about organizational structure and managing people and processes (**Exhibit 1-7**).

In the past, organizations were built on the Newtonian principles of mechanistic functioning, compartmentalization, and vertical control (**Exhibit 1-8**). The dominant theme of Newtonian thinking is that the universe is simply one vast machine. In fact, Newton saw the universe as a sort of giant clock that could be explained in mechanistic terms, and he and his followers took the goal of physics to be the discovery of the laws that supposedly govern the parts of the

CHAPTER ONE   A New Landscape for Leadership: Changing the Health Script in an Age of Value

---

Exhibit 1-7 The Major Tasks of the Value-Driven Healthcare Leader

- Deconstructing the barriers and structures of the 20th century
- Alerting staff about the implications of changing what they do
- Establishing safety around taking risks and experimenting
- Embracing new technologies as a way of doing work
- Reading the signposts along the road to the future
- Enumerating and evaluating small tests of change
- Translating the emerging reality of health reform into language staff can use
- Demonstrating personal engagement with the creation of sustainable value
- Helping others adapt to the demands of a value-driven health system
- Creating a safe milieu for the struggles and pain of changing practice and service
- Enumerating small successes as a basis for supporting staff
- Celebrating the journey and all progress made
- Enabling others to act

Exhibit 1-8 Newtonian Characteristics

- Vertical orientation
- Hierarchical structures
- Focus on control
- Reductionistic scientific processes
- Top-down decision making
- Mechanistic models of design
- Process-driven action

> **Key Point**
>
> People no longer undergo a hospital stay to obtain most medical services. Innovative treatments, evidence-based practice implementation, and service-based care management provide value to stakeholders without requiring hospitalization.

universe (material particles and the bodies of which they are constituents). Almost all scientific progress of the late 19th century and the first half of the 20th century was grounded in Newtonian concepts.

The kind of mechanistic explanation favored by Newtonians has not accounted for human behavior and other patterns of activity in the universe, however. Even in the early decades of the 20th century, questions were raised about the adequacy of Newtonian physics to explain the incongruous and apparently messy underpinnings of the universe. Biology perhaps has offered the best evidence that not everything works mechanistically and that the universe is rife with chaos and incongruities.

Quantum theory and other more recent scientific theories have had a large impact on contemporary theories of leadership. Many of the elements of traditional leadership grew out of a Newtonian/industrial framework, especially those focusing on hierarchical control. Indeed, during the 20th century organizational leaders tended to rely on vertical hierarchies and compartmentalization of activities to manage people and productivity, and the structures of their

---

Exhibit 1-9 Quantum Characteristics

- Multifocal characteristics
- Nonlinear structures
- Focus on relatedness
- Relational designs
- Multisystems scientific processes
- Center-out decision making
- Complexity-based models of design
- Value-driven action
- Deliberate, sustained focus on engagement and burnout reduction

---

organizations reflected this tendency. The rise of quantum theory and the new appreciation of complexity and complex adaptive systems as foundational characteristics of the universe have changed our views of science and of life (**Exhibit 1-9**). Many mistakenly believe that all that has occurred has been a shift in focus from physics to biology, but this way of looking at matter itself reflects a kind of compartmentalism. Rather, what people are beginning to understand is that all elements of the universe are a part of a broad system of intersections and relationships.

> ## Group Discussion
>
> Describe the core concepts of Newtonian thinking and how these concepts were manifested during the 20th century. Consider, for example, how social institutions and structures reflected the commitment to Newtonian thinking, and how Newtonian thinking influenced the leadership role.

The major shifts in scientific thinking challenge all our current theories of leadership. What we once thought were the foundations of leadership are now being subjected to further exploration and clarification. Vertical control and managing ritual and routine, for instance, are no longer seen as effective processes for leadership. Rather, relationships and interactions within organizations should focus on diverse teams and collective leadership (Duncan, 2019). Further, we now recognize that the patterns of relationships in an organization are just as important as the relationships themselves or what lies within the related elements. Leaders must understand the importance of empowering knowledge management that generates new ideas that may promote institutional knowledge and lead to internal and external organizational prosperity (Lunden et al., 2017).

New Framework, New Models of Leadership

The current literature on leadership contains a large array of concepts that suggest a whole new framework for action. Foremost among these is the concept of complexity and the view that everything is related. In this view, the interactions among the parts of a system are critical to the system's productivity, and ultimately its sustainability (Gros, 2015). The main leadership

> **Key Point**
>
> In the emerging age, a large part of the leadership role will involve facilitating the transition to a new way of living and working. Leaders will increasingly devote their energies to helping others adapt to the new conditions and principles for thriving in the emerging world of work.

task, then, is not so much to manage function or work, but instead to coordinate the elements (e.g., the workers) and facilitate the relationship between work and worker at every organizational level.

Leaders must maintain a panoramic view of the world to discern the direction their efforts should take. Their ability to see intersections, relationships, and themes ensures that the organization will undertake the activities it needs to thrive.

In the Industrial Age, leaders were concerned most of all with function and operation. The work was compartmentalized, and the focus was on the activities of the individual employee. The employee's work life was regulated by a set of job obligations, and by meeting these obligations the employee was able to advance upward, receive better pay, or obtain other rewards. A performance evaluation system might have been in place to assess the employee's proficiency, and any rewards given to the employee were based on the quality of the work, not on whether the work made a difference to other employees or to the organization as a whole. Work processes have historically been treated as having more value than their collective and relational impact.

In this new age, the ordering is reversed. The most important question is not "What have you done?" but "What difference did it make?" The former question reflects the Judeo-Christian tradition that work is inherently valuable, whereas we now view work as valuable to the extent it achieves the purposes toward which it is directed. Consequently, leaders need to consider the relationships among the work, the worker, and the purpose of the work as a dynamic that continuously drives value. Further, they need to understand that the relationship is cybernetic, which means that each element supports and feeds the others in a seamless connection.

In fact, this notion of connectivity and relationship is the predominant driving framework for constructing the future of human organizations, communities, and global relationships (called connectography). The leader of today and tomorrow will need to incorporate a broad array of relational, interdisciplinary, collaborative, generational, and cultural management tools to address the increasing complexity of human communication and interaction. Relational work will grow in intensity and will continue to comprise an ever-increasing percentage of the leader's skills and energies. The ability to manage relational complexities will increasingly be a normative set of expectations in leadership expression and will require a maturing facility for building the collective enterprise, establishing common frames for teamwork, crossing traditional boundaries and limitations, moving work continuously across and around the enterprise–community–globe, and managing work and relationships virtually 24 hours a day. Connectivity will be the condition that informs the leader's work; connection will be the driving force for advancing the work (Khanna, 2016).

Within this larger context for work and relationship, the interaction between process and outcome is clear, but it is not always simple or direct. Many circumstances and variables, including inherent and contextual influences, as well as unplanned factors, are embedded in the process and affect the relationship between each element of the work and outcomes of the work. These variables interact with the work process and influence both the process and outcomes. It is in these places where complexity is embedded.

The new age commitment to focusing on process from the perspective of outcome/value creates havoc among health professionals. Leaders must be fully aware of professionals' intractable attachment to process and the functional activities that comprise it. People generally come to prize particular work activities once they become expert at and are rewarded for doing them. They find it a challenge to adjust or even eliminate what they do in the face of a lack of evidence that it produces anything meaningful or sustainable (valuable). Indeed, simply getting folks to the table to discuss the product/impact of their activities can be difficult. Yet this is what leaders must do if they are to change the content of the work, make it more meaningful, and determine its essential value.

Group Discussion

Explore the notion of goodness of fit between processes and the achievement of value. In particular, discuss how a leader's expectations of staff would likely change if the leader looked at service and care from the perspective of achieving value. As part of this discussion, describe what steps the leader can take to get staff to focus on value rather than function (process). What changes would occur in the provision of healthcare services as a result of this focus on achieving value for the user?

Everything Is Part of One Comprehensive System

Formerly, it was believed that three types of functional relationships existed: any two things in the universe were independent of each other; they were interdependent; or one was dependent on the other, but not the reverse. In the quantum age, however, we realize that all things are interdependent, and indeed intertwined (**Exhibit 1-10**). That is, all things are tied together in a wide variety of refined and sometimes inexplicable ways; some obvious, and some all but invisible at any level of observation.

Exhibit 1-10   Interdependence

In nature everything is interdependent and intertwined. There is an ebb and flow, a dependence among all the elements of life. Leaders must see their role from this perspective. Most of the work of leadership will be managing/facilitating the interactions and connections between people and processes. Leaders must keep aware of these truths:

- Action in one place ultimately has an impact in all other places.
- Fluctuation of mutuality means authority moves between people.
- Interacting properties in systems make outcomes mobile and fluid.
- The value of an action drives its meaning and informs its content.
- Relationship building is the primary work of leadership.
- Trusting feeling–gut–sense is as important as valuing thinking.
- Acknowledging in others what is unique in their contribution is vital.
- Supporting, stretching, challenging, pushing, and helping are part of being present to the process, to the players, and to achieving value.

> **Key Point**
>
> Chaos is the essential energy driving all change. It works to take apart and challenge whatever is impeding movement. Chaos challenges us to simultaneously let go and to take on. It reminds us that life is a journey of constant creation, not simply a series of tandem events.

Leaders now must carry out their tasks with an awareness of the relatedness of processes, actions, behaviors, and functions. No act is independent, and no act adds to the viability of an organization independent of its relationship to every other element in the system. Every element interacts with every other element in some meaningful and measurable way, and all the elements together constitute an essential, yet complex, mosaic of movement and intersection. When looked at as a whole, the picture the elements present—and the information they impart—is entirely different from how they are viewed separately. Indeed, looking at the parts independently of each other may lead one to draw conclusions that might impede the progress of a whole process or prevent its completion, with lasting and perhaps limiting results.

To help readers adopt the proper perspective, this text demonstrates the principles of complexity and chaos theory and explains the various operations of complexity and how it affects work, relationships, organizations, and interactions. It also discusses many of the new skills and talents that leaders must acquire, as well as new metaphors and terminology better suited to describe work-related interactions and processes. By attaining a deeper understanding of the implications of systemness and complexity, leaders can relate to and interact with others in new ways and be challenged to develop a new foundation for their role as leaders and toward the creation of more relevant and effective systems.

Planning for the Trajectory, Not the Goal

In the Industrial Age, it was believed that everything should be outlined and planned down to the smallest detail toward some idealized future goal. The expectation was that by planning future activities with great specificity and a clear notion of the endpoint, an organization could respond to the current situation accurately and effectively on its way to a defined goal. This notion of clearly defining a specific future goal and planning to the last detail assumes much more control over circumstances than, in truth, we actually have. New thinking in complex adaptive systems tells us that far more vagaries influence planned action than we can anticipate. It is wiser to understand the trajectory of change than it is to know the specifics of that change (Storkholm et al., 2019).

When a plan is constructed, the future looks a certain way at that moment in time, and the context at that moment creates the field of vision for what is anticipated. However, because change is constant and the greater environment is forever in a state of chaos, flux, and creativity, the context is never stable. The reality at the planning stage (at any given moment), quickly gives way to a new emergent reality that could not have been anticipated at any previous time in the planning stage. And, of course, this cycle is continuous and never-ending, making it impossible ever to plan for some predetermined endpoint with broad certainty.

Leaders now must incorporate the vagaries of complexity and chaos into the process of anticipating and planning for the future. Detailing the specifics of some future state in absolute or predictable terms has been proven not to be a viable means of planning (Storkholm et al., 2019). Discerning environmental and contextual shifts, or "good signpost reading," is a better skill to have than those related to narrowly defining specified goals or endpoints. Leaders must realize that no real-time insight is permanent, nor is it entirely accurate. These notions or insights are simply a reflection of the particular point a person or organization is at a given moment in time in the longer, more continuous, and relentless unfolding and becoming that is the future.

Good leaders can read the signposts generated in the larger environment that suggest a change is imminent and can discern the direction of the change and the elements indicating its implications and impact on the trajectory of the organization or system. Good leaders synthesize rather than simply analyze, and view changes thematically and/or relationally, drawing out of it what kind of relevant action or strategy should be applied or trajectory embraced; that is, the response that best positions the organization to thrive in the emergent circumstances. Good leaders are adept at sensing changes in the external environment, indeed, even anticipating them, and using those insights to determine what adjustments or course shifts must occur in the planned trajectory to ensure that the organization remains relevant and viable.

For leaders to act as a strategist today means not detailing the organization's future point in time, but rather analyzing the relationship of the system to its external environment, determining the ability of the system to respond and adapt in a sustainable way, translating that relationship and capacity into language that has meaning for those who must do the work of moving the organization, and disturbing ingrained assumptions (Brandenburger, 2019). Translating the signposts into understandable and inspiring language for the people of the system is more critical than almost any other strategic task. It is vital that a change have implications for the stakeholders doing the work. Another way of saying this is that it must have meaning to each and every stakeholder within the framework of their work activities so that they can commit to it, which they must do if they and the organization are to adapt to the change successfully. The leader's job is to describe the change with language that engages and inspires the workers to understand its value and how it will positively inform and impact their own efforts.

In this new complexity framework, leaders need insights about contextual themes rather than step-by-step guidance on how to implement a minutely defined vision. They must understand that their organization is on a journey, and that they need to peruse the influencing external landscape continuously for directional guidance rather than create a list of steps through which the organization will move on its way to a preset goal. Becoming aware of the themes and undercurrents and reading the contextual signposts regularly is a wiser and more effective strategy for the complexity leader than is laying out an itemized plan that may or may not correspond with future conditions.

Adaptation and Complexity

Central to the concept of adaptation is the understanding that all sustainable systems respond collectively to changes in their environment. It is important in this understanding to recognize that systems have an intelligence that reflects a continual and dynamic interacting between all of the persons and processes that compose the system and the system with its external environment. These ever-interacting change phenomena emerge and reemerge between a system

> **Point to Ponder**
>
> Good leaders know how to integrate the rational and the intuitive because both are equally important to thriving. They often conflict with each other, but also complement each other. Consequently, leaders must know when they complement and when they contrast with each other, influencing and informing the underlying flow of change.

and its external environment and within the life of all the elements inside that give the system form. In fact, in all human dynamics, transformation and reproduction, and change and stability, are intrinsically intertwined. The wise leader understands these interactions and sees them as central to the effort of recognizing change and both embracing and engaging it (McKimm & Till, 2015).

Historically, leadership has emphasized rational and operational science skills and functions at the expense of insight, intuition, and feeling. In most workplaces, the former, seen as more masculine and rational, is prized, whereas insight, intuition, and feeling, which are often viewed as feminine, are taken to be less applicable in the historically masculine corporate world.

Even in health care, caregiving and relational behaviors are more often viewed as OK for nurses and doctors to express but as having little place in the business end of service delivery. The principles of quantum science, chaos, and complexity theory, however, warn that failure to incorporate these behaviors into the operations of an organization—in addition to rational, hard-driving, objectified behaviors—reduces the organization's awareness, availability, and sensitivity to its environment. In addition, too much of the rational and hard-driving can alienate people and distance them from personal ownership of their work process, reducing their energy, their creativity, their commitment to the organization, and their ability to perform their roles effectively.

Simply being capable and competent in form and function is not enough; leaders must also exhibit the ability to balance a complex range of skills and system resources to develop workers' capabilities and grow the organization. They must know how to create a balance between means and meaning and enter into the relationships among all the elements at the personal level and at the organizational level. Incorporating their vast array of behaviors and skills into the mosaic of interactions creates resonance between the functional and the relational, both of which are essential for developing and maintaining the vitality of person and system.

Finding the Right Balance

Weighing the various structures and influences in a work system and finding just the right mix of elements is challenging work. Yet that is exactly what leaders must learn to do. And they must learn to do it with a minimum of artificial supports.

Throughout most of the healthcare system, the various infrastructures are so burdensome and complex that they now actually interfere with the ability of organizational leaders to nimbly and precisely do what they now need to do. Because of widespread bricks-and-mortar infrastructure, most organizational leaders would not know how to challenge and change the structural elements that encase every function and activity in the current system. This is of special concern in a time of value-driven health reform. Much of the traditional tertiary care architecture and infrastructure must now give way to a more strongly developed

> **Point to Ponder**
>
> Information and data are tools for decision making. Because information can be collected ad infinitum, but still never be enough of the right information, the critical issue for leaders facing decisions at a given moment is at what point there is sufficient information to make a reasonably informed decision. Of course, the circumstances determining the amount and type of required data will always change. Therefore, information needs are dynamic, not stable, and the leader will need to make the choice regarding how much information is enough to decide and to act.

primary health core. A primary health core requires deconstruction of the past brick-and-mortar and system infrastructure to make way for a more mobile and portable, decentralized, and user-driven delivery system that responds to a stronger demand for population and community health practices.

In this age of value, we must realize that there should be just enough structure to support the integrity of the organization, and not an ounce more. The more structure an organization has, the more that structure demands from the organization, and the more resources are drawn to support it and away from the service system. Too much structure is actually an enemy of work and effectiveness. Under the rubric of "good order" and operational routine, too much structure drains the energy and creativity from a responsive system and obstructs relationships and interactions necessary for the system's nimble change and sustainable functioning. Too much structure ends up crippling the system's ability to transform its work and to continuously fulfill its purposes, now reinforced and in need of redesign. The goal of an organization's leadership should be to reduce structure to only that required to advance the purposes of the systems and the essential processes of work in a way that ultimately ensures that the system can synergistically respond to its environment quickly, fluidly, and effectively.

Information, like structure, can easily be overvalued. Clearly, information should play a vital and central role in decision making. Yet there will never be enough of the right-configured information to guarantee that any decision is the best one in given circumstances. Furthermore, an organization can strangle itself with data in an effort to know everything pertinent to a critical decision before actually making the decision (a virtual impossibility). Leaders need to accept that they will never have sufficient information to guarantee the correctness of their decisions, and that information is simply a useful tool that offers a glimpse into relevant factors at a given point in time. Because conditions are constantly in flux, too much dependence on information alone can lead to poor decisions just as easily as a total lack of information can.

For information to be valuable, its quantity is not as important as its relevance, and its volume is not as important as its utility. Leaders must know how much information is enough, how accurate is it, what its focus is, what it indicates, and what its bearing is on the decisions that need to be made. They also must know when the use limits of information have been reached, and when its application requires discernment, deliberation, and judgment. The similarity between information and structure is obvious: the right amount of the right kind of information is critical to organizational effectiveness. Yet, for all leaders, there is a point in time when the risk must be taken and a decision made.

Every level of activity in any system has a complex recurring geometric pattern. Quantum scientists often identify this pattern in the language of fractals, previously discussed in this chapter. Fractals are represented in every element and process of life. Although complex, they exert a simple and direct influence on order and chaos in the universe and are evident in the action of planets and stars, plants and animals, and even in the rhythm of a human heart and the cellular work of mitochondria. Our understanding of fractals and their application to organizations flies in the face of every traditional organizational model. True fractal organizations generally represent minimal and simple hierarchies (vertical and horizontal), and both, in the continual dance of balance, generate

> **Key Point**
> The leader is a primary facilitator of the journey to a new way of thinking and working. The leader's role is to keep people on the journey of which they are all part, and to help them understand what that means to them going forward.

and distribute accountability and performance strategically and equitably throughout the organization. In more traditional models, including the organizational charts and job descriptions associated with them, a more concerted effort is made to exclude from organizational life the normative disorder, fluidity, and chaos that lies just below the surface. Yet no matter how rigorous the structure, turbulence, fluidity, and even chaos burst through and generate creative discordance and confusion, making nonsense of any effort to control it.

It is impossible to codify all the activities in an organization. How many healthcare facilities, in an effort to truly control circumstances, implement innumerable policies and procedures that then are promptly neglected until the next accreditation visit? It is simply not possible to codify all the elements, interactions, and relationships necessary for the care of human beings. The vagaries of the human condition block organizations' ability to create formats or structures stable enough to set adequate behavioral or procedural parameters for treating medical conditions. The foundations of action are rooted in the principles of care and service, but although the principles are constant, the context within which they are applied is not.

Here again, it is the relatedness among factors that should drive a leader's response in these complex systems. Because the elements, behaviors, and variables affecting action are inconstant, the leader's task is to achieve as much balance as the circumstances allow. And because this balance is fluid, leaders must act to adjust it in response to changes in circumstances, including internal and external influences. Leaders are always interpreting, explaining, adjusting, and applying the issues and dynamics affecting the drivers–character–content of the work and the integrity of the workplace.

Group Discussion

In a fractal, the whole is replicated in each aggregating part. Each branch of a tree, for example, shows the same pattern as the whole tree, as does each leaf. The indentations and projections in a few feet of shoreline may mimic those in a 100-mile stretch of coastline. Apply the notion of a fractal to organizations, groups, and teams. For instance, how does the notion of a fractal apply to the design of an organization? To the relationship among leaders? To point-of-service clinical teams? To individual roles? How does it impact the design of an organizational chart for a healthcare system?

Besides being an explicator of complexity wherever necessary, leaders must be present to the staff in a way that assures them of positive connection, understanding, and experience. Leaders must show that they are as vulnerable to the vagaries of circumstance as anyone, and can live with chaos and constant movement comfortably and knowledgeably. Still, it is difficult at best to deal with normative chaos embedded naturally yet deeply within every system. People fundamentally crave order and want their leaders to deliver a sense of stability and "normality." Despite this fact, leaders, rather than insulating people from innate complexity, uncertainty, or even disorder, must instead help people to embrace these factors, understand them, harness them, and develop the personal skills necessary to positively use them to transform themselves and the systems within which they live. It is to that end this book is designed (Porter-O'Grady & Malloch, 2016).

The Effects of Chaos and Paradox

At every level of existence, chaos and complexity are fully present. Creatures as small as one protein are constantly undergoing both accidental and transitional modifications and adaptations that give them a better chance of thriving. It is a basic requisite of all life to adapt to changing conditions. The demise of the dinosaur is a good example of what happens when living beings fail to adapt to changes in their external environment.

The age within which we currently live is vastly different from the age within which most of us grew up and reached maturity. Science and technology continue to alter every aspect of our lives. Our challenge is to embrace the new circumstances and sort out their implications and applications as we go. For the person who says, "I don't want to learn about the digital world and how to use advanced technologies," the best response may be, "You can't survive for long living only in your past; to thrive, you must fully engage the creation of your future." Although challenging, that piece of advice reflects an element of truth. Technological advances and the need and capacity to adapt to them are not going to go away.

As the age continues to unfold, leaders will be called to tell the truth, teach coping and adaptation skills, learn new skills, and apply them in new ways in new settings. The infrastructure that generated past leadership roles is disappearing, and the new circumstances demand new roles and challenge everyone to respond to an entirely new set of questions.

Furthermore, the new age will open the door to uncertainty and a general lack of "rightness." The prevailing principles will be open to interpretation and will be applicable in a host of ways. No one response to a change or answer to a question will be clearly the only one or the best one. There might be a variation of correct responses depending on the cultural, social, economic, and intellectual context. Leaders must respect the diversity embedded in every condition or issue (**Exhibit 1-11**).

Every leader is now required to know the techniques for finding common ground, for sorting through the various landscapes representing the diversity inherent in each issue. Also required are consensus-building and group-process skills, because a leader's job is to get people to come together around issues and help them determine appropriate responses within the context of their own roles. This is especially true in the age of growing interdisciplinary decision making and action where clinical alignment now includes collaborative practice around "bundles," episodes of care, services to populations, and interaction along the continuum of care. Leading this value-grounded foundation for care, communication, and integration is a challenge that cannot be met by establishing standardized job procedures or rules. Indeed,

---

Exhibit 1-11 Paradox

Many paired elements of life appear contradictory but at a deeper level are in fact complementary. These include the following:

- *Chaos and order*: There is order in all chaos, and vice versa.
- *Creativity and tension*: Tension leads to creativity, and creativity causes tension.
- *Conflict and peace*: Conflict is necessary to peacemaking, containing in it the elements upon which peace must be built.
- *Difference and similarity*: Difference seen at a great distance appears as an integrated whole.
- *Complexity and simplicity*: Complexity is simply the visible connection between aligned simplicities.

competent leaders must be able to "set tables" wisely and carefully to ensure that the right people are engaged in the right way around issues that are central to their role and essential to their adaptability and sustainability.

Leaders must develop an affection for legitimate risk and for life at the boundaries of agreement and understanding. They must be able to "push the river" so that the mental models people bring to the resolution of concerns or the determination of strategies and actions are shifted or even fundamentally altered. There is nothing worse in deliberation than using a mental model or frame of reference that does not fit the prevailing circumstances. As we move inexorably further into this new age, we must try to understand its characteristics within the context of its "becoming" rather than of the past. Peter Drucker (2009) said it best when he suggested that we must all close the door on the Industrial Age and simply turn around.

It is in turning around to face the future that we begin to confront the inadequacies of our historic mental models. We begin to see the future unfold within its own context rather than one we bring to it informed only by our past experience. We look over the landscape of our becoming and are stimulated to go to those places that least fit our prevailing mindset and that challenge what we understand and the language we bring to the journey.

Leaders need to be called out of certainty into experimentation. They must take smaller steps and let the measured consequences of each step suggest the best direction in which to move next. It is in the steps of experimentation—of testing and evaluating—that their direction and its appropriateness can be discerned most easily. Finally, leaders stand to gain most information about what is viable and sustainable by bringing a variety of testing procedures together and using them jointly.

Pay Attention to the Informal Network

In every organization there is a formal structure and process and an informal network. The informal network is primarily relational and carries most of the information about how people in the organization think or feel and what their sentiments are regarding almost anything in the system. It is as vital and valid a part of the system as any other, and it requires attention because, among other things, it typically contains essential pieces of the dynamic that have been overlooked or missed as well as the "undiscussables," issues that are too sensitive to lay on the table and opinions that do not reflect the prevailing point of view. Embedded here, too, are some of the most dynamic notions of what should happen or what should be done.

> **Key Point**
>
> All decisions and actions are rife with risk. Risk cannot be eliminated and should not necessarily be decreased, because courses of action that possess great value tend to be associated with higher risk. What is important to determine is not whether the risk can be eliminated, but whether the level of risk is appropriate for the actions undertaken, and, if so, what strategies can be used to manage risk.

All organizations, large and small, have a small number to hundreds of informal networks that operate as peer groups, colleague networks, service teams, care communities, long-term employee groups, task forces, and so forth. Huge inflows and outflows of information, sharing, and knowledge move dynamically through these matrices and informal groups in ways that have a significant impact on organizations and systems. Indeed, much more of the real daily work, relationships, and interactions are expressed in informal networks than is seen in the more formal structures of organizations. Leaders generally fail to recognize the power and influence of these informal networks and use them far less than the capacity and value they bring to organizations warrant. Although these informal networks are powerful, they represent a level of complexity and relational density that is difficult to manage in formal and systematic ways. However, through leadership recognition, access, and interaction within the context of these informal networks, much can be accomplished and a great deal of the dynamics of change can be effectively harnessed to enhance quality and improve service.

The power of the informal infrastructure is going to become increasingly important as healthcare institutions and structures continue to move into broad-based formal service networks. These networks will have significant implications as institutions move from predominantly vertically designed and structured formats to much more integrated, horizontal, and relationally driven organizational partnerships and service networks. The growing emphasis on an effective, health-based continuum of healthcare services and early engagement of users will radically alter structure and will accelerate demands for systems and clinical partnerships, care teams around a wide variety of models of health service along the care continuum, and integrated clinical actions around a variety of specific value equations and the service algorithms that support them.

Group Discussion

Karen Weiss, RN, is the leader of the nursing department in a medical clinic. The staff members like her because she can get things done and keep things moving. Although she has a highly developed sense of order, recent dramatic changes in how care is rendered in a population-based approach are making it harder for her to stay "in control." She feels as though things are getting ahead of her now, and she is losing her touch. Others are not as satisfied with her performance as they once were. Discuss the following: What is the real issue in this case? How does Karen's need for control conflict with the principles of complexity? Who is accountable for decisions? Should Karen change her manner of leading? If so, how should she change it, and what does she need to do to change it? How does Karen ensure that staff members are more involved in decisions that affect their own lives?

All elements of the system, whether formal or informal, are a part of the dynamic of change in the organization. Each can be a vehicle for action and even transformation. Leaders need to notice all the informal pathways and networks of communication and relationship, from hallway conversations to lunchtime discussions, from whispered comments to sarcastic asides—each plays a role in the complex web of interactions necessary for sustaining the organization. Taking an opportunity to hear, communicate, or interact is never inappropriate. All means are legitimate and deserve attention. Each, when joined with the others, contributes to discovering the state of the organization and determining the proper actions to take to redirect and strengthen it.

Simple Systems Are Linked to Create More Complex Systems

The universe operates in a web of simple and discrete networks that continually interface, confront, and intersect and interact with each other. Complexity is the sum of simplicity. Each is intrinsically linked with the other. Simple systems seek each other in a mysterious dance of self-organizing and join with each other at appropriate intersections to facilitate continuous and dynamic change and configure a larger whole. Called *chunking*, this process is similar to fitting together pieces of a child's erector set to build a structure. Each element has its own purpose and meaning, but its purpose remains unfulfilled until it interacts with the other elements. In short, their linkage, connection, and interactions demonstrate a synergy (and sometimes a divergence) of energized interfaces and relationships that can define the operation of the whole only when seen acting in relationship to each other, each doing its part in the "dance of change" that ultimately leads to some shifting impact or transformation.

The implication for human organizations and behaviors is that all things begin with the simple. Sustainable change rarely operates from the top of a system; instead, it usually is initiated and lives at the center and works its way outward. For instance, the purpose and meaning of a service organization are generated over the places where the staff does its work, closest to where the services are provided, which is also where the organization's value-grounded, dynamic growth, adaptability, and creativity originate and are sustained.

Leaders need to understand that sustainability comes from the places where the organization lives out its life and meaning—converging around its points of service. There, the pieces of the organization come together to fulfill the organization's purpose. Providers and clients come together to carry out the processes toward which the organization's infrastructure and operations are directed.

Although leaders profess to recognize the importance of the point of service, traditional organizational design does not reflect its key role in deciding and acting. The organizational hierarchy typically strangles the essential inclusive dynamics of the point of service and creates an artificial and unsustainable framework for decision making and action that happen at places far away from the point of service, often independent of the implications for action that ultimately must generate from the point of service. Individuals not at the point of service take responsibility for strategy, policy, and direction setting and, by so doing, exclude those whose obligation it is to carry out work and actions to fulfill strategy, policy, and organizational direction. A universal principle of system effectiveness states that the farther away from the point of service a decision is made about what goes on there, the higher the risk, the greater the cost, and the less sustainable the decision. Sadly, many organizations increase their risk and their costs and fail to attain their objectives as a result of failing to incorporate this principle into their way of doing business.

> **Point to Ponder**
>
> Traditionally, knowledge has been viewed as something that can be possessed. Today, however, it is viewed as a utility—something not possessed, but accessed. People who want to use knowledge should know how to access it, how to apply it, and when to let it go.

Staff, in constructing the correct complex relatedness and infrastructure, must be free to chunk from their center and create linkages with the strategic, financial, and support structures that facilitate their work. Here again, tearing away much of the unnecessary intervening infrastructure and the organizational layers and compartments serves to free the organization to enter into the more fluid and variable relationships it needs to provide stakeholder engagement in a way that advances health care. Then, those who own the work and its outcomes can join the simple, essential components of local locus of control and systems strategy to other essential components to construct a web of intersections and resonating connections that hum with the life and meaning underpinning sustainability.

The operation of digital equipment perhaps best exemplifies these forces at work. Software code defines functions but must interact with other pieces of data before it is useful to the technology user. A certain segment of code might have application value, but it must interact with other segments before this value can be realized. In other words, each segment has value in virtue of its contribution to the whole.

Learning occurs in the same way. Simple concepts lead inexorably to understanding other simple concepts, and when they are all ultimately tied together, the learner understands the interdependence of different simple processes and thereby achieves knowledge. Furthermore, the learner recognizes that knowledge, rather than being valuable in and of itself, is valuable to the extent that it can be applied in action.

What complexity teaches us about knowledge is that it is not so much a capacity as it is a utility. It has relevance at a particular moment or in a specific situation. A shift in the context, an increase in understanding, or new information affects the elements of knowledge and challenges the person to "move on" and adjust what is known, valued, and applied. In fact, an endless dynamic is composed of the aggregating of knowledge, the letting go of what is no longer valid, and the reaching out for what is next and expands the endless journey of learning. The critical point here is that what is relevant or irrelevant, adequate or inadequate, at any given moment is not the whole of a person's knowledge but rather developing and adapting pieces or elements of knowledge (chunks). Persons move in and out of these chunks and, in so doing, alter the relationship between themselves and the whole complex of knowledge.

In systems thinking, leaders are aware of the importance of intersections. At intersections much of the work of leadership unfolds. The interface between the elements of a system is where the challenge and the work of effectiveness occur. The problem of creating good fit between the pieces of a system requires focus and effort on the part of leaders and serves as the place where most of the "noise" and confrontation between people and systems unfold.

Good leaders understand this and can use it in the interests of others and the organization. They never become so attached to any specific item, process, or activity that they treat it as permanent and/or unchanging. Each item, process, or activity is part of a mosaic and comes and goes depending on demand at various times. Good leaders know to let go when that is appropriate and to take on and adjust when that becomes necessary. Furthermore, they know that the organization's complex and chaotic circumstances require them to keep an eye on the larger picture, read the changes (in the constant interface between environment and organization) that are occurring or that are about to occur, and make the necessary adjustments at the appropriate time.

Good leaders know that a complex, adaptive system works when the simple systems work. If something is wrong at the point of service, the system as a whole is affected. Because the interdependence between simple components is so tight in an effective and viable complex system, any break in the simple (or local) systems leads to breaks at all levels of the complex system. By ensuring the effectiveness of the simple systems, good leaders facilitate the integrity and efficiency of the whole system (**Figure 1-4**).

Systems Do Not Compete with Each Other, but Instead Simply Seek to Thrive

Chaos theory and quantum theory both hold that competition is anomalous (Vakili et al., 2013). Still, current literature on organizations and their management contains numerous

Figure 1-4 Point-of-Service Systems Design.

discussions of the viability and importance of competition (Westra et al., 2017). This is a simplistic and often uninformed notion of the conditions and circumstances of thriving and advancing both as individuals and as communities. The old-fashioned and unidimensional notion associated with using a competitive model to thrive and advance holds sway among the most powerful in the business and political communities to the detriment of those communities they lead.

All living systems seek to thrive (Ford et al., 2013). At a fundamental level, they are not concerned with each other's survival unless it is somehow related to their own need to thrive. To this end, all life has a complementary and interdependent relationship with other life rather than a competitive one. Adaptation is not about competition between the fittest but about survival of the fittest, and the survival of a system depends more on its inherent adaptability to its environment and its ability to build community response than on anything else. To thrive, the system must have beneficial interactions with its environment, universal internal response to the environment, and the capacity to adjust to the prevailing conditions quickly and effectively. A system is fundamentally in competition with itself to thrive, not with anyone or anything else (**Figure 1-5**).

Generally, the concept of being in competition with oneself is foreign to unilateral capitalistic ways of thinking (as opposed to collateral capitalistic notions). Still, even unilateral capitalism treats competition as fundamentally a personal exercise—a contest between oneself and

Figure 1-5 Structural Integrity and Interdependence: Functional Components of a Health Structure.

others for profitability and success. What this approach fails to recognize is that success has less to do with one's competitors than with one's own adaptability, creativity, energy, and commitment to succeed. In other words, the pursuit of success should not be viewed as a contest with others but as a personal effort to give one's best and to thrive in the environment one has chosen to live in.

In the emerging age, persons and organizations will be challenged to adjust to a new context with a new set of rules. Those who thrive will be those who can read the signposts of environmental shifts quickly and effectively and apply the resulting insights to their own lives and operations. Organizational leaders need to learn the fundamentals of thriving in the new age of fast-paced technology drivers. They must make a diligent effort to keep up with the transformations in technology, global communications, information infrastructures, and social conditions and the drive for sustainable value. Here again, reading the signposts to create a tight fit between the demands of environmental changes and the system's capacity to embrace and adapt becomes a very important skill. Paying attention to indicators, monitoring innovations, experimenting with new and unfamiliar approaches, and living comfortably in the space between ambiguity and clarity, and the noise of constant change, are all essential skills of good leaders of the future.

The Compression of Time Will Affect How Work Is Done

There simply cannot be a leader anywhere on the earth who has not noticed the not-so-subtle change in our sense of time and space. Most people have noticed how time has sped up and how radically its quickening has affected the content and flow of work. Leaders can turn anywhere and hear others in the organization suggest that there is insufficient time to do all that is required. Leaders themselves are aware of how very little time they seem to have to meet a growing set of demands.

Technology, including the prevailing methods for purchasing and shipping material goods, is primarily responsible for the compression of time and work. For example, LASIK surgery, a type of corrective eye surgery, takes only 7 or 8 minutes to complete; internet grocery stores deliver groceries within 2 hours of order placement; and communication by email and text message is virtually instantaneous. Quick transmission of information and quick delivery of goods and services are increasingly normal in our global society.

The need for narrow hierarchy—for many layers of decision making and management—has all but disappeared from the business world. In the late 1980s and early 1990s, business leaders reconfigured their organizations to eliminate management structures that had long been part of organizational culture. The goal for organizations was to become nimble and fluid, and whatever impeded their achievement of this goal was either cast off or reconceived.

Today, healthcare organizations are experiencing a similar crisis. The growing demands of a value-based approach to health reform and system transformation require a complete reconceptualization of the design and infrastructure of healthcare delivery. The need to move from tertiary, process-heavy health service delivery to a more nimble primary healthcare model that advances the net aggregate health of American citizens creates new pressures for deconstructing, reconceiving, and recalibrating contemporary health service designs and models. Impeding this transformation is tertiary care–driven, fee-based, brick-and-mortar infrastructure that supports a delivery system that is no longer relevant (this infrastructure hinders the system's survival). Changes in technology, service structure, clinical models, consumer demand, and healthcare economics coalesce in response to the need for value-driven healthcare organizations that possess the same fluidity and nimbleness required of technology-grounded businesses.

> **Key Point**
>
> There is never enough time. Technology has compressed time so that what once was enough is now insufficient. Leaders must help others see their work from the perspective of compressed time. For example, now that clinical interventions require less time, practitioners and patients must shift their expectations to fit the narrowed time frame.

> **Point to Ponder**
>
> Over the next decade, as healthcare reform advances and services and interventions become more mobile, organizational leaders will be engaged in the deconstruction of the institutional infrastructure of health care—the bricks and mortar—and create a more network-designed model of integrated service delivery.

The current chaos in the health system arises from conflict between leadership commitment to an outmoded infrastructure and a system design that reflects value. The myriad stakeholders in the healthcare industry—administrators, nurses, doctors, hospital trustees, pharmacists, and so on—struggle to hold on to their piece of the healthcare pie without realizing that the pie is now being sliced in an entirely different way. The emerging healthcare system demands a significant change in the intersections of professions and their relationship to the health system and the individuals and populations it serves.

The compression of time works inexorably to reconfigure the context for health care and restructure its framework—often without consent from participants. Healthcare leaders must focus on interpreting external demands and translating them into internal actions. They are being called into the chaos of creativity to produce a good fit between the value framework and the infrastructure that must support it.

Much of the current work of healthcare leaders involves deconstructing existing health service models. The current infrastructure must be deconstructed so that it can be replaced by the more relevant, value-driven models of service and support. Leaders must perform a range of activities in reconfiguring health care to fit the clinical value work, where space and time will be even further compressed, services are more fluid and mobile, and the locus of control will shift from the provider to the user. The changes that will occur include these:

- *The hospital bed has ceased to be the main point of service.* During the next 2 decades, the number of hospital beds will decline by approximately 25%. Indeed, in the current healthcare paradigm, admission to hospital bed–based services is an indicator of the failure of the health system to provide health-based services that circumvent inpatient services.
- *The service structure will continue to be decentralized.* The healthcare system will deliver small, broadly dispersed units of service across the continuum of care.
- *Increasingly, services are moving out of the hospital.* By the end of the next decade, more than 70% of the medical services currently provided in hospitals will be provided in clinics, community settings (including pharmacies), health homes, advance practice provider and physician primary care offices, and virtually or digitally, with users remaining in their own environment.
- *The core practices of the professions are now being substantially altered.* The institution-based late-stage services that once predominated will be replaced by high-intensity primary care–based interventions that do not require hospitalization. These interventions will transform the roles of the various health professionals.
- *Users of health services will become more accountable for their own health.* Providers have the major job of helping to transfer the locus of control of medical decision making and life management to individuals, who have never had it and do not yet know what to do with it. Healthcare providers' work over the next 2 decades will include educating the users of health services and assisting them in acquiring the necessary skills to manage their own health through health management and preventive healthcare programs.
- *The users of health services and the technology of health care continue to progressively interface.* Virtual and technical interaction and communication will increasingly become the norm of health service provision. Connection between providers and patients will necessarily be virtual and seamless, with supporting technology enabling the provision of clinical services to patients remotely.

For the deconstruction of health services to be effective, leaders must know that this value-driven transformation is taking place and agree to lead the effort. The conditions are already in place, but the work of making the change meaningful and feasible is in its first stages. If a leader is opposed to the transformation or is unable to acquire the necessary skills, both the leader and the transformation will suffer.

One responsibility of leaders is to help others mourn the loss of practices and roles that are becoming irrelevant. Many popular reasons people have entered the health professions will no longer apply to their emerging roles. Despite this, health professionals continue to believe that their initial intent for entering their profession is still valid. Or they simply refuse to acknowledge that their idealization of the past might be keeping them from embracing the emerging and far different future of health service, to their own detriment.

One way to aid health professionals in mourning their losses is to help employees enumerate these losses and determine what they must let go to obtain the skills and master the roles they need to function in the emerging reformed and transformed healthcare system. Employees must individually voice their losses and symbolically let them go to turn in the direction of change and meet the challenges ahead. By doing this, employees become free to explore innovations and ultimately design a personal strategy to accommodate their profession and its role in transforming health care and improving the experience for people and communities.

Death is part of the cycle of life and is a requisite of all change. Not everything in the universe that thrives today will always do so. When circumstances change radically, some formerly vigorous systems fail. In some cases, the demands are beyond the system's capacity to adapt; in other cases, the changes call for a new work format that cannot be achieved simply by altering some of the characteristics of the workplace.

Leaders are obligated to help those whose work should change or be extinguished to do so quickly. Leaders are expected to make it clear to the staff that the process of bringing something to an end is as necessary as any other organizational process. A part of the tough work of facilitating necessary change is altering staff attitudes about the permanence of work. Employees get stuck in rituals and routines. Their attachment to these routines may be the only point of security they have in this quickly changing world. What employees might not know is that holding onto practices that are no longer relevant endangers their ability to succeed in the future. Leaders must "truth tell" to keep staff in mind of the fact that work effort and function are transitory and that a mindless attachment to the work itself may be the greatest impediment to their own success and that of the system.

Group Discussion

Thirty years ago the average length of stay in a hospital was 5.7 days. In the coming decade, the average procedure will require a stay of only 4.5 hours or fewer. These two different circumstances indicate the extreme shift in the nature of clinical services. Discuss how the new value-based service model will change the way healthcare providers work. What tasks will cease to possess value? What are emerging value-grounded functions? How can leaders convince staff to abandon old practices that are no longer relevant? And what are the implications for patients?

Leaders must keep their eyes fixed on the work and on how changes might affect the ability of staff members to do the work. The function of work continually changes, and attachment to work routines simply slows individuals' adaptation. A refusal to adapt does not diminish the demand for change; it just makes the adjustment to unrelenting change increasingly more difficult for the individual.

Change and Effectiveness

As Stephen Hawking has eloquently stated so many times, "Change is." Chaos, complexity, and change are not things but forms of dynamic activity. According to Hawking, they are the only constants in the universe (Hawking & Mlodinow, 2009). They will never cease because their end would be the end of everything. Perpetual dynamic movement is what underpins every action and process. This aspect of reality is less understood and less often made use of than physical laws, but it exists nonetheless.

Leadership is mainly concerned with adapting to change, and all the leadership functions and activities outlined in this and other contemporary leadership texts are informed by this understanding. In fact, theorists are inclined to be less definitive than they once were in their statements about the attributes of leadership and in their recipes for leadership success. Instead of being guided by an unchanging set of principles, leaders need to be fluid and adaptable because their role changes in concert with the changing conditions.

Leaders are aware that it is in the pursuit of meaning that the direction of a change can best be discerned. They continually look past the real and the present toward the unformed and potential to better evaluate the present and the direction of transformation (assessing how changes in the external environment create a demand for personal and organizational change). The subtle themes and ebbs and flows that lie just beneath the surface of events and experiences have more to say to leaders than do the events themselves.

Leaders know that much of what is seen and experienced is a metaphor for the operation of the infrastructure of change. The chaos so often represented in the change process is a cover for an explicit and elegant order that can be perceived only by focusing on the whole rather than on the parts. Indeed, looking at only the individual parts makes it almost impossible to see the integrity, order, and beauty embedded in an elegant web of flow and linkage. Staff is hungry to obtain from the leader this insight about the operation of the whole and how changes at this level of the system affect the choices and actions of persons at the system's points of service.

Leaders are encouraged by the connections that give meaning and value to the current and the real (**Exhibit 1-12**). The rules that guide the journey of change are both simple and complex, and the full set is not fully comprehensible all at once. An important task for any leader is to discern the predominant operating variable(s) affecting the journey at any given moment. Using insight, leaders can apply value to the predominant operating variable(s) represented and use them as a window for viewing the next factors, principles, or interacting forces pushing toward the changing next steps in any transformation.

Leaders are forever caught in the "potential" of life and experience. The ability to thrive in this "potential" place distinguishes good leaders from the rest. Good leaders are always on the edge of chaos, looking over the horizon, looking just beyond the precipice of the current, the "now." Located there, they can read, interpret, and express what they discern. Living in the "potential" suggests a capacity there to observe the trajectory of change, the unfolding conditions and circumstances embedded in environmental shifts and the convergence of circumstances that create a new or emerging reality. Their real gift, after having spent time in this

---

Exhibit 1-12   Unmotivated vs. Motivated Leaders

Unmotivated	Motivated
• Focus on the present.	• Focus on the potential.
• No time for the work.	• New kind of work.
• Things are getting worse.	• Things are different.
• Cannot do the work any more.	• New mental model for work.
• No one knows . . .	• How can I get to know . . . ?
• It is too much for one person.	• Share the work.
• This too shall pass.	• It is a journey I lead.
• Doing more with less.	• Doing different work differently.

"potential" place, is their ability to backtrack to where those they lead are living and working and translate what they have seen into a language that has force and meaning for those who can hear it. They then have the job of getting behind the staff and pushing them into their own conceptualization and definition of response to the emerging reality, allowing the staff to own what they see and act on it in a responsive and viable way.

Conclusion

Leadership skills are learned skills, and their mastery requires neither magic nor an untenable level of intellectual capacity. Leaders emerge in a wide variety of circumstances and reflect a broad range of talents and personalities. There is no one pattern of behavior or personality type that is most suitable for the leadership role. In short, leaders come in every size and shape.

What leaders must possess is the ability to understand the vagaries and complexities of human interactions and relationships. In their role as leaders, they must take into account chaos and complexity as these do their work and create their inimitable patterns of adaptation and growth. Good leaders live in the edge land between now and the very next thing and can engage folks in the journey of the whole across the landscape of a preferred and optimistic future.

Leaders in the coming age will need new skills and new insights about leadership and the preferred methods of "journeying." New skills and insights can be learned, adapted to current conditions, and applied in a variety of ways to meet the demands of the journey. In their application, individuals may come to discover the leader in themselves, feel the excitement of leadership work, and inspire others in the journey of discovery and advancement.

Chapter Takeaways

1. Change is not a thing or an event but is rather a dynamic that is constitutive of the universe. Change is always, everywhere, endless, and conditional. Change is the one single constant in the universe.
2. The primary and transformative work of leaders is embedded in their availability to the requisites of change, the opportunity to discern and respond to the change dynamic, and the capacity to guide and lead others in both forming and moving the change in a way that advances the human condition.
3. Leaders must not just close the door on old models of healthcare delivery and clinical work, they must also turn around and face the future with a view to the emerging landscape and a commitment to develop a workable vision and to implement it.
4. The most radical shift informing the role of leaders is the move away from mechanistic (Newtonian) and reductionistic models of thought and action toward integrated, multilateral, and multidimensional whole systems (quantum) models exemplified by complexity and continuous innovation.
5. The rise of quantum theory and the new appreciation and application of complexity and complex adaptive systems as foundational characteristics of all human action have altered our view of leadership and life. The role of leaders is now informed by the dynamics associated with complexity and call for new leadership thinking and acting.

Case Study 1-1

Transforming Leaders

Cameryn is the vice president for professional development at a large metropolitan hospital in the Midwest. She has been in her role for 6 years and has accepted new responsibilities over the years, widening her scope of work to include the direction of all of the clinical nurse specialists (CNSs), the new graduate residency program, and the research- and evidence-based practice initiatives. She also oversees the Magnet program, which strives for continual readiness for redesignation.

Cameryn and some of the other leaders in the organization have become concerned about the competence level of some nurse managers and their assistant managers, clinical leads, and shift supervisors. The managers and others "get the job done," but they do not seem to be focused on inspiring the workforce to achieve excellence in their work or preparing potential leaders for succession. In fact, some managers seem to be threatened by informal leaders who excel in the clinical setting; they fail to encourage them to develop their skills and competencies to assume direct leadership roles in the future.

For all in manager and supervisory roles, the hospital provides a quarterly leadership educational event with motivational speakers. The feedback regarding the leadership event is positive, and managers are expected to share with their staff the new knowledge gained from the motivational speakers and presentations. How this new knowledge is shared and disseminated is not assessed. Cameryn wonders whether it is shared at all and questions how well the leadership messages are integrated into the daily behaviors and activities of the managers.

Cameryn has been reading about transformational leadership and how one of the characteristics of a transformational leader is to inspire others to achieve what they previously thought was impossible. Cameryn reflects on those in her own career who inspired her to return to school for further education and ultimately to seek roles where she could influence nursing practice and patient care. In her heart, she wants to provide the same experience for all developing nurse leaders in the clinical setting and also in beginning-level management positions. She believes that management is far more than "getting the job done and completing tasks" and needs to include behaviors that transform individuals into those who have a thirst for new knowledge and quest to constantly change the status quo to achieve excellence in their work.

Cameryn is inspired to do something about the development of the nurse managers. She realizes that the first step would be to inspire her colleagues to embrace the same vision for nursing leadership at all levels within the organization, especially with their focus on managing budgets and meeting organizational priorities. Cameryn is convinced that with better prepared frontline managers, many of the organizational priorities could be achieved more expediently. She wants the group to examine the current roles expected of clinical leads, shift supervisors, nurse managers, and their assistants and the personal and experience requirements for the roles. She also wants to impress upon her colleagues that their own behaviors strongly influence those who are watching their interactions with others and daily behaviors in their roles. She realizes that this is a sensitive subject, and she decides to develop a strategy to informally lead her colleagues on a journey for their own improvement and to influence them to improve the experience of their direct reports. She realizes that the interconnection between her colleagues and their direct reports is critical for the changes that she envisions to transform every nurse manager and supervisor into true inspirational leaders.

Cameryn decides to move beyond the occasional inspirational speaker and elects to empower the management team at all levels with as much information as possible about transformational leadership, workplace empowerment, healthy work environment, and nursing excellence. She works with the Collaborative Governance Council for Professional Development to initiate a leadership journal club for clinical leaders and all levels of management. The journal club is led by the members of the Professional Development Council who choose the journal articles to read and review. The council also establishes group meeting norms, leads the discussions about the articles, and creates a short summary of the articles for all of the nursing staff to read in the Magnet Nursing Newsletter.

Cameryn also decides that it is important to determine the actual learning needs of those in management positions, so she develops a self-assessment tool using the leadership domains outlined by the American Organization of Nurse Executives and the Benner levels of competency as the response set. The new assessment tool provides information as to how each manager, assistant manager, clinical lead, and shift supervisor perceives his or her level of competence in each of the leadership domains. From that information, Cameryn plans to develop educational content and experiences that are targeted to areas where managers perceive themselves to be least competent. She also meets with those who are more expert in the leadership domains and discusses their mentoring those who are less experienced and competent and presenting some of the formal content needed for development of the frontline leadership team.

Recognizing that professional development is a very complex and multileveled task, Cameryn also plans to develop educational content and experiences for the more expert group to teach them how to mentor others and how to prepare and present educational content using teaching methods that are innovative, engaging, and inspiring to the learners. Cameryn realizes how interconnected each level of the plan is and how necessary it is to create a fluid and adaptable project management plan to guide the various stages of development to transform nurse managers into true leaders.

She soon realizes that in her work with the collaborative governance councils to develop an educational intervention for the frontline managers she has forgotten to engage the Human Resources department, which is also responsible for leadership development. There are many indications of their discontent with her new leadership development program. When Cameryn recognizes their concern, she meets with them to discuss ways that Human Resources could be instrumental in the assessment and development of frontline managers.

Needless to say, not all of her colleagues embrace her vision to transform the leaders in the organization. Many barriers emerge that would dissuade most from continuing to achieve their vision, and Cameryn is disappointed at times and must continually refocus her energies to remain on course despite the barriers. When she recognizes that one of her colleagues or one of the nurse managers is not "on board," she spends personal time talking with that person and helping to translate the vision so that it could become his or her reality as well. She is continually engaged in dialogue with others to support the change effort, and she formally recognizes the actions and efforts of those who are involved in mentoring less experienced nurse leaders and those who are involved in the educational activities.

The transformational process has taken several years, but reflecting on the progress, Cameryn and her colleagues believe that significant changes have occurred in the organization and that nurse leaders at every level have benefited from the efforts to enhance the competencies and skills of the frontline managers. The benefits of the program are validated with significant improvements in employee opinion surveys and in surveys to assess healthy work environment.

Questions

1. How do you think that complexity science and quantum leadership systems thinking provide a framework for an initiative to advance the competencies and skills of frontline managers and to change the management culture to a leadership culture in an organization?
2. How effective do you think Cameryn was in transforming the leadership culture in her organization? What might she have done differently to facilitate the change process?
3. One of the roles of the quantum leader is to read the signposts that give direction and feedback regarding the change process. What were some of the signposts that Cameryn encountered during the development of the frontline manager group, interactions with her colleagues, and the encounter with the Human Resources department?
4. In your opinion, what effect will advancing the frontline managers, her own colleagues' competence, and transformational leadership culture have on the organizational climate, nursing satisfaction, and even patient outcomes?

Case Study 1-2

Inspiring Greatness

Lynn has been the dean of the College of Nursing at a prestigious university for the past 2 years. Others describe Lynn as having incredible energy and vision, and being someone who is in constant motion, leading and transforming the college into a powerhouse among the other colleges at the university. It would seem that Lynn knows no limitations or boundaries to her visions. She is recognized as an extraordinary leader by her colleagues at the university, and she is known as a national and international expert in her clinical area of expertise as well as in her direction for the development of many interdisciplinary programs within the College of Nursing. Lynn has multiple appointments to national advisory boards and is a fellow in the American Academy of Nursing as well as a number of other nursing practice academies. She sits on several interdisciplinary strategic planning expert panels for national healthcare reform and other health initiatives. Clearly, she is recognized as one of the top leaders in nursing and health care.

Lynn is the first to recognize and acknowledge that being a national expert does not make it any easier to initiate and execute change within one's own organization. Even though Lynn is acknowledged as an external leader, she is continually challenged internally with the same barriers of resistance that less recognized experts encounter when they try to initiate change within their organization. Although Lynn has boundless energy and is motivated to help others make a significant difference in their work and contributions, she also struggles with how to manage those who do not embrace her vision or have the same passion for accelerated change. When asked how she manages her feelings related to the naysayers in her life, she states that she seeks to listen carefully to the message that they are trying to impart and understand their perspective on the matter and their concerns and fears. From that framework, she tries to find a connection between her own vision and the vision of those who oppose her, realizing that a shared vision is the beginning of all successful change. She then seeks to find a way to focus their attention on what is shared in common in their visions and highlights areas where they are interdependent or mutually dependent on one another to achieve their visions.

The nursing and healthcare literature is replete with evidence and opinions about the need for interdisciplinary collaboration to ensure optimal patient outcomes, professional role satisfaction, and healthcare excellence. With this in mind, Lynn proposes to develop an interprofessional curriculum for colleges of nursing, medicine, pharmacy, and social services. Lynn develops a proposal for the intercollege planning committee and provost that outlines a number of courses that could be taught with an integrated curriculum to students from each of the colleges. She also includes how the proposed integrated curriculum could be budget neutral or actually realize a cost savings because classes presented to each college in duplicate would be eliminated and integrative classes would be developed using fewer faculty and facility resources. Lynn supports the proposal with evidence about the positive effects of an interdisciplinary approach in improving relationships among professionals and the recommendation from the Institute of Medicine and Robert Wood Johnson Foundation report on the future of nursing.

Lynn is not an inexperienced leader, so she anticipates that there will be resistance to her proposal. She tries to prepare herself for all the voices that will say, "It can't be done. We've never done it before. We are successful with the current curriculum structure," and offer a host of other objections. Some of the loudest voices of opposition justify their position by stating that the social power imbalance between nursing and the other healthcare professions is a reason why the integrated curriculum should not be implemented. Some mention that the intellectual level of the medical and pharmacy students is far different from that of the nursing and social work students and that the nursing and social work students would not be able to manage the rigor of the courses needed to educate future physicians and pharmacists.

Some of the meetings are intense, chaotic, and filled with motion as the curriculum committee discusses the pros and cons of having an integrated curriculum. At times Lynn is very discouraged with the progress, but she keeps focused with positive energy and strong belief that her proposal is critical to improving patient care. She recognizes that the simple proposal is loaded with complexity and the discord that is happening is an important part of the process as participants reflect on their beliefs and values. On the one hand, Lynn wishes that the provost would simply step up and direct the group to develop an integrated curriculum because Lynn realizes that the provost supports the proposal. On the other hand, she realizes the value of the change process and how the participants' values and beliefs will morph over time as a result of the discussions, readings, and continual analysis of the pros and cons of the proposal.

Lynn recognizes the need to be patient and not push the change, but rather to quietly influence others on the merits of interprofessional education. She provides a number of articles from reputable journals, arranges for speakers on the topic, and even creates an all-day workshop to bring in national speakers and participants to discuss strategies to develop interprofessional curricula. Of course, she arranges the workshop around the availability of the other deans so that they can attend the workshop as well. She even arranges for a few of the more forward-thinking deans to present at the workshop. She invites one of the other deans to co-present with her at an international conference focused on interprofessional education. Lynn acts as if they have already accepted the idea even though she knows that part of her strategy is to convince them to accept the proposal.

Within the year, the curriculum committee not only accepts the proposal for an interprofessional curriculum to begin the next year but actually acts as if the notion was their idea to begin with. At this point, Lynn realizes that she has successfully managed the change.

Questions

1. Identify the elements of complexity in this case study.
2. How effective do you think Lynn is in managing the conflict, complexity, and the chaos that emerges around her proposal to develop an interprofessional curriculum?
3. How well does Lynn read the signposts and develop strategies to manage her vision?
4. What processes might have been used to help the curriculum committee to accept the proposal and move beyond their personal agendas, values, fears, and doubts about the importance of interprofessional education?
5. What role do you feel a quantum leader needs to play in developing consensus around decision making?
6. What quantum leader characteristics does Lynn portray in leading the group to embrace her vision and to change and adapt the curriculum to an interprofessional focus?

References

Aarons, G., Ehrhart, M., Farahnak, L., & Hurlburt, M. (2015). Leadership and organizational change for implementation: A randomized mixed method pilot study of leadership and organization development intervention for evidence-based practice implementation. *Implementation Science, 10*(11), 1–12.

Ash, A. S., Mick, E. O., Ellis, R. P., Kiefe, C. I., Allison, J. J., & Clark, M. A. (2017). Social determinants of health in managed care payment formulas. *JAMA Internal Medicine, 177*(10), 1424–1430.

Bennis, W. G., Sample, S. B., & Asghar, R. (2015). *The art and adventure of leadership: Understanding failure, resilience and success.* Wiley.

Bilal, M., Iqbal, H. M. N., Guo, S., Hu, H., Wang, W., & Zhang, X. (2018). State-of-the-art protein engineering approaches using biological macromolecules: A review from immobilization to implementation view point. *International Journal of Biological Macromolecules, 108*, 893–901.

Birk, S. (2013). The future of physician leadership: Physician leaders and the changing healthcare landscape. *Healthcare Executive, 28*(1), 8–10, 12–14, 16.

Brandenburger, A. (2019). Strategy needs creativity. An analytic framework alone won't reinvent business. *Harvard Business Review, 97*(2), 58–65.

Brill, S. B., Moss, K. O., & Prater, L. (2019). Transformation of the doctor–patient relationship: Big data, accountable care, and predictive health analytics. *HEC Forum, 31*(4), 261–282.

Costich, J., Scutchfield, F., & Ingram, R. (2015). Population health, public health, and accountable care: Emerging roles and relationships. *American Journal of Public Health, 105*(5), 846–850.

Drucker, P. (2009). *Management.* Harper Collins.

Duncan, M. (2019). Integrated care systems and nurse leadership. *British Journal of Community Nursing, 24*(11), 538–542.

Edersheim, E. H., & Drucker, P. F. (2007). *The definitive Drucker.* McGraw-Hill.

Flury, C. G. (2017). Social media as a leadership tool for nurse executives. *Nursing Economic$, 35*(5), 272–275.

Ford, L., Seers, A., & Neumann, J. (2013). Honoring complexity. *Management Research Review, 36*(7), 644–663.

Gros, C. (2015). *Complex and adaptive dynamical systems: A primer* (4th ed.). Springer.

Hawking, S., & Mlodinow, L. (2009). *A briefer history of time.* Bantam.

Kane, S., Gandidzanwa, C., Mutasa, R., Moyo, I., Sismayi, C., Mafaune, P., & Dieleman, M. (2019). Coming full circle: How health worker motivation and performance in results-based financing arrangements hinges on strong and adaptive health systems. *International Journal of Health Policy and Management, 8*(2), 101–111.

Khanna, P. (2016). *Connectography: Mapping the future of global civilization.* Random House.

Lunden, A., Teräs, M., Kvist, T., & Häggman-Laitila, A. (2017). A systematic review of factors influencing knowledge management and the nurse leader's role. *Journal of Nursing Management, 25*(6), 407–420.

McKimm, J., & Till, A. (2015). Clinical leadership effectiveness, change and complexity. *British Journal of Hospitals Medicine, 76*(4), 239–243.

Meissner, P. (2018). LADDERS: A dynamic paradigm for planning, implementing, and evaluating sustainable change in learning health systems. *Learning Health Systems, 2*(3), e10058.

Newell, S., & Jordan, Z. (2015). The patient experience of patient-centered communication with nurses in the hospital setting: A qualitative systematic review protocol. *JBI Database System of Systematic Reviews and Database Reports, 13*(1), 76–87.

Porter-O'Grady, T., & Malloch, K. (2016). *Quantum leadership: Building better partnerships for sustainable health* (3rd ed.). Jones & Bartlett Learning.

Ricciardi, W., Pita Barros, P., Bourek, A., Brouwer, W., Kelsey, T., Lehtonen, L., & Expert Panel on Effective Ways of Investing in Health (EXPH). (2019). How to govern the digital transformation of health services. *European Journal of Public Health, 29*(Supp. 3), 7–12.

Souba, W., & Souba, M. (2018). How effective leaders harness the future. *Academic Medicine: Journal of the Association of American Medical Colleges, 93*(2), 166–171.

Souba, W., & Tsai, A. (2019). Beyond better, safer, cheaper health care: What's ultimately at stake? *Academic Medicine: Journal of the Association of American Medical Colleges, 94*(11), 1679–1684.

Storkholm, M. H., Mazzocato, P., & Savage, C. (2019). Make it complicated: A qualitative study utilizing complexity framework to explain improvement in health care. *BMC Health Services Research, 19*(1), 842.

Uhl-Bien, M., Marion, R., & McKelvey, B. (2007). Complexity leadership theory: Shifting leadership from the industrial age to the knowledge era. *The Leadership Quarterly, 18*(4), 298–318.

Vakili, G., Tabatabaee, F., & Khorsandi, S. (2013). Emergence of cooperation and peer-to-peer systems: A complex adaptive system approach. *Systems Engineering, 16*(2), 213–223.

Volti, R. (2017). *Society and technological change* (8th ed.). Worth.

Westra, D., Angeli, F., Carree, M., & Ruwaard, D. (2017). Coopetition in health care: A multi-level analysis of its individual and organizational determinants. *Social Science & Medicine, 186*, 43–51.

Suggested Readings

Arnold, R. D., & Wade, J. P. (2015). A definition of systems thinking: A systems approach. *Precedia Computer Science, 44*, 669–678.

Basole, R., & Rouse, W. (2008). Complexity of service value networks: Conceptualization and empirical investigation. *IBM Systems Journal, 47*(1), 53–70.

Best, A., Greenhalgh, T., Lewis, S., Saul, J. E., Carroll, S., & Bitz, J. (2012). Large-system transformation in health care: A realist review. *Milbank Quarterly, 90*(3), 421–456.

Bryman, A. (2011). *The SAGE handbook of leadership.* SAGE.

Cardiff, S., McCormack, B., & McCance, T. (2018). Person-centered leadership: A relational approach to leadership derived through action research. *Journal of Clinical Nursing, 27*, 3056–3069.

Erickson, J. I. (2013). Reflections on leadership talent: A void or an opportunity? *Nursing Administration Quarterly, 37*(1), 44–51.

Everett, L. Q., & Sitterding, M. C. (2013). Building a culture of innovation by maximizing the role of the RN. *Nursing Administration Quarterly, 37*(3), 194–202.

Malloch, K., & Porter-O'Grady, T. (2009). *The quantum leader: Applications for the new world of work*. Jones & Bartlett Learning.

Orlando, R., III., & Haytaian, M. (2012). Physician leadership: A health-care system's investment in the future of quality care. *Connecticut Medicine, 76*(7), 417–420.

Pati, S., Reum, J., Conant, E., Tuton, L., Scott, P., & Abbuhl, S. (2013). Tradition meets innovation: Transforming academic medical culture at the University of Pennsylvania's Perelman School of Medicine. *Academic Medicine, 88*(4), 461–464.

Porter-O'Grady, T., & Malloch, K. (2009). *Innovation leadership*. Jones & Bartlett Learning.

Spaulding, A., Kash, B. A., Johnson, C. E., & Gamm, L. (2017). Organizational capacity for change in health care: Development and validation of a scale. *Health Care Management Review, 42*(2), 151–161.

Watkins, M. D. (2012). How managers become leaders. The seven seismic shifts of perspective and responsibility. *Harvard Business Review, 90*(6), 64–72, 144.

Quiz Questions

Select the best answer for each of the following questions.

1. For the past 30 years, we have been leaving which of the following ages?
   a. The Middle Ages
   b. The Age of Technology
   c. The Information Age
   d. The Industrial Age

2. What is the primary vehicle moving us out of the past age?
   a. Economics
   b. Technology
   c. Satellites
   d. Politics

3. As we get closer to fully living in the new age, the pace of change:
   a. quickens.
   b. slows.
   c. becomes unstable.
   d. stays about the same.

4. Adaptation means:
   a. adjusting to the current reality.
   b. accommodating the emerging reality.
   c. bringing the past reality forward.
   d. living fully for today.

5. What happens in the process of autopoiesis?
   a. Living systems seek to continually reinvent themselves.
   b. Living systems leave behind forms they do not like.
   c. Living systems maintain their stability throughout each change.
   d. Living systems end themselves because they have no other role.

6. What is accountability a matter of?
   a. Using good work processes
   b. Acting responsibly
   c. Performing efficiently
   d. Achieving desired work outcomes

7. Systems thinking identifies which of the following as an essential characteristic of all systems?
   a. Codependence
   b. Predictability
   c. Interdependence
   d. Incrementalism

8. Chaos is essential to all change. What is the primary purpose of chaos in the change process?
   a. To confuse people enough to make them change
   b. To challenge people to see the changes that are coming clearly
   c. To cut people's attachment to the past and engage them in the "noise" of change
   d. To get people to identify the characteristics of a particular change and to respond specifically to those characteristics

9. What is the primary role of the leader during a time of great change?
   a. To help people embrace and adapt to change
   b. To explain the kind of changes people can expect
   c. To minimize the pain points of the change process
   d. To push people into necessary changes and help them cope

10. Chaos theory and complexity science require leaders to alter their understanding of how change works. To develop a new understanding of change, leaders must first see their role in relationship to which of the following?
    a. The changes that are occurring in the workplace
    b. The whole system and its place in the change process
    c. The staff's issues and their responses to the demands of change
    d. The challenges that lie ahead in implementing new changes

11. Which of the following statements about living in "potential reality" versus "actual reality" is true for leaders?
    a. Living in actual reality allows leaders to deal with chaos in a structured way
    b. Living in potential reality promotes guessing the future and preventing chaos
    c. Living in potential reality allows leaders to predict a path of future change
    d. Living in actual reality promotes attention to emerging uncertainty

12. A fractal is critical for comprehending the order that exists in chaos because:
    a. it is the largest unit of organization that describes all elements that are subsets of something larger than itself.
    b. it is a pattern of precise detail that appears repeatedly in the same pattern at every scale in a web of forever-expanding symmetry.
    c. it is an unnatural and chaotic discordant pattern of differentiation that does not repeat itself over time and space.
    d. it is the smallest unit of organization that defines how all other units will operate and represents a fixed notion of system function and design.

13. *Value* can most correctly be defined as:
    a. the number of dollars attached to a service or product.
    b. a numeric indicator of significance or importance.
    c. a subjective determination of significance that changes based on perception.
    d. an objective determination of relative worth, merit, or importance.

14. The fundamental substantive change in American health care over the past decade has been driven by:
    a. a reduction in the total number of financial resources available for the provision of healthcare services.
    b. a decreasing number of physicians and nurses, creating an increasing level of stress in the capacity to provide services.
    c. a fundamental shift from volume to value in both paying and providing for healthcare services.
    d. insurance companies increasing the price of healthcare insurance coverage and reducing the number of benefits available to users.

15. Which of the following is one of the major tasks of 21st-century healthcare leaders?
    a. Creating a safe milieu for the struggles and pain of changing practice and health service
    b. Assuring that all health professionals are doing the same work in the same way with the same measures of excellence
    c. Maintaining a strong vertical alliance in health organizations to ensure that every level of the organization is focused on doing the same work
    d. Separating and clarifying the role of professions and departments in order to more clearly define their unilateral work functions and performance in the organization

16. One of the central skills reflecting a new framework for 21st-century leadership is:
    a. strengthening the ability to see intersections, relationships, and themes, which ensures that the organization will continue to undertake the activities necessary to thrive.
    b. ensuring that operations and functions that clearly defined the organization are strengthened and reaffirmed so that each department is clear about its specific work in the organization.
    c. refining employee job descriptions and performance expectations to be clearly defined and stabilized to facilitate employees' ability to understand work requirements.
    d. developing an excellent employee performance evaluation system that assesses individual employee proficiency and rewards individual employees for complying with requirements.

17. The notion of interdependence is critical to understanding complexity. Which of the following statements is correct?
    a. In any system, action in one place has an effect in all other places.
    b. Fluctuation of mutuality means authority does not move between people.
    c. Trusting feeling (or having a gut-sense) is less important than valuing thinking.
    d. Interacting properties in a system make outcomes fixed and finite.

18. Planning is an important leadership skill set. Which of the following statements is true with regard to contemporary planning activity?
    a. Plans always look at a fixed point at some time in the future.
    b. Plans are a certain commitment of the organization and must remain stable to their completion.
    c. Contemporary planning requires an understanding of the trajectory of change.
    d. Planning assumes that strategies are clearly and finitely determined and are changed only when completed.

19. Central to the concept of adaptation is the understanding that all systems respond collectively to change in their environment. Which of the following relates to this statement?
    a. These noninteracting change phenomena remain stable between the system and its environment.
    b. All systems have an intelligence that reflects a continual and dynamic intersecting between all persons and processes in the system.
    c. Rational and operational science skills and functions are more important to organizational effectiveness than insight, intuition, and feelings.
    d. Being capable and competent in form and function in a system is enough for the leader to provide clear and meaningful direction in the system.

20. For information to be valuable, its quantity is not as important as its relevance and timeliness. With regard to information, leaders must know:
    a. all recently published information available on themes that affect their work.
    b. any information that other leaders in the organization expect them to know.
    c. how much information on a theme is sufficient to determine its bearing on decisions.
    d. what is important to the department but not necessarily important to other leaders.

21. Chaos is continually at work in all systems. One of the elements associated with complexity is paradox, which is often evident in paired elements of life that appear on the surface to be contradictory. Which of the following is *not* one of those paired elements?
    a. Chaos and order
    b. Creativity and tension
    c. Conflict and peace
    d. Difference and diversity

22. Effective systems do not compete with each other; instead, all systems simply seek to thrive. Therefore, chaos and quantum theory hold that competition is:
    a. synonymous.
    b. unidimensional.
    c. antediluvian.
    d. anomalous.

23. Going forward, the health system will change significantly enough to alter existing structure in the health system. Six projections were offered in this chapter. Which of the following is *not* one of these projections?
    a. The hospital bed will cease to be the main point of service.
    b. The service structure of health care will be further decentralized.
    c. Users of health services will become more accountable for their own health.
    d. The core practices of the professions will remain substantially unaltered.

24. In this chapter, it was suggested that leadership skills are learned. What particular leadership ability or understanding was identified as critical to the contemporary role of leaders?
    a. Giving employees clear and precise direction.
    b. Predicting strategy and objectives when identifying future work.
    c. Understanding complexities of human interaction and relationships.
    d. Creating fixed points of reference to define and guide change.

25. What is one of the best ways leaders can discern the potential direction of change?
    a. Understand the present, live fully in it, and help people accommodate reality.
    b. Look toward unformed possibilities to better understand their meaning.
    c. Develop clearly defined operational realities of current work processes.
    d. Manage signposts to enhance stability, thereby increasing employee confidence.

CHAPTER TWO

Ten Complexity Principles for Leaders Advancing Value in the Quantum Age

Do not go where the path may lead, go instead where there is no path and leave a trail.

—*Ralph Waldo Emerson*

Chapter Objectives

At the completion of this chapter, the reader will be able to:

- Analyze the key characteristics of complexity and their impact on the leadership role.
- Evaluate personal characteristics and their fit with the leadership skills needed in all complex systems.
- Formulate personal goals for adapting to the leadership role in the presence of chaos and complexity.
- Summarize the principles of complexity and describe their practical implications for the leadership role.
- Apply the principles of complexity theory to the personal exercise of leadership.

Ours is a time of continuous significant social, cultural, economic, and health transformation (Thakrar & Bell, 2017). New scientific foundations grounded in the concept of complexity and its impact at every level of existence have altered our understanding of the leadership and management of change (Gergen, 2015). The growing understanding and explication of quantum theory and the subsequent application of complexity and chaos theory to human organizations have altered the nature of leadership forever. Leaders must now more deeply understand the implications of complexity theory for the leadership role and for processes associated with transforming work and the workplace. Principles of complexity theory largely determine how best to help others own their own change, undertake the right change processes, and understand the rules of engagement in the postindustrial age.

The emerging constructs of complexity associated with human dynamics and the multifocal interface and myriad of intersections in human systems is reinforcing the very foundations of effective leadership. Building on the previous 5,000 years of unfolding leadership thought and theory, complexity leadership pushes beyond the functional, two- to three-dimensional foundations upon which leadership roles have been examined. The emergence of a deeper understanding of the influence of the dynamics of complexity applied to human activity reflects a deeper understanding of the "dance" of interaction, interface, and relationship at every level of human dynamics and in every place in the social system. The capacity to lead now must reflect these emerging insights and realities and describe a different format and forum for leadership expression.

Throughout the world, healthcare personnel are overwhelmed by their work, the pace of change, limitations on their time, the endless advance of technology and related social changes (de Jong et al., 2016; Lal, 2019). Especially now, health care is experiencing increased demand for value and, thus, transformation in an environment of severely diminished resources. Reflecting the many demands of health reform, the pace of change is so rapid that many healthcare leaders have left the field and many health professionals are considering whether to follow. Several factors drive this situation:

- *Change is endless.* In the "good old days," it seemed as though changes came in an ordered fashion and with enough time between them to allow people to adjust to the new demands. Indeed, because changes came so rarely and moved so slowly, people almost believed they created them rather than responded to them. Today, changes come so quickly that it is difficult to know when one change ends and another begins. Further, five or more changes may be unfolding at one time, and because people must deal with these changes simultaneously, they often do not know how they are doing or if any of the changes are sustainable. They may be confronted by so many changes, and be making so many changes, that they wind up changing the changes. Stephen Hawking stated, "Change is," by which he means that change is a constant. Change is not a thing, but a dynamic, a context for everything that happens in the universe. During a time of transition, forces converge to make it possible for many changes to occur simultaneously. What is most striking about the nature of change today is the large number of forces converging and the large number of changes unfolding at the same time.
- *The growing social, political, and economic forces driving contemporary health reform and transformation to reflect a stronger value orientation accelerate the requirement to embrace and engage entirely new notions of healthcare service and value.* The transformation of the healthcare system requires movement out of a predominantly tertiary care model of service delivery toward more general use of value-driven models of episodic, population, and continua of care services. Approaches to accountability, value, and affordability require a new level of consciousness between provider and user and significantly different approaches to designing health care, providing service, advancing health-based outcomes, and creating a sustainable and affordable framework for health delivery in the United States. All of this requires the capacity to reconceptualize approaches; define new methods and models of care delivery; evaluate effectiveness, value, and sustainable health outcomes; and reduce the untenable cost of health service. When linked and integrated, the degree of complexity and intensity invested at every level of leadership and service in health care has few historic parallels. Challenges associated with this major transformation are constant and operate at both the collective and individual levels of leadership.

- *Information is remarkably more available than in the past.* Previously, the amount and kind of information needed at work were rarely readily available. Today, the vast amount of data on hand makes it very difficult to distinguish what is relevant and valuable. The goal is not simply to find the right information, but to find it at the right time, in the right form. Indeed, too much information is just as much a hindrance as too little. Making good decisions is still a matter of choosing data carefully. Further, this is the Information Age, which means that information is the key to sustaining integrated activities and assessing their value and impact. The importance of information has, in turn, affected the content and manner of decision making. Clinicians, for example, rather than depending solely on traditional medical principles and human judgment, now must draw from increasingly complex categories of evidence-grounded information in their decision making.
- *Knowledge is more a utility than a capacity.* In the 20th century, knowledge was treated as a possession—one had knowledge or gained knowledge. The process of learning was essentially a process of "stuffing" facts into one's head. As a result of this process, the knowledgeable person possessed knowledge and could draw from it when necessary. Today, however, from the quantum perspective, we see knowledge as a utility. Because so much information is available, no one has sufficient capacity to acquire all the knowledge needed. Thus, the focus has shifted from possession to access. To use knowledge appropriately, people must be able to access the right knowledge at the right time in the right way for the right purpose, apply the knowledge wisely and well, and then let knowledge go when it is no longer relevant (Lunden et al., 2017). The current challenges for leaders are to recognize that knowledge is a utility; to develop skills needed to access, promote, and manage knowledge; and to use knowledge in organizational learning (Lunden et al., 2019).
- *Technology is changing the character and content of the service relationship.* Virtually nothing has changed the circumstances of life as radically as the application of new technologies. Most of us confront technologies that we read about in science fiction novels and assumed we would never live to see. Thirty years ago, the average length of stay for hospital services (the only healthcare services available) was 5.7 days. Today, the average length of stay for many high-tech services is 4.5 hours. What a dramatic change for providers and users! Technology affects all elements of service. Procedures once done only in a hospital under close supervision can now be done in a clinic or even at home. Laser therapy, CT scanners, nanotherapy, DNA-moderated interventions, microtherapeutics, 3D printing, and learning healthcare systems derived from big data, to name just a few technologies, are signs of the radical shift occurring in the delivery of services. The shift is still in its formative stages, with much more to come as a result of improvements in pharmaceuticals, technotherapeutics, and the application of genomics.
- *Wireless technologies now operate in a way that defies boundaries.* We live in a boundary-less world, with all that implies. This sense of universal collectivity changes the perceptions of differences, boundaries, and barriers and allows each of us to remain connected to anyone, no matter where in the world we live. We can take our technology into any location, no matter how isolated, and still be connected to every other part of the world. This sense of the world and our connection to it has led to global communities

of work, entrepreneurship, innovation, communication, and social enterprise (Knight et al., 2018). New kinds of international partnerships and models that connect people and systems and challenge old constructs of boundary, be they national, regional, work related, organizational, or social, are emerging.

This list merely indicates the dramatic changes that are affecting health care and other arenas of social existence. Further, the pace of these and other evolving and revolutionary changes is not likely to slow any time soon. The quantum, complex, even chaotic nature of change and the convergence of forces periodically brings about an age of transition, and that is exactly what we are living through now.

Chaos and Complexity and the Drive for Value

The interacting and intersecting character of complexity draws us into a web of relationships and interactions that will ultimately change our way of living. From strange attractors to webs of influence and relatedness, elements of complexity theory alter the rules of work and interaction by giving us a deeper understanding of the relatedness of things and the role of change and discernment in human progress.

The strange characteristics of complexity are embedded in human activities as well as physical processes. An item at one level of reality is affected by everything else at all other levels. Sometimes we can see and understand the causal process. In most cases, however, the cause is not transparent and requires special knowledge to be understood. In addition, because of the connection of all elements of any process, the observation of the process affects what takes place, as evidenced by the wave–particle duality of electrons, which explains how electrons exhibit wave characteristics or particle characteristics depending on the experimental arrangement.

The impact of leadership often depends on the amount of time the leader spends living in the potential. Schrödinger's cat, a famous thought experiment intended to illuminate the difference between actuality and potentiality, helps us understand the importance of leaders applying the principle of the potential to their own role. In 1935, Schrödinger used an imaginary scenario to illustrate a quantum mechanics problem. He posited that a cat might at one time be both alive and dead depending on an earlier random event. In the experiment, a cat, a flask of poison, and a radioactive substance are placed in a sealed box. If an internal monitor detects radioactivity, the flask is shattered, releasing the poison that ultimately kills the cat. Schrödinger's interpretation of quantum mechanics implies that, after a while, the cat is simultaneously alive and dead, yet when we look in the box, we see the cat either as alive or dead, not both. The question is: When exactly does quantum supposition end and reality collapse into one possibility or the other? These rather complex notions indicate that things

> **Key Point**
> Understanding complexity is requisite for understanding relationships. Complexity science teaches us that everything is related at some level.

> **Point to Ponder**
> How many leaders realize that their primary work is to help others deal with the changes that affect their lives and their work? Living in the potential for change is focusing on the "journey" of work rather than on the "events" of work. This journey should be a leader's primary focus.

Exhibit 2-1 Actual Versus Potential Reality

Living in the Actual
- Focus on the present.
- Living the experience now.
- Focus on good process.
- Key is work quality.
- Emphasis on current activity.
- People focus on their own work.

Living in the Potential
- Inclusion of coming events.
- Seeing the work as journey.
- Focus on good outcomes.
- Key is optimal results.
- Read "signposts" of change.
- People focus on team.

---

are not always what they appear to be. In a state of quantum entanglement, the states of two systems that once interacted and then separated may not be divided each into their own definitive state. This interpretation of quantum mechanics implies that the states of two systems collapse into a definite state when either one of the systems is measured.

Actual reality is the state in which most of us live; it is where we perform our actions out of awareness of the present. We live actively in the present and attempt to meet the demands that lie right in front of us and that define our experience in current time and space. Potential reality, though just as real and current as actual reality, has different characteristics (**Exhibit 2-1**). Living in the potential means being aware of a reality that is not present but that is inevitable because of the prevailing circumstances or the force of its trajectory. A good example is the standard stop sign placed at intersections. When a driver sees the sign, he or she understands what it means and is willing to respond to it appropriately. However, the driver does not stop immediately because that would be an inappropriate (or untimely) response. The sign is a symbol of potential reality in play; action is inevitable but does not occur instantly.

Group Discussion

Sue Craft loves the details of managing her department and tends to focus on the staff issues of the day. She seems able to handle just about any problem, and follow-up is her specialty. Sue has noticed, however, that more problems than usual are emerging. Although she is not certain where all of them are coming from, a lot more changes are originating "up there" than usual, creating more daily problems. She is beginning to feel overwhelmed. Discuss the options available to Sue for dealing with the increase in problems. Consider the following questions: Is her focus on the problems that arise daily appropriate for someone managing a department? How might her leadership role be altered to help her handle the large number of changes being handed down by higher levels of management? How might Sue change her orientation to be better in touch with future issues?

Leaders are good signpost readers. They understand what the signposts indicate about the journey and act on them only as the circumstances dictate. Good leaders have what is called predictive and adaptive capacity. This is the ability to see and understand the interface among environment, organization, and persons and to predict the impact that interface has on action. From the perspective of action, leaders can predict the trajectory that lies ahead and adapt practices and behaviors that best demonstrate the convergence between the demands of the environment and the trajectory of the journey. Leaders' ability to anticipate which actions will be needed, through accurate reading of the signposts (predictive and adaptive), is one of the keys to good leadership. It also demonstrates living in the potential (**Figure 2-1**).

How many organizations have been led by people who live so thoroughly in the actual that they are unable to anticipate events far enough ahead of time to allow for an effective or timely response? How many organizations merely react to one crisis after another because the power of the potential is not incorporated into the leadership role in a way that enables it to be applied properly and at the right time?

Living in the potential requires leaders to recognize that they are managing a journey and thus need a specific set of predictive and adaptive skills. On the one hand, predictive skills are more linear in their application in that leaders look at current conditions, environmental factors, and suggestions for change that indicate and generally prompt a particular necessary response or action. Adaptive capacity, on the other hand, allows for a tremendous range of flexibility that comes from the need to respond to the more incremental and serendipitous characteristics embedded in the change process that may be the result of predictive elements or the impact of the unpredictable and "emergent" characteristics of continuous change. Leaders who have been raised on the 20th-century model of leadership tend to focus on the goal or endpoint and implement activities that will get people to that goal. In the true or more chaotic process of change, where deconstruction occurs at the same rate as construction, or even faster, the opacity and chaos of momentary change makes it difficult for leaders to see the goal. Instead, leaders must read the signposts of the change continuum, understand how the signposts indicate the trajectory of decisions and actions, explain to others what the decisions

Figure 2-1 Seeing the Journey into the Future.

and actions mean, and engage others in activities that move the organization in the direction indicated (Lal, 2019; McKimm & Till, 2015). Two skills are critical here. First, leaders need the ability to read where changes are occurring in the present environment and determine the right responses. Second, leaders must anticipate the next signpost (the trajectory) early enough to evaluate current progress and determine one signpost's relationship to the next one in order to inform current action (adaptation). In short, leaders need to respond fluidly to current demands and changing circumstances, remain open to the messages carried by longer-term indicators, and act in accordance with these messages (Marshall & Broome, 2016).

Many leaders get sucked into the concerns of daily work (actual reality) to such an extent that they lose sight of the potential (the emergent). When leaders focus their energies on daily activities, they are not able to discipline these activities in the light of imminent unfolding influences or circumstances. In many, if not most, organizations, the ability of leaders to engage their own future at the right time is frequently compromised by the fact that they never saw it coming. In this case, all eyes were on the activities of the moment, which consume everyone's attention and prevent anyone from seeing the emerging shifts and circumstances that will ultimately affect the organization's ability to thrive.

Many authors, including Ulh-Bien (Ulh-Bien & Marion, 2008; Uhl-Bien et al., 2007) and McKimm and Till (2015) have delved into the dynamic of complexity to make it understandable and applicable to human enterprises. They derived certain principles for and a number of insights about the coming age and how to navigate it. The remainder of this chapter presents rules that can help leaders consider the leadership role in a complex environment and separate out the activities that best match the demands of this new world of work.

Principle 1: Wholes Are Not Just the Sum of Their Parts

Wholes are made up of smaller units that interact with each other to sustain the whole.

In the 20th-century organization, managers believed they had to focus simply on the units of work for which they were responsible. They were evaluated within the context of their own units of service, and if they did well in those units, managed the workforce well, and advanced productivity and profitability, they were rewarded and sometimes even promoted.

In a systems mindset, any service unit is looked at as a part of a broader context that gives the unit direction and purpose. A unit does not simply provide services independently of its relationship to other parts of the organization. Each unit, at some level, is required to ensure that what it does fits well with the activities of the other units. According to systems theory, the fit between the components of a system is as critical as the work of any one component. This notion of goodness-of-fit is what drives the understanding of the relationship between the whole and its parts. The whole is not simply the sum of its parts; it is instead the representation of the interface and coordinated interaction and integration of all of the parts in a synergy and fluidity of relationship, interdependence, and collective support essential to sustainability of purpose and achievement of outcomes.

The most common problem in systems is that a unit and the people that make it up get co-opted by their work and their intentions. Because they leave

> **Key Point**
> Leaders need to focus on issues of "fit." They live in the "white space," the connections, most of the time, and must constantly attempt to see where the intersections are and how they facilitate the work of the system.

their work and relationships within the context of the unit, they forget that whatever they do has a broader frame of reference that must be taken into account in assessing the viability of their work.

An organizational leader must always keep the focus on the organization's broader purpose. The leader's role is to ensure that there is a goodness of fit between the activities of those at the point-of-service and the overall work of the organization. This takes considerable doing, especially when the leader also must pay attention to the kind and quality of work done at the point-of-service. Being singularly present at the point-of-service can cause the leader to get caught up in the day-to-day activities of the service and to forget the ultimate and broader systems goals toward which these activities are directed.

Leaders are responsible for seeing and living "systemness." The differences between institutions and systems are significant (**Exhibit 2-2**). In institutions, most of the work is compartmentalized and organized vertically, which, together with the focus on process, creates a clear separation among the various loci of work. Because the focus is on results at the point of productivity, special roles are created to address the issue of fit. Yet those responsible, from managers to specialty engineers, are not located where most of the work is done, and those who do the work are fully engaged in the tasks to be done and the processes to be undertaken and often not thinking about where these tasks came from and why or why not they should do them. What results is a clear and obvious disconnect between the broad directional strategies of the system as a whole and the specific and narrow work activities of those at the point-of-service.

Group Discussion

Systems are different from institutions. Systems thrive on relationships and intersections, and models of systems reflect relationships rather than control. Discuss the effect that a systems orientation would have on the design of a healthcare facility. Draw an organizational chart to reflect relationships instead of functions, including relationships to the community, other services, other health systems, and so on. Finally, discuss the differences between leading a facility that is a system and leading a facility that is an institution.

Exhibit 2-2 Institutions Versus Systems

Institutions	Systems
• Unilateral interests/goals	• Multifocal interests/goals/values
• Nonaligned	• Strong alignment of stakeholders
• Driven by self-interest	• Collateral interests
• Focus on structure/function	• Focus on relatedness
• Highly competitive	• Outcomes driven
• Survival focused	• Centered on thriving
• Vertically integrated	• Horizontal/vertical linkage

In most organizations, the organizational chart speaks volumes about the structuring of work and the value placed on it. Lines and boxes enumerate the various functional capacities expected within the context of each role. The reporting infrastructure is critical to the structuring of work, and clear lines and patterns of interaction are important—but only with regard to communication about work activities.

Workers at the point-of-service generally have not been concerned with value, linkage, and integration. Instead, they are busy performing the routines of daily work and perfecting these routines so that the work gets done effectively, is of high quality, and is completed within the allotted timeframe. As a result, on the one hand, work may be viewed as more important than its purpose. Workers may become caught up in the politics and process of the work itself, which impairs their ability to embrace change and adjust their activities in response to new demands driving the work.

In systems, on the other hand, the real work of management and leadership is to refocus work and place it into its appropriate context. To do this, however, leaders must avoid being equally co-opted by the work and thereby prevented from identifying its relationship to other factors that influence it. Imagine, for example, how challenging it is for leadership and staff today to reconfigure the work they do and the service they deliver within the context of a value-driven framework for health care. Different from functional, volume-driven, and process-based focuses, where the emphasis is on the quantity of the work, value-based practices center on the intensity and integrity of the relationship between the work, its purpose, and the achievement of a sustainable health outcome.

Many of the problems in organizations arise from the inability of leaders to think and act horizontally or collaterally. In other words, leaders must be able to see the whole and characterize each of the units of work within the context of its contribution to the whole. They must also be able to see how the units work together to advance the purpose and value of the whole. The interface and the intersection of work in all the various locations in a system are as critical to the success of the system as is the quality of any individual effort in the system.

In fact, this capacity to see all of the corelationships and interactions between loci, disciplines, stakeholders, and users (patients) is fundamental to the foundations of nursing practice and the expectations of the nurse's role. This text emphasizes equity and partnership between all participants in the clinical process. It should be noted, however, that the predominant foundational characteristic of the role of the nurse is to coordinate, integrate, and facilitate the integration, relationship, and collaboration; indeed, the collective enterprise in order to assure all of the elements (the whole) come together to accomplish their mutual aims and impact users with anticipated and expected legitimate outcomes.

In essence, good leaders, regardless of their location, see all work from the perspective of the whole system. Indeed, they analyze each work activity in terms of the function it plays in achieving the purpose of the whole. The leader's role is based on the system's imperatives and how the individual and collective work activities operate in concert to achieve them. At the same time, the structure of the system enables leaders

> **Point to Ponder**
>
> Everything in our society reflects a vertical orientation, including organizational hierarchies. Leaders now must complement vertical thinking, which is about control, with horizontal thinking, which is about relatedness. Both are necessary, yet leaders, because of the prevalence of vertical thinking, must concentrate on building horizontal connections.

to see and act out of systemness and keep in touch with the demands of the whole. A part of constructing more effective organizations is the consideration that the compartmentalization and isolation of leader and staff action in departments, services, and units limit their ability to connect. More value must be attached to individual effort to seamlessly connect it to the purposes of the system. The reverse is also true: infinitely challenging for executive leaders is the capacity of leadership to connect the strategic imperatives of the system in a meaningful way to the individual work activities unfolding in departments, services, and units.

Systems operate more as biological units than as mechanical structures. They are the sum of all the dynamics that drive them. Therefore, they are best viewed as a set of relationships and intersections rather than as a mere collection of components. In systems, the intersections between the elements are as critical as what goes on within any single element. The goodness of fit between the actions and processes of a system is what ultimately creates the fluidity that is the essence of the system's capacity to identify, engage, and adapt its operations and functions to an emergent and/or prevailing reality. Goodness of fit is much more important than any element by itself. Effective leaders always examine the activities of members to determine their goodness of fit with each other. One of the leader's challenges is to bridge the dichotomy between the workers' focus on good "task" and their need to focus on good "fit."

Leaders and staff need to recognize that no one person can make a sustaining contribution though his or her own efforts alone. Although an individual's efforts can achieve incremental improvements, sustainability of improvements depends on the degree of interface and integrity (goodness of fit) between the individual's efforts and the consolidated and aggregated efforts of the whole. The ability of leaders to make this fact clear to the staff is critical to the effectiveness of their activities.

As noted previously, work is not inherently valuable. Instead, its value lies in its purpose, and the efforts of leaders should reflect this reality. Yet decades of process and functional orientation at every organizational level have made a belief in the value of work effort alone a fundamental part of every worker's belief set. Just observe the reaction of healthcare workers to the myriad work-related changes that, in their view, prevent them from effectively doing the activities with which they have become most familiar. In addition, many workers are mourning the fact that they are no longer performing the tasks they had come to know so well. What they have forgotten is that many tasks have been made obsolete by changes inside and outside the organization, and leaders now have the major challenge of reintroducing staff, as well as other leaders and managers, to the concept of "system" or "network" and then convincing them of the importance of fitting the organization's work to its changing purposes. This is especially true as leaders attempt to create the change context that translates the national imperative to move health care out of volume constructs and into a much stronger value framework.

During the 20th century, various healthcare disciplines, out of a need to find meaning in their professional work, tried to define themselves and to devise and promulgate practice parameters. Indeed, one of that century's achievements is the contribution of many healthcare disciplines, from nursing and medicine to pharmacy and nutrition, to the improvement and elaboration of health services, leading to a broader and more complex array of services than has been available at any time in human history.

Today's challenge for the health professions is to make their boundaries more fluid and to renegotiate their roles to create a comprehensive continuum by better integrating the health services they provide. Value-based health care now demands that the professions find the interface between their roles and construct the collateral and collaborative network of relationships and interactions that best meet patients' needs and advance the quality and value of health service. The professions now must find what connects them rather than focusing on what separates them. In other words, here again the components (the professions) must converge to address the whole (the public's health). Further, technological tools now make it possible to do this—and make it necessary, at least if the health professions are to ensure the health of people over ever-increasing life spans.

> ## Group Discussion
>
> Discuss the healthcare professions as they are currently configured and predict their likely future. Are they going to continue to function effectively in the 21st century as they now exist? If not, how will they have to be revised to remain relevant in the new age of health care?

Principle 2: All Health Care Is Local

The integration and effectiveness of health services ultimately depend on local relationships, not centralized authorities.

Everyone has heard at least once that all health care is local. As Martin Buber would have said, all health services are provided within the context of the "I and Thou" relationship. In healthcare language, someone provides a service, and someone receives it. Through this fundamental human equation, care and healing emerge, and everything from structure to equipment, competence to relationship, is reflected in it. When two or more parties interact, the result is always an intimate bond represented through the exchange of feelings, thoughts, expectations, conversation, and action (I and Thou) (Richards, 2011). From a systems perspective, most of the other components of the system converge at some level to support this exchange, and those that do not ultimately will impede it (Hannah et al., 2013).

The function of structure in a service system is twofold: (1) to ensure the integrity of the system and the ability of its components to work in concert to achieve its ends efficiently and effectively and (2) to facilitate the work of the system. In

> **Key Point**
>
> All health care is local. A system operates from its point-of-service outward. If healthcare providers are not directly giving care to a patient, they are serving someone who is.
>
> In a system, everything operates from the center out. Systems are organic in shape and design. The most obvious configuration for a system is a circle. That this is so indicates that systems are more about relationships and intersections than about anything else. Systems possess flow and fluidity and are more dynamic than static. They encompass interactions and relationships in a continuous and vibrant interplay that results in the fulfillment of their purposes. All activities of a system work together to help the system adapt to changes, meet its goals, and ensure its survival.

health care, the purpose of a health system is to address the needs of the community. The system, of course, cannot serve its community without also serving individual members of the community at the point-of-service; although at the governance level, the system serves the community as a whole. Both levels—the point-of-service level and the governance level—are essential, and each supports the other.

The main implication of this principle is that each element of the system must serve to empower those at the point-of-service and allow them to provide care to the community through their individual acts. In an effective system, 90% of the critical decisions are made at the point-of-service, and the life of the system is always primarily lived out there as well. At the point-of-service is the intersection between the purpose of the system (strategic) and the place where the meaning and the life of the system is expressed (the work).

An effective system has no more structure than is absolutely needed for its work. When unnecessary structure exists, it tends to suck resources and work away from the point-of-service. The more structure a system has, the more likely the system will support its structure rather than its services, the more money the structure will cost the system, the fewer the resources the system will have available for its work, and the less able the system will be to thrive and fulfill its purpose.

Every system takes its life from the places where it intersects with the greater community. In particular, a health services system is directed toward advancing the health of the community where it is located, and there is obviously a tight relationship between the system and the receivers of its services. The system must therefore make sure that its services reflect the community's culture. The leader's role is to ensure that the purposes of the system and the needs of the community are congruent and that everything the system does is directed toward meeting those needs in a culturally appropriate manner.

All other components of a system are intimately connected to its center—the place where it carries out its mission. At this place, the point-of-service, the provider and the receiver of services meet, the community is served one member at a time, the life of the system is expressed, and the value of the system is realized. All the system's other components should be configured to support the activity that occurs at its center. It is here where the direction, strategy, goals, and the life of the organization are fully expressed in the work of the people who do it.

The point-of-service is also where the majority of conflicts occur and where a poor structure, inadequate strategy, poor direction, and ineffective leadership has the largest impact. If the processes at the point-of-service are not structured with this goodness of fit in mind, the system will begin to break down. Eventually, its purpose will become lost and its ability to thrive will be compromised.

> **Point to Ponder**
>
> Culture rules. The point-of-service is driven by the culture of the patient population. The system is defined by the culture of its community, which gives it purpose, and the culture of its members or workers, who give it focus. These constituencies converge to drive the system to thrive.

The vast majority of the work done by system leaders involves building sustainable relationships, driving innovation, and keeping the system intact and on course. Because a system is a membership community, it can easily disseminate and lose sight of its purpose and forget what its real work is. Leaders seek congruence between the system's purpose and the work of its members, and in doing this, leaders face the challenge of overcoming the ever-present conflict between personal and system agendas. Leaders must remain aware that the system is an inclusive membership community and remind others of this fact as well. Good leaders realize that the system's survival depends on the dance between good structure and good process, the members' focus on the product of their work, and the positive impact the system has on those it serves.

Good leaders also ensure that the structure of the system does not impede the system's fluidity and flexibility—its ability to quickly adapt to changing conditions. To do this, leaders must revise the structure as the system grows to position the system to better serve the community. Leaders also must be sensitive to the tightness of fit between the system's structure and its purposes, because the structure has the potential to obstruct the work processes rather than support them. When the structure acts as an obstacle and draws to itself unnecessary resources, it must be reconfigured.

Point-of-service workers must be able to act so as to meet the demands of the culture of those they serve. For example, they should have few constraints placed on their ability to make decisions and construct appropriate service arrangements and processes. Of course, their actions should be informed by principles and practices worked out in advance by the stakeholders at the point-of-service.

The configuration at the point-of-service must, at some level, reflect the character and content of the work. Here the issue of differentiation becomes critical. Each population-based service configuration is unique because it represents the characteristics of the specific population served. The 20th-century addiction to organizational sameness must be overcome. The rules that govern the functioning of each service must be derived from the service's relationship to those served, not just its relationship to the prevailing structure of the system. Although a heavily fixed structure is critical at other places in the system, it is not appropriate at the point-of-service because there the culture of the population is more important than the needs of any other element of the system.

The elements of the point-of-service are dramatically changing as the various components of health reform are translated into action in an accountable care continuum-based format. Value-based care along an episodic or population continuum demands much more fluid, portable, and variable approaches to both designing and delivering healthcare services. Point-of-service that reflects patient-centered, holistic care includes a stronger orientation to user-driven, home-based, community-centered service delivery approaches that move

Group Discussion

The point-of-service drives approximately 90% of the decision making in a healthy and effective system, and therefore most decisions should be made by workers located there. For example, the Ritz-Carlton Hotel is well known for allowing its point-of-service workers to make service decisions to enhance guest experiences. Discuss the effects on a health system of moving 90% of the decisions made to the point-of-care. What impact would this have on the authority structure of the system? What changes would have to occur to make the transfer of decision-making power sustainable? How would staff have to change to manage the additional decision-making responsibilities?

providers out of an institutional frame of reference into a service-based frame of reference. The service delivery shift represents a stronger grounding in community- and population-specific models of care delivery. Service providers are much more mobile and adaptable at the point-of-service in a clinical model that addresses the cultural and structural issues of users more than the institutional structural formats of providers (Armstrong & Mullins, 2017).

The preceding makes clear the importance of the point-of-service and the need for structural independence and functional liberty at the point-of-service. Each point-of-service worker has an obligation to ensure that the decisions and activities that unfold are congruent and that each is informed and disciplined by the system's purposes and direction as it addresses the needs of the community. Furthermore, decisions made at the point-of-service should predominate because they give form to the work of serving the community one person at a time. Out of this dynamic—consisting of the interplay of the system's purposes with the worker's decisions and activities—comes the seamless and symbiotic relationships between the system and the workers that create the place where the system lives out its purposes and makes a difference in the lives of those it serves.

Principle 3: Value Is Now the Centerpiece of Service Delivery

Anything that adds value to any part of a system adds value to the whole system. The sustainability of the system requires the aggregation of numerous additions of value.

In the Industrial Age, assessments of value were often based on volume. One of the most common measures of the value of work, for instance, was the quantity of work done. Even the language of health care reflected a volume orientation: nurses, physicians, and other health professionals often spoke of wanting to do the "most" they could do for their patients. The processes associated with work were viewed as almost more important than the work's purpose, and there was a sense that the activity of providing health care was inherently valuable. The orientation toward process was almost sacrosanct, and much attention, even in the quality movement, was devoted to establishing good processes for delivering services.

Users of health service have the right to know about the services they are provided, including quality and cost. Increasing emphasis on healthcare transparency requires that users of health care have the information necessary for good decision making and can choose health services and providers based on some objective, measurable notion of value. Providing reliable value, including cost and quality information, helps inform user choice. Users use this information to make particular choices in a way that is consistent with their values and their resources. Over time the use of user-modified cost and quality information informs more effective thinking and appropriate resource use.

Good value is driven by a notion of high-level interoperability. Interoperable systems (integrated or converged) are deeply embedded in the DNA of effective service systems. Integrity and integration of processes, functions, and structures necessary to support effective service are essential. Smartphone technology is perhaps one of the best sources of evidence of interoperability. Thousands of functions, components, and elements converge to create an instrument that can be used for multiple purposes, such as list making, purchasing of goods and services, or accessing information and entertainment, etc. Accessibility and high levels of integration and interoperability in the health system facilitate user choice, utility, effectiveness, and, ultimately, good experiences and positive health impact.

Although process integrity is vital, it does not in itself create or add value. Work processes are always disciplined by and gain their meaning and value through the purposes toward which they are directed. Any activity, to be meaningful, must at some level advance some purpose; unless work is directed toward purpose, the worker actually takes value away from the enterprise. Even if the worker does nothing, the action of doing nothing is actually drawing value away because purpose could have been positively advanced by almost any activity—an activity that is thereby not being performed and a contribution not made. Work, then, either adds value or reduces it. It adds value when it advances the purposes of the system, and it takes value away when it fails to advance these purposes.

In a true system, all activities, roles, and functions, no matter how large or small, have value. Each, when working in concert with the others, does something to advance the system's purpose and has an impact on the system's vigor and viability. For this reason, careful selection of every role in the system is essential to the system's ability to thrive. This ability depends, in part, on the goodness of fit between roles and functions, not simply on the roles and functions themselves.

Value, however, is not just tied to the persons who do work. Value is more closely linked to the products of that work. Increasingly, there is a demand for transparency between process and product so that this fit is continually assessed and evaluated to determine the efficacy of the relationship between process and product. Users expect to have the right and the capacity to make value decisions based on data that reflect the effectiveness of health work through the lens of its impact on health (Davidson et al., 2017). Increasingly, government entities, insurers, and advocates require that accountability-driven evidence-based data be constructed and made available to enable users to make wiser health service choices. Data/metrics become the public representation of value that allows users to make effective judgments related to health service comparability, costs, quality, and sustainable impact. Through this mechanism, both the form and action of value become drivers of choice based on measures of quality, cost, and impact (Zhang et al., 2019).

The triadic relationship among purpose, person, and performance is the cornerstone of any measure of vitality in any kind of system. Effective leaders understand this relationship almost intuitively. It is so embedded in the dynamics of the system that almost nothing can be accomplished if it is not used as a framework. The whole is a reflection of the fit between its parts—of the congruity and resonance of the many functions that make up its infrastructure. As these elements join in a seamless dance of intersection and interaction, each individual element becomes invisible, but all of them together, at least in a true system, work so harmoniously and are so tightly interwoven that they are perceivable only as a whole. In ineffective systems, the parts and pieces are easy to see because of their incongruence and lack of flow or fit and because they appear out of context. Rather than contribute to the whole, ineffective systems draw resources, energy, and attention away from the whole, impairing system integrity. Being drawn away from the whole can cause a system to break down and fail to achieve its purpose.

Contemporary thinking about evidence-based practice reflects a focus on essential systemness. Evidence of making a difference in the lives of those served cannot be determined unilaterally. Isolating individual action from the intersection with other forces and actions simply does not tell us whether any sustainable difference has been made and whether our actions had anything to do with

> **Key Point**
>
> Everyone in a system is obligated to add value to it. Everyone is doing something, even if it is negative. When people are not adding value, they are taking away value.

Figure 2-2 The Value Equation.

the difference or change. Only when integrated and synthesized, if you will—with other related and connected efforts—does the convergence of the effort produce anything meaningful. The convergence of efforts, related and linked together, drives evidence of contribution and sustainability of effort and outcomes (Melnyk et al., 2017). In current efforts to establish evidence-based clinical processes as a foundation for clinical decision making, success is limited to the extent that system connections between stakeholders are made and the interface of collaborative efforts is established. Evidence of making a difference is also evidence of collaboration, integration, and systemization of all the related contributions.

Leaders must operate out of an understanding that each component of a system is a microcosm of the system. To lead any one component, leaders must direct their vision from the perspective of the whole toward the component part and its contribution to the whole. The focus should be on how each component contributes to the integrity and action of the whole. From this perspective, leaders diagnose the element and evaluate its goodness of fit with the other elements as they contribute to the whole. Leaders also attempt to keep value, which depends on the congruence of work, quality, and resources, at the center of everyone's sense of relationship to their work and to the workplace (**Figure 2-2**).

Leaders are always aware of the connection between the elements of the system and the fluidity and "tightness" of the intersections between elements, where the life of the system is most evident. Questions related to interface, connection, integration, communication, and interaction are the driving concerns of the leader. If there are problems in a system, even if they originate in inadequate or failed processes, they are ultimately expressed as brokenness between the elements and in their failure to exhibit the flow, seamlessness, and linkage essential to the system. For the system to advance, individual contributions must be woven together in a way that achieves substantive consonance.

Principle 4: Simple Systems Aggregate to Complex Systems

Simple systems combine with other simple systems to form more complex systems. Complexity grows incrementally through the interconnection of smaller, simpler systems (i.e., chunking).

To understand complexity, we need to look for the simplicity that is generated from its center. Everything is related to everything else in some way. This concept lies at the center of any understanding of how systems operate and thrive. The task of system leaders is to delineate the linkages and intersections among all elements of the system. Leaders identify the common elements present everywhere in the system and those unique contributing elements that are located at critical places in the system and contribute to the effectiveness of the whole.

Every element of a larger system is a system itself. It has its own simplicity, complexity, integrity, and chaos. If the component system is viewed only as something simple, its fit and contributing purpose remain invisible. System components are disclosed when the system is seen in the appropriate context (i.e., as part of the larger system).

Each component system abides by the same rules as the larger system. The component system must have fluidity, fit, and integrity, and its parts must intersect and operate in a way that advances its contribution and value to the whole system. The component systems' substantial and continuous interaction maintains the integrity of the larger system (Parolini et al., 2019; Pepler & Martell, 2019).

> **Point to Ponder**
>
> Leaders who are heads of a particular service or department must see their role from the perspective of the whole system. In fact, the best way for leaders to look at matters is as if they are leading the whole system from the perspective of the particular service or department. Each leader's commitment to the system gives other leaders, no matter where they are located, focus and a framework for the expression of their roles.

With regard to component systems, there are two basic requirements. First, each must have well-integrated components and function well internally. Second, the systems must intersect and interact with other related systems to make up the larger system and ensure its effectiveness (**Figure 2-3**).

In the past, leaders have not always paid attention to these two requirements. Many organizations have suffered from the narrow focus of leaders who concentrate on their area of responsibility to the detriment of other component systems and the enterprise as a whole. Even reward systems sometimes encourage people to excel at the expense of others, destroying relationships, obstructing interaction, and skewing the distribution of the available resources. Whole organizations are held hostage to these highly unilateral decision makers and never fully achieve their potential. The glue of trust is never established, precluding the level of productivity that can result from a truly resonating system.

All leaders of a component of larger systems must ensure that the component operates effectively. The effectiveness of a component system, however, cannot be achieved simply through having an internal locus of control. For example, in an organization that provides health services, although the point-of-service drives the content and culture of the entire organization, the point-of-service must also reflect the obligations and operations of the entire organization. Each smaller system should mirror the larger system, although it is refined in its specific manner of representing it and doing its work. Anyone who comes directly to the smaller system should see a picture of the whole system, including that system's mission, service, quality, and outcomes, all of which should be manifest in the smaller system's work.

Too often, healthcare organizations have components that do not fit together well. Think how typical it is for people seeking healthcare services to be asked the same questions over and over again as they move through the system. From admissions to treatment, a patient may face five or more points of query simply because the components do not interact seamlessly

Figure 2-3 From Simplicity to Complexity: Aggregation Across the System.

enough to eliminate the need for them. Although there are papers on how to systematize healthcare, the perceived cost of allowing simple systems to operate independently rather than together has never fully been measured. Complex systems work because they act interdependently, representing their synthesis at every point in the continuum. Without this synthesis, systems break down and ultimately fail, affecting everything within them and everything to which they are connected.

Group Discussion

Sam Casey, as head of his department, has consistently looked out for the interests of his department and its staff. Occasionally, he has had to fight other departments to get what he wanted for his own. According to him, that is all part of being a good leader. Discuss whether he is right. Among other things, consider Sam's approach from the perspective of systems thinking. What problems is his approach likely to create? What advice could Sam be given to help him improve his leadership? How should a departmental leader balance the system's needs and the functional needs of the department?

Principle 5: Diversity Is Essential to Life

Diversity is essential to life on every level. Only where diversity is present is the capacity to thrive ensured. Diversity makes chaos visible because it pushes systems to forever adapt to changes in their environment.

It is common wisdom—at least if you believe the literature on leadership—that conflict should be avoided and that processes must be in place to reduce conflict to a minimum. Unfortunately, nothing could be further from the truth.

Diversity is the visual manifestation of the normative chaos that exists within all systems. That chaos is the energy that arises from the confluence and conflict among the elements of a system as they intersect to create the conditions necessary for the system's adaptation. Diversity is a characteristic of the endless dance of design and configuration as the elements of strategy and creativity confront each other and sort out a way of fitting together.

In creating an effective and meaningful workplace, leaders must attend to a number of issues. First, they must understand that diversity is necessary for a system to thrive—it is an essential element in the movement and adaptation of any system (Hamadi et al., 2019). Essentially, a wide range of views and roles is essential for determining the direction the system should move in and for establishing the common ground necessary for leading the participants and elements in that direction. Homogeneity is the enemy of success because it represents the unilateral, the stable, the inert. Missing from homogeneity is the contrast, conflict, accommodation, and interfacing among elements and their sorting and reconfiguring around ever-changing circumstances as the system keeps rhythm with the constantly moving environment within which it must thrive.

The presence of conflict indicates that a system is healthy and energetic. It enables the leader of the system to see the differences that exist and challenges the leader to sort through the differences to determine what they indicate. Embedded in these differences are the many varieties of influence that, when viewed together, tell the leader where the organization is, what the issues are, and what the organization's responses might be.

Leaders must recognize that their main work is interpreting present activities in light of their potential to create the future. The future does not simply happen. Each future moment is part of a flow of activities moving from the "now" toward a completion where lies the foundation for the next set of activities arising in the next moment. Each present moment encompasses indicators of the next moment and of the changes that will occur then. To influence the future, therefore, leaders must be able to see the vortex of ever-conflicting and converging elements in motion to get a sense of the trajectory of these forces and what their convergence tells about the context and content of potential change.

Leaders must be able to harness chaos through its visible conflicts and divergences because these reveal the direction of any changes that are occurring. For this reason, the role of leaders in today's world is more similar to that of being a gatherer than a director. In the old Newtonian model, leaders of an organization were expected to determine the organization's strategic endpoint and direct the organization toward it through personal influence. Today, the leader's strategy should be to connect with the diverse components of the organization to engage the collective synergy that yields insight about the appropriate and right choices for the system's trajectory. In doing this, leaders should capitalize on the strengths, skills, insights, and wisdom that are located in these diverse participants. Only by embracing and engaging the diversities and conflicts within the organization are leaders able to discover the actions most likely to keep the organization thriving.

> ## Group Discussion
> Charles Frederick has been the chief operating officer of a health clinic for 2 years. He is nice enough, but hates to have his views or leadership questioned. Therefore, although he hires bright people like himself, he tends to favor those who think like him so that he will not have to fight to achieve his goals. In time, his staff have come to understand this and have stopped offering different insights and points of view. Discuss what happens when leaders hear only what aligns with their own thinking. What is missing from the decision making in such a situation? What are some of the problems that arise? Among other issues, what are the effects on accountability?

Here, both the value and the meaning of conflict become especially important. Conflict is a vehicle for discerning the proper direction for the organization to take. In particular, it is the strongest indicator of where to begin the work of determining the most appropriate actions at any given time. Leaders both honor the essential differences that exist and use them to reach clarification. Essential differences include cultural differences as well as the diversity of insights, opinions, and skills possessed by members of the organization. No one person has all the knowledge and abilities necessary to adequately "see" the patterns of emergence embedded in diversity, complexity, and chaos. Only through processes that actualize the disparate potentials present in the full range of participant contributions can the signs of change and its themes be found. Good leaders can tap into diversity by using effective methodologies. Through dialogue, for example, leaders pull out the premises, themes, and signposts that indicate the best direction for the organization to move in and actions most likely to lead it in that direction. The goal for leaders, in short, is to utilize collective wisdom and, through the coalescence of this effort, establish the foundations for organizational common ground.

Principle 6: Error Is Essential to Success

Both random error and conscious error are essential to the process of creation. In fact, error underpins all change.

Historically, leaders have been taught that error, especially in health care, is harmful and must be avoided at all costs. And of course, in the clinical sense, for the most part that is true. However, what we have now come to understand is that error is an essential constituent of all change. Further, error can be used as a measuring device to indicate where people are currently located on the pathway to some desired impact, endpoint, or outcome. Therefore, leaders must value error as a useful leadership tool.

Error is present everywhere in the universe. It is embedded within systems and contributes to their adaptation and thriving. Error indicates where a system has to adjust to new circumstances. It forces people to stop a process of change long enough to assess the situation and make the necessary

> **Key Point**
> Error is essential to all progress. Far from being a deficit, error indicates where someone is on the journey. The only unacceptable error is the error that is repeated.

modifications before resuming the process. It informs the agents of change of where they are in the change process and what is actually happening (Erwin, 2009). It alerts them to a change in conditions or a breach in the process or a demand for a different response. Error indicates where and how the system is in relationship to a process or an initiative. It alerts people to the convergence of incongruent variables that led to the mistake or flaw and that indicate their presence or impact on the flow of events.

Error is an essential teacher. At varying levels of complexity, error indicates a break in the confluence and congruity of processes in a way that causes participants to note the break, assess the situation, and take action. Although some errors are certainly undesirable, such as those resulting in death or severe damage, they serve as indicators of critical problems and as incitements to action. They teach, inform, advise, warn, and alert by showing that the current circumstances vary dangerously from the norm or from expectations. Errors point dramatically to important lessons and ensure that these lessons are, in fact, learned (Porter-O'Grady & Malloch, 2017).

Error plays a critical role in learning and in developmental activities. When error fails to teach, the negative energy embedded deep within begins to emerge, operate, and create problems. The only inappropriate error is the error repeated, as it indicates that the relevant lesson has remained unlearned (**Exhibit 2-3**).

Leaders can use error, as a constituent of change, to evaluate a change process and determine the best activities for advancing the system and preventing the same mistakes or flaws from recurring. A leader's attitude toward error determines how he or she addresses individual errors. If leaders value errors as tools, they tend to use each individual error as a guide to improving performance. If leaders treat errors solely as a cause for punishment, individual errors will never be able to serve as indicators of problems and as stimulators of corrective action, to the organization's detriment.

> **Point to Ponder**
>
> Risk can never be fully eliminated. Indeed, risk should be viewed as a resource that simply requires good management. It is inherent in all human activity and must be accommodated in any plan. Planning for error makes room for risk and provides the space to learn from it.

Of course, some errors must be controlled. Life-threatening or risk-intensive errors must be managed in a way that reduces their incidence and impact, even though these also have the capacity to teach. Error cannot, however, be eliminated entirely. Concerted efforts to eliminate all error and strive for 100% error-free processes and environments defy reality. Error is the universe's mechanism for ensuring change, adaptation, and advancement. Error is always present at some level. The total absence of error serves as a metaphor for death. How error is

Exhibit 2-3 Mistakes Versus Errors

Mistakes
- Are nonrandom
- Are repeated
- Do not result in learning
- Impair sustainability

Errors
- Are random
- Are repeatable
- Contain lessons
- Foster sustainability

managed and used, where it occurs, how risk is strategically handled, and how improvement results are the keystones for effective error management processes.

Leaders must remember that there is a certain randomness to error and that all the good planning and control in the world cannot eliminate every mistake and defect. Errors can be reduced by a high degree of management and control, as demonstrated in the redundancy approach: redundancy, standard processes, protocols, routines, algorithms, and so on compensate for inherent error by making multiple and organized options available to anticipate and respond to the errors that do occur. For example, the airline industry (and increasingly, health care) is built on good error management, which accounts for the fact that the level of risk from errors in flight is lower than the risk present in almost any other business activity.

Healthcare organizations also have a large capacity for reducing risk from errors. Because of the focus on value as an outflow of health reform, more attention is being paid to risk and error systems in healthcare organizations. Indeed, many errors and risks are still not discussed, and may even be ignored or overlooked because of the legal implications of exposing clinical errors with their attendant risks. In recent years, however, the unacceptable level of risk resulting from medication and medical procedure errors has brought about a renewed emphasis on risk reduction and error management activities. Healthcare leaders use error as a tool in managing behavior and as a vehicle for change rather than as a cause for disciplinary action. Consequently, leaders should become familiar with the new science developing around the management of human error. As comparative effectiveness becomes a more important part of measuring and evaluating essential clinical value, increasingly sophisticated digital processes and tools become a common part of clinical leadership decision making.

Principle 7: Systems Thrive When All of Their Functions Intersect and Interact

Systems thrive when their functions and dynamics intersect and interact in a continual dance of relationship and transformation.

Newton once described the universe as a great machine. Einstein said it was more like one great thought; his point is that nothing in the universe is mechanical or organized in a machine-like structure. Modern notions of thinking and behavior are based on the emerging scientific principles and observations of our time and guide the management principles of the 21st century. An outdated Newtonian management perspective is that the purpose of workers is to accomplish the economic and production goals of the organization, generally through monetary, coercive, and control mechanisms.

More recent discussions of leadership in organizations represent later Western philosophical thought (generally that of Kant) and indicate the belief in the paradox of being subject to nature but also free from it. This move away from scientific rationalism deepens the understanding that people are both subject to the laws of nature yet free to set their own direction and goals. The product of disbelief generates a deeper understanding of self-organizing systems (instead of the notion of systems driven by an external, objective force living outside of the force's impact and therefore not influenced by it), demonstrating a growing knowledge of the action, interaction, and interdependencies of "wholes" generally understood in the concepts of formative teleology. The notion that humans are a part of nature as well as observers of nature makes them full participants in a way that cannot separate them from what

Principle 7: Systems Thrive When All of Their Functions Intersect and Interact

they observe and participate in. Human beings are essentially free to act but are inextricably entwined with the nature of which they are a part, subject and mover at the same time (thus, humans' actions have consequence and interact with other actions that also generate consequences). The contemporary struggle in this formative teleology is that the "agent" of change must use objective notions and ideas in a way that incorporates them inside of the "experience" of any change. The leader then allows this dynamic interplay to unfold in innovative and creative ways that generate new ideas, processes, and products that push the human experience continuously forward. In this scenario, effective leaders are more often facilitating a dance of interaction than directing a series of processes or functions.

Systems science posits that the universe operates as a set of interacting forces and interdependent relationships. Everything in the universe is in some way acting on or interacting with something else. Because interdependence is an essential characteristic of systems, the leadership role in a system operates critically different from the leadership role in institutional models of organization. An essential ebb and flow enables complex interactions that flow out of a constant energy that represents an essential disequilibrium out of which streams novelty, innovation, creativity, and highly dynamic relationships and interactions. This text rests on a foundation represented by this complex, emergent, and multifocal role of leadership, which reframes a conception of leadership that can be both formal and emergent (Weberg, 2017).

Traditional theories of leadership—those that informed the work of leaders and organizations in the 20th century—reflected both linear and vertical thinking (**Exhibit 2-4**). This mechanistic and highly structured approach to leadership favored the use of compartmental, formal, structured, and definitive work formats and processes to organize and codify work and its products. Workers were considered subsets of the work and were organized and treated accordingly. Much of what defined work was both developed and owned by the organization and those who directed it.

In the latter part of the 20th century and the beginning of the 21st century, the very foundations of work and the workplace began to change as a result of the emerging scholarship around complex adaptive systems and the subsequent complex responsive processes. Newer models evolved because of the advent of computers, chips, and information technology and their impact on every aspect of society. Knowledge work became increasingly important to the workplace, and organizations now require substantial knowledge capacity, most of which they could not own separate from the human beings who create it. The emergence of the knowledge worker changed the relationship between the worker and the work and also between the worker and the workplace. In today's world, workers typically acquire skills and knowledge

---

Exhibit 2-4 Linear Versus Collateral Thinking

Linear Thinking (Industrial Age)	**Collateral Thinking (Information Age)**
• Vertically oriented	• Multidirectional
• Hierarchical	• Horizontal
• Mechanistic	• Whole oriented
• Reductionistic	• Integrative
• Compartmental	• Intuitive
• Controlling	• Relational

needed for a certain type of work in an academic setting or the workplace. In complex thinking, knowledge workers are essentially "freed" from the organization by virtue of their own knowledge creation, generation, and utilization capacity, which operates independently of the structural constraints of the organization. In fact, knowledge workers and their capacity have become an economic value center, and systems and organizations compete to access resources that they feel they traditionally or historically "owned." This has turned the understanding of work and value on its head and changed the fundamental complex of relationships, interactions, intersections, and values in the social and economic enterprise.

Accelerated digitalization of work and relationships has allowed workers to become much more mobile and portable because their skill sets have much broader utility than they did in the past. Knowledge has become a resource in extreme demand; it is in essence a scarce resource, and consequently workers now are more important to the workplace than the workplace is to workers. Because knowledge has great utility, portability, and transferability, workers have many more employment and value options.

Although the worker has been changing, so has the workplace. In local enterprises as well as global entities, the organization and design of work have been radically altered. Organizations at all levels have had to create tight, efficient, nimble, and quickly adjusting work units (just-in-time models) to thrive in the more fluid, horizontal world of digital and wireless communication, fiber-optics, nanostructures, and other highly sophisticated technologies.

In this new world of intersections, interactions, interdependencies, and horizontal linkages, the entire infrastructure of work has been altered, as has our understanding of the mechanics necessary to facilitate effective work. The movement from institutions to systems has created a foundation for a new characterization of work and the worker.

Systems encompass closed and open components. Closed components are predictable, efficient, and ordered. They are the parts of a system that are constant and remain unaffected, at least directly, by external influences. The open components are adaptable and change in response to the constantly shifting demands of a dynamic environment. All functions and relationships in a system interact with and are dependent on the intersecting actions and processes in the system. Components such as production, service, management, governance, support, and locus of control are all included, according to common understanding, in the set of system functions. Of course, the relationship between the elements of process and outcome, as well as the relationships between structural and process components, is complex and as changing as technology and environment demand. In a complex system, no one element remains inert as other elements adapt to internal and external forces or leads the process of adapting to these forces.

> **Point to Ponder**
>
> Advances in technology have made work more portable. Knowledge workers, because of their high-level skills, have gained substantial control of the work they do and have also become more mobile. Unlike the previous generation of workers, they are not faithful to the workplace. Instead, they are faithful to the work, moving anywhere the opportunity to do it appears.

This constant wave or flow of change and adaptation operates as the undercurrent of every system. The action never stops. Leaders of a system, always aware of this movement and the constant exchange of energy among all the components, look for the drivers and receivers of action and change (agents). Leaders' attention must be on the ebb and flow of the cycles and the vortex of change as the system interacts with external sociopolitical, economic, and technological forces. The object is to discern the effects of these forces and to judge which actions will maintain the system's integrity, adaptability, and viability.

Leaders of the system, of course, cannot perform these tasks unilaterally. All leaders of system components must be made aware of the processes and skills necessary to manage systemness and of the interacting elements that make systems thrive. Any system is negatively affected if single leaders act in the best interest of their component and without consideration for the impact of their behavior on the integrity of the whole. Single leaders actually hold the system "hostage" to their own component.

Component-centered behavior is common in traditional organizations. Various units, services, or departments of an organization might operate over long periods of time either independently or at the expense of other parts of the organization, especially if great sums of money can be produced as a result of their unilateral behavior. However, component-centered behavior is not sustainable. The dynamics of shifting information, service, and technology interacting with constantly changing demands of the environment creates the conditions that change strategy, trajectory, technology, resources, and the nature of work. Ultimately, the day always arrives when the organization has to pay substantially for its unconnected behavior, and the organization's ability to thrive will likely be threatened.

Leaders of a system component must recognize that their proper role is not simply to make the component thrive but to help make the whole system thrive. Every leader's main attention of course is on their functional obligations to the component, but their real work is to ensure the fluidity, interface, connectedness, and flow of the component with the full range of system interactions (goodness of fit).

Over the years many theoretical approaches have emerged to try to define the structure and processes associated with an organization's work. From bureaucratic theory, the human relations school, and the contingency and resource-dependent approaches to the strategic, population, and institutional models, theorists have written extensively on how and why organizations function as they do. According to the complexity approach, any element may act at any given time in an organization, and the interaction of forces will tell the leader how the organization is behaving and what the implications of its behavior are for its work and its transformative journey. Every system must possess structure and cultural foundations and must be able to respond flexibly to the environment and relationships, create value, improve itself, and interface directly with the external processes that influence its future. In other words, each theoretical approach contributes at some level to our understanding of how systems operate and how to make them effective (Arnold & Wade, 2015).

Biological metaphors frequently have been used to characterize the activities of systems, and each metaphor can assist leaders to focus on the functions and relationships that must work in concert. Signs point to an increase in complexity as a fundamental part of the evolutionary process. This complexity is an intrinsic force of evolution toward more complex organisms. In addition, general complexity is advanced by the astronomically large number of simple organisms that, although they are simple, establish complex interactions and relationships with each other in the larger environment (Weberg & Fuller, 2019). These simple organisms must work inside a complex network of interactions and partnerships in a way that facilitates balancing the whole environment, which is their medium for thriving. These multilevel, multilateral, simple organisms, when aggregated, create an integrated and collaborative collective that must maintain a tenuous balance and whole systems integrity to support the general thriving of each species and all species.

The analogy of a hologram is helpful in understanding organic complexity. In each part of a hologram, regardless of how many times it might be divided, the whole is always present. In short, the whole is always present in each of its parts. In this analogy, a whole system is reflected in each of its parts, and the relationship between the whole and each part is critical to both thriving, one with the other and in the other. The role of leaders, in this perspective, is to keep focused on both the whole and the parts of the hologram—the constant interchange between the parts and the whole and the impact of the parts on each other and on the operation and integrity of the whole.

Leaders must pay special attention to the points of interaction among the various components because therein lies most of the action, energy, and noise of a complex system, as well as most of the relationship, goodness-of-fit, and workflow problems. Because of the intensity of the dynamics there, sometimes problems and issues are not resolved or are "turfed" outside the locus of accountability that exists at these connective points. Examples include physicians taking their problems to the "administration," managers letting relationship problems "hang," and staff members refusing to deal with other staff members because the interactions would be too painful. Indeed, in any human system most activities, perhaps as much as 90%, reside at the point-of-service (the dynamic intersection) and the boundaries between the various services.

Group Discussion

The Industrial Age saw the emergence of a whole host of schools of leadership thought. Discuss the various approaches to leadership advocated by these schools (e.g., bureaucratic, human relations, behavioral, contingency, and situational). Then, reflect on the type of workplace that is emerging and discuss the implications for leadership style. As a help, consider which approaches to leadership might be appropriate or sustainable in the new age of work.

Key Point

The primary job of a leader is to manage relationships and interactions, mostly at the intersections of the system. Seeing the organization holographically (i.e., in three dimensions) can help the leader detect the interactions and processes that occur there.

Because these locations are where the applied work of a clinical system gets done, most of the issues affecting the work arise here. Problems are exacerbated if they are not resolved where they arise.

As principle 7 states, a system thrives to the extent of its intersections and interactions of its functions and actions. The best metaphor here is that of a continual, dynamic dance of interaction. The leader's role is to act as choreographer and ensure that the parties and the parts resonate with each other in a seamless contributory partnership to sustain the energy of the system.

Principle 8: Equilibrium and Disequilibrium Are in Constant Tension

A constant and permanent tension exists between equilibrium (stabilizers) and disequilibrium (challenges). This tension is essential to life and reflects the fact that disequilibrium is the universe's natural state. For leaders, it is important to continually investigate and to understand how the relationships among parts of a system generate the collective behaviors of the entire system and how that whole system interacts and relates with the environment of which it is a part.

Although it is normal for the universe to live on the edge of its own chaos, a certain amount of stability is necessary for change and for undertaking action. The role of leaders in this delicate equation is to find the points of stability and use them as places where evaluation and action can occur. The notion of variation is central to the balance between stability and instability. Agents of change (e.g., individuals, families, businesses, communities, countries, and computer programs) interact continuously with the variables and elements affecting events and direction of movement. Through use of their skills, knowledge, mental and physical properties, and location, leaders, among other agents of change, can take the best path to achieving improvements.

Leaders understand the dynamic interaction between stability and change and walk the narrow way between them with consciousness and purpose. Leaders are constantly opposing the normative forces of entropy and dissipation, even as those forces manifest in organizations and people, to ensure that the human system remains dynamic, active, and changing positively. They understand that absolute and continuous stability is synonymous with death. Recognizing this, they know the value of chaos and the necessity of harnessing it to improve the circumstances and processes of work and productivity.

People do not make change. Instead, like disequilibrium, change is universal. This fact is at odds with the usual desire of people for stability and quiet in their personal lives. Leaders understand both the prevalent human wish for stability and the universe's tendency of continuous movement toward the creative and the chaotic. They know that they must develop strategies for addressing the conflict between equilibrium and disequilibrium—strategies that take into account both the environment and their own goals. Further, they know that not all strategies work as planned, and they periodically evaluate every strategy in use to make sure it is having the desired effect and revise it as necessary.

Time and shifting circumstances, often in part created by earlier strategies, have an impact on the chance of success of current strategies and on the formation of future strategies. A strategy that has stood the test of time can suddenly become unavailing. Changes in people and conditions can converge or act independently to influence what will work and what will not. Leaders must understand that wide variation in the effectiveness of a strategy over time is normal, and they must keep this fact in mind as they attempt to lead change and help people adjust to the inevitable adaptations that are a constant part of life.

The fluctuating effectiveness of strategies is one reason that measures of success are so critical to making judgments about what works. By using structured approaches to evaluating success, leaders

> **Key Point**
>
> In systems language, *stability* is another word for death. Absolute stability is the absence of life. The leader always walks a tightrope between stability and chaos, tending to favor the latter.

can better determine what is working, what is not, what is shifting, what is emerging, and what adaptations need to be implemented. Measures do not have to be perfectly accurate; they simply have to say something about where changes are occurring and what adjustments are indicated. In a complex system, an apparently "wrong" outcome is as significant as a "right" measure might be. In other words, in the chaos of change, it is as important to know the wrongs as it is to know the rights.

Changes in people or populations may create a need for changes in process and approach. A change may alter people's circumstances, even their behavior, resulting in a need to alter the strategy or approach for the next stage of change. For example, people are affected by using the internet, and thus those who use the internet will likely require a process and mechanism of change that accommodates their new "position" as internet users. For example, in pre-internet times, "presence" meant that you were geographically located in relationship to another; in the digital experience of the internet, "presence" has no geographical requirement. This digital notion of presence is now changing how we make and keep relationships, connect personally and emotionally, learn, communicate, and manage knowledge. If any approach to change does not accommodate or use these emerging digital realities, the adaptations implemented will have limited success. In general, the changes people undergo must inform the strategy used by leaders to guide further evolution. Here it is important to emphasize the concept of relevance and change. The relevance of a change is directly related to its timeliness and appropriateness within the context of the environment (e.g., the digital universe) at any given point in time. There is nothing worse for an organization than to retain a strategy that lacks currency or to suggest a strategy that lacks timeliness and relevance.

Group Discussion

Margie Smith likes to have all of her ducks in a row. She believes that good order indicates good leadership. Her office is clean and orderly, and her life is highly structured. Margie hates when people clutter up their lives and are unable to think logically or act rationally. She works hard to make sure that her staff know what she expects and do everything as she thinks it should be done. Recently, though, the pace of change has picked up, and new programs and technologies are being implemented faster than Margie can handle. She has become less orderly, less comfortable, and, at times, short with staff. She occasionally speaks negatively about some of the changes, she has asked her supervisor whether the rate of change could be decreased, and she has even begun to think about looking for another job, one that would give her more control. Discuss what Margie needs to do to cope better. What changes should she make in her role as leader? What is the chaos she is experiencing trying to tell her? Is changing jobs going to be an effective solution to her current discomfort?

Leaders look to people as both designers of change and vehicles of change. Although leaders are interested in changing people, they must be aware that people are a source of their own change because they are sources of learning and adaptation for each other, they act as initiators and/or recipients of change or improvement, and they are part of an environment that is itself always in transition (Babalola et al., 2016; Hoch et al., 2016). Good leaders are aware that the

Principle 8: Equilibrium and Disequilibrium Are in Constant Tension

people with whom they work are virtual experts on their insights, position, and condition relative to a desired or needed adaptation. By looking at the population, leaders determine where they are in relation to any given change and use their observations as a template for evaluating measures and indicators of the external forces of change. The general behavior of a population always influences its specific behavior, just as any specific behavior might inform leaders about the best methods for altering the population's general behavior. For example, if a population uses a specific tool, such as a handheld digital device, for managing personal information and communication, it will more easily adapt to using such a device for communication, documentation, and interaction in the clinical setting. People's individual behaviors serve as both signposts and templates for broader and further adaptation in other settings and circumstances. Thus, as noted, leaders must be good signpost readers and translators and must use their interpretive skills to facilitate further change and adaptation.

Leaders must also understand that complexity and chaos represent inherent energy. Although leaders do not generate the energy, they harness it in support of a particular form and direction. This energy is always swirling in human circumstances—it never stops. Leaders discipline the energy, driving it in a direction that results in desirable or congruent changes. The interaction between energy and effort is what gives the changes their form, and it is the substance that can be defined and measured.

Leaders must be able to discern the interaction patterns in the energy and flow of a change because these patterns are most indicative of the context and content of the change. The interaction among forces, agents, and environment is the substance of the change and informs leaders about appropriate responses. Leaders look for the convergence of these forces and elements. The "story" that they contain, when well read, tells leaders what responses are likely to lead to specific outcomes or products. From this set of responses, leaders select those that are likely to move the system in the direction that is needed or desired.

Not all selections will be correct. Leaders will choose ineffective responses as often as effective ones. Here again, it is not the selection that is critical to the change process but what the effect of the selection tells leaders and what their responses are. When a strategy is correct and does result in a preferred behavior or condition, adaptation is said to have occurred, and this adaptation forms the foundation for the next change. For example, particle-beam CT scanners were highly successful as diagnostic tools, yet they also formed a foundation for future improvements and refinements. Electron-beam whole-body CT scanners currently provide more detail and accuracy and have broader diagnostic and clinical utility, but these scanners could not have been developed until the earlier scanners had been devised and used. Adaptations often build on previous adaptations. In fact, all adaptations are temporary and merely serve as the foundation for future adaptations.

> **Key Point**
>
> The leader lives in the space between action and potential, anticipating the next step and translating the process for others.

Leaders are constantly aware of the intense interactions of complexity. These interactions are often represented in a chaotic vortex of energy that on the surface looks undecipherable. Yet when critically "read" and put into context, the vortex often reveals the "stuff" that will ultimately influence the next stage of change. Leaders are always pushing up against this potential energy, and good leaders are those who can translate it (context, systems, processes, and structure) into concerted actions. When an action joins with other related actions, the entire set creates the foundation for meaningful change. This can be viewed as a process of harnessing complexity. Through understanding and using complex interactions and intersections, through recognizing that all this is clothed in complexity and chaos, good leaders act to create the future.

Principle 9: Change Is Generated from the Center Outward

> **Key Point**
> A system thrives only when those at the point-of-service own the decisions that are made there.

Effective change generally moves from the center of a system to all other parts, influencing everything in the system. Successful and sustainable change is rarely ever driven from the top of any system.

Every system has a unique life that reflects its meaning and value and gives it an individual character. Within the system are all the activities that create balance among the work of the system, the internal demands, and the external requisites for thriving. Because every system is part of a larger system, there is an ever-evolving dance or interchange among the activities inside the system and between the system and the larger environment of which it is a part (**Figure 2-4**).

The "center" (i.e., the point-of-service) is where the system lives the majority of its life, and the workers at the point-of-service are especially critical to its ability to adapt and thrive. However, many components of a system contribute to its integrity and allow it to function and adapt, and many types of personnel, from managers to staff, play a role in advancing the work of the system.

In a service system, the value of the system is determined by the character and content of the services offered. The services have value when they are provided in a manner that satisfies

Figure 2-4 Out of Simplicity: A View of Complex Health Systems.

APP, advance practice providers; CC, care coordinators; MD, medical doctors; NA, nursing assistants; RD, registered dietitians; RN, registered nurses; RT, respiratory therapists; SW, social workers.

those who use them. In addition, the services contribute to the system's ability to thrive by demonstrating that the system provides valuable, high-quality services. Even more than the activities of marketing and business planning, the delivery of services creates the system's reputation; thus, the people who deliver the services are critical to the ability of the system to thrive. They are, in fact, much more critical to the system than any other single role or factor, although this statement should not be taken as denigrating the value of any of the intersecting roles that make up the system. We should be reminded at this point that all life and action in any system converges at the intersection of this life where the energy of all the agents that reflect the action of the system converges in a way that sustains change and advances the purposes of the system.

No service system can be sustained if the point-of-service does not deliver. Although this truth is easy to state, in many, if not most, service organizations, the power, independence, flexibility, and locus of control necessary to respond immediately and appropriately have been designed out of the system's point-of-service. These organizations have a vertical array of controls, hierarchical structures, and processes that obstructs decision making where the pertinent issues most often arise—at the point-of-service. The ascending ladder of control moves the authority for decision making away from the point-of-service, and the farther away the locus of authority is, the less likely the decision will meet the need that motivated it. In a typical example, a physician on a unit who has a problem with a staff member might take the issue to the administrator to make sure that the highest level of authority is brought into play. But if the problem is to be solved permanently, the solution must involve those who are located where the problem originated, and so action on the solution must ultimately be returned to the point-of-service.

Systems develop dynamic and cyclic patterns. In a typical pattern, there is a core or center point where the pattern either originates or culminates. The mosaic of activities ultimately builds on or supports the center point (**Exhibit 2-5**). In a service system like a healthcare organization, all structure that is sustainable builds on the service configuration, and the system's sustainability depends on the degree of congruence between the prevailing service structure and the supporting structures. If the system is well designed, most of the organizational configurations advance the freedom of activity and judgment at the center point (i.e., point-of-service). If they do not, they increase the chance that the supporting systems

---

Exhibit 2-5 Mosaic of Decision Making in a System

Point-of-Service Decisions
- Individual
- Service driven
- Judgment based
- Highly variable

Team-Based Decisions
- Team defined
- Group standard
- Protocol driven
- Agreement based

Unit or Service Decisions
- Coordinated
- Support based
- Standards driven
- Resource related

System Decisions
- Integrated
- Collective
- Direction setting
- Resource generating
- Support systems based

become the center point and therefore draw energy away from the proper locus of control, creating a framework that demands attention and resources that should be focused on the point-of-service.

The more the focus of a service system is drawn away from the point-of-service, the more expensive the structure of service becomes. Specifically, when patient-centric healthcare decisions are made at the point-of-care, the greater the likelihood of integrating evidence-based interventions, clinical expertise, and patient preferences (Taylor et al., 2016). In a system in which those responsible for structuring the system are not dedicated to enabling the locus of control to remain at the point-of-service, the tendency is for more and more decisions to move away from the point-of-service and for more infrastructure to be built to compensate for the lack of control. In addition, the more infrastructure that is built, the more extensive (widely dispersed) the lack of control becomes. When locus of control does not remain at the point-of-service, relationships may be harder to build, organizational priorities may not be aligned, and efficiencies are lost (Nguyen et al., 2020).

Leaders of a service system labor to fully comprehend the essential interactions among the system elements and assess the degree to which those interactions facilitate the work going on at the center point. Leaders must also assess the degree to which the system's configuration supports the openness and ownership of decisions and actions at the point-of-service and the amount of compensation necessitated by inappropriately made decisions. Leaders judge the level of skills at the point-of-service and look at the support structures necessary to ensure that the level of competence there is right and in the right configuration to meet the needs of those served. It is not just what leaders know about the people, services, or the system that matters, it is also what the point-of-service workers know.

> **Key Point**
>
> When any system has too much structure, the energy of the system begins to support the structure rather than accomplish its objectives. Unnecessary structure draws resources away from the system's services and interferes with its ability to do its work. The same holds true for unnecessary management.

> **Point to Ponder**
>
> The only difference between revolution and evolution is the time and pain it takes to make a sustainable change.

The effectiveness of the system is directly related to the system's support of decision ownership and application at the point-of-service. In addition, when structure at the point-of-service supports decision making and action there, less infrastructure must exist at other levels of the system. Financial and professional costs accelerate when the legitimate locus of control shifts to other places in the system. To avoid fostering illegitimate loci of control leaders must ensure that most decisions and actions remain at the point-of-service. A shift in the locus of control away from the point-of-service causes a misfit between decisions and the specific situational needs of the services and their providers. It also obstructs the provision of competent, skilled, high-quality services and the workers' sense of ownership of their work.

Leaders are fully involved in setting up and assessing the adequacy of the support structures of the overall system. Support structures must be configured in a way that does not take from the point-of-service what belongs there. Functions of strategic, operational, and service support must also be configured in a way that allows them to be understood and implemented.

The goodness of fit between the contextual activities of the strategic and support systems is vital because all the processes that unfold in the structure of the overall system must ultimately contribute to the provision of services. Leaders' understanding of the impact of structure is critical to informing the database of the point-of-service workers that guide their decisions and actions. Leaders act as moderators of the relationship between those in strategic and support systems and those at the point-of-service. Keep in mind that support structures serve as a vessel for organizational behavior. Whatever the structure facilitates or permits in relationship to organizational behavior influences what the system obtains. If leaders seek a change in patterns of behavior but do not make a concomitant change in the structure of the organization to support new patterns, the existing and prevailing structure will extinguish new behaviors in the system.

Principle 10: Revolution Results from the Aggregation of Local Changes

Revolution (hyperevolution) occurs when many local changes are aggregated to inexorably alter the prevailing reality, called the *paradigmatic moment*.

> ### Group Discussion
>
> New sciences such as genomics and complexity science, advances in older sciences such as pharmacology, and technological developments are conspiring to change the health services format. What is currently in place will be deconstructed, and newer structures and models need to be conceived. Brainstorm the dramatic changes affecting health care at this time. Then discuss how they will alter the design of health services. What might some of the new designs be, and how will they change the use and location of healthcare providers in the health system?

Most changes that occur are progressively evolutionary; that is, they happen in a continuous and dynamic process over a period of time—most often over a very long period of time. Included are many iterations of evolutionary dynamics within which change can occur (coevolution, punctuated equilibrium, mutation, adaptation, speciation, etc.), yet all of them lead to a change of some kind. As Darwin pointed out, the evolution of species is a dynamic process in which the living creatures best able to adapt to the changing environmental circumstances survive and thrive. This is no less true in the human enterprise.

A revolution, however, is a dramatic, almost instantaneous, change in conditions, and it presents living creatures with the challenge of adjusting quickly. In a revolution, many events converge to create a situation in which life can no longer be lived in the same way.

A revolution usually occurs in a system when the components converge to make sufficient demand for significant change. This demand is usually a result of the components being acted upon by the external or internal environment or by natural, sociopolitical, economic, or technical transformations. To thrive in the face of the demand for change, the system must quickly alter its structure and behavior to operate effectively under the new conditions.

Much of what is happening in health care is revolutionary in nature. The very foundations of health care are being transformed by the impact of new technologies, in the realm of computers and the internet, robotics, pharmaceuticals, genomics, and sociopolitical and economic reforms. Technological advancements are so pervasive and influential that, in concert, they are fundamentally altering health therapeutics as well as the delivery of health services. The same can be said for the sociopolitical and economic forces. In particular, health services are less "bed based" than they were previously, the structures of hospitals and other healthcare organizations are being radically transformed, and providers must seek new ways of offering services that demonstrate effective health outcomes within a cost- and service-value chain.

The role of healthcare leaders is to focus on the implications of the revolutionary changes of health reform, including the implications for the behavior of those who work in the healthcare fields. Leaders must help other healthcare professionals to adapt to the changes and must position healthcare organizations to continue to thrive in an emerging value paradigm. They must discern the new roles, processes, and behaviors that will be necessary for future success.

The current transformation in health care is attended by changes in other conditions that challenge healthcare organizations to alter their way of business. For instance, the environment will require these organizations to reconfigure supporting structures and finances because the older configurations have become severely stressed in a way that threatens them. A further threat is presented by the fact that while the supporting infrastructure of economics, policy, and work is being reformed, the existing structures and behaviors will be even less relevant than they were previously.

Here again, leaders of a healthcare organization must recognize the critical nature of the shift and undertake the dramatic and sometimes perilous process of quickly revising structure, processes, and behaviors to become more congruent with the emerging demand for sustainable health value (**Figure 2-5**). Besides reading the signposts of the change accurately, leaders must begin to create a sense of urgency about change in the minds of those who will live in this new world. The issue that creates drama and suspense is whether everyone's responses will be timely and appropriate. Leaders must move people quickly through mourning the loss of established rituals and routines and raise the stakes for thriving and advancing the work in the context of a new set of reforms.

In a time of revolution, all the principles of adaptation and complexity management come into play. The leader's ability to apply these principles and bring the elements of complexity and chaos together determines whether the organization thrives. As an agent of change, leaders know that a variety of "agents" in a system can stimulate action or change. Leaders are always looking for how these agents act to create the critical events that lead to an adjustment or a transformation.

Leaders also know that there is a variety of choices and strategies that can create a good fit between the demand for reform and our response. Leaders look for the relationships in the demand for change. By paying attention to the issues, themes, and mosaic that best demonstrate the flow and impact of the patterns, leaders can facilitate the making of good decisions and the undertaking of effective actions.

Principle 10: Revolution Results from the Aggregation of Local Changes

Organization
- Committed leaders
- Credible measures
- Good infrastructure

Group
- United vision
- Good conflict
- Shared decisions

Individual
- Collaboration
- Stakeholder
- System view

Figure 2-5 Organizational Levels and Associated New Age Characteristics.

There is substance, artifact, hidden agendas, and opinions in all change. The leader's role is to sort through the options and determine which elements are evidentiary and which are simply "noise" representing the change itself. Leaders do not discard the artifacts of change. Instead, leaders determine their value and use them either as tools of change or symbols of the journey itself. Artifacts may tell participants where they are in the journey and may also provide help in getting through the journey's various stages (Nguyen et al., 2019).

Testing the way of the transformation is as important as any other activity. Although many things that occur during a revolution are important, equal amounts of "stuff" are unhelpful or even obstructive. Furthermore, it is important to determine where the system is in the process of change—what has been accomplished and what has yet to be done, what the deviations are, and what the successes are. Consequently, a means of measurement is needed so that the agents and strategies selected can be validated against the distance traveled and so that the expectations can be compared with the reality (**Figure 2-6**).

Exploration and experimentation are essential elements of any major change. The context is often significantly different from what was previously experienced or lived, and as the context changes, so, too, do the rules. Both the journey and the way of living that results from the journey are so different from the past that previous experience is inadequate to meet the new demands. The script gets written as part of the journey itself. This means that most of the change agents are learning about the change at the same time as they are leading the adaptation to it. This is especially true during a postparadigmatic change where the script is essentially new to all the players. Here, leaders must successfully demonstrate their own capacity to learn, predict, and adapt as discernment, experimentation, application, and short-term evaluation yield data not previously available. A certain level of leadership vulnerability is essential to demonstrating individual capacity to discern, question, and explore new ways of thinking and responding to dramatic change events. When the script is written as it is lived, the collective wisdom garnered from the active engagement of all participants is critical to the assessment of effective progress.

> **Key Point**
> Leaders are agents of change. They bring the vision and context of change to the stakeholders so that the latter can develop the content of change.

Processes:
Signposts
Concepts
Innovation
Patterns

Processes:
Knowledge
Technical
Procedural
Intellectual

Results of change

Congruence

Distance traveled

Changes implemented

Processes:
Passion
Rewards
Outcomes
Environment

Figure 2-6 Evaluating Transformation.

Choosing strategies that fit the circumstances is not always easy to do. Because the ground shifts as people try to learn to live on it, the leader must have an open attitude regarding what is to be discovered. Leaders must understand what is meaningful and sustainable on the journey thus far and how it has been experienced. A leader's experience forms the database for the next stage of the journey.

At the same time, leaders experiment with actions. Because leaders do not know what the sustainable or valuable actions are until they are applied, they recognize that there is an element of risk that must be embraced. All actions are prone to error. Indeed, the very risk of error advances the opportunity for learning and adaptation. Any particular error may contain the answer to a problem or at least be a signpost that could not be discerned in any other way, making the error a tool for the evaluation of direction and goodness of fit.

In short, leaders see everything within the context of systemness. All elements of a dynamic system are related and interact with each other, and the interactions, when aggregated, are what create the conditions for the system's adaptation and ability to thrive. When internal need and external conditions converge, they create the demand for change and adaptation.

Leaders see systemness everywhere and recognize that they can play a major role in the system's ability to adapt and improve (**Figure 2-7**). Leaders' decisions to adapt and improve largely depends on their ability to anticipate, live in the potential of, and embrace each change at the right time. In addition, leaders must realize that they are important change agents, and must always act out of that understanding.

To ensure that the system adapts appropriately to changes and continues to thrive, leaders need to keep in mind the following:

- They must apply the skills of exploration and exploitation, and know when to apply each skill set.

Principle 10: Revolution Results from the Aggregation of Local Changes

Elements of systemness
- Internal integrity
- Goodness-of-fit
- Seamlessness
- Open boundaries
- Team based
- Point-of-service driven
- Measures of value
- Coordinated effort
- Sustainable change

Surrounding context: Unplanned challenges, Shifting realities, Sociopolitical challenges, Innovations, Changing technology

Figure 2-7 A System and Its Context.

- Throughout a period of change, leaders must know which processes accommodate and use inherent variation and which processes maintain stability and good order, and then use these processes appropriately. Some level of inherent stability and some normative forces help to reinforce adaptation, and yet innovative and creative solutions and strategies often are embedded in the chaos and variance. In other words, both stability and variability are essential for adapting to change.
- Knowledge of the inherent interactions of elements in the system can direct leaders to build on those intersections that bring coherence, integrity, and trust into the system. These features of systemness can enhance people's ability to change and adapt quickly and well.
- All strategies have consequences. Leaders must determine the appropriate strategies for guiding the system in the right direction. Implementation of strategies must take into account that random influences may lead to valuable insights not available in any other way.
- Systems are membership communities. They operate through the consent of their members. Relationships among the members, including their communication with and support of each other, are as critical as any other factor for ensuring sustainable adaptation.
- Failure can be an important measure of direction and change. It should not, however, be an uncontrollable factor and should operate within the context from which it emerges. Small changes should not contain large failures. If they do, it indicates that the associated strategies are ineffective or misconceived.
- The team is the basic unit of work, and the relationships among the core members drive all successful change. Here is where change gets lived out and applied. The interaction, relationship, and competence of the team members are essential to the viability of the team's work and the sustainability of the system. In human systems, all else exists to support the work of this unit.

- Small changes lead to big changes. Further, all changes affect the system as a whole, either individually (evolutionary change) or in the aggregate (revolutionary change). It is not possible to affect any part of a system without ultimately affecting the whole system.

Crisis and creativity frequently emerge in unanticipated places and ways. Often in the act of achieving something else, the creative and innovative arise. Leaders must always be open to serendipitous and emergent forces that arrive unexpectedly.

Conclusion

The presentation of principles in this text is neither exhaustive nor fully developed. This chapter serves merely as an introduction to concepts important to leaders in the Digital Age, who must operate using different ideas than those common in the Newtonian-inspired Industrial Age. Leaders must review the adequacy of their skill sets in light of the realization that the era of unilateral and vertical orientation of functions is quickly passing.

Dramatic and dynamic changes continue to affect the leadership role. To understand this role in the new age of work and reform, leaders must learn about quantum principles and how they are to be applied. They must also become adept at understanding biologic metaphors, which are much stranger tools of thought than the old machine- and building-based metaphors. Permanent structures are no longer good models for work, especially in health care, and the architectural infrastructure characteristic of the coming age has a value-based format within an information infrastructure. Leaders must devote their full energy to pulling people out of work and service models that no longer operate efficiently and placing them in a context that demands thinking and acting in radically new ways.

It is interesting to note that, in recent times, people have not become more isolated. In fact, the opposite has occurred. Human beings have more potential for relationship and connectivity than at any time in history. The tools of connection and communication are creating linkages that were once only dreams. Living in this kind of a world, however, brings its own set of challenges and requires a different way of relating and behaving.

Leaders have an obligation to move people and structures into the new framework for work and leisure. To do this, they need a different mental model, new tools and skills, and a genuine desire to move both themselves and others into the new age. They need new knowledge, true enough, but they also need excitement so encompassing that others can see it and feel it, be energized by it, and develop the hope and enthusiasm necessary for creating a sustainable future.

When all is said and done about leadership—and these days much is said about it—it is important for every leader to engage with and embrace the script of life and to get others to do the same so that the conditions of life are improved. Through discernment and exploration, design and formation, experimentation and application, leaders can help foster the richness of experience that enhances the quality of life for all. The effort to make life better and the chaos out of which improvements emerge give form to the leadership role. The process of discerning and drawing from the complexity of all systems the simplicity that lies at their center and applying that simplicity to the lives of others gives critical substance to the work of every leader.

Chapter Takeaways

1. Leaders must now more deeply understand the implications of complexity theory and its application, especially in relationship to the leadership role and for all the processes associated with transforming work and the workplace in this postdigital age.
2. The principles of complexity applied largely to organizations and leadership determine how best to transform systems, people, and work and to undertake the appropriate sustainable change processes understanding these new rules of engagement in the new age for work.
3. The interacting and intersecting character and foundations of complexity draws us all into a web of relationship, interaction, and systemness and the level of understanding that will ultimately transform our work and our lives. From strange attractors to webs of influence and relatedness, to relationship and interaction at the system intersections, the principles and elements of complexity alter the rules of work and all of the relationships and interactions embedded within it. The principles of complexity give us a deeper understanding of how these relationships operate in the role of substantive change in discerning and directing human progress.
4. Understanding the 10 principles of complexity and their applications outlined in this chapter deepen the leader's insights about their elements and content, their applications, and how to navigate them as tools of sustainable change. The 10 principles outlined in this chapter help leaders consider the leadership role within complex systems and separate out those activities that best match the demands of 21st-century work.
5. Dramatic and dynamic changes will continuously affect and transform the leadership role. Leaders must continue to learn about quantum (complexity) principles and how they are to be applied and translated into strategies, processes, and actions that will radically transform the future of health care.

Case Study 2-1

Creating Change in the Midst of Chaos

Nancy has been the chief nursing officer (CNO) at Shady Point Hospital for 15 years, but this last year has been the most difficult for her. It seems as if there has been one change after another this year, and Nancy is tired of trying to lead the nursing staff through the changes, making sure the physicians are satisfied, and ensuring that the patients receive the best possible care. It seems that the staff are fatigued with all the changes and meetings as well, and some have said, "We just want to be nurses and take care of patients." It was easier in the past—the hierarchy and structure of the hospital seemed to provide some stability. Nurses were content to work at Shady Point for their entire careers, and nearly 50% of nurses had been there 15 years or longer. Some nurses had actually trained at Shady Point's nursing school, a diploma school that closed 25 years ago.

Feeling the pressure from other hospitals' CNOs in the Northwest Healthcare System, Nancy has been investigating what it will take to commence the Magnet journey. In preparation, she has hired a director of professional development and research who has a doctoral degree from a respected university. Although it seemed like a great idea in the beginning, she notices now that the nonproductive education hours are completely over budget, and the CFO is pressuring her to correct the problem. The new director of professional development is encouraging nurses to develop career plans, return to school, and become certified. Now, many nurses who feel like they should return to school to get a bachelor's degree or become certified in their specialty are demanding more support for tuition reimbursement, increased pay after they obtain their specialty education, and some paid hours for attending classes. Nancy is overwhelmed with all the demands, changes, and pressures she feels from the rest of the executive team to stay in budget and to improve nurses' satisfaction levels. The entire organization seems to be in a state of chaos under demands to reduce operating expenses while the staff and physicians are demanding more and more. Nancy typically holds things "pretty close to her chest" and tries to manage the nursing department on her own without sharing many of the details with her team of directors.

At wit's end, Nancy seeks the counsel of a colleague in a neighboring state who has led his hospital through complex times and even led the nursing staff to Magnet designation. He advises her to reach out to her colleagues on the executive team because the nursing department is core to the business of the hospital. He thinks that she needs to create a shared sense of responsibility for changes that are occurring in the hospital and in nursing and to work toward a better understanding of how a satisfied nursing staff influences patient outcomes, physician satisfaction, and departmental relationships. He also advises her to develop her own directors to work together as a high-performing team and to be more transparent about the pressures she feels to meet operating targets. They talk about her adjusting her own attitude to the job with a goal of creating new mental models about the demands. Perhaps she could consider them more as challenges that need to be solved rather than impossible situations.

Just talking about all that she has faced seems cathartic, and speaking out loud about the problems seems to give her new direction. She realizes that some people would have simply entered into her negative feelings and either advised her to seek a different job or pitied her situation. Nancy is grateful for her colleague's honesty, and she tells him how much she appreciates his boldness and encouragement of her reaching her full potential. They agree that she will keep in touch with him and that he will mentor her over the next few months. She takes some time off to relax and think things through, and she is actually surprised to feel excited to return to work again.

Nancy arrives at work with a new sense of commitment and resolve. She calls together the directors of the various nursing departments and the director of professional development and research and talks with them about her vision to transform the nursing division. She shares her concern that obtaining Magnet designation will be a huge challenge in the economic climate of the hospital. She is very frank with the directors about all that needs to occur and asks them to join her in this endeavor. Some of the directors are very excited about the possibilities of changes in organizational structure, advancement of the staff capabilities, and transformation of the organization to a high-performing one. Nancy asks the director of professional development and research to do a gap analysis of the organization's current capabilities in comparison to the Magnet requirements. She also asks that the directors work together as a team to identify strong nurse leaders among the staff who can compose a new Magnet steering committee. Nancy shares her vision that the Magnet steering committee should design the collaborative governance structure for the nursing division, and that the directors should act in roles as consultants instead of designing the structure themselves. The director group soon realizes that Nancy's style of leadership has changed dramatically since her vacation, and they are excited and uneasy about the changes she outlines.

Nancy also meets individually with the COO, CFO, and her CEO to share her concerns about the across-the-board budget cuts that negatively affect the nursing division and, ultimately, patient-care quality. She shares a plan of how to reduce expenses while preserving the professional role of the nurse as the team leader in the planning and implementation of patient care. She tries to develop a shared vision among her colleagues so they will be invested in her plan to develop and advance the nursing division but also see her as responsible and accountable for the financial integrity of the overall organization. Nancy also meets with the other divisional leaders to discuss how their roles intersect in meeting the organization's goals and financial targets.

As part of the transformation of the nursing division, Nancy works with her direct reports to discuss different leadership styles and leadership theories. She introduces them to concepts such as the servant leader, transformational leadership, and motivation and change theories. She recommends that the directors who do not have master's degrees in nursing leadership consider returning to school, and she offers them 1 day off per week to attend classes. She still expects them to meet their productivity and financial targets and other quality indicators, but she sees the potential in each individual and is confident that the directors will be able to accomplish their roles at the hospital and their new student roles. All the while she is speaking, she is constantly observing the directors' body language, facial expressions, and reactions to her thoughts on expanding their knowledge, skills, and capabilities in leading high-performing teams. Although she realizes that there is some risk in asking her direct reports to return to school while working full time, she is confident that their exposure to new knowledge will also expand their success at work. She reassures them and lets them know that she is available at any time to talk with them about their fears and concerns. She also encourages them, and particularly the director of professional development and research, to motivate the staff nurses with diploma and associate degrees to also continue their education toward the bachelor's degree. Nancy indicates that she is in negotiation with one of the local universities to provide some of the education on site at the hospital to facilitate the nursing staff and directors furthering their education. She shares that she is also working with Human Resources, her executive colleagues, and the Shady Point Foundation to develop nursing scholarships and tuition reimbursement up to $1,000 per person per year.

After a few months, Nancy reflects on all the changes that are occurring at Shady Point Hospital and the pressures she continues to feel to be a good steward of the hospital's resources. She feels excited about the transformation she is witnessing in her directors and the staff as a whole. She also feels more connected with other divisional leaders and the executive team, and although they don't always agree on solutions to problems, they do agree to work as a team to accomplish their shared goals. Changes are coming fast, but Nancy has found strength within herself and her director team that she never dreamed possible.

Questions

1. Who are the stakeholders in this case? Analyze the case by taking on the role and perspective of each stakeholder.
2. How can Nancy possibly lead Shady Point to thrive in the face of the organizational chaos and complexity?

3. What strategies would you use to prepare the nursing team for a Magnet application?
4. What should Nancy do to sustain the gains she has seen in teams at Shady Point?
5. What strategies can a leader employ to create a shared vision?

Case Study 2-2
Developing Service Lines in a Healthcare System

Ella has been the executive director of the Women's and Children's Hospital for the past 10 years at Best Health Memorial Hospital, which is the flagship hospital in a major healthcare system. Five other hospitals in the healthcare system are located within a 50-mile radius of Best Health Memorial Hospital. As executive director, Ella provides leadership to approximately 600 professional staff members who report directly to 12 different managers. The managers also report to 5 directors who provide leadership for the women's surgical areas; labor, delivery, recovery, and prenatal services; maternal and infant services; and neonatal intensive care services. In addition, one director is responsible for professional development and research and supervises the clinical nurse specialists who are assigned to each of the clinical areas.

Ella reports directly to the CNO, who also is responsible for executive directors of other major divisions, including acute care (including oncology, orthopedics, and general medical-surgical care), critical care and emergency services, rehabilitative services, and home health and hospice services. Ella is one of four nurse leaders who direct women's and children's services for the hospital in the Western Regional Health System. The Women's and Children's Hospital at Best Health is the largest in the healthcare system, and the other hospitals include the following: (1) one suburban hospital with a small delivery rate of approximately 900 annual deliveries; (2) one urban hospital with an annual delivery rate of approximately 1,500; (3) an urban hospital with an annual delivery rate of approximately 3,500 and a level II neonatal intermediate intensive care nursery; and (4) one suburban hospital located approximately 50 miles from Best Health with a strategic plan to develop a new maternity service line with a level II neonatal intermediate intensive care nursery. All of the other hospitals have transfer agreements with Best Health's Women's and Children's Hospital for high-risk perinatal and neonatal transports for tertiary care. Beyond the transfer agreements, there is very little coordination of efforts or sharing of resources among the five hospitals.

Ella has assumed the informal leadership among the other directors of maternity and newborn services at the other hospitals, and she is respected for her national reputation as a leader in women's and children's services. Ella is a frequent speaker at national conferences associated with maternal newborn health and children's health services. She has recently attained her PhD in nursing with an emphasis on nursing leadership, is certified by the American Nurses Credentialing Center (ANCC) and the American Organization of Nurse Executives (AONE) in nursing leadership, and is certified in high-risk perinatal services by the Association of Women's Health, Obstetric and Neonatal Nurses (AWHONN). Ella is also a frequent contributor to journals specific to maternity, newborn, and women's services.

The president of Western Regional Health System and his executive team have decided to develop specialty-focused service lines for women's and children's services, cardiac services, orthopedic services, and cancer services. Other service lines will be developed in the future depending on the effectiveness of these four service lines in reducing variation in care, redundancy of services, and costs associated with patient care protocols. It is also hoped that the service-line structure will improve market share and recognition for excellence with improvements in quality outcome indicators, physician and patient satisfaction, and coordination of care across both inpatient and outpatient services related to each of the specialties. To initiate the vision for service-line integration, four corporate vice president positions are announced with star performers in each of the service lines selected for the new role.

Ella, the star performer for women's and children's services, was appointed as the corporate vice president (VP) for women's and children's services. Although surprised and excited about this new role, Ella had mixed feelings about leaving her executive director position at Best Health Memorial Hospital's Women's and Children's Hospital. She and the other newly appointed corporate vice presidents will be relocated to the corporate offices rather than having an office at any one of the five health system hospitals. A new executive director will be recruited for Best Health's Women's and Children's Hospital. The president of Western Regional Health System announced the new organizational structure, vision for system integration, and a newly appointed senior vice president for Service-Line Integration position. The new senior VP is a physician who was recruited from an academic position on the East Coast and who has some experience with a large healthcare system developing a service-line structure. All of the new corporate VPs report directly to Dr. Thomas, the new senior VP.

Needless to say, these organizational changes created absolute chaos among each of the entity hospitals' executive and leadership teams because they were uncertain how the new system structure would affect their strategies and decisions related to the service lines within their own entities. Some of the executive and leadership teams are fearful that they will lose autonomy in decision making related to the service lines. The leaders of the smaller hospitals are pleased that they might have more resources allocated to them as a result of the system change because they often did not receive as many resources as were allocated to the larger hospitals in the system.

There is significant scuttlebutt around the organization as to how the corporate VPs were chosen independent of the usual process of opening positions and allowing inside and outside applicants to be considered. The unilateral decision by the president and his executive team upset many of the leaders in the healthcare system, who voiced concern that this same process might be used for other key positions in the future. Several are concerned that their own power and authority base will be undermined by these newly appointed corporate VPs, and ultimately by the senior VP for Service-Line Integration. The entity leaders are also concerned that their roles and responsibilities in physician recruitment, program development, financial management, and philanthropy will be minimized with the new service-line structure.

The chaos and confusion regarding the new organizational structure are often blatantly apparent at the system-wide executive meetings chaired by the president of Western Regional Medical Center. He finally informs the CEOs of each of the entities that they must put a positive spin on their communication to their leadership teams as well as the staff at each of their hospitals. He provides as much information as possible regarding the position descriptions for the senior VP and the corporate VPs and has several open discussions about his vision for service-line integration across the system. He also suggests that the CEOs read several articles written by national leaders in healthcare integration and authors of books on "systemness." Over the next months, the president invites national speakers to present at Western Regional Healthcare System's corporate offices with invitations for the entity leaders to attend and discuss system integration that has been successfully implemented at other major healthcare systems throughout the United States.

Ella becomes excited about her new role, and she reads everything possible about vertical and horizontal integration of healthcare systems. She begins to meet with the new senior VP and the other corporate VPs who are now her peers. Her position description includes service-line development, integration, and innovation with an emphasis on improving quality and financial indicators by reducing variation and redundancy. She also meets with data analysts to assess the volume, financial, and quality outcome data for each of the entities. Because she had enjoyed a very positive relationship with each of the entity's directors of Women's and Children's Services, she expected to continue this positive relationship in her new role. She also meets with the CNO who was involved in the development of new women's and children's services at the outlying hospital.

When she meets with each of the directors at the respective entities, she is surprised to receive a less than positive reception. Suddenly, her colleagues who had worked with her so well in the past seem distant and negative in their interaction toward her and her ideas related to service-line integration of women's and children's services. With the exception of the CNO who was developing women's and children's services from scratch, the others strongly emphasize their desire to maintain their autonomy in the direction of their services instead of centralizing decision making related to women's and children's services. It seems to Ella that they have no concept of the president's vision for service-line integration or what systemness would look like. Despite her frequent meetings with them and developing an organizational structure for women's and children's services with them, she seems to receive only cordial and superficial coordination of services rather than a commitment to true integration.

Ella's experience is not unique, and the other corporate VPs report similar reactions with the exception of the orthopedic service line. In one of the service-line meetings, Ella mentions that the hospitals are acting more as a confederation of hospitals rather than as a healthcare system. Each of the entity hospitals struggles to maintain as much autonomy in decision making as possible while the corporate system leaders attempt to integrate service lines to create a total and comprehensive system of care for the community with branding of the Western Regional Healthcare System as a name for healthcare excellence.

The orthopedic service line seems to be more advanced in its integration of services because there are few threats among the orthopedic surgeons and nursing leadership at each of the entity hospitals. They see system integration as an opportunity to obtain more resources for capital equipment, marketing and promotional services, and specific leadership for the specialty beyond the current immersion in general acute care services at each of the entities. The cardiac service line struggles with the system integration initiative because each of the entities desires to be named the premier cardiac center within the healthcare system, and several of the interventional cardiologists are direct competitors for market share within the region. Because there are two cancer centers in the healthcare system, the cancer service line also struggles with how to manage competing centers of excellence with physicians and leaders who have no incentive to integrate their services or referral systems. In fact, physician and entity leaders for the cancer service line voice their discontent with the system initiative, stating that it reduces their ability to enhance their market share coming from the smaller hospitals within the system.

Ella continues to review the literature related to the development of systems in general and healthcare systems specifically. She realizes that for the women's and children's service line, she needs to demonstrate the value that could be added by the integration of services across the entities in contrast to each entity acting alone. She also realizes that it is important to identify areas where autonomy in decision making is legitimate and to support each of the entity leaders in their efforts to maintain entity autonomy in their specific region within the city. She recognizes that it will be difficult for each of the entities to give up its respective individual branding within its community, so she advocates at the system meetings for the development of a system brand that also allows for entity branding as a developmental step in the overall goal of system integration. Because each of the entities also provides services to different cultural groups, Ella suggests that these diverse cultures be highlighted in the branding of each of the entity's programs and services. This action recognizes each of the entities for a unique contribution to the system as a whole.

Several different actions and initiatives to develop system integration are tried, and many succeed, whereas others are not so successful. Ella tries to analyze the forces at play in each of the successes and failures. One area that is very successful is the development of a system organizational structure for women's and children's services for the service line that was designed by the entire group of entity leaders. System-wide councils were developed using successful models of shared governance reported in the literature. The following councils were developed: (1) Operations Council, which focused on financial and productivity goals and supply and capital acquisitions; (2) Quality Council, which focused on nurse-sensitive indicators and other quality outcome indicators; (3) Professional Development and Education Council, which focused on integrating orientation and on-boarding, professional development courses, and preparation for specialty certifications; (4) Research and Innovation Council, which focused on developing system-wide research projects, evidence-based practice projects, and new innovations that could be shared among the entities; and (5) Patient and Family Education Council, which focused on the integration of all educational materials for patients and families and the standardization of clinical protocols for patient education across the system.

Ella led the process of developing each of the councils with respective charters, deliverables, and reporting structure to a system-wide steering council composed of physician leaders in women's and children's services and the entity directors at each of the hospitals. It seems that over time the entity directors moved from simply coordinating efforts at each of the hospitals to actually working toward integrating some of their professional education offerings and patient education materials and activities. They also began to assume responsibility in developing a new women's and children's service program at the outlying hospital. Ella begins to realize that system integration could not simply be mandated by system leaders but rather that systemness is a developmental process. Reflecting over the past few months, Ella notes that moving toward systemness has several identifiable steps that include developing trust among the service-line and entity leaders; sharing information and resources across the hospitals; coordinating services and programs across the system; and, finally, developing strategic thinking from a systems perspective instead of the individual entity level.

Questions

1. How do you think that the president's announcement to move to a service-line platform and the centralized decision to appoint service-line vice presidents in contrast to an open recruitment process affected the system service-line initiative?
2. What do you perceive the differences are between a confederation of hospitals and a fully integrated healthcare system?

3. How would you strategize to minimize the fears and anxiety of entity leaders in the development of a system-wide service line?
4. In this case, what are the apparent barriers and contributors to system integration for the service lines?
5. In your opinion, how much autonomy in decision making and marketing and promotions should each entity have in an integrated healthcare system?
6. What are the factors that might affect the decision to honor entity autonomy in contrast to system integration and centralization of decision making and marketing and promotional activities?

References

Armstrong, M. J., & Mullins, C. C. (2017). A value assessment at the point of care: Incorporating patient values throughout care delivery and a draft taxonomy of patient values. *Value in Health: The Journal of the International Society for Pharmacoeconomics and Outcomes Research, 20*(2), 292–295.

Arnold, R. D., & Wade, J. P. (2015). A definition of systems thinking: A systems approach. *Procedia Computer Science, 44*, 669–678.

Babalola, M., Stouten, J., & Euwema, M. (2016). Frequent change and turnover intention: The moderating role of ethical leadership. *Journal of Business Ethics, 134*, 311–322.

Davidson, S., Weberg, D., Porter-O'Grady, T., & Malloch, K. (2017). *Evidence-based innovation in nursing and health professions.* Jones & Bartlett Learning.

de Jong, T., Wiezer, N., de Weerd, M., Nielsen, K., Mattila-Holappa, P., & Mockałło, Z. (2016). The impact of restructuring on employee well-being: A systematic review of longitudinal studies. *Work Stress, 30*(1), 91–114.

Erwin, D. (2009). Changing organizational performance: Examining the change process. *Hospital Topics, 87*(3), 28–40.

Gergen, K. (2015). *Invitation to social construction* (3rd ed.). SAGE.

Hamadi, H., Tafili, A., Apatu, E., Park, S., & Spaulding, A. (2019). Medicare' hospital-acquired condition reduction program and community diversity in the United States: The need to account for racial and ethnic segregation. *Hospital Topics, 97*(4), 148–155.

Hannah, S. T., Balthazard, P. A., Waldman, D. A., Jennings, P. L., & Thatcher, R. W. (2013). The psychological and neurological bases of leader self-complexity and effects on adaptive decision-making. *The Journal of Applied Psychology, 98*(3), 393–411.

Hoch, J. E., Bommer, W. H., Dulebohn, J. H., & Wu, D. (2016). Do ethical, authentic, and servant leadership explain variance above and beyond transformational leadership? A meta-analysis. *Journal of Management, 44*, 501–529.

Knight, A., Fouyaxis, J., Jarrad, G., Beski, K., Cho, G., & Bidargaddi, N. (2018). Systems to harness digital footprint to elucidate and facilitate aging in place. *Studies in Health Technology and Informatics, 246*, 91–101.

Lal, M. M. (2019). Leading effectively through change. *Journal of Nursing Administration, 49*(12), 575–576.

Lunden, A., Teräs, M., Kvist, T., & Häggman-Laitilia, A. (2017). A systematic review of factors influencing knowledge management and the nurse leaders' role. *Journal of Nursing Management, 25*(6), 407–420.

Lunden, A., Teräs, M., Kvist, T., & Häggman-Laitilia, A. (2019). Transformative agency and tensions in knowledge management: A qualitative interview study for nurse leaders. *Journal of Clinical Nursing, 28*(5–6), 969–979.

Marshall, E. S., & Broome, M. E. (2016). *Transformational leadership in nursing: From expert clinician to influential leader* (2nd ed.). Springer.

McKimm, J., & Till, A. (2015). Clinical leadership effectiveness, change and complexity. *British Journal of Hospital Medicine, 76*(4), 239–243.

Melnyk, B. M., Fineout-Overholt, E., Giggleman, M., & Choy, K. (2017). A test of the ARCC© model improves implementation of evidence-based practice, healthcare culture, and patient outcomes. *Worldviews on Evidence-Based Nursing, 14*(1), 5–9.

Nguyen, A. M., Cuthel, A., Padgett, D. K., Niles, P., Rogers, E., Pham-Singer, H., Ferran, D., Kaplan, S. A., Berry, C., & Shelley, D. (2020). How practice facilitation strategies differ by practice context. *Journal of General Internal Medicine, 35*(3), 824–831.

Nguyen, H. B., Thomson, C., Jarjour, N. N., Dixon, A. E., Liesching, T. N., Schnapp, L. M., Madison, J. M., Murin, S., Glenny, R., Kaminiski, N., & Leadership Working Group of the Association of Pulmonary, Critical Care, and Sleep Division Directors. (2019). Leading change and negotiation strategies or division leaders in clinical medicine. *Chest, 156*(6), 1246–1253.

Parolini, A., Tan, W. W., & Shlonsky, A. (2019). Decision-based models of the implementation of interventions in systems of healthcare: Implementation outcomes and intervention effectiveness in complex service environments. *PLOS One, 14*(10), e0223129.

Pepler, E., & Martell, R. C. (2019). Indigenous model of care to health and social care workforce planning. *Healthcare Management Forum, 32*(1), 32–39.

Porter-O'Grady, T., & Malloch, K. (2017). Failure and resilience: The lifeblood of innovation. In S. Davidson, D. Weberg, T. Porter-O'Grady, & K. Malloch (Eds.), *Evidence-based innovation in nursing and health professions* (pp. 335–365). Jones & Bartlett Learning.

Richards, G. (2011). *Psychology, religion, and the nature of the soul a historical entanglement. Library of the history of psychological theories*. Springer.

Taylor, M. V., Priefer, B. A., & Alt-White, A. C. (2016). Evidence-based practice: Embracing integration. *Nursing Outlook, 64*(5), 575–582.

Thakrar, S. V., & Bell, D. (2017). Sustainability and transformation plans: Translating the perspectives. *British Journal of Hospital Medicine, 78*(10), 580–583.

Uhl-Bien, M., & Marion, R. (2008). *Complexity leadership: Conceptual foundations*. Information Age.

Uhl-Ben, M., Marion, R., & McKelvey, B. (2007). Complexity leadership theory: Shifting leadership from the industrial age to the knowledge era. *The Leadership Quarterly, 18*(4), 298–318.

Weberg, D. (2017). Innovation leadership behaviors: Starting the complexity journey. In S. Davidson, D. Weberg, T. Porter-O'Grady, & K. Malloch (Eds.), *Evidence-based innovation in nursing and health professions* (pp. 43–76). Jones & Bartlett Learning.

Weberg, D. R., & Fuller, R. M. (2019). Toxic leadership: Three lessons from complexity science to identify and stop toxic teams. *Nurse Leader, 17*(1), 22–26.

Zhang, H., Cowling, D. W., Graham, J. M., & Taylor, E. (2019). Five-year impact of a commercial accountable care organization on health care spending, utilization, and quality of care. *Medical Care, 57*(11), 845–854.

Suggested Readings

Berwick, D., Nolan, T., & Whittington, J. (2008). The triple aim: Care, health, and cost. *Health Affairs, 27*(3), 759–769.

Foti, R., & Hauenstein, N. (2007). Pattern and variable approaches in leadership emergence and effectiveness. *Journal of Applied Psychology, 92*(2), 347–355.

Juarrero, A., & Rubino, C. (2010). *Emergence, complexity, and self-organization*. Emergent Publications.

CHAPTER TWO   Ten Complexity Principles for Leaders Advancing Value in the Quantum Age

Malloch, K., & Porter-O'Grady, T. (2009). *The quantum leader: Applications for the new world of work.* Jones & Bartlett Learning.

Yang, A., & Shan, Y. (2008). *Intelligent complex adaptive systems.* IGI Publishing.

Quiz Questions

Select the best answer for each of the following questions.

1. Change can be defined as a dynamic rather than as an event. This means that change is:
    a. cyclical.
    b. periodic.
    c. timely.
    d. continuous.

2. Complexity science is based on a new understanding of the operation of the physical world. What is this understanding referred to as?
    a. Newtonian physics
    b. Quantum mechanics
    c. Universal science
    d. The Einstein principle

3. A number of converging forces have ushered in the new age. The three main forces converging are sociopolitical, economic, and:
    a. technological.
    b. international.
    c. scientific.
    d. commercial.

4. Systems are dynamic entities driven more by relational elements than by functional processes. In this way, which of the following do they resemble?
    a. Biological structures
    b. Business structures
    c. Social structures
    d. Information structures

5. In a healthy system, 90% of decisions are driven by which of the following?
    a. Top of the system personnel
    b. Bottom of the system personnel
    c. Point-of-service personnel
    d. Managers

6. According to complexity theory, anything that adds value to a part of the system adds value to the whole system. Which of the following is an implication of this principle?
    a. Each part of the system drives the work of the whole system.
    b. The whole system is the only legitimate source of sustainable value.
    c. All real value derives from the work of the people in the system.
    d. Every component of a system contributes to the integrity of the whole system.

Quiz Questions

7. In complexity theory, how is *chunking* defined?
    a. It is the support provided to a complex system by the operation of simple systems.
    b. It is the formation of a complex system through interdependent simple systems.
    c. It is the operation of a complex system consisting of independent parts.
    d. It is the dynamic relationship between independent simple systems.

8. Diversity is essential to change for which reason?
    a. It creates the variety required by change.
    b. It accentuates the similarities that exist through change.
    c. It makes chaos visible and underscores the need for adaptation.
    d. It highlights the difficulty of reconciling differences.

9. Error is essential to change. Not all errors are acceptable, however. Which of the following errors are to be avoided?
    a. System-based errors
    b. Errors in judgment
    c. Repeated errors
    d. Human errors

10. Systems are driven by different rules than are functional institutions. Which of the following are the cornerstones of systems design?
    a. Relationships and intersections
    b. Functions and actions
    c. Policies and processes
    d. Rules and regulations

11. To ensure the system's vitality, the leader of a system must pay special attention to which of the following?
    a. Stability
    b. Chaos
    c. Form
    d. Function

12. When does revolution in a system occur?
    a. When the pace of evolution is insufficient for the necessary changes
    b. When things cannot continue to operate in the same way
    c. When violence is introduced into the system
    d. When many local changes occur at once

13. Leaders now must more deeply understand the implications of which of the following in order to apply the contemporary role?
    a. Economic theory
    b. Sociopolitical theory
    c. Complexity theory
    d. Atomic theory

14. Knowledge has historically been treated as a capacity. From a quantum perspective, knowledge should be treated as a:
    a. possession.
    b. utility.
    c. toolset.
    d. vehicle.

15. The impact of complexity leadership often depends on the amount of time the leader spends:
    a. illuminating the difference between actuality and potentiality.
    b. addressing the day-to-day problems that affect the leadership role.
    c. developing policies and procedures to guide the function and actions of work.
    d. managing and disciplining people to ensure that their actions are aligned with work expectations.

16. Living in the "potential" means:
    a. successfully meeting the demands of the present.
    b. translating prevailing circumstances for worker understanding.
    c. identifying real-time problems and helping others develop effective solutions.
    d. expressing awareness of an inevitable emerging reality within the context of a change trajectory.

17. In systems the real work of leadership is to:
    a. see that work gets done appropriately and effectively.
    b. help focus workers on the relationship between the work and its outcomes.
    c. refocus the elements and processes of work toward its larger organizational or systematic context.
    d. strengthen the functional and process-based focus of work to meet work needs.

18. The function of structure in a service system is:
    a. to ensure the integrity of the system in achieving its goals.
    b. to empower the board to set and meet operational and functional requirements.
    c. to ensure that executives and managers make the right decisions about work at the point-of-service.
    d. to ensure that activities of work are controlled by finances and resources.

19. The necessary drivers of good value are:
    a. clinicians who are committed and work hard at delivering service and addressing outcomes.
    b. good quality processes and well-developed quality metrics directed to achieving outcomes.
    c. strong managers who really believe in quality and require quality performance from staff.
    d. high-level integration and integrity of value-based processes, functions, and structures.

20. The measure of vitality in any kind of a system is:
    a. the relationship between work and the principles that guide it.
    b. the interaction between management and staff around good work.
    c. the triadic relationship among purpose, person, and performance.
    d. the resources, energy, and attention toward doing good patient care.

21. Diversity is:
    a. the elements of sameness across all kinds of people.
    b. the visual manifestation of the chaos and energy that arises from conflicts.
    c. the homogeneity necessary to accomplish meaningful work.
    d. the seamless thread of elements found between and among all populations.

22. *Error* can be defined as:
    a. a break in the confluence and congruity of processes that causes participants to assess the situation and take action.
    b. a deficit that requires retrenchment, correction, discipline, and a renewal of effort in achieving objectives.
    c. a negative change in conditions or an unnecessary breach that impedes achievement of goals.
    d. failure of the organization to achieve planned objectives, priorities, direction, or activities.

23. Systems thrive when:
    a. leaders make sure that actions are consistent with leadership priorities.
    b. they limit the number of negative forces impacting goals and operations.
    c. their components are clearly defined and each have unique contributions.
    d. their functions intersect and interact in a continual dance of transformation.

24. There is a constant and permanent _____ between equilibrium (stabilizers) and disequilibrium (challenges).
    a. balance
    b. tension
    c. interface
    d. state

25. A revolution occurs in any system when:
    a. sufficient evolution has occurred over time to create a seminal event.
    b. many components converge to make a significant demand that prompts life-altering change.
    c. a component of a system no longer functions and creates "noise" to the other functions of the system.
    d. a system's essential functions have grown old and need to be changed.

CHAPTER THREE

Innovation Leadership and Professional Governance: Building the Structure for Transformation

> Man's mind stretched to a new idea never returns to its original dimensions.
> —Oliver Wendell Holmes

Chapter Objectives

At the completion of this chapter, the reader will be able to:

- Explore professional governance as a vehicle for structural empowerment and innovation.
- Define key concepts and terms associated with innovation and innovation leadership.
- Identify the rationale for innovation in healthcare organizations.
- Compare and contrast the work of innovation with the work of routine operations.
- Describe the role of leaders in advancing the integration of innovation into the work of healthcare organizations.
- Evaluate multiple metrics for the measurement of innovations.

Shared governance models for structural empowerment are transitioning to professional governance models in which the nursing profession continues to increase accountability to the profession, recognize the obligations of professional membership, strengthen partnerships with key stakeholders, and advance evidence-driven decision making (Clavelle et al., 2016). Advancements in the profession of nursing reflect maturation of the shared governance model as well as the engagement and contributions of nurses in regard to advancing healthcare innovation, new knowledge, and best practices.

Traditionally, the emphasis of healthcare organizational structures has been on stability and goal achievement. Experimentation with patient care processes was discouraged (or minimized) to avoid additional expenses and to ensure that safe and effective patient care occurred. Leaders tended to delay process modifications until there was significant research and high-quality evidence for new processes or the current processes failed abruptly. The traditional approach was typical even when current processes were known to be only marginally successful in providing safe and effective patient care. Maintaining the status quo, where cost and outcomes were known, was preferred to taking risks in which costs and outcomes were not clearly known.

Nearly 30 years ago, Wheatley (1992) challenged leaders to think differently about leadership. She challenged leaders to search for new ways of understanding leadership. Professional governance now requires innovation. Integration of innovation into the leadership paradigm provides an objective marker of Wheatley's challenge (Stuke, 2013; Wheatley, 1992). To be sure, the traditional approach is understandable, but it is shortsighted. Adopting a leadership mindset that actively supports both innovation and effective operations is important for organizations to grow, sustain new practices, and excel in the future healthcare marketplace.

In today's healthcare environment, leaders and managers need a wide and varied range of competencies to manage not only the operations of the organization but also the work of continually adapting to new evidence, technology, and processes. The work of adapting to new approaches requires knowledge specific to creativity and innovation. This chapter presents the concept of innovation leadership, the rationale for innovation, leadership expectations, organizational structures and strategies to advance and integrate innovation, and metrics to measure innovation. The work of innovation is served and supported both within and independent of a professional governance framework. The 21st-century leader must develop skills to lead in a world in which innovations are the lifeblood of the organization (Bates et al., 2017). Further, leaders must foster and nurture a culture of innovation and the individual innovations that emerge.

The seemingly contradictory nature of healthcare leadership, which requires both sound business practices to create real value for the organization and a designing eye on the future, is an increasingly difficult challenge. Healthcare, behavioral, and education scientists, rather than software engineers, must create innovative environments that use many forms of health information technology–based communication, including artificial intelligence, social media platforms, robotics, augmented and virtual reality, electronic health record, and healthcare database software, all of which are constantly evolving. Leaders have always been involved in adopting new work processes; however, the current intensity and frequency in which messages are received can have a negative effect—too much incoming communication at one time, and without time and knowledge to ascertain their value to the organization. Ultimately, a focus on work that is known is much less stressful than working to modify or eliminate current work in favor of the unknown and untested. The risk-adverse mindset of traditional organization leaders too often leads to continually reworking ineffective established processes—much like the metaphorical rearranging of the deck chairs on the *Titanic*! Thus, the balance of continuing with known initiatives and cultivating and implementing innovations is a challenge to contemporary leaders.

With a shift from shared governance to professional governance, nursing is well-positioned to contribute substantively to systems, structures, processes, and outcomes that reflect value-based

> **Key Point**
>
> Professional governance is foundational to autonomous practice and achievement of exemplary empirical outcomes via accountability to the nursing profession, recognition of professional obligations, development and maintenance of collateral relationships (partnerships), and involvement in decision making based on evidence (Clavelle et al., 2016).

care. To get from innovation to value-based care, leaders need to support the conduct of research, process initiatives that involve implementation of innovative interventions, translation of evidence-based research into practice, utilization of team-based care models in population health, equitable interprofessional relationships, and uptake of opportunities for innovations in health practices (Clavelle et al., 2016).

Definitions and Concepts

Innovation is not a magical, fog-laden concept. The two essential ingredients are *novelty* (or creativity) and *value* (having a purpose and important outcomes) (Endsley, 2010; Ness, 2012). Novelty can have a wide scope, from original, fresh, never seen before, or different. An innovation must be applied and its value must be obvious or shown in quality improvement or research findings to garner the term. Value can mean that the innovation is useful, an improvement, or that it makes something better. Getting to common ground on what innovation is and what it is not serves to minimize confusion and chaos. An improvement to a process or product that is already in place or commercialized can be an innovation if the improvement is novel and adds new value by making the process or product better. Consider the improvements in cell phones that led to smartphones (and that had new value)—camera, apps, storage, music, global positioning systems, and other features. A *disruptive innovation* is defined as an innovation that initially is considered inferior until the quality increases and people are willing to switch to it. Thus, it generally cannot be used by customers in mainstream markets. It defines a new performance trajectory by introducing new dimensions of performance compared to existing innovations. Once a disruptive innovation goes to market, it generally pushes the incumbents out of the market (Christensen et al., 2015; Fuller & Hansen, 2019).

When exploring specific innovations, consider definitions and descriptions such as the time parameters, levels of change, drivers of change, and agency (individual, team, or population). Attention to these components is helpful when an organization is creating or adopting a definition of innovation and may help to distinguish between an idea, innovation, or improvement. In health care, innovation can be seen as new knowledge that solves a problem; the creation of new resources or improvements to existing resources; or implementation of a new idea, product, service, structure, business model, or device that is recognized internally or externally as important.

Innovation leadership is a term used to describe a philosophy by leaders that influences, supports, and facilitates the production, cultivation, and development of shared objectives via novel concepts, algorithms, products, services, and technologies, despite potential risks. Essentially, nursing leaders who are innovation leaders support ideas and innovations that will design the future of nursing and health care (Weintraub & McKee, 2019). Innovation leadership makes it possible for leaders to address the challenges of meeting current and traditional operations that result in profitability, and simultaneously to work to recreate the future as new developments emerge in health care and as local stakeholders develop and present novel ideas and concepts with value. Weberg (2017) believes that innovation leaders have seven characteristics, many of which are meant to be practiced in cooperation with others, not as individual or isolated activities. First, innovation leaders span boundaries that may have been previously reserved for top leaders. Second, they take risks in regard to experimenting with untested processes, technologies, systems, and products and have a vision of how innovation will create the future. Third, innovation leaders have vision. At the macro level, they consider their influence on innovation during strategic planning, even if leading change is not part of their formal role. When visioning, innovation leaders collaborate with others to build strategy that will aid the success of an innovation. Fourth, innovation leaders leverage opportunities. They volunteer to test creative solutions and look for funding to bring innovation forward. Fifth, innovation leaders are adaptive. They may take on roles as opportunities emerge and use their roles to drive adaptations. Sixth, innovation leaders are coordinators of information flow. They not only influence how information is shared and interpreted, they may champion innovation and take actions that enable behaviors. Finally, innovation leaders are facilitators. They help others understand the relevance of innovation, and they understand how their behaviors can influence the system.

Superior innovation provides organizations with opportunities to grow faster, better, and smarter than their competitors—and to ultimately influence the direction of its industry. To initiate or expand a culture of innovation, chief nursing leader behaviors should include assessing the environment for an innovation orientation, assuring that leaders understand their responsibility for creating a culture and an environment that allows innovation to thrive, educating and building skills that promote openness to new views, and practicing solving big problems through innovative solutions, knowing that failure is a part of innovation (Weatherford et al., 2018).

> **Key Point**
> When complex innovations are introduced into an organization, expect that active coordinated actions by multiple stakeholders are needed to achieve organizational benefits (Rangachari, 2018).

Innovation is more than just creating new technology or a gadget or process; it is about continual adaptation to the changing healthcare environment and available resources. Innovation includes creating new business models and strategies for the organization to survive and thrive into the future. Innovation leaders balance the need for value/profit and the creation of new and improved approaches to health care. An infrastructure that supports rapid, evidence-driven, and effective outcomes at the point-of-care may be reflected in job descriptions of personnel who are indirect leaders, for example, clinical nurse specialists.

This chapter provides a new perspective and overview of innovation leadership as an essential competency of quantum leaders, those who approach the work of health care from a systems perspective, continually recognizing the importance of sustainability, growth, and renewal for survival. The reader is encouraged to delve further into the rich and extensive writings on innovation.

Rationale for Healthcare Innovation

The rationale for innovation in health care is multifaceted and was initially driven by the explosion of information on the internet and then by the explosion of electronic health records. Variations in care, medical errors, fragmented services, ineffective processes, patient safety concerns, and consumer expectations have contributed to the need for change in the system. The transformation to a knowledge-based digital world demands that leaders move faster, get optimized, and go global—all sooner rather than later. Further, in today's healthcare environment, in addition to a focus on health information technology, there is a growing focus on improving healthcare quality. Organizations are investing funds to promote product and technology innovations that improve care processes and enhance consumer convenience, value, and access, as a commitment to the future (Bates et al., 2017; Samet & Smith, 2016). Contemporary leaders recognize that organizations cannot grow through cost reduction and reengineering alone. Nor can they survive when there is continual chaos and changing processes at the expense of providing value-based service. Organizations of the 21st century must be focused and create flexible structures that meet the new demands of the technology age in a way that supports the introduction, testing, and integration of new ideas and novel solutions. Asking individuals to think outside the box is insufficient for integrated innovation; principles, behaviors, and metrics for success are needed to support innovative thinking. Most important, new mindsets are needed for leaders to manage these seemingly contradictory expectations of stability and uncertainty.

Group Discussion

Is there any process, product, or technology that should not be changed or viewed as an opportunity for improvement? Is there any truth to the adage, "If it's not broken, don't fix it"? Identify examples of areas that are believed to be immune to change. If appropriate, describe strategies to gain support for evaluating opportunities for new and better approaches.

Healthcare innovation is limitless. It is about rethinking and recreating methods of healthcare delivery that are scalable and impactful and that include preventive, diagnostic, and prognostic approaches; interdisciplinary communication methods; documentation of services' billing and payment services; and solutions that enhance healthcare provider efficiency and effectiveness. Healthcare leaders are called to reinvent a healthcare system that was designed without safety in mind and without ensuring organized and defined processes that support patient and provider safety and minimize adverse patient and provider outcomes. Innovations are needed to correct system inefficiencies. Interestingly, as leaders integrate the work of innovation into their organizations, they are also challenged to identify processes and treatments that lack evidence of efficacy and to eliminate them.

In the last 45 years, biotechnology has transformed the healthcare industry, as well as the way people are treated for disease. The convergence of biotechnology, information technology, and nanotechnology has transformed the way in which health care is provided. Biologics—drugs that target specific diseases—and biomarkers—tests that predict presence of disease and/or clinical responsiveness to treatments—are now available to treat allergic and respiratory conditions and some chronic diseases (Casale, 2017; Koch-Nolte et al., 2019). It is possible to improve treatment because biologics target specific ion channels, cells, and diseases, turning many fatal diseases into chronic conditions and helping those with chronic conditions to live with reduced symptoms. Biologic innovations, although unequivocally beneficial for health, are not always welcomed and easily integrated into the existing healthcare system, which was designed for different products, services, and roles.

Innovation is rapidly changing the scope and methods of health care for both consumers and providers. Innovation is impacting patient care delivery processes (e.g., digital health tools, virtual house calls, medical homes, health hubs within retail locations, and hospital at home), technology that alters the methods used to educate healthcare providers and patients (e.g., virtual and augmented reality headsets), technology for patient record keeping (e.g., speech recognition for clinical documentation), information integration (e.g., integration of brain assessment tools from multiple disciplines to advance neuropsychological assessment), and the overall business model for health care (e.g., mobile health clinics and strategies that reduce unnecessary services in primary and specialty care). Healthcare consumers demand care that is local and immediately available and that does not require complex invasive processes and long recovery times. Providers of health care expect computerization, internet access, and increasingly interconnected applications that foster patient–provider communication and integrate best practices and alerts to identify patient-risk situations. Healthcare leaders and policymakers continue to expect more streamlined processes and expeditious communication of costs and transactions within the system.

Innovations related to methods of patient care delivery to consumers has been a focus of the Health Care Innovations Awards program led by the Centers for Medicare and Medicaid Services (see https://innovation.cms.gov/initiatives/Health-Care-Innovation-Awards/). The program aims to discover innovations that deliver better health, improved care, and lower costs. In one meta-analysis of 43 ambulatory programs, models that included health information technology or community health workers achieved the best cost savings, and models aimed at clinically fragile patients (those with complex conditions or at high risk for disease progression) had moderately large cost savings (Smith et al., 2017). **Exhibit 3-1** lists examples of areas for healthcare improvement that are needed within three categories: methods of patient care delivery to consumers, selection and integration of technology, and business models that support the entire healthcare system.

Group Discussion

Innovation is often confused with creativity, continuous improvement, or quality (performance) improvement. In a small group, compare and contrast the definitions and expectations of each of these four concepts. Consider also the advantages and disadvantages of each. Is there a difference in sustainability for each concept? How is each of these supported and funded in your organization? Based on your discussion, what recommendations would you make to advance innovation in your organization?

Innovation and the Quantum Leader

The role of the quantum leader is to create an infrastructure that integrates innovation into the overall work of the organization. Innovation leadership is about creating conditions, securing resources, and providing rewards for innovative work (Malloch, 2010). The desired supportive culture of innovation is one in which employees are encouraged and valued for challenging existing work processes and providing services that ensure organizational viability. It is important to note that advancing one's culture to embrace innovation can be paradoxical—it takes time to shift a culture to support innovation (as it involves a change in values, norms, and assumptions) *and* the marketplace demands speedy changes (Miller &

Exhibit 3-1   Healthcare Challenges

Patient Care Delivery
- Less invasive
- Less painful
- More convenient
- Less costly
- Increased consumer control

Technology
- Pharmaceuticals
- Diagnostic methods
- Patient record keeping
- Interconnected/integrated information

Business Models
- Less fragmentation of processes, providers, payers, settings, vendors, suppliers
- Increased vertical and horizontal integration

Wedell-Wedellsborg, 2013). Innovation leadership requires continually transforming and remaking structures and processes of the current system to integrate new processes and technology so that systems do indeed perform more effectively (Weberg, 2017).

The system complexity that accompanies healthcare innovation is a source of accelerated uncertain expectations. Of significant concern for the contemporary leader is how to determine and manage the uncertain expectations associated with innovation, the speed at which change occurs, and the anticipated outcomes of new knowledge, technology, and process interactions with as little negative impact on the organization as possible.

By its very nature, there is no evidence for innovations in the making, only expectations. This reality does not deter most leaders from continuing to expect assurances and metrics for success. Risk taking is not viewed as a classic leadership behavior, and it is not traditionally welcomed and encouraged. Instead, risk taking is viewed negatively. It increases the organization's exposure to unforeseen hazards and to the loss of net income. Playing it safe and being a hardworking employee leads the organization nowhere because the intent is to sustain the past and to continue the practices that have been deemed to work yesterday.

Taking the initiative to advance innovation, rather than clinging to the same old routine, is the work of contemporary leaders. Innovation requires that leaders expose themselves to failure, avoid mediocrity, and embrace opportunities rather than retreat from them. The role of leaders is to inspire creativity and hard work and to challenge the past as the means to a better future. The work of inspiration requires not just inspirational phrases but inspirational behavior. Risk-disposed leaders motivate others by showing what can be done, not merely by sermonizing about opportunities. They also exhibit candor and vulnerability, identify value in marginally successful efforts, and allow others to take risks and experience success and failure.

Innovation Leadership Is Not . . .

Innovation leadership is about integrating innovative ideas into the operation of an organization. Often, when an individual assumes the responsibility to manage the implementation of a technology product, the perception is that this work is innovation leadership. Innovation leadership is not project management. Innovation leadership is about who the leader is and how the world of work is approached. Project management is about the dissemination of processes using a top-down approach. Traditionally, the work of project management is done by a manager who is following and guiding the implementation of a clearly defined plan. However, as the healthcare industry works to better integrate innovation and operations, an innovation leader can also be a project manager for selected projects. This approach increases cross-fertilization of innovation and operations, and at the same time, it provides real-time opportunities for the innovation leader to correct course or modify the project plan to ensure optimal results.

Strategies to Integrate and Advance Innovation

The following considerations are suggested for leaders interested in advancing the work of innovation in the culture of the organization:

- Integrating mission, vision, and values within an innovation paradigm
- Assessing community and team needs
- Evaluating organizational structure
- Supporting organizational processes
- Measuring results

Integrating Mission, Vision, Values, and Innovation

The first consideration to advance innovation is a clear statement within the organization's mission, vision, and values. It is important to formally define the organization's commitment to innovation as an integral part of the work of the organization. Using the previous list of definitions and descriptions of innovation, leaders can adopt, modify, or create their own definition to reflect the mission, vision, and values of the organization. The mission incorporates the desire to provide a service or product that is continually viable and able to meet defined goals. The vision statement continues the expression of the desired service and the level of achievement necessary to achieve the mission. The values selected are those that support behaviors necessary to achieve the mission of value and innovation. **Exhibit 3-2** is an example of innovation-based mission, vision, and values statements.

Assessing Community Innovation

The second consideration is the identification of the needs of the community for innovation within the confines of the mission, vision, and values. Each organization is challenged to identify the unmet needs of the organization and its customers, the obstacles to excellent patient care, and the bottlenecks for efficient throughput as considerations when integrating the work

---

Exhibit 3-2 Innovation-Based Mission, Vision, and Values

Mission: To provide excellent patient care that provides value and makes a difference in people's lives.

Vision: To be the market leader of quality, service, and cost-effectiveness in health care.

Values: Participation, multiple intelligences, creativity, risk taking, respect for chaos, vulnerability leadership, evidence-based processes, and measurement.

of innovation with operations. Strategies that can improve the culture of innovation within the community are (1) providing education on innovation and leading innovation, (2) creating strong linkages, (3) supporting competitions that promote innovation and entrepreneurship, (4) developing policies that support innovation based on national/international standards, and (5) developing an entrepreneurship ecosystem (Househ et al., 2015). Ultimately, the organization leaders need to create a focus for innovation and avoid the temptation to work on a great idea that is not consistent with the community's or organization's needs.

Assessing Team Innovation Skills

In addition to knowing community and organizational innovation needs, it is also important to know the innovation skills of team members in the organization. Knowledge of comfort levels with different innovation skills can assist leaders in the reinforcement of existing skills and the development of new ones. The essence of innovation should be integrated throughout educational offerings. Opportunities to explore mental models associated with skill updates can be especially helpful.

Evaluating Organizational Structure

It is not enough to hold a 1-day retreat and ask others to think outside the box. Structure and support are needed to fully embrace and realize the work of innovation. Interestingly, some believe that structure and process are the natural foes of creativity. Leaders often treat innovation as if it were magical, not subject to guidance or nurturing, much less planning. In actuality, there are times, places, and conditions under which innovation does indeed flourish. However, innovation and creativity require some restraint. Creativity with a vision, rules about how to get there, and deadlines support rather than hinder new ideas.

> **Key Point**
> Certain types of individuals, physical facilities, authority designations, decision-making expectations, and systems to document and measure results are essential elements of an organizational infrastructure. An organization's infrastructure is a reflection of its mission, vision, and values. Innovation leadership is about embedding support for innovative thinking in the mission, vision, and values, and from there throughout teams in the organization. Organizational structures are continually evaluated and reshaped to better match the work to be done. Roles are added, modified, or eliminated to improve performance and outcomes. More recently, advancements in professional governance have provided new expectations for optimizing the organization's infrastructure. Each change is accompanied by anticipated but unknown outcomes.

Supporting Organizational Processes by Valuing Natural Tensions

As one considers innovation structure, it is important to recognize the natural tensions and competing priorities that exist in a complex organization. There is a natural tension between being creative and delivering value from being creative. Leaders are very experienced in exploiting existing and known processes and less experienced in exploiting new opportunities for growth. Both the lack of time and the intense pressures within the existing work contribute to the limited attention and effort given to innovation. O'Reilly and Tushman (2016) challenge organizations to become ambidextrous organizations, or those that emphasize balance between creativity and value capture so that the company generates successful new ideas and

> ## Group Discussion
>
> To increase comfort with innovation thinking, begin small. One example is relooking at the impact and value of continuing education programs. Consider two approaches to creating a continuing education program. In scenario A, the designer will use an established continuing education set of rules or guidelines. In scenario B, the designer will use principles; that is, the expectation that knowledge will be integrated into practice and change behaviors. Compare and contrast the advantages and disadvantages of each approach.

gets the maximum return on investment. Balancing these two seemingly disparate processes requires leaders to think differently and to continually develop the skills of middle managers to balance these same processes.

The tension between stability and innovation is especially notable in the area of patient safety. Serious efforts are in place to support high-reliability processes in which there is consistency and redundancy to ensure safe outcomes. Standardization is the goal. What is also known is that despite standardization many patient care processes do not result in safe outcomes. Patients are injured from falls, medication errors, wrong-site surgical procedures, and malfunctioning equipment. Processes to test, innovate, validate, and ensure safety can be achieved through the lens of innovation leadership, organizational resources, and a strong commitment to excellence and continual course correction.

Two basic approaches have been developed for organizational structuring to support innovation. The first approach is to develop leaders and managers who have the ability to be rigorously dedicated to value and to support the work of innovation. With this option, the balancing of goals and priorities is much more complex than the balancing required for two distinct groups.

The second approach is to develop two distinct but collaborative groups in the organizational structure: one group focusing on current business value and the other group focusing on potential business. This approach deliberately secludes new ideas and intellectual property until the organization determines they are appropriate to release. With two distinct groups, role confusion is minimized. Interestingly, this model is effective in the short term, but separate innovation efforts and structures are at risk in times of economic stress.

Regardless of the approach taken by an organization, the leadership team must support operations that are multifocal in nature. The difference between the two options is in the amount of emphasis and time required to support each approach. The skill to operate multifocally is necessary to effectively sustain business while exploring the future and minimizing organizational chaos. Choosing an approach is directly related to the levels of innovation anticipated by the organization and the available skill sets of employees. The integrated approach requires higher levels of leadership skills to plan, collaborate, negotiate, and synthesize business. The distinct group approach requires parallel systems and processes for current business and potential business. Seldom does an organization choose an all-or-nothing approach. Rather, a combination of focused and integrated approaches is selected.

The anticipated expectations for innovations in the future should be considered in creating the structure. Levels of innovation range from minimal innovations to entire system innovations. Lower levels of innovations are described as incremental or partial and do not completely disrupt the work of an organization. Incremental innovations are introduced using project management methods and change management principles; then, they are woven into the fabric of existing systems—into the core of the organization.

Disruptive innovation, a concept identified by Christensen and colleagues (2015), is a unique approach to introducing innovation. The innovation focuses on disruption to the competitive landscape rather than incremental, semi-radical, and very radical innovations that affect both technology and the business model. A healthcare example of disruptive innovation occurs when a large system builds a new healthcare facility that is designed to transform the healthcare experience. New technology, state-of-the-art technology, computerized patient records, and evidence-based architecture meld to create the backdrop for a culture revolution. Every work process and worker role is examined and remodeled to fit with the innovative healthcare facility. Not surprisingly, the work of design and construction is only the beginning. Identifying, role modeling, and sustaining new practices are the work of change management, negotiation, and teamwork.

Innovation Label Versus Innovation Role

Another consideration is the use of the innovation label. The label *innovation* can have both positive and negative effects on the organization's intended goals. Some believe that using the innovation title should be avoided because it further separates the work of innovation from the traditional work of creating value and profit for the organization. Labeling a new team, department, or individual with the innovation label separates business from design. The designers or innovators are frequently perceived as better or different from those in routine operations. In contrast, when senior leaders are able to value and function in both the business and the design worlds, the innovation label recognizes that innovation work is different, is funded differently, and is an important segment of the organization in addition to operations. The goal is to select a title that is consistent with the mission, vision, and values; does not induce hostility or divisiveness among coworkers; and invites as many as possible into the processes of innovation (**Exhibit 3-3**).

Exhibit 3-3   Innovative Leader Titles

Chief Marketing Officer
Director of Design and Brand Experience
Chief Innovation Officer
Champion of Innovation
Chief of Design
Director of Global Innovation
Director of Strategic Marketing
Innovation Champion
Vice President, Enthusiast Services
Vice President, Strategic Leadership and Competency Creation
Chief Technology Officer

Supporting Innovation Processes

Walking the talk of the innovation mission, vision, and values requires specific behaviors that reflect the value of innovation for the organization. Several considerations should be kept in mind when supporting innovation. Although it is clear that the traditional culture is one that supports stability and safety, this rationale cannot be used to avoid innovations. Leaders need to be aware of the culture but not blame the culture for failure to advance. Three processes can assist leaders in transforming the current healthcare culture from a risk-averse model to one that balances both value creation for net income in the present and designing for the future—support, measurement, and continual modifications. These three processes are necessary to ensure ultimate integration and value production. If the three processes do not occur, innovations die a slow, sometimes painful, sad death.

Interestingly, some organizations find that coming up with a great idea is the easy part; the more difficult work is selecting the right ideas and implementing them. There is no template or road map for innovation sustainability. What are available to leaders are the guiding principles of change management and conflict utilization, along with previous experiences in the integration of new processes and technology. Process activities that continually link innovation to the organizational mission through appropriate metrics and rewards reaffirm the commitment of leaders. Given the complex and multifaceted nature of innovation, no two innovation integration situations are identical.

Integrating innovation behaviors into the organization does not require a revolution inside of an organization. When leaders create a culture of innovation success and encourage and reward risk-taking, success is more likely (Weintraub & McKee, 2019). Innovation requires thoughtful construction of solid management processes and an organization that can get things done. Employees want problem solving and innovation to be valued and supported (Snow, 2019). Innovation should be routine rather than random, central rather than marginal, and exciting rather than scary. Efforts to integrate quality assurance and performance improvement into the basic structure of healthcare organizations have been successful; those efforts can be examined to assist in the integration of innovation work. Innovation leadership is about integrating two seemingly disparate worlds of business and design, and about integrating the need for safety and stability with the need to test innovations designed to improve safety, quality, and value.

Operationalizing Innovation

A consideration of integrating innovation is to operationalize it within the organization. Innovation needs to be demystified, and individuals need to respect and value innovation as a core value and process of the organization. Operationalizing innovation is not unlike the efforts of national quality or patient safety initiatives—there is a commitment to adopting proven best practices, and the work is not isolated to a specific department but rather is a core competency for all employees. Elemental and global infrastructure and processes rely on leaders who assert that they are committed and accountable supporters of innovation as defined by the organization, and of the adoption of specific innovations as a first step of diffusion (Albert, 2018). Greater numbers of colleagues dedicated to innovation create a critical mass of energy and effort dedicated to thriving in uncertainty—uncertainty that is channeled into the productive work of confronting, monitoring, and modeling innovative behaviors whenever possible.

Expect Evidence-Based Processes

Another consideration is work based on evidence. Evidence-based practice and innovation may seem contradictory on the surface. Practice based on evidence seeks consistency and standardization, whereas innovation is about creating new and different processes and products. An inherent relationship exists between evidence and innovation, one that is dynamic and, at the same time, rigorous and structured. Indeed, innovation and evidence are essential to each other because innovation frees evidence to alter the trajectory of our practice and evidence disciplines innovation to affirm the veracity of practice (Porter-O'Grady & Malloch, 2017). **Figure 3-1** depicts the cybernetic interface of evidence and innovation (Porter-O'Grady & Malloch, 2017) that reflects their dynamic nature. Information is always in process, either as evidence at some level or as an innovation needed to close identified gaps in research, outdated information, expertise, and/or clinical values.

Significant work has occurred in developing a commitment to providing patient care services based on evidence from research, clinician's expertise, patient's values, and other recognized sources of knowledge (e.g., ethical knowing, sociopolitical knowing, and aesthetic ways of knowing) (Dols et al., 2017). The relationship between evidence-based practice and innovation is apparent when there is a gap between research evidence and patient values. Recommendations from valid randomized clinical trials are seldom appropriate for every patient;

Figure 3-1 The Cybernetic Interface of Evidence and Innovation.

rather, research recommendations are generalizable to patient clinical conditions. Implanted defibrillators, insulin pumps, and transdermal medications are specific to patient clinical conditions and must be examined for appropriateness prior to individual patient application. When a patient has difficulty functioning effectively with these recommended treatments, other ideas and issues need to be explored to discover innovative solutions that are more likely to achieve desired outcomes.

Valuing Multiple Intelligences

Successful innovations result from a unique combination of ideas, perceptions, beliefs, and skills. Innovation leaders create conditions for the expression and valuing of many intelligences and wide diversity as sources of new ideas. In addition to the traditional valuing of linguistic and mathematical intelligence, additional intelligences are supported and encouraged.

Intelligence theorist Gardner (1993) posited that most theories of intelligence, singular and multiple, assume that intelligence is simply a biological entity or potential and exists in the brain distinct from context. Gardner's theory of multiple intelligences is helpful for innovation leaders. The seven intelligences identified by Gardner recognize other spheres of knowledge and intelligence that could be supportive of creative thinking and the work of innovation (**Exhibit 3-4**). These intelligences each describe ways of knowing the world and how different individuals perceive the world. Each individual's perspective is rich with perceptions, ideas, and potential ideas to transform current realities. Additional intelligences from other authors contribute further to recognizing the wide and varied perceptions from individuals that leaders can access.

Provide Time for Reflection and Idea Generation

The work of the leader is to continually challenge the status quo to encourage new ideas and better ways to provide health care. Most work processes have limited effectiveness times; new technology quickly renders them ineffective and costly. The challenge is to determine which processes are the most obsolete and in need of replacement or elimination. Idea generation requires time and an open mind. Brainstorming, mind mapping, identifying what-ifs, model building, and future-state mapping are strategies to support idea generation. Directed creativity and codesign sessions are essential strategies to assist individuals in bringing forth their creative skills and knowledge. Innovation laboratories also serve to intensely focus efforts on product idea generation from concept to reality. Leadership innovation laboratories are less

---

Exhibit 3-4   Seven Intelligences

1. *Linguistic:* The capacity to use language to express ideas and understand others.
2. *Logical/mathematical:* The capacity to analyze problems logically.
3. *Spatial:* The capacity to recognize and use patterns of pictures and spaces in one's mind.
4. *Musical:* The capacity to think in music, to hear and recognize patterns.
5. *Bodily/kinesthetic:* The capacity to use all or parts of one's body to solve a problem.
6. *Intrapersonal:* Having an understanding of oneself and one's limitations.
7. *Interpersonal:* The capacity to understand other people.

Source: Gardner, H. (1993). *Frames of mind: The theory of multiple intelligences.* Copyright © 1985. Reprinted by permission of Basic Books, an imprint of Hachette Book Group, Inc.

obvious and are traditionally integrated into executive leadership programs in which leaders are continually asked to integrate new knowledge, challenge assumptions, and redesign leadership processes. Leadership of the 21st century demands new processes and outcomes. The 21st-century leader works to find the appropriate amount of time and frequency in which idea generation can occur.

> ### Group Discussion
>
> Using the seven intelligences, examine the innovation of the 3D printer and identify how each of the intelligences is realized in this innovation. Are some intelligences more prominent than others? Less prominent?
>
> For more information on 3D printing, see https://en.wikipedia.org/wiki/3D_printing.

Recognize the Value of the Anomaly

Not everyone is ready and willing to explore and consider new ideas. Resistors to innovation or process modification can be hostile and totally unwilling unless there is an overwhelmingly compelling reason to change. The greatest obstacle to innovation is people and their comfort with existing and known processes. Although is it unrealistic to expect all individuals to embrace innovation at the moment of introduction, the opportunity to recognize and value the anomaly is present. Innovation leaders necessarily work to neutralize the organizational resistance that kills off good ideas because they are different from the norm and work to transform the resistance into a meaningful phase of the innovation process. New ideas are anomalous to the norm and require individuals to behave differently. The anomaly, a deviation from the common order, is typically addressed in one of three ways: it may prompt mental stimulation (to create solutions that resolve it), mental manipulation (which could lead to ignoring it), or comparison (Trickett et al., 2009). Anomalies present both challenges that are inherent in the nature of the change process and opportunities to design and mold future systems.

Innovations, in their purest form, represent anomalies to the individuals and to organizations presented with the new idea or process. Some individuals will embrace the novelty, whereas most will respond along the innovation–adoption continuum. When faced with an innovation, five characteristic behaviors are present in individuals: innovator, early adopter, early majority, late majority, and laggards. Rogers (1995) described the innovators as venturesome, educated, needing multiple sources of information, and having greater comfort with risk taking. The early adopters are social leaders, popular, and well educated. The early majority are more contemplative and have many social contacts. The late majority are typically skeptical, more traditional, and in lower socioeconomic groups. The laggards get information about innovations from friends and neighbors and worry about costs. From an organizational perspective, innovation adoption theories are prevalent, and when compared, authors describe the constructs of leadership, innovation fit with norms and values, operational size and structure, attitudes and motivation toward innovations (Wisdom et al., 2014), organizational climate, and readiness for implementation (Allen et al., 2017) as commonalities.

> **Key Point**
> Be cautious that creative zeal does not crowd out the reality of organizational effectiveness and survival.

> **Point to Ponder**
> Innovation implementation is a crucial component for the future success of health service systems.

Crucial strategies to persuading others of the value of an innovation are providing information about the innovation, supporting a decision to put the innovation to use, and finally, accepting it. Resistance to anomalies is not uncommon. The digital world could be considered an anomaly as the move from paper to electronic documentation emerged. Virtual healthcare services, in which there is no physical contact between the patient and provider, are another. Once the anomaly gains acceptance and is believed to be the preferred way to do work, leaders begin the adoption process, using sound change management strategies to integrate the anomaly into the emerging paradigm.

Develop Capacity for Rational Risk Taking

Another consideration is proactive support for risk taking. Leaders' decision-making styles vary widely, from very decisive to more contemplative. The risk of failure is ever-present for all leaders and manifests in a variety of ways. Regardless, the risk of failure must not be paralyzing and counterproductive to organizational success. Rational risk taking is a skill to be learned and practiced within existing organizational structures.

Shifting the notion of risk taking as negative and costly to one of essential work in a complex and rapidly changing organization requires major organizational change in mission, role expectations, rewards and recognition, and measurement of outcomes. Traditional organizations view errors and negative outcomes as costly to the organization from both a quality and a financial perspective. Innovation leaders integrate the work of unsuccessful occurrences into the design work of the organization. These occurrences are viewed as opportunities for discussion and evaluation of the existing system structure and processes.

Rational risk taking is designed to enhance the organization, to support innovative processes, and to avoid obvious negative outcomes. Examples include advancing the organization and skill development. Adding new programs, expanding services, selecting equipment and technology, and setting priorities are rational and minimize risk when choices are made on the basis of core values, respect for others, the safety of individuals, strategic goals of the organization, and available resources. Another example is developing the skills of employees. Gaining new knowledge and skills is considered a rational risk when those skills are needed to improve job performance or to develop abilities for anticipated opportunities. Examples include developing computer application, public speaking, sports, creative arts, and personal protection skills.

Risk taking is considered irrational in several situations. The first situation is when there is a history of failure and oppression. If a previous attempt at innovation implementation did not work and there is little interest in repeating the process, the risk should be questioned. Although it is important to recognize that something that was not successful previously could be successful in the future under the right conditions, continuing to push an idea or product with new energy, new rationale, and new value may be irrational. The second situation is poor judgment. Walking in traffic is an example where the risk of injury to oneself and to others is present and probable. This action is irrational and similar to the leader who continues to hire employees in the midst of a financial crisis. The organization incurs additional financial obligations, and the positions of new employees will most likely be eliminated. The third irrational risk is in situations where there are unrealistic expectations or very little potential for success. Attempting to implement one more program when the staff is already overwhelmed and frustrated is not rational.

> ## Group Discussion
>
> Artificial intelligence (AI) systems that can assign a risk score for diagnosis, prognosis, or worsening of a medical condition are contributing to new ways of assessing and treating chronic conditions. For example, in heart failure, internal monitoring devices in the pulmonary artery or left atrium of the heart can quantify risk of a future hospitalization due to fluid overload. As AI tools gain increasing acceptance, their utility seems obvious and irrefutable. Reflect on the use of AI innovations in health care and identify at least five obstacles that were offered to resist them. Consider the resistance from providers of medical care, policymakers, insurance companies, potential users, and family members.

Form Uncommon Partnerships

Another consideration to advance innovation is the creation of partnerships that include individuals from diverse backgrounds and disciplines. Innovation requires teamwork and strategic partnerships that are in-person, verbal, and virtual online relationships. Networks of stakeholders are the building blocks for innovation. Strategic partnerships serve to allow organizations to create value that no single individual or organization could create alone. Innovation ecosystems bring both opportunities and risks (Silva & Ramos, 2018). New partnerships include risks specific to creating an initiative, ongoing coordination of activities, and adoption strategies to ensure the initiative is commercialized and then fully integrated into the system. Further, as fewer academic patents are commercially available, organizations have a greater need to engage with industry partners to leverage their innovative assets (Silva & Ramos, 2018).

Multiple levels of collaboration and teamwork are needed to support innovation. Internal stakeholders, those who touch the innovation in any way, and others external to the process should be considered for brainstorming and idea generation. Often, those external to the process who could provide new insights are not easily identified. Many successful innovation leaders deliberately invite colleagues with differing viewpoints and points of reference to form a more complete approach. Examples of colleagues external to the process include stakeholders responsible for the location of services, payments, ownership and oversight of the processes, profit status, patient advocacy, technology development, legal accountability, policymaking, and quality measurement.

Measuring Results: Innovation Metrics and Evaluation Strategies

New metrics are needed when innovations are introduced. In most cases, multiple interrelated metrics are required to adequately reflect the value of the innovation. Measurement of an innovation, both qualitative and quantitative, is essential and fundamental to the work of the organization. What is different about measuring innovations is that initially only historical and anticipated metrics can be selected to examine. Innovation leaders select a group of metrics knowing that they must be routinely evaluated for comprehensiveness and sensitivity and updated as needed as new and unexpected changes occur with an innovation (**Exhibit 3-5**).

Numerous organizational metrics specific to broad operations, human resources, supplies, technology, and patient outcomes are available. Often, single metrics are selected to evaluate effectiveness to simplify the measurement process. The disadvantage to single-metric evaluation is the loss of information specific to interim achievements that may ultimately affect the selected single metric. For example, selecting hours per patient day as the single metric to

---

Group Discussion

Blogs, social networking, and podcasting are recent modes of electronic communication. Your organization is looking for ideas on how to improve patient throughput in the emergency department. How could each of these modes of communication, or a combination of the modes, be used to obtain ideas and provide new strategies to improve throughput? Consider who should be involved and create a problem statement and measures for success.

- *Blog:* A weblog, usually shortened to *blog*, is an online publication with regular posts.
- *Social networking:* Internet-based programs used to make connections with others.
- *Podcasting:* A method of distributing multimedia files across the internet. A podcaster creates content for an audience that wants to listen when they want, where they want, and how they want.

Exhibit 3-5 Guidelines for Selection of Innovation Metrics

1. Select metrics to assess innovation progress and costs in advance. Incremental benchmarks are especially important to track progress and identify trends. Different sets of funding, testing, and performance criteria for incremental, experimental, and potentially disruptive innovations are needed.
2. Aim to identify early successes. Major initiatives often require significant time to realize the full benefits. Interim achievements are necessary to demonstrate progress and the likelihood of achieving the full potential of the innovation.
3. Get data to back up your gut. Successful innovators begin with the "gut feeling" and must move quickly to develop the quantifiable supporting data.

evaluate an innovative model for patient assessment would not consider the quality and completeness of the assessment data. Incomplete data could result in an extended length of stay and patient complications.

> **Key Point**
> Innovation never occurs in isolation or by a single individual—it requires a team of dedicated individuals passionately committed to making a difference.

When different metrics or different groups of metrics are selected for analysis, additional uncertainty is introduced, and the number of potential conclusions increases. The work of leaders is to identify the metrics that reflect the true value of the work.

The greatest difficulty is to identify and measure what really matters—which metrics are the critical variables that indicate value, service, and cost outcomes accurately and comprehensively. Multiple related metrics are required to explain the causality of relationships; seldom does one variable explain one outcome. By its very essence, the complex and dynamic nature of health care renders it resistant to simple linear cause-and-effect metrics. For example, no one intervention is accountable for the resolution of a patient's pneumonia; diet, fluids, medications, and activity all contribute to the resolution of chest congestion. Similarly, the metric of hours per patient day cannot be simply linked and traced to the activities of a single unit leader; the competence of staff, level of illness of patients, number of interventions required, and availability of equipment and supplies all affect the level of hours per patient day used. With each modification of work, the outcome expectations change. New mindsets, new approaches, and new resources also evolve as expectations change. Consider the evolution of two processes: creating and managing one's personal calendar and the documenting process. It is important to note that as the innovation evolves and becomes more defined, expectations evolve reflecting the intent of the innovation. Evolution of expectations is an integral part of the process of adopting innovations (**Exhibit 3-6**).

Not all innovations require new metrics. Some changes in healthcare work result in new expectations for greater involvement of individuals or higher performance targets while the specific metric remains the same. For example, changing from nurse-administered pain medication to

Exhibit 3-6 Personal Calendar: Evolving Expectations and Metrics

Innovation	Expectation (Intent)	Metric
Handwritten calendar	Summary of information	Appropriate space allocation for entries
Computerized calendar	Automated, editable, accessible by multiple individuals, able to archive and retrieve information	Real-time availability, accessible to selected individuals to facilitate scheduling, decreased time in calendar management
Interconnected internet-accessed calendar	Wireless, internet access	Accessibility from multiple devices and multiple locations

patient-controlled analgesia pumps does not change the expectation for pain control; rather, the intent of the change is to improve the level of achievement or performance of the specific metric. Patient satisfaction with pain control and comfort should be better with the patient-controlled analgesia than with nurse-administered pain interventions (**Exhibit 3-7**).

Course Corrections

Expectations for success are not realized for a variety of reasons. Wise leaders work to minimize time spent ruminating about unsuccessful events and focus on developing new solutions and course corrections to achieve desired outcomes. Change often fails if the culture is not supportive or if leaders are not qualified to lead innovation. Lack of urgency or passion by and of the innovator, poor communication, or lack of teamwork are common obstacles. According to Rogers (1995), rejection of an innovation may occur any time along the adoption process, which includes awareness of the innovation, interest, evaluation, trial, and then adoption. Discontinuance is a rejection that occurs after adoption of the innovation. Further, there are two types of discontinuance:

> **Point to Ponder**
>
> An innovation that meets criteria for novelty and value does not guarantee its successful implementation or uptake, once implemented. Innovation leaders need to be passionate about the innovations created within their healthcare system and persistent in providing guidance, including course corrections.

1. Disenchantment discontinuance, which is a decision to reject an idea as a result of dissatisfaction with its performance.
2. Replacement discontinuance, which is a decision to reject an idea to adopt a better idea.

Given the inevitability of rejection or discontinuance of a new work process, the emphasis first needs to be on making course corrections with evidence and rationales, and then on realizing the information and lessons that can be learned from the experience (**Exhibit 3-8**). Before implementing course corrections or new strategies, the team must once again be sure that the values of the work continue to be congruent with the organization, and then the team can challenge the assumptions of work processes that went awry and clarify expectations that new processes have a high degree of potential for success.

Exhibit 3-7 Barriers to Effective Innovation Measurement

1. The business model is flawed, resulting in selection of the wrong levers of value creation.
2. Subjective (qualitative) measures of effectiveness are excluded or are inadequately designed.
3. Available information technology for data mining and analysis are not used, terms are not clearly defined or measured consistently, or there is a high missing data rate for important variables.
4. Information technology replaces analysis and judgment.
5. The right question is not asked about what is being measured.
6. Expected outcomes of the actions of the innovation are not clearly articulated.
7. Budgetary concerns are overridden.
8. Staff participate in measurement but lack full awareness of the initiative.
9. A sufficient sample size is not achieved to evaluate the innovation rigorously.

Exhibit 3-8 Common Causes of Failure and Strategies to Get Great Ideas into Practice

Getting great ideas into practice is often a challenge and requires several course corrections to achieve the desired result.

Common causes of failure
1. Inadequate preparation.
2. Lack of pretesting.
3. Lack of engagement of key stakeholders.
4. Lack of support for the new idea (including failure to adequately communicate value).
5. Poor timing.
6. Rigid implementation rules.
7. Incomplete or inconsistent implementation due to innovation complexity, multiple steps, or lack of instructions or education.
8. Idea fragmentation: New idea not integrated into the system of care.
9. Lack of evaluation of implementation processes that might require tweaking to optimize performance or use.

Strategies to increase success and avoid failures
1. Prepare with those involved in the implementation and with longtime users.
2. Pretest or pilot the idea.
3. Engage and communicate the value to users.
4. Support the implementation and follow-up.
5. Practice good timing.
6. Be open to flexibility in implementation.
7. Integrate accountability into the system.
8. Learn from past efforts.
9. Harness the economic and political power to meet the innovation's needs.

Conclusion

Innovation leadership is essential when attempting to implement innovative processes that improve performance or business outcomes. An assessment of current ways of doing business, including identification of the unwritten rules about how work is accomplished and how processes enable or inhibit innovation, is an essential process that begins the transformation to a balanced value-innovation culture.

Chapter Takeaways

1. Innovation is an essential component of healthcare organizations.
2. Professional governance advances the clarity and quality of nursing's collaborative work in health care.
3. The leadership of innovation includes the following competencies: engaging others, thinking differently, and creating the business case for innovation.
4. Course corrections to new ideas are an essential part of the innovation process.
5. Rational risk taking should be encouraged to continue the growth of the organization.

CHAPTER THREE Innovation Leadership and Professional Governance: Building the Structure for Transformation

Case Study 3-1
Innovative Strategies to Prevent Hospital Readmissions

Mission Medical Center is a 700-bed hospital in an urban city in the Southwest. Mission is part of a vertically integrated healthcare system with a number of physician medical groups, ambulatory care settings and surgical centers, a psychiatric hospital, an orthopedic specialty hospital, and a children's specialty hospital. All hospitals are within a 50-mile radius of one another. At Mission Medical Center, the nursing division is organized under a chief nursing officer (CNO) who is also the designated chief operating officer (COO) for the medical center.

John has 25 years of experience in nursing leadership, and for the past 10 years he has been the CNO for Mission Medical Center. Six nursing directors report to John and provide supervision and direction to Medical-Surgical Services, Surgical Services, Maternal-Newborn Services, Rehabilitation Services, Intensive and Emergency Services, and Professional Support Services. John meets with the directors once a week for a Nursing Operations Council that focuses on the operational aspects of providing and coordinating patient care with other professional disciplines. Once a month, John meets with the directors and the clinical nurse specialists (CNSs) for the Nursing Executive Council. The purpose of the Nursing Executive Council is to promote the professionalism of nursing, advance strategies and initiatives to improve patient care outcomes, promote research and evidence-based practice, and ensure a healthy work environment that attracts and retains nurses. Mission Medical has been designated as a Magnet organization and is currently working toward redesignation, which is scheduled in approximately 2 years.

As an organization, Mission Medical is very forward-thinking and is considered to be one of the top hospitals in the state. One of the reasons that Mission has earned its reputation is because of its recruitment of top medical specialists, attractive new patient bed tower, state-of-the-art capital equipment for patient care and surgical services, and a strong financial foundation. Whereas Mission Medical has strategically sought to advance its market penetration into competitor territory, it has also been thoughtfully conservative not to overbuild beyond its financial capacity. The strategy to emphasize excellence in patient care services, excellence in the work environment, and excellence in medical staff has attracted a growing market share of insurers that wish to contract with Mission Medical and individuals in the community who have elected to purchase medical care through the Mission Medical Plan.

At one of the Nursing Executive Council meetings, a discussion ensues about changes that may need to occur as a result of penalties incurred from the Affordable Care Act and stagnation in the 30-day readmission rate over the last few years. John and the directors realize that reimbursement has been strongly tied to patient outcomes, readmissions to the hospital within 30 days, and other operational metrics. Although the nursing-sensitive indicators, Hospital Consumer Assessment of Healthcare Providers and Systems (HCAHPS) scores, and satisfaction levels of patients, physicians, and nurses are extremely high, the directors realize that they must somehow motivate nurses to identify new ways of providing patient care that will minimize redundancies and maximize workflow. They also realize that they must ensure that every patient is ready to be discharged and able to care for him- or herself at home to prevent readmissions within 30 days of discharge. The directors and clinical nurse specialists discuss a number of ideas. John encourages the open discussion and listens to each of the ideas with interest. While he quietly listens to the input from the nursing leaders, he considers the various organizational structures and processes that might need to change to support some of the ideas. He realizes that he must also encourage nurse leaders to consider how they will measure the effect of the changes that they would like to implement, but he does not want to discourage the open dialogue and freethinking during the initial stages of the discussion.

One of the major points of discussion is about lowering readmissions within 30 days of discharge. Because of the major financial impact that this issue has on the hospital's bottom line, John and the nurse leaders are keenly interested in any innovative thinking as to how to reduce occurrences. After several hours of open dialogue, John asks the CNSs and the nursing directors to divide into three teams and challenges them to work together in their teams to identify a strategy around reducing readmissions. To incentivize the groups, John states that the team with the best idea will be rewarded with a prize for their respective areas. He also tells them that their ideas must include not only the intervention but also methods of measuring the effect of the intervention on reducing readmission rates. He suggests that the directors work with the chief financial officer (CFO) to develop a return on investment (ROI) on their respective ideas. The group agrees that they will reconvene in 1 month for each group to present their ideas.

Three groups return a month later with posters to illustrate their respective plans, formal PowerPoint presentations, and supporting evidence to substantiate their innovative thinking. Group 1 recommends developing a role in each unit for a discharge resource nurse, who would not be counted in the daily staffing, but who would be responsible for reviewing each patient's status for discharge. The discharge resource nurse would coordinate a patient's needs with social services, the discharge planner, the physician, and the patient's family to ensure that all of the resources that the patient needs after discharge would be readily available upon arrival home. In addition, the discharge resource nurse would assess patients' understanding of their illness each day and their knowledge of their medications, required therapies, and appointments with their primary providers. A significant part of the discharge resource nurse's role would include patient and family education and assessment of the patient's readiness for discharge. Group 1 suggests that they would measure success by reducing the number of readmissions per quarter from the existing baseline. They estimate that the cost savings from potential losses in reimbursement without the intervention would more than pay for the expense of the new discharge resource nurse position.

Group 2 proposes a very similar intervention; however, they based their proposal on evidence that demonstrated the effectiveness of a patient-centered approach to care in improving patients' knowledge and ability to care for themselves prior to and after discharge. Group 2 proposes defining "patient-centered care" to be patient empowerment, engagement, and activation in their care. The new definition of patient-centered care would reflect nursing's involvement in educating the patient and empowering patients with knowledge to be completely engaged in decisions related to their care, and thereby activating patients' own resources to care for themselves at home. Group 2 presents the notion that every nurse believes that he or she provides patient-centered care without fully understanding the concept or realizing the nurse's role and responsibility in ensuring patients' involvement in their own care. The CNSs in Group 2 propose an educational platform for nurses to promote the new definition of patient-centered care and provide standardized educational plans for high-risk conditions that have been correlated with readmissions in the past. The CNSs propose that they would measure the effectiveness of their plan by having patients and/or their families complete a readiness for discharge assessment tool that they had reviewed in the literature and to measure the patients' knowledge and abilities to follow up with their proposed treatment plan during hospitalization and after discharge.

Group 3 recommends a collaborative, interprofessional approach using team rounding with patients each morning to ensure that patients and family are knowledgeable about the plan of care. In addition to the team rounding, Group 3 suggests changing the unit structure to include a clinical nurse leader (CNL) who would be assigned to approximately 12 patients with a team of primary care nurses. The CNL would coordinate each patient's care among the various disciplines and ensure that patients were instructed in self-care and engaged in their care. In addition, the CNL would coordinate with the discharge planner, social services, and other specific disciplines to meet with the patient each day of his or her hospitalization in preparation for discharge. Group 3 also proposes adding a responsibility to the primary nurse's role to call each of the discharge patients 1 week after discharge to ensure that they are adequately cared for and following up with medications, therapies, and provider appointments. Group 3's proposal includes the addition of several new positions. They present several studies where the role of the CNL saved money in other organizations and improved patient satisfaction, physician satisfaction, and nurse satisfaction rates as well as patient outcomes.

John invites the CFO, the CEO, and a guest consultant to hear each of the proposals and to provide feedback to each of the teams. It is a time of great excitement because of the competitive nature of the presentations, but also friendly engagement in discussions about the merits of each of the proposals. It is suggested that the best intervention would be a combination of all three proposals with the development of the CNL who would act as a patient care coordinator and a resource nurse to support direct care providers. In addition, it is suggested that the discharge nurse coordinators assume a greater role in assessing patients' readiness for discharge and that the CNS group and nurse educators assume a greater role in assessing patients' level of knowledge and ability to care for themselves and to follow up with the proposed treatment plan during hospitalization or after discharge. It is decided that a previously published instrument, the readiness for discharge assessment tool, would be used with all patients to assess their level of empowerment through education, engagement in decision making and planning, and activation of their own skills for self-care. It is also decided that the readiness for discharge assessment tool would be used again in a follow-up phone call by a discharge liaison nurse (new role) who would contact each of the discharged patients for the unit on day 2, day 5, and then weekly for a month after discharge. In addition, the group decides to develop a "Call a Nurse" hotline to facilitate decision making among discharged patients relative to their questions about their health status, follow-up instructions, or care questions.

The CFO offers to work with the directors to estimate the expense of the new positions and the return on the investment for minimizing the number of readmissions each quarter. All participants realize the risks involved in adding new full-time equivalents (FTEs), but also realize the potential loss of revenue that would result from failure to reduce readmissions within 30 days of discharge. The CEO and CFO are particularly impressed with the evidence shared from other hospitals that had implemented the CNL role and subsequently reported positive outcomes from having nurses with master's degrees coordinating the care, discharge, and after-hospitalization experience of a small group of assigned patients. This idea coupled with the other support roles seems to be the best innovation to address the problem of loss of revenue related to readmissions within 30 days of discharge.

Questions

1. What are your thoughts about John's approach to using friendly competition among the three groups to motivate them to think creatively about solving the problem?
2. Of the three possible proposals, which proposal do you think has the greatest merit in reducing readmissions?
3. Because the three groups were charged with designing an innovative solution to the problem, how do you think that the morphing of their proposals into a fourth solution affected the nurse leaders' motivation to think creatively in the future?
4. What would you add to the final solution to ensure its success in decreasing the readmission rate for Mission?
5. What barriers, if any, do you think that the nursing leaders will encounter when implementing the final proposal to reduce readmission rates?
6. What stakeholders do you think should be involved in developing implementation and measurement strategies in the adoption of this new innovation?

Case Study 3-2
Using Innovative Strategies to Correct Unit Problems

There seems to be a serious problem among the nursing staff on the acute care unit at West Memorial Hospital. The unit manager has just received the employee opinion survey results for the past year and is shocked to find that the questions related to "respect among employees" and "open communication among employees" were scored in the 45th percentile. The nursing satisfaction scores on the NDNQI survey are also extremely low in comparison to other nursing units at West Memorial Hospital and regional and national hospitals of the same size. The unit manager realizes that something needs to be done to improve the scores, but most importantly to improve the morale of the nursing staff and their satisfaction with the work environment. The unit manager shares the results with the clinical nurse specialist (CNS) and enlists his help in determining the root of the problem. The two decide to talk with some of the informal leaders among the nursing staff to ask their perceptions of why nurses would rate their satisfaction level and their respect and communication among their colleagues so low on the two surveys.

While talking with several other nurses, it becomes readily apparent that they are not willing to talk or share their feelings with the unit manager or the CNS, and in fact it seems as if some of the nurses are actually fearful of talking at all about the situation. One or two of the more courageous nurses who are interviewed share that they are fearful of reprisal from some of their colleagues. They share that several of the nursing colleagues on both the day and night shifts would refuse to talk with them or help them when they tried to approach them about improving communication among the nurses. The unit manager and the CNS are quite concerned about the situation but are uncertain how to approach correcting the problem.

Not long after the survey results are available, there are two reportable patient falls. When the nurses who were involved in the care of the patients are interviewed, they indicate that in one case the nurse did not ask for assistance from any of the other nurses to get the patient out of bed for the first time because there had been recent occasions when some nurses were openly hostile when asked to assist in patient care. In the second patient fall, the nurse involved indicates that she had asked for assistance from her colleagues, but they had openly refused to help her. Therefore, she tried to ambulate the patient on her own and was unable to prevent the patient from falling. These two incidents confirm in the minds of the unit manager and the CNS that something needs to be done quickly to correct the attitudes and behaviors of the nursing staff on the unit. Patient safety was at risk, and nursing morale was at the lowest it had ever been.

Although the unit manager tries to discuss the situation in staff meetings and asks the staff to be more collegial with one another, it seems that this message falls on deaf ears. It is quite obvious that the nursing staff are unwilling or fearful to speak to anyone about the specifics of the situation. It is also obvious that there were informal leaders among the nursing staff who may have instigated the bullying behavior toward some of the less experienced and younger nurses. The unit manager invites a human resources representative, a counselor from the employee assistance program, the CNS, and a member of the Lean/Six Sigma team to a meeting to discuss the situation and to identify possible interventions to address the problem. The group decides to call themselves the "Innovation Team" and decides to use an innovative approach to solving the problem because the traditional method for a quick resolution had failed. After discussion among the Innovation Team, it is decided that a more detailed assessment needs to be done to determine the actual issues among the staff. Because talking with the nursing staff was not effective because of the fear factor, the employee assistance program counselor suggests having a series of education and discussion sessions regarding the importance of a healthy work environment, collegiality, and open communication among the nursing staff for their own well-being and for patient safety. She volunteers to develop a content outline that could be presented to the group at their next meeting. She also offers to have more time available for individual counseling should any of the nurses elect to participate. The CNS offers to do a literature search to find a survey or instrument that could measure nursing attitudes more specifically so that a definitive action might be taken. The Six Sigma representative reviews the problem using an A3 diagram to mind map all possible scenarios that could be causing the problem and also a fishbone diagram identifying the desired outcome and all of the potential barriers that are preventing the desired outcome in the current situation. The group realizes the severity of the problem and the potential for other patient issues; therefore, they place the actions in the high-priority category for implementation.

The CNS discovers several survey tools to measure collegiality, communication, trust, and respect among nurses and prepares a formal institutional review board (IRB) proposal to measure these attitudes and behaviors before and after the educational series. The series would be presented by the employee assistance program (EAP) counselor to raise the staff awareness and knowledge about the benefits of a healthy work environment and the risks of a negative, hostile, and uncooperative work environment to their own health and to the safety of their patients. It is decided that after a few of the educational sessions, the Six Sigma representative would engage the staff in conversations using the mind-mapping technique and fishbone diagrams to openly discuss some of the issues that the staff were obviously feeling. It is felt that this step cannot be taken until more trust is developed among the staff, which is expected after the educational series is presented.

After IRB approval of the proposal, the CNS posts flyers on the unit and announces in the staff meetings that a survey would be available for the staff related to developing a healthy work environment. He also announces that a series of educational classes would be presented by the EAP counselor on developing a healthy work environment, and that he hopes that as many staff as possible would participate by completing the survey and attending the classes. It seems that the nursing staff feels safe in recording their perceptions of the communication, respect, and cooperation on the survey instruments when they were not at all expressive of their feelings in individual meetings or group settings. After the presurvey is completed, the CNS tabulates the results and shares the findings with the nursing staff in the staff meetings. It seems as if the staff are shocked at the level of discontent that is revealed in the survey results. Perhaps these findings motivate the staff to attend the educational sessions offered by the EAP counselor, which focus on crucial conversations, crucial confrontations, collaboration, respect in the workplace, and attributes of a healthy work environment. It is stated in the classes that every employee has a right to feel safe in the work environment; supported by their unit manager and colleagues; respected for their individuality, knowledge, and skills; and accepted as a valued team member. Each class also includes time for discussion; however, in the initial classes most of the participants are absolutely silent. As they receive more content, many of the staff begin to participate by sharing their personal feelings and hopes that a healthy work environment could be achieved. By the end of the educational sessions, it is apparent that the staff are engaged not only in the class content but also in a newly found commitment to improve the unit culture. Informal leaders with negative attitudes suddenly lose their power base and followers as many of the staff begin to demonstrate behaviors that they are more willing to place their affiliation with the group who wants to make a more positive work environment.

After the classes end, the EAP counselor keeps her promise and offers 1 hour of individual counseling to any employee who wishes to meet with her. Many of the staff accept that offer and meet with the counselor. The Six Sigma representative also meets with some of the more positive staff members, and they begin to identify specific causes of some of the issues and identify possible behavioral changes that could create positive changes.

Several months later the CNS readministers the postsurvey, and the findings reveal significant improvement in the staff's perception of open communication, respect among coworkers, nurse satisfaction, and perceptions of cooperation in patient care. Needless to say, the Innovation Team is excited about the findings and develops a strategy for sharing these findings with the staff. Tables and graphs of the improvements are prepared, and the findings are shared in a special staff meeting on both day and night shifts. The EAP counselor is on hand to facilitate discussion among the staff, who also seem excited about the results. Many of the staff comment that the changes on the unit are palpable and that coming to work is a much more pleasant experience. It seems that the staff are engaged in resolving the issues and committed to making the work environment more pleasant.

The unit manager and the CNS are excited about the positive changes that they could see on the unit for themselves and that are reported to them by individual nurses who comment on how appreciative they are that steps were taken to change the work environment. The unit manager and the CNS decide to write an article about how their unit's culture changed once the staff realized how the problem was affecting them personally as well as negatively affecting their patients. Increasing the staff's awareness about the potential for a healthy work environment and the behaviors that would be required of them to create such an environment made a significant difference in their overall perceptions of the relationships with their colleagues. The Innovation Team also prepares an abstract for presentation at a national nursing conference on Innovations in Nursing Practice and is selected to share their process of problem identification, problem solutions, and measuring the outcomes of the innovative interventions.

Questions

1. What are your perceptions of the methods used by the unit manager and the CNS to resolve the unhealthy work environment on the unit?
2. What might have been some of the barriers that could have been anticipated by the Innovation Team in resolving the negative work environment?
3. What are the factors that might affect the adoption or rejection of the innovation that was used to improve the work environment?
4. How did the Innovation Team engage the staff in resolution of the poor unit morale?
5. What might you do as an innovation leader to ensure that this change was sustained over time?

References

Albert, N. M. (2018). Operationalizing a nursing innovation center within a health care system. *Nursing Administration Quarterly, 42*(1), 43–53.

Allen, J. D., Towne, S. D. Jr., Maxwell, A. E., DiMartino, L., Leyva, B., Bowen, D. J., Linnan, L., & Weiner, B. J. (2017). Measures of organizational characteristics associated with adoption and/or implementation of innovations: A systematic review. *BMC Health Services Research, 17*(1), 591.

Bates, D. W., Sheikh, A., & Asch, D. A. (2017). Innovative environments in health care: Where and how new approaches to care are succeeding. *Health Affairs (Project Hope), 36*(3), 400–407.

Casale, T. B. (2017). Biologics and biomarkers for asthma, urticarial, and nasal polyposis. *Journal of Allergy and Clinical Immunology, 139*(5), 1411–1421.

Christensen, C. M., Raynor, M. E., & McDonald, R. (2015, December). What is disruptive innovation? *Harvard Business Review.* https://hbr.org/2015/12/what-is-disruptive-innovation

Clavelle, J. T., O'Grady, T. P., Weston, M. J., & Verran, J. V. (2016). Evolution of structural empowerment: Moving from shared to professional governance. *Journal of Nursing Administration, 46*(6), 308–312.

Dols, J. D., Muñoz, L. R., Martinez, S. S., Mathers, N., Miller, P. S., Pomerleau, T. A., Timmons, A., & White, S. (2017). Developing policies and protocols in the age of evidence-based practice. *Journal of Continuing Education in Nursing, 48*(2), 87–92.

Endsley, S. D. (2010). *Innovation in action. A practical guide for healthcare teams.* Wiley-Blackwell.

Fuller, R., & Hansen, A. (2019). Disruption ahead. Navigating and leading the future of nursing. *Nursing Administration Quarterly, 43*(3), 212–221.

Gardner, H. (1993). *Frames of mind: The theory of multiple intelligences.* Basic Books.

Househ, M., Alshammari, R., Almutairi, M., Jamal, A., & Alshoaib, S. (2015). Building a culture of health informatics innovation and entrepreneurship: A new frontier. *Studies in Health Technologies and Informatics, 213*, 237–240.

Koch-Nolte, F., Eichhoff, A., Pinto-Espinoza, C., Schwarz, N., Schäfer, T., Menzel, S., Haag, F., Demeules, M., Gondé, H., & Adriouch, S. (2019). Novel biologics targeting the P2X7 ion channel. *Current Opinion in Pharmacology, 47*, 110–118.

Malloch, K. (2010). Innovation leadership: New perspectives for new work. *Nursing Clinics of North America, 45*(1), 1–9.

Miller, P., & Wedell-Wedellsborg, T. (2013). The case for stealth innovation. *Harvard Business Review, 91*(3), 91–97.

Ness, R. (2012). *Innovation generation. How to produce creative and useful scientific ideas.* Oxford University Press.

O'Reilly, C., & Tushman, M. L. (2016). *Lead and disrupt: How to solve the innovator's dilemma.* Stanford University Press.

Porter-O'Grady, T., & Malloch, K. (2017). Evidence-based practice and the innovation paradigm: A model for the continuum of practice excellence. In S. Davidson, D. Weberg, T. Porter-O'Grady, & K. Malloch (Eds.), *Leadership for evidence-based innovation in nursing and health professions* (pp. 3–41). Jones & Bartlett Learning.

Rangachari, P. (2018). Innovation implementation in the context of hospital QI: Lessons learned and strategies for success. *Innovation and Entrepreneurship in Health, 5,* 1–14.

Rogers, E. M. (1995). *Diffusion of innovations* (4th ed.). The Free Press.

Samet, K. A., & Smith, M. S. (2016). Thinking differently: Catalyzing innovation in healthcare and beyond. *Frontiers in Health Services Management, 33*(2), 3–15.

Silva, P. J., & Ramos, K. S. (2018). Academic medical centers as innovation ecosystems: Evolution of industry partnership models beyond the Bayh-Dole Act. *Academic Medicine: Journal of the Association of American Medical Colleges, 93*(8), 1135–1141.

Smith, K. W., Bir, A., Freeman, N. L., Koethe, B. C., Cohen, J., & Day, T. J. (2017). Impact of health care delivery system innovations on total cost of care. *Health Affairs (Project Hope), 36*(3), 509–515.

Snow, F. (2019). Creativity and innovation. An essential competency for the nurse leader. *Nursing Administration Quarterly, 43*(4), 306–312.

Stuke, K. B. (2013). Understanding leadership through leadership understandings. *Journal of Leadership Studies, 7*(2), 55–61.

Trickett, S. B., Trafton, J. G., & Schunn, C. D. (2009). How do scientists respond to anomalies? Different strategies used in basic and applied science. *Topics in Cognitive Science, 1*(4), 711–729.

Weatherford, B., Bower, K. A., & Vitello-Cicciu, J. (2018). The CNO and leading innovation. *Nursing Administration Quarterly, 41*(1), 76–82.

Weberg, D. (2017). Innovation leadership behaviors: Starting the complexity journey. In S. Davidson, D. Weberg, T. Porter-O'Grady, & K. Malloch (Eds.), *Leadership for evidence-based innovation in nursing and health professions* (pp. 43–76). Jones & Bartlett Learning.

Weintraub, P., & McKee, M. (2019). Leadership for innovation in healthcare: An exploration. *International Journal of Health Policy and Management, 8*(3), 138–144.

Wheatley, M. J. S. (1992). *Leadership and the new science: Learning about organization from an orderly universe.* Berrett-Koehler.

Wisdom, J. P., Chor, K. H., Hoagwood, K. E., & Horwitz, S. M. (2014). Innovation adoption: A review of theories and constructs. *Administration and Policy in Mental Health, 41*(4), 480–502.

Suggested Readings

Davidson, S., Weberg, D., Porter-O'Grady, T., & Malloch. K. (2017). *Leadership for evidence-based innovation in nursing and health professions.* Jones & Bartlett Learning.

Dy Bupin, J. J. (2016). Differences in innovative behavior among hospital-based registered nurses. *Journal of Nursing Administration, 46*(3), 122–127.

Joseph, M. L. (2015). Organizational culture and climate for promoting innovativeness. *Journal of Nursing Administration, 45*(3), 172–178.

Middlebrooks, T. (2013). Introduction: New perspectives of leadership. *Journal of Leadership Studies, 7*(2), 32–34.

White, K. R., Pillay, R., & Huang, X. (2016). Nurse leaders and the innovation competence gap. *Nursing Outlook, 64,* 255–261.

CHAPTER THREE   Innovation Leadership and Professional Governance: Building the Structure for Transformation

Quiz Questions
Select the best answer for each of the following questions.

1. Which of the following best describes innovation?
   a. Out-of-the-box thinking
   b. Something new or different
   c. A process that requires brainstorming, modeling, and testing
   d. A product that succeeds soon after introduction to the marketplace

2. Which of the following characteristics demonstrates the optimal organizational structure for innovation?
   a. It includes the traditional work of operations.
   b. It includes both departments of innovation and operational departments.
   c. It requires verbal support from the chief executive officer.
   d. It considers the innovation work to be done and the skills of leaders.

3. What is the primary purpose of a department of innovation?
   a. To support creativity as an integral part of the organization's mission
   b. To promote creativity among scientists and leaders dedicated to innovation
   c. To silo innovation resources and be the warehouse of all innovation
   d. To promote idea generation; regardless if ideas are cultivated

4. Which of the following best describes disruptive innovation?
   a. It is work that does not support required healthcare services.
   b. It is work that requires new thinking by all stakeholders.
   c. It is an innovation that cannot be used by customers in mainstream markets.
   d. It is work that has been terminated because of poor outcomes or dissatisfaction.

5. When is rational risk taking appropriate?
   a. When new skills are being developed
   b. When there is adequate insurance coverage
   c. When no obvious changes are anticipated
   d. When team members support the risk

6. Which of the following best describes opportunities for innovation?
   a. They are limited to organizations focused on technology.
   b. They can be found in all walks of life.
   c. They are present in healthcare delivery systems.
   d. The best healthcare arena is in the technology field.

7. Which of the following best describes entrepreneurship?
   a. It is the creation of a personal business using company funds.
   b. It is the organization and management of an enterprise with both initiative and risk.
   c. It is an innovation laboratory developed by an innovation leader.
   d. It is when employees exercise independence in an initiative.

8. Metrics for measuring innovation should include which of the following?
   a. Cost of technology and personnel needed to maintain operations
   b. Those that determine a global impact on the organization
   c. Important components of the condition being assessed
   d. Variables that reflect the intended value of the innovation

9. Which of the following describes course correction for organizations committed to integrated innovation?
   a. Used to achieve desired outcomes
   b. Used when implementation plans failed
   c. Used to cover up negative outcomes
   d. Used to garner new ideas

10. Resistance to innovation is generally *not* due to which of the following?
    a. Personal discomfort with new ideas
    b. Lack of understanding of the goals of the innovation
    c. Excellent performance in one's current role
    d. General belief that "I am not an innovative person"

11. Professional governance:
    a. is built on shared governance.
    b. has the potential to advance the quality and prestige of nursing.
    c. emphasizes accountability to the profession of nursing.
    d. replaces shared governance.

12. Creating a unique definition of innovation for your organization can result in:
    a. greater engagement and understanding of innovation.
    b. distortion of the published definitions of innovation.
    c. increased collaboration among employees.
    d. time wasted in light of the available definitions.

13. The impact of minimizing change and innovation in an organization can result in:
    a. increased stability and safer patient care.
    b. more cost-effective patient care.
    c. increased employee satisfaction, as changes in routines are minimal.
    d. stagnation and missed opportunities to improve care.

14. System complexity that accompanies innovation in health care can result in which of the following?
    a. High levels of turnover in support staff
    b. Multiple new technology products
    c. Uncertainty of healthcare funding
    d. Interactions between employers, patients, and the environment

15. Most organizations experience multiple ongoing tensions. These tensions between stability and innovation:
    a. should be minimized quickly to achieve organizational stability.
    b. should be valued as necessary for creativity and growth.
    c. should be valued in order to learn more about employee interests.
    d. should be expected in complex organizations.

CHAPTER THREE   Innovation Leadership and Professional Governance: Building the Structure for Transformation

16. Open, user-driven innovation:
    a. minimizes the role of evidence-based practice in complex environments.
    b. recognizes the importance of the gap-analysis process when developing solutions.
    c. uses a comprehensive framework to integrate evidence and innovation.
    d. provides a comprehensive view of knowledge development.

17. An anomaly in a healthcare organization is often considered:
    a. an opportunity to consider a new way of doing things.
    b. an abnormality that needs to be corrected or eliminated.
    c. an error in employee performance.
    d. an opportunity for innovation.

18. Which of the following is *not* correct regarding risk taking in healthcare organizations?
    a. Risk taking is commonplace and is seen as a workaround.
    b. Risk taking is usually avoided due to believed risks to patient safety.
    c. Risk taking is avoided to focus on operations and organizational stability.
    d. Risk taking is considered appropriate when risks advance skill development.

19. Selecting metrics for an innovation in staff scheduling would ideally include:
    a. the cost of the system and staff satisfaction.
    b. differences between the current and new systems.
    c. wireless access and ability to accommodate staff requests.
    d. the unique characteristics of the new system.

20. Clinicians in the organization believe that the admission process is adequate and are not open to innovation. Which criteria or evidence could you present to engage clinicians to consider an innovative virtual model?
    a. All clinical processes can be improved upon.
    b. Data from the current system is not integrated into a unified document.
    c. Resistance to changing individualized forms can be overcome with incentives.
    d. Inconsistencies in documentation have rendered the data unreliable.

21. Sources for innovation are everywhere. Which of the following is the best source of innovation in health care?
    a. Persistent problems or errors that negatively impact care quality
    b. Employee performance review recommendations for improvement
    c. Recommendations from healthcare technology experts
    d. Patient satisfaction ratings below the desired target

22. A community organization has requested your healthcare organization to participate in an innovative approach to cardiac care. Which of the following is the most appropriate response?
    a. It is not within our mission to provide cardiac care services.
    b. A partnership should be explored because the community identified this need.
    c. Invite community representatives to join the organization's innovation team.
    d. Take no action.

23. An organization can be considered ambidextrous:
    a. when competing priorities are identified and addressed separately.
    b. when innovation is recognized as important to the organization and located in a special department.
    c. if operations and patient safety are at the top of the priority list.
    d. if the natural tensions between operations and innovation are optimized to create value and support creativity.

24. Knowledge creation and research in an organization are:
    a. foundational to the interface of evidence and innovation.
    b. distinct from innovation gaps specific to clinical values.
    c. strongly influenced by economic factors that impact policy.
    d. primarily concerned with evidence-based practices.

25. Support for innovation in healthcare organizations requires all of the following, *except*:
    a. individuals from diverse backgrounds.
    b. internal and external stakeholders to do the work of innovation.
    c. experts in the creation of innovative products.
    d. effective teamwork competencies.

CHAPTER FOUR

Innovation and Opportunity: Leading Through the White Water of Change

> The great use of life is to spend it on something that will outlast it.
> —*William James*

Chapter Objectives

At the completion of this chapter, the reader will be able to:

- Identify three key contextual characteristics necessary to create an organizational frame for innovation.
- Name the central obligation of the critical roles of leadership in creating a context for innovation.
- Outline the various role obligations of leadership in building a structure of innovation across the network.
- List the components and elements of the innovative infrastructure of the organization that supports the activities of innovation at every place in the organization.

With all the sociopolitical, technological, and economic shifts affecting our society, leaders are likely to find themselves in the midst of major social transformation. The postdigital and postreform age increases the demands on organizations and systems to engage and embrace essential structural and technological shifts that alter the foundation of their work. Leaders must create strategic and structural imperatives that incorporate new and emerging technologies and innovations in the evolving "way of doing business" (Wiljer & Hakim, 2019). The almost daily impact of emerging and new technological applications makes it nearly impossible to conceptualize or even afford all of them. Today, technological applications are continuously altering how healthcare services are being delivered, and for technologies that have been adopted by many organizations, such as electronic health records and telemedicine, late adopters need to move quickly (Rumball-Smith et al., 2020). Technological innovations have become their own "disruptive technologies" insofar as each succeeding generation of clinical technology makes the preceding generation obsolete (**Exhibit 4-1**). In addition to making technological innovations available to

---

Exhibit 4-1 Disruptive Technologies

Disruptive Technology Features and Themes

- Innovations
- Unanticipated
- Threaten existing products/realities
- Represent unexpected competition
- Fill previously unfilled roles
- Revolutionary and often destructive

Communication and Treatment Systems: Technology Themes

- Point-of-care diagnostic applications (e.g., ultrasound plug-ins for smartphones)
- Wireless body area network (WBAN) for sensor devices
- Artificial intelligence healthcare practices that include expert systems, robotic process automation (e.g., used in social robots in dementia and autism disorder), natural language processing, machine learning– and deep learning–assisted decision making
- Mobile health (mHealth) applications with patient-reported outcomes
- Speech recognition in the electronic health record
- Genome-wide sequencing and other genomic technologies for screening, testing, and treating disorders
- Personalized digital health technologies

---

providers and patients, healthcare leaders need to understand that when technologies are complex, challenges and lessons learned need to be expected (Businger et al., 2020) so that they are prepared for their commitment to the future. This is the state and these are the conditions that healthcare leaders and providers must function in every day.

Driving the Culture of Innovation

Elements and requisites of innovation require a cultural context that is unique from all those that have previously existed. The compartmentalized, hierarchical, rigidly ordered, unilaterally medically controlled hospital and healthcare service model is no longer relevant as a frame for sustainability in contemporary healthcare service structures (Malloch & Porter-O'Grady, 2017). The complexity and breadth of knowledge that are now inculcated within a wide variety of clinical practices in health care call for reconceptualization of the infrastructure and framework that have historically defined and directed the actions and relationships between and among the various key players in health service delivery. In addition, the demands of health reform require a total reconceptualization of health care, the way it is offered, and the way it is funded. The configuration and trajectory of health services have been forever changed by the introduction of value-driven financial and service models for health care and the requisite that citizens' health (patient-centered care and personalized medicine) be the ultimate attainment.

The historical culture of medical subsidiarity and subordination that has driven health care for the past 100 years clearly delineated the primacy of the physician's role and both legally and functionally limited the role of other provider disciplines. Although physician supremacy did much to strengthen the scientific and academic bases of clinical practice and create a positive trajectory for clinical science, invention, and applied technology, it has also had negative side effects. Three major negatives persist: (1) a lack of interdisciplinary collaboration, linkage, and interaction; (2) unilateral educational pathways for each discipline that duplicate

Exhibit 4-2 Focus of Work

Historic and Current	**Future**
• Emphasis on function	• Emphasis on outcomes
• Driven by policy and procedure (slow process)	• Evidence driven (quick process post publication of high-quality new knowledge)
• Characterized by control	• Characterized by autonomy
• "Employee" oriented and managed	• Make own decisions; manager supports
• Active, not reflective	• Reflects on value of practice
• Treatment/intervention centered	• Patient-centered, personalized care
• Hospital focused	• Focused on continuum of care

content and resources; and (3) social, cultural, and professional barriers and boundaries between disciplines that result in both identity and relational conflicts. Each negative is a precise social and cultural constraint that impedes the creation of a dynamic and responsive organization available and ready for innovation (Minvielle et al., 2014; Porter-O'Grady & Malloch, 2016).

The historical culture of functionalism and process-fixed notions of work has also created an existing frame that makes it virtually impossible to embed a dynamic of innovation that is represented by high levels of integration, interaction, and relationship. Collateral and interactional collaboration among disciplines based on equity and value is now a fundamental centerpiece essential to the success of health reform. Indeed, the historical focus on functionalism and work processes actually removes the more professionally driven urge toward sustainable impact, outcome, and evidence of making a difference so important in reform (**Exhibit 4-2**; Porter-O'Grady, 2019b). These latter characteristics are more commonly associated with the social mandate of professionals rather than the functional processes of an "employee workgroup" orientation. The historically delineated "external" (independent) role of the physician and the predominantly "internal" (employed) orientation of other developing disciplines created a significant wall between them.

Because medical professionals have maintained their independence and unilateral locus of control, they have been able to develop based on the separate and unique needs of members (Saxěn, 2018). The nursing profession and other emerging disciplines, in contrast, have not had the same opportunity by virtue of their more dependent positions as both subordinates and employees (Garcia-Sierra et al., 2016). Although the nursing profession has led the way in creating a unique body of knowledge and an academic frame for knowledge creation and utility, it has not moved forward with the same degree of dispatch toward professional independence by virtue of its two historically subordinating factors: it is predominately composed of women, and it has been historically employee based (Setoodegan et al., 2019). Both of these circumstances have been well documented, and the conditions parallel the historic journey to equity of women and of the profession of nursing (Keynejad et al., 2018; Rounds et al., 2013).

> **Points to Ponder**
>
> To drive a culture of innovation, leaders must be able to diversify and adapt when making decisions aimed at filling gaps. "The way it was" will not guide you toward the future. Diversification and using innovative products, services, methods, or systems may be the best strategic fit for the organization.

Equity and Partnership

Creating a culture amenable to innovation is necessarily based on the relative understanding and application of equity within an organizational framework. Equity is a statement of value and suggests to all the specificity and clarity of value that each role plays in contributing to the life and integrity of an organization. Equity assumes equality, but it bases that assumption on notions of value. Equity suggests that in any membership community the members are there because of their unique capacity to contribute to the effort of the community as a whole (**Exhibit 4-3**). Indeed, the whole community is defined by the aggregate contribution of each of its members. In the case of professionals, it is not the obligation of the community to demonstrate unilateral value for members, rather it is the obligation of individuals to demonstrate their specific and unique contribution to the aggregate contribution of the whole. This classic interdependence between members of the community sums the value of this contribution in a way that demonstrates the significance of the community. In short, the professional community represents the sum of the value of the contributions of each member. It is vital for professional communities to recognize the centrality of value to the life of the profession (Wong et al., 2015).

Further, it is important for each profession to recognize its unique and significant contribution to the life of the system in concert with other disciplines and workgroups. Sustainability depends on the notion of value between disciplines as much as within them. Equity suggests that each discipline represents its essential interdependence with the other disciplines necessary to the achievement of impact and outcome (Liu et al., 2016; Porter-O'Grady, 2019a). In contemporary health care, no single discipline can operate effectively and achieve sustainable value independent of its relationship with other disciplines, which it depends on for its own contribution or success (Franklin et al., 2015; Sangaleti et al., 2017). This intensity of interface and degree of interdependence are the earmarks of contemporary healthcare service. However, to make these essential principles live in current healthcare service systems and networks, organizational infrastructure and leadership capacity must be constructed to reflect these more relevant tenets.

Equity, therefore, suggests that the following considerations be reflected in the organizational constructs necessary to establishing a creative and innovative organizational infrastructure:

1. Each discipline makes an intentionally equal and unique contribution to the work of other disciplines and to the evidence and impact of patient care.
2. Accountability is the centerpiece of the role and obligation of each discipline and demands clarity of understanding regarding ownership and expression of it.

Exhibit 4-3 Equity

- Value based
- Reflects accountability
- Characterized by equality
- Horizontal relationships
- Inclusive, suggesting ownership

Exhibit 4-4 The Professional Mandate

For the professions, the direction of obligation is from the professional to the professional community. The profession is not obligated to the member. It is the members who owe obligation to the profession, enabling and sustaining it in its value and work. The profession is defined by the collective action of each member, committed in his or her own life to represent its values and social mandate in every thought, action, and impact.

---

3. Partnership, not subordination, represents the essential character of horizontal connection necessary to determining and obtaining value and for the synthesis of effort necessary to sustain it.
4. The fact that nursing as a discipline is located at the center (nodal point) of the clinical network is a statement of location, not of control. However, the centrality of the nursing role in coordinating, integrating, and facilitating both the structure and the continuum of care within the organized healthcare system must be acknowledged.
5. Each discipline must know the contribution it makes in relation to other disciplines and its contribution to equity. It is the aggregation and mutuality of the unique contribution of each discipline that create the aggregate of effort that is ultimately more viable and sustainable.
6. Contemporary health systems are networks, not hierarchies. They are successful to the extent that relational clarity is established between them. Positional control (lines and boxes on organizational charts) no longer adequately describe the nature of the relationship or the interaction among elements of the network and players in the system.
7. Evidentiary dynamics drive clinical actions and relationships and demand the synthesis and integration of interdisciplinary effort to legitimately define and sustain clinical value and viability.

Creating an equitable clinical infrastructure demands an understanding of how networked professional organizations operate and function effectively (**Exhibit 4-4**). When using shared decision-making principles and practices within a professional governance model, organizations must reject approaches based on positional control and, instead, build on a decisional locus of control (Clavelle et al., 2016; Porter-O'Grady, 2019a). For the foundations enumerated here to become a normative part of organizational dynamics, the healthcare system must confront, resolve, and better identify a structural frame based on decisions rather than positions (Porter-O'Grady, 2019a).

Decisions and Structures

One of the first steps necessary to building a context that truly stimulates and sustains innovation is the reconfiguration of infrastructure based on decisional accountability rather than positional authority (**Exhibit 4-5**). The traditional hierarchical organizational structure created positional management structures that authorized the manager to control and administer components of the organizational structure. Although that traditional business construct brought order and form to the delivery of healthcare services, it did so at

Exhibit 4-5 From Position to Decision

Positional Control	**Decisional Control**
• Hierarchal	• Relational
• Reductionistic	• Multilateral
• Vertical	• User driven
• Locational	• Value centric
• Directive	• Direct impact

Staff engagement levels in succeeding initiative efforts

Figure 4-1 Trajectory of Diminishing Successive Initiative Efforts.

the expense of staff decisional ownership, investment, and appropriate locus of control. It invested in the manager accountabilities that rightfully belong to the disciplines; when the disciplines surrendered them, the ownership necessary to achieve and sustain value disappeared. Indeed, it created an illegitimate locus of control for authority and autonomy that should rest with the professions who own it. Once divorced from this accountability, the professions lost legitimacy (some suggest they may have never obtained it), and the managers to whom these accountabilities had been assigned could never achieve legitimacy because their role could not obtain or sustain the outcomes attendant to legitimate ownership. Such outcomes could only be achieved and sustained by the disciplines that owned these accountabilities (Crow & DeBourgh, 2017).

This management-driven illegitimate locus of control is evident in the endless cycles of new initiatives that become necessary to engage workers. Because of the intense effort of managers to obtain ownership from staff in the interests of the organization, managers must create a culture of "buy-in" both to get and keep workers interested in the goals and initiatives of the organization as defined, directed, and controlled by the management structure. The problem with these initiative-driven activities is that they become increasingly more difficult as more effort is directed to them. Staff demonstrate decreasing interest in investing in an endless array of new initiatives and become less excited and interested as more of these initiatives are created for them (**Figure 4-1**). The result is that buy-in is never achieved. Buy-in is not ownership. Investment is not simply engaging staff in issues with which they do not personally identify. *Engagement* means empowering people by incorporating their perspectives and personal values in decisions and actions that affect their lives over which they have clear ownership (Crow & DeBourgh, 2017).

Personal value means more than just pay and benefits. Pay and benefits certainly are addressed through the foundations and basics of work activity. Beyond that, there is no evidence to suggest that interest, ownership, or investment can be obtained or sustained through those same means (Mazhindu et al., 2016; Yarbrough et al., 2017). A stronger connection between personal values and goals and those of the organization must be made in a manner that evidences and represents a convergence of meaning and value between the organization and those who compose it. This is especially true for professionals. Because professionals see their work as a social mandate rather than as an employee-driven activity, the kind of engagement necessary to sustain them cannot be obtained simply by order, initiative, and hygienic incentives (Yarbrough et al., 2017). As indicated earlier, if professionals are seen and treated simply as an employee workgroup, their commitment to the values of the profession as well as their interest in the external goals of the organization will diminish (Davidson et al., 2017). Loss of professional identity has a great impact in ways other than that they are simply becoming another employee workgroup. Loss of professional attachment and value is accompanied by a loss of meaning, commitment, and purpose—a loss that ultimately affects their relationship to the workplace, to each other, and to the work of the profession (Read, 2014).

This focus on alignment of decisional structures with appropriate locus of control for the decisions is a critical element in the configuration of structure in a way that supports creativity, innovation, and professional commitment (Porter-O'Grady, 2019a). Locating decisions in the places where they are most effectively exercised and then configuring them in a way that represents the expectations and activities unfolding at that place in the organization are critical pieces in the alignment of structure and process with work systems. Some of the greatest impediments to creativity and innovation are the organizational and structural barriers that limit this sense of ownership and that have control over decisions that directly affect what people do (Zuber & Moody, 2018).

In relating to professionals, the notion of locus of control is a critical factor for leaders. *Locus of control* simply means that decision and action are located at the most legitimate place, where information can most effectively be deliberated, decided, and acted on in a way that specifically advances purpose and, ultimately, success. One of the greatest problems in complex organizations is related to decisions being made by people and in places where they cannot most effectively be acted on in an efficient and effective way. Perhaps one of the greatest errors in organizational leadership is exemplified by decisions made by leaders who are not positioned appropriately to make such decisions or who do not demonstrate the relevant content competence necessary to make such decisions effectively and to translate them into viable and sustainable implementation processes for those who must both implement them and live with the consequences. Innovation demands the kind of infrastructure support that allows ownership, freedom, and investment on the part of innovators (Crow & DeBourgh, 2017; Zuber & Moody, 2018). Innovators must be allowed to control their circumstances, undertake creative processing, and maintain dynamic interaction in ways that can yield genuine benefits unconstrained by illegitimate control that is exercised from outside the immediate "circle of innovation" (Malik et al., 2016; Pines et al., 2014).

> ## Group Discussion
>
> Differentiating professions from employee workgroups is an important consideration for leaders as they work to more clearly establish the relationship between the organization and the professional. Professionals are driven by accountability, which incorporates the elements of autonomy, authority, and competence. As you refine your understanding of the role of the professional, consider and discuss the following key questions:
>
> - What do professionals need that is different from the needs of employee workgroups?
> - Name at least two leadership behaviors that are essential to lead professionals versus employee workgroups.
> - Identify at least two structural changes in the organization necessary to adapt to the needs of professionals as differentiated from employee workgroups.
> - Is it possible to be both employed and professional in the contemporary healthcare workplace? What might have to change to make the organization more supportive of the life and action of a professional?

Figure 4-2 Circle of Innovation.

The circle of innovation is simply a context in which the innovative dynamic unfolds in a way that eliminates the traditional structural impediments, operational practices, traditional processes, and operating role expectations that preclude the necessary flow of interactions that feed the innovation process (**Figure 4-2**). Line controls and positional decisional authority and expression do little to facilitate the out-of-the-box constituents necessary to innovation and do much to shut down those very processes. Certainly, leaders must be aware of the necessary constraints and parameters that influence the dynamic of creativity and innovation. However, these realities are incorporated into the innovation process itself and are not successfully managed in an innovative organization outside the circle of innovation. When exercised outside the circle of innovation, the only outcome is to shut down the innovative process, turn off the innovators, and reestablish rote, ritual, and routine (Malloch & Porter-O'Grady, 2017).

Innovation is by definition unsafe. Not unsafe in the traditional sense, but in the sense of being willing to undertake risk, to open doors not previously opened, to threaten processes hanging on the edge of irrelevance, and to create possibilities not previously perceived as a part of the emergent reality of the organization. To address these characteristics, the historical and traditional structural frames need to be seen as a part of the control mechanisms of the traditional system. A more effective perspective representing the networked mosaic of intersections and interactions that sustain a dynamic and responsive human system (organization) needs to emerge (Weatherford et al., 2018).

At the same time, innovation builds on a solid foundation of evidence. The relationship between evidence and innovation demonstrates a cybernetic or continuous feedback communication control framework that reflects both the interactive and continuous relationship and the dynamic influence evidence and innovation have on each other. All innovators understand the need to lay firm foundations in principle, protocol, and appropriate sustainable standards, which compose the evidentiary floor for all innovation. Subsequent good practice is simply a reflection of what is known and demonstrates and explicates the foundations laid for those practices. It is out of that bedrock the seeds of innovation emerge.

The Centrality of the Point-of-Service

Networked organizations and system constructs are more relational entities and less organizational hierarchies. Hierarchies are always present, and their value should not be diminished: They represent breadth of relationship rather than intensity of control. In all living systems, homeostatic mechanisms represent and demonstrate the essential linkage between smaller elements and larger systems elements to which the interaction and convergence of the smaller elements contribute (Bucknall & Hitch, 2018). This hierarchy is a representation of relatedness, interdependence, and synthesis rather than compartmentalization and control, as has been evident in traditional organizational structure. The control in networks is exemplified by the enumeration of their points of intersection and the nature of their interdependence (**Figure 4-3**). These factors contribute to each element's definition of its value and significance as well as its specific role in contributing to the accelerating value of the whole as visualized in the integrity and operation of the network. The saying "a brokenness in any part of a network is a brokenness in the entire network" is the best definition of this principle of synthesis. All networks and organizations represent the sum of the integration and synthesis of the efforts of each of their parts and their convergence, where individual contribution joins with the whole to create truly symphonic action (McCovery & Matusitz, 2014; Schultz et al., 2013).

This notion of the centrality of value from the point-of-service or point-of-productivity is critical to understanding the distribution of decision making in a way that best exemplifies both the kinds of decisions that need to be made and the nature of the resulting actions that need to be taken. Seen from the perspective of the whole (the network), each point of action recognizes its unique function and contribution within the mental model of the whole (**Figure 4-4**). In this way, no compartments, departments, services, or local actions can ever be undertaken without a clear sense of the effect such action will have on the integrity of the

CHAPTER FOUR   Innovation and Opportunity: Leading Through the White Water of Change

Figure 4-3 Networked Organizations: Multiple Points of Intersection and Interdependence.

network. This perspective sees decisions distributed in a way that represents the appropriate loci of control so that people at key "nodes" or locations in the system know what decisions belong to them and the effect those decisions have on the network. "Value" is simply the product of the linked and synchronous efforts of all stakeholders who contribute to it at a level of understanding and intent that indicates conscious partnership, concerted action, and a common contribution to sustainable outcome. Part of the real work of leadership, therefore, is to clearly and appropriately delineate a "grid of accountability" that carefully enumerates the location of specified decisions in a way that creates a mind map of the decisional loci of the network (Fleiszer et al., 2016). In this way, leadership creates a view of the mosaic of decision points across the network that represents the relational, interactional, and synthesis dynamics of the system; best shows the integrity of the system; and demonstrates the concert of actions converging to meet goals, advance purpose, and strive to succeed in the larger environment.

Wise executive leaders understand that human systems operate in this manner, and they recognize the importance of creating the structural configurations within the context of the dynamic vision of a network. The executive, rather than looking for control or to manage organizational ego (line hierarchy), seeks integrity, convergence, and synthesis of the entities of the network around mission, vision, purpose, and strategy—all the components necessary for the system (network) to thrive in the larger, ever-changing environment. In such an organizational view, those in the executive suite effectively see themselves as purveyors of the goodness-of-fit between the ever-moving demands of the external environment and the operating and internal dynamics of the organization. The innovative element embedded in this scenario is demonstrated in the organization's ability to create new responses, processes, and products when innovators challenge the realities of the external environment and create conditions and configurations that can push the edges of new thinking and generate opportunities to redefine action and outcome by what they create from within (McKimm, 2015).

The effective and wise leader of innovation recognizes that the life of the system operates predominantly from its point-of-service. At the heart of the system is where the intensity of the life

Alignment, Not Motivation

Nodes **Nodes**

Links

Figure 4-4 Network of Intersecting Nodes and Links.

of the organization is best visualized. It is here that the executive recognizes that all prevailing structure and support converge either to advance or impede life lived at the point-of-service and system effectiveness. This leader recognizes that purpose and organizational life are not sustained at the top or at the periphery of an organization. Certainly, the goodness-of-fit between the internal life and dynamics of the organization and its appropriate and sustainable interface with the external environment is managed, facilitated, and refined in the executive suite. However, if the system is to live and be sustained, the determining factor is demonstrated by how well strategy is transformed into action at the point-of-service and lived out by those who work there and how this action drives the tactics and actions that lead to organizational success (**Figure 4-5**).

Alignment, Not Motivation

Leaders of innovation see the critical value of good alignment between the various loci of control and decisions in the organization. Leaders seek to ensure that the greatest degree of empowerment is enabled close to the various points of service so that as much freedom, ownership, and investment in the life and work of the system can unfold in those places. Leaders of innovation see the organization as a membership community and have a high level of understanding of the rights of membership and the obligations of ownership. In this frame, leaders of innovation are constantly building partnerships, interfaces, relationships, and points of convergence in the network that, when aggregated, move the system effectively in a direction that ensures its long-term viability (Willis et al., 2016).

> **Key Point**
>
> Alignment is the key element in the leader's role in motivation. Aligning staff motivation with organizational goals is the only sustainable way of ensuring staff investment and ownership. It is more work, but motivation lasts longer.

Core of the network: The point-of-service where all structure and effort converge to fulfill the purposes of the system.

Figure 4-5 Network Convergence at the Point-of-Service.

Alignment is a critical element of creating context for innovation; when refining and restructuring, it is important to "make it fit" (Batras et al., 2014). The alignment of motives is a much more powerful and viable strategy for engagement than is the constant leadership emphasis on motivation. Much has been written about motivation, very little of it factual. Often, when one reads and researches motivation, a heavy emotional overlay begins to appear. Usually, the suggestion is that if leaders can only help staff feel more excited, energized, and spirited, these workers would demonstrate more investment, engagement, and commitment (Marciano & Wingrove, 2014). If leaders could only make workers feel better, they could make them produce more. Although it is important that workers feel good and be happy, much of what produces those feelings comes from them, not from leaders or the workplace. It is the height of hubris to suggest that leaders are so influential and demonstrate such exceptional persuasiveness that they can permanently excite and motivate others by force of personal charisma. These perspectives that underpin much of what is written on motivation remain essentially invalidated by any real, disciplined, or formal research. In fact, research demonstrates that motivation is internally generated (intrinsic), controlled by the individual, and reflected by personal perspectives, experiences, challenges, and opportunities. Motivation cannot be externally mandated; it must be generated from within, connected with a set of values and intentions derived from an individual's life and linked and connected to organizational life.

Simply said, it is not possible to externally motivate anyone to do anything in the long term. In organizations enamored with the idealization of motivation, so many organizational resources, such as time and effort, are wasted on motivating individuals to undertake activities that organizational members have no interest or investment in or ownership of. Each time an organization attempts to stimulate worker excitement over a new initiative that was originated

Exhibit 4-6 Elements of Motivation

- Internally generated.
- Consistent with personal values.
- Characterized by engagement.
- Connected with personal ownership.
- Gains are mutually advantageous.

---

with little investment or participation from the staff, workers demonstrate decreasing interest, involvement, and excitement. More often than not, many of these ideas intended to motivate staff originate in the minds of those who do not have to implement them, add them to their own workload, or even devote the necessary time and energy to them. Adding a new initiative is like grinding salt into the open wounds of failed past initiatives from which workers have not yet fully recovered. Clearly, it is no wonder that so many initiatives are either short-lived or fall short: they fail to understand the real elements of engagement and use the mechanics of motivation inappropriately (**Exhibit 4-6**).

Alignment, on the other hand, is an entirely different leadership skill that yields infinitely more viable outcomes and value. Leadership alignment creates a context for innovation by suggesting the necessary configuration of personal response to the demands of the external environment and the need for personal ownership of that response. In the process of alignment, leaders see the demand for change through the perspective of ownership and engagement. Leaders recognize that any demands for change have a dramatic and immediate impact on all elements of the organizational network and require the configuration of responses that integrate and link every component of the network in a consonant and collaborative process that adequately addresses the challenges and growing demand of the change process.

> **Key Point**
>
> Leaders cannot motivate anyone to do anything. Motivation is internally generated. The role of a leader is to create congruence between external realities and internal motivation. To do this, the leader focuses on creating good alignment between personal motives and organizational goals.

For leaders, the much harder work of sustaining organizational effectiveness and integrity is looking from the perspective of goodness-of-fit between the demand for significant change and the responses necessary to address it effectively. In the management discipline of alignment, leaders constantly look at issues of impact and effects of change on the community and individuals. Here, leaders look at change from the perspective of the various constituents by asking questions such as the following: How does this change affect them, inform them, challenge their current circumstances and conditions, and call them to action in a way that has meaning for them? Furthermore, leaders are concerned with using the most appropriate language to present issues and needs so that responses reflect the values of those who must respond.

When alignment has been established, leaders become concerned with how the language of issues that drive change best fit the involved constituents. In addition to alignment at the operational level, leaders can use second-order cognitive and cultural levels of alignment in discussions with community constituents or individuals to identify and personalize change. Within this frame of reference, leaders, having established alignment, can engage those who feel the impact in a way that challenges them to reflect, respond, and act (Hilligoss et al., 2017).

In creating alignment, leaders never divest ownership and partnership in change issues or events from any member of the community affected by the change. The assumption of alignment does not reflect divorce of ownership from stakeholders in the network (organization). This basic understanding of membership in the work community drives the leadership mental model and expression in a way that includes all members of the community sharing a stake in its life, direction, and decisions. Although decisions are differentiated by their characteristics—strategic, tactical, process, and personal—leaders recognize that every member of the community has a stake in all decisions and, ultimately, plays some meaningful role in the exercise of any of them. In the process of alignment, leaders understand that participation in decisions is differentiated by role, not by position. Each player in the membership community (network) plays some role in relationship to every decision.

Through this application of alignment, differentiation in role and decision making requires a different set of competencies, not a different level of engagement and ownership. In creating a context for innovation, the leader in this set of circumstances recognizes community ownership of the work of the system and further acknowledges the need to clearly delineate the attributes, skills, content, processes, and actions of the various stakeholders based on the expression of their stake holding represented by their locus of control. Leaders understand it is appropriate for the board to make decisions about strategy; it is necessary for executives to make decisions about priority; it is essential for managers to make decisions about tactics and budget; and it is required for staff to make decisions about process and action. Each member of the network has his or her own role, yet the role of each is cross-referenced and intersects with others' roles. Each member informs the roles of others and is represented in others' decision making so that the decisions are fully informed in regard to their impact on the system, including the effective challenges and opportunities related to successful implementation. This is especially true in organizations predominated by professional workers (knowledge workers), where every decision at any place in the system has an impact on the integration and activity of each discipline. Understanding of alignment of stakeholders drives many of the principles and structures of professional governance that have been detailed and articulated in other works (Clavelle et al., 2016; Porter-O'Grady & Malloch, 2016). Although creating structures and processes that represent the principle of alignment requires organizational competence and management talent, it yields relevant and sustainable results.

To create a context for an energizing and innovative workplace, leaders need to articulate the foundational principles that guide the constructs necessary for point-of-service ownership and investment in the innovation process. Not considering the principles associated with good alignment considerably challenges the leader's ability to create a context for innovation and to sustain the innovation dynamic as a way of doing business in any setting. The following are the key foundational principles related to creating this framework:

1. It is virtually impossible to undertake the activities of innovation in a "closed" environment with rigid hierarchy, tight control, compartmentalized structure, and narrowly vertical organizational structures.

2. Creativity and innovation are stimulated and encouraged in environments where network configurations predominate, reflecting strong horizontal alignment, relational configurations, decisional synthesis, and a highly collaborative organizational construct.
3. In work environments predominately composed of professionals (knowledge workers), shared governance structures that ensure that stakeholders are represented and engaged in decision making provide the strongest opportunity for involvement, creativity, and innovation.
4. Effective innovation occurs closest to its point of impact. The context for innovation reflects this understanding and makes it possible for the structural elements that support innovation to operate effectively in the places where innovations are created.
5. Innovation is a dynamic with clear components and processes. Leaders must understand the elements necessary to advance innovation and competently create conditions that make the innovation dynamic possible in their settings.
6. Motivation occurs where good alignment is established. Leaders, therefore, must focus on creating an understanding of alignment between required change and appropriate response to it. Ownership of the response to change is directly related to the perceived value of that change and the effect it has on the life of the community and its individual members.
7. Successful alignment occurs when individuals, struck by change, can demonstrate their ownership of change with language and action that reflect the personal impact of the change and their engagement.
8. Innovation is also a discipline. It is important that innovation be appropriately supported with sufficient resources, time, technique, and focus in a way that ensures that the activities of innovation have a place in the work of the organization. Innovation is not just a process; it produces a product, change, and outcome.
9. Sustainable innovation demands good leadership. Every leadership role in the organization should have as a part of its performance expectations the facilitation, coordination, and integration of innovation processes at every point of decision making in the system.
10. Innovation is driven from every place in the organization. The organization's contextual framework for innovation must be reflected in the decisions made and processes implemented, from the board room to the patient. Innovation should reflect the requisites of good strategy and demonstrate its contribution to advancing the interests and sustainability of the system. All stakeholders in the organization must see themselves as a part of the dynamic of innovation that defines the organization and provides for a sustainable future.

These foundational principles provide the content and contextual frame necessary for innovation to become a way of life in the organization. Each comprises a portion of the elements necessary to attain and sustain an innovation framework that leads to a continuum of successful responses to the demand for innovation. What is important for leaders to keep in mind is that innovation is merely the response to the constant demand for adjustment and reconfiguration of the relationship between the eternally changing external environment and the organizational and human response to this demand for change.

> ## Group Discussion
>
> If motivation primarily comes from within and is generated by individuals, leaders must use different strategies for engaging staff. The leader's charisma and personality are not sufficient to create the context for consistent and constant staff engagement. Aligning staff members' personal motivation with organizational goals is critical to generating investment and ownership by the staff. It is important for leaders to take time to delineate the drivers of staff self-motivation to help staff align their personal drives, insights, and goals with the goals of the organization. As a group, discuss how this can occur as you respond to the following questions:
>
> 1. What techniques might the leader use to get a sense of individual staff members' personal work motivation?
> 2. How might the leader determine what themes or consistency exists between individual motivators and the capacity to align staff motivation as a group?
> 3. What information must the leader delineate or make available to staff about the organization and organizational decisions as a first step in engaging with them in both responding to the organization and advancing personal and organizational agendas?

Creating Stakeholder Value

As health reform leads us into a deeper understanding of the demand for value, leaders must now be aware of the need to emphasize value-driven processes at every level of the system. The traditional, all-encompassing volume-based approaches to care and service delivery in the health sector have created a mental model at every level of delivery that is difficult to dismantle. The notion of value is a critical element in the consideration of innovation. Stakeholder value is of special concern. Organizations are made up of structures, processes, and persons in a networked mosaic of interdynamics that operate in a way that sustains the action of each element and the synthesis of the whole (Rubin & Abramson, 2018). This reality provides the frame for understanding the operation of value in the organization. A fundamental underpinning of the notion of value is the reality that each element of the enterprise must be a part of both the experience and the expression of value. People especially look for meaning in what they do as a reflection of their place in the world. This need for value operates in every individual, and therefore is present at every place in the organization.

The central tenet of value recognizes that every human being is involved in personal activity that seeks to validate and even extend his or her value in the world. In the search for personal meaning, individuals seek a means of expression of who they are or what they do. This, of course, is no less important in the workplace. The historical and industrialized notion that workers are subsets of the work, and therefore either do not reflect or give up their personal identification of value when they walk through the workplace doors, is simply unsupportable. The basic need for meaning and its expression and value exist in the hearts and minds of people regardless of where they may be located and is simply not surrendered when they enter the organization. Furthermore, the idea that individuals surrender personal identity, desires, and goals and

Figure 4-6 Creating Sustainable Value.

subordinate them to the externally determined values, strategies, and actions of the organization as defined by select others is also invalid. It is simply not possible to give up personal identity, meaning, and value and mindlessly subordinate them to those constructed by others for a salary and prestige. Yet, in the vast majority of work organizations in the United States, this has been precisely the expectation and framework on which workplaces have been traditionally organized (Lynch & Verner, 2013; Thompson et al., 2018). The idea that organizations are membership communities made up of a diversity of individuals, each with a unique set of values, has simply been a foreign notion in the traditional construct of organizations.

Wise leaders understand that individuals need to find meaning and express value, even in the workplace. Leaders know that relationships at work are a constant and dynamic negotiation between individual values and choices and the strategic imperatives of the organization. In this regard, good leadership is simply a successful effort to converge these forces into a synthesis that represents organizational mission and strategy and individual value and purpose. This "dance" between the individual and the organization reflects the essential skill sets of alignment that are critical to the success and sustenance of an entrepreneurial and innovative organization. In short, leaders work to create equilibrium, a "value equation" that represents the effort to coherently link and integrate the personal and organizational variables in a way that sustains both the organization and the individual (**Figure 4-6**). In health care, this value equation demonstrates a transdisciplinary commitment to advancing the interests of the health of the community, ensuring the foundations of practice with viable quality metrics, and undertaking all health practices within the context of a cost-effective pricing framework. This triple aim of satisfaction, quality, and price is part of the driving infrastructure for contemporary efforts at reforming American health care.

The Contextual/Strategic Role of the Board

Each role in the organizational network is a unique set of characteristics and functions that must be performed effectively to create a sustainable context for innovation. As previously stated, every level of the organization is required to demonstrate its obligation of creating a context sufficient to support and sustain innovation throughout the organization. The role of the organization's board is unique in this regard because it must not only be responsive to the external demand for creativity and innovation, but it must also make that demand operate as a key component of organizational life (Bates et al., 2017).

The board is obligated to create the strategic fit between the external demand for change and the internal organizational response. Using corporate governance of healthcare quality as an example, leadership makes decisions about the unique characteristics of the organization, its mission, purpose, and strategic response to its place in the broader social context (Brown, 2019). The focus on mission, purpose, and strategy provides the peripheral frame of the organization in regard to its place in a larger social and economic context. Through the strategic process, decisions about the response of the organization to collaboration and compatibility with external demands versus decisions related to stretching the mission and parameters of the organization to push into unexplored territory fall under the capacity for innovation coming from the board.

In the innovative organization, the board ensures that its members have access to and are aligned with external and internal stakeholders. At the board level, alignment with appropriate stakeholders represents a critical contextual accountability within an innovation framework. In this dynamic, the board seeks to include members and stakeholders from the larger community as well as those from within the membership community. Effective innovative boards create a fluid relationship between board membership and other stakeholders within the organization. An effective innovative board seeks to create a dynamic connection between the point-of-service stakeholders and those operating at the governance level. In this way, the board seeks to connect strategy and innovation as a way of doing business. Innovative boards recognize the need to be informed from a variety of real perspectives: those that reflect environmental concerns and the internal responses to them related to social, economic, budgetary, and process realities. In addition, the board recognizes the need for interaction and communication with those from the points-of-service who share the board's perspectives with an eye to translation, design, processes, and application realities that can only be articulated from their perspective.

> **Key Point**
> The innovative board recognizes its central role in linking the system or organization to the external environment, which influences its ability to thrive and sustain. The board constantly works to translate circumstance into action through its capacity to predict environmental changes, directly confronting challenges with a carefully constructed and relevant response.

Those composing the board must be skilled and experienced in being able to evaluate environmental indicators and benchmarks that inform them of particular and significant changes in the environment. An environmental awareness of significant contextual changes creates a requisite for the board to respond in a timely fashion in a way that best informs strategic decisions and guides organizational direction. The innovative capacity embedded in this role is exemplified by the board's ability to predict changing environmental conditions, encourage a culture of continuous improvement, and make an impact on the organization far enough in advance so that the organization can competently and comprehensively respond.

An effective innovative board overcomes the historical isolation of board members and the practice of decision making that references only the most senior levels of the organization. The historical justification for this has been to maintain the board focus on governance, not operations, as though exposure to other members of the organization would somehow taint their ability to uphold this obligation and diminish its "purity." Of course, nothing could be further from the truth. Exposure to essential stakeholders who share information that cannot be as effectively communicated through other means does not diminish the obligation of the board to act in the strategic best interests of the organization. In fact, engagement with essential stakeholders, especially active clinical leadership, emphasizes the obligation of governance. It is imperative to design mechanisms that promote communication of information to the board that it needs to hear in a language that represents the people and places in the organization where strategy formation becomes real, is translated, and either succeeds or fails. Ultimately, the board must be exposed to reliable, longitudinal data if they are to have an evidence-informed governance system (Bismark & Studdert, 2014; Jones et al., 2017).

> **Points to Ponder**
>
> No matter how brilliant an innovation or invention seems when envisioned or created by the designers, implementers are not the designers. Leaders must ask key questions during assessment to ensure that the innovation creates sustainable value. Consider questions related to perceived outcomes and also those related to time, resources needed, changes in routines, and other factors associated with implementation and achieving outcomes over time.

Group Discussion

Much discussion takes place regarding nursing membership on boards of trustees of organizations and systems. Discussions often reflect the historical perception and relationship of nurses to the healthcare organization, a frame of reference that challenges notions of nurses at the governance table. Yet nurses are more than 60% of patient care providers in healthcare organizations, representing the largest single stakeholder group offering healthcare services. Tradition allows that physicians are at the governance table, yet nurses are excluded. As a group, and in recognition of the significance of the profession of nursing in healthcare organizations, it is now time for you to make the argument for nursing representation on your healthcare system's board of trustees. Respond to the following questions to help construct your argument:

1. What unique value does the nurse representative bring to the board different from what is already present?
2. What area of expertise would you expect the nurse to contribute as a member of the board?
3. What skills and credentials would you suggest the nursing board member bring, and how would you make sure this nurse represents the larger community?

Innovative organizations are well recognized by the ease of access to information, individuals, and ideas. This fluidity is represented in a strongly horizontally oriented organizational construct that diminishes the impact of positional hierarchy and extends the exposure to broad-based role differentiation and accountability. In horizontal constructs, power is differentiated by roles, not by positions. Relational power and access to power in innovative organizations are more highly valued than positional or control power. Here again, in innovative organizations, leaders' build and extend relationships to create stronger role accountability, impact and intersection, and have ready access to people and processes that facilitate both creativity and work effectiveness.

Because the board creates the contextual framework for innovation, it needs the opportunity to consider strategy and the organizational constructs necessary to support dynamic innovation. If the board is to make accurate and appropriate strategic and directional decisions, it should understand the management approach to building in organizational and resource supports for innovation in a way that exemplifies innovation as a mechanism that stimulates creativity in health service provision. There has to be some assurance at the board level that the approaches and processes used in the organization make it possible for those strategies to succeed. Connecting board strategic initiatives to point-of-service processes and actions helps ensure positive outcomes that advance the organization with congruence between board direction setting and point-of-service design and implementation.

Construct and context for innovation originates at the governance level of the organization. By defining relationship and access expectations and setting the decision-making table to include relevant stakeholders prior to making strategic decisions, the board creates both the frame and the behavioral pattern for innovations that can be replicated throughout the organization. The board simply sets the tone for both the expectations and behaviors of the organization it governs. As the organization demonstrates creativity and innovation in its own structure and processes, the board serves to evaluate its effectiveness and efficacy through the strategic lens.

The C-Suite and the Context for Innovation

Senior executives must lead the translation of strategic imperatives into tactical obligations. Officers and agents of the board link strategic decision making with tactical response and join strategy with the operating life of the organization. Senior executives are uniquely located between governance and function to ensure effective translation of strategy and incorporation of strategy into the life of the organization. This ensures that the organization can meet external demands for continuous change and relevance and implement an internal design that ultimately aligns with strategy and action.

In the preparation of strategy, the senior team informs the board of the external and internal factors influencing priority setting and decision making, helping to guide decision makers with information and tools that represent the most accurate and relevant data available. A part of constructing information and a support network that validates recommendations for strategic priorities is the development of an engagement mechanism/process that includes key stakeholders from all levels of the organization, especially those from the point-of-service where the greatest likelihood for innovation and insight can be generated (Murray, 2015). Once strategic decisions are made, the senior team is obligated to connect the links and nodes in the network in a way that effectively and successfully translates strategy into decisions and

> **Exhibit 4-7** Central Role of C-Suite Leaders
>
> - Link and bridge between the board and staff.
> - Inform the board and translate strategy to the system.
> - Provide good linkage between the "nodal" loci of control.
> - Create a positive context for worker relationships.
> - Build the infrastructure for decisions and action.
> - Be transparent and honest about changes ahead.
> - Embrace optimism during change.

actions that move the organization toward a positive and successful response to strategic choices (**Exhibit 4-7**).

The senior team is the first link in the chain connecting organizational alignment to the strategic goals. Executive leaders focus specifically on the linkage and connections among key stakeholders and the nodes and networks in the system. Executive leaders seek to "set the table" and connect key stakeholders whose role is to engage particular strategic goals and translate them into operational decisions and actions (Cochrane, 2017). In the innovative organization, executive leaders primarily provide access, linkage, forums, and format for connecting critical stakeholders in a way that invests ownership at the appropriate locus of control and engagement with the various decisions and actions necessary to successfully design and implement them.

Unlike traditional allocations of executive skills, in the innovative organization, executives are primarily seen as points of linkage, intersection, and connection between the various constituencies and nodes of the network. They ensure that the essential and appropriate stakeholder structures, resources, and processes are aligned so that the strategic effort is in the right hands and that stakeholders have what they need to succeed. The oversight role at the executive level is responsible for determining and evaluating whether the right focus, relationships, infrastructure, resources, and processes have aligned appropriately to ensure that the elements necessary for successfully translating strategy into action are in place and operating effectively. In the innovative organization, the executive continually asks the following question: Is the right decision being made by the right person in the right place at the right time, and is it fulfilling the right purpose? From a quantum systems perspective, the senior executive is interested in the effectiveness of the system of decision making and action, not the decisions and actions themselves (that is a first-line leader role). From the executive perspective, if there is alignment between the infrastructure and systems supporting effective translation of strategy into action, the outcomes of innovation should be evidenced in the successful products of innovation (**Figure 4-7**).

First-Line Leaders: The Catalyst for Innovation

The most important and most highly skilled management leader lives at the intersection of the system and its point-of-service. Here, translation meets reality and the critical interface between design and action occurs. Here, the most dynamic evidence of lived innovation must be most visible, and here the skill sets necessary to ensure that innovation occurs are most apparent. From a quantum systems and innovation perspective, the first-line leader is often the unsung hero. The need for effective and successful leadership skills is most critically evidenced

Cycle of executive accountability:
- Inform the board
- Translate strategy
- Infrastructure for innovation
- Resource allocation and budget
- Complex adaptive network structure
- Empowerment and relational leadership

Figure 4-7 C-Suite Roles.

in this role. This role defines the location that represents the interface between the structural and process dynamics of the system and the functional and action dynamics of those who do its core work.

The first-line leader is obligated to create an operating milieu, a context, that most evidences the frame and its interface with the action of innovation. It is here where the dance of stability, risk, and the challenge of change is most difficult, yet it is here where the most opportunity lies. Here, the leader must demonstrate the skills necessary to facilitate the creative impulses and activities that push the parameters of stability, yet still ensure that those processes can be translated into action that makes a difference and gives life to the organization's strategic imperatives. Here, the leader can ask the strategic and the tactical questions, translate them to the actionable, and help ensure that the translation works, demonstrates real value, and is sustainable.

> **Key Point**
>
> The first-line leader is the key leadership role on which the organization or system most depends. In this role the strategic, tactical, and actionable converge. Here, the symphony of the organization and its members is constructed and conducted by the only leader who has both place and capacity to ensure its success.

The first-line leader needs to establish real and effective partnerships between stakeholders, set the right table for deliberation and design, ensure the right configuration and mix of stakeholders at the table, and determine appropriate human dynamics and group processes to move innovation from the table to the workspace. Ultimately, these elements ensure that timely, appropriate, effective, and viable outcomes are achieved (Valaitis et al., 2016). This leader is most fully connected to the points of service and, horizontally, to the nodes and networks in the system that reflect the points of reference and intersection necessary to creating the linkages and partnerships essential to successful design and action. The first-line manager must demonstrate the ability to manage uncertainty, diversity, and differing degrees of stakeholder diligence and drive momentum for achieving success.

Especially important to the first-line leader is the talent associated with selecting and setting the deliberative table where stakeholder partners will engage each other in the innovation process, using a discipline that guarantees results. Skill sets related to strategic translation, group construction, deliberative dynamics, the creative use of the tools of innovation, and the disciplines of decision making are all essential to the role of the first-line leader.

All too often in traditional healthcare organizations, the first-line leader role has been understated and under-resourced. Often the most skilled clinical provider, without the requisites to excel, has been appointed to this role. The results of this rather serendipitous and relaxed selection process have been disastrous to both the advancement of the role of leader and the competencies necessary for engagement and innovation. The truth is that this is perhaps the most important role in the organization and the one that demands the greatest skill capacity and maturity. Selection here cannot be incidental or accidental. Preparation for this role should include the most critical elements of skill development and the greatest focus of succession planning. In an innovative organization, this role becomes critical to the vitality and the success of the innovation process.

In addition to basic skill, development of the following additional requisites of the role of the first-line leader in the innovative organization is mandatory:

- The first-line leader has an ability to identify the creativity in others and to recognize the unique characteristics of the out-of-the-box thinkers, those who challenge current notions—the idea generators, the tinkerers, the first engagers, and the persons who seem to live in the question "why?"
- The first-line leader possesses leadership skills of curiosity and information gathering that are reflected in the ability and willingness to read broadly, listen carefully, perceive subtleties in the changing environment, recognize and take advantage of good timing, challenge and raise questions that generate new insights, and willingly engage others who do the same.
- The first-line leader is able to set aside real time for conversation and exploration that challenge ritual and routine, barriers, inadequate or unnecessary processes, and ideas that raise issues about being or doing differently.
- The first-line leader can create a safe space for debate and dialogue to engage differences in insight and align differing notions in a way that both translates and transforms them into positive and actionable items.
- The first-line leader is determined and focused on pursuing the innovation process through its various stages, helping stakeholders successfully move idea to action and process to outcome.
- The first-line leader recognizes the value of incremental failure in any innovation undertaking as a learning opportunity, not a mistake. Innovation is a nonlinear process, and the opportunity for ultimate success is moderated by the number of failures necessary to arriving at a viable outcome. Making space for failure and defending the processes that

Exhibit 4-8 Creating a Context for Innovation

Old Models of Work	New Models of Work
• Passive	• Ownership
• Obedient	• Participation
• Compliant	• Challenged
• Ritual	• Engaged
• Routine	• Experimental
• Policy	• Seeking evidence
• Process driven	• Inquiring
• Manager dominated	• Relating
• Job oriented	• Stretching

inevitably include failure are part of the leadership requisite to advocate for, defend, and articulate the value of innovation and the vagaries it incorporates.
- The first-line leader articulates the "why" and keeps employees informed and updated on innovative strategies and their rationale.

An important part of creating a context for innovation at the point-of-service is the character and behavior of the first-line leader. Leaders, by virtue of their role, create the context for worker experience. The leader can either make it exciting, interesting, and challenging work or simply represent and reflect operational focus and the status quo. In a time of great change such as is currently occurring in health care, the status quo—although all too common—is not sustainable. Each category of leader must do his or her part in creating context for innovation, from the places where strategies are formed to the places where they are transformed into action and outcome. In a networked organization, each player must do her or his part to fulfill the accountabilities of each role, creating the interfaces and synthesis in roles that are necessary to generate a living and sustainable context for the innovation dynamic (**Exhibit 4-8**).

Creating a Context That Supports the Innovator

Innovation is essentially a point-of-service activity. Everyone has a role to play in the processes associated with successful innovation. Although the innovator is often perceived as a person who stands out by demonstrating a unique personality, role characteristics, and patterns of behavior, this is rarely correct. Invention is often mundane and serendipitous. Invention most frequently generates out of frustration, the unworkable, and barriers to successfully doing what one thinks is necessary. The notion of the innovator and inventor as a dreamer or mad scientist working alone in some dark and chaotic space creating something out of nothing is more myth than reality.

Innovation is ultimately a collaborative effort. The vast majority of innovations are the products of the collective wisdom and effort of many stakeholders gathered together around the commitment to produce something new or different (Berry et al., 2019; Chan et al., 2018). It takes a community of diverse and committed individuals to create a truly viable innovation. This reality is what most drives the demand for effective leadership and coordination of stakeholders in both the creation of a context that makes it safe for innovation and the generation of a process that actually produces innovations. The leader's ability to obtain the best thinking and most committed processes within an innovation dynamic is the best indicator of the existence of an appropriate process supporting innovation in the workplace.

Innovators must have a sense that it is safe to innovate. *Safety*, in this case, means that the environment for work reflects an abiding respect for the individual and an opportunity for individuals to hear and fully engage in the decisions and actions of the unit or service. In creating a context for innovation, the importance of engagement cannot be understated. The leader's ability to shape an environment of ownership and investment in the decisions and actions of the workplace lays the critical foundation upon which safety and openness depend.

This is especially true in working with professional and knowledge workers. These individuals already have a sense of ownership with regard to their knowledge and the work they do. If the workplace environment and the leader behaviors understate or undervalue that sense of ownership, the knowledge, energy, and commitment necessary to translate that into deliverables are simply missing. If they are missing long enough, both the creativity and inventiveness associated with them go missing as well. And once lost, it takes a great deal of effort to reengage ownership and to generate the potential value embedded in it. This is one of the classic challenges of contemporary clinical organizations. Many clinical professionals do not have a sense of partnership, engagement, and ownership sufficient to respond with enthusiasm, interest, and creativity to the huge number of initiatives generated by organizations without their consent, involvement in design, and commitment to the additional activities necessary to obtain the outcome.

Group Discussion

Building a community of innovation requires significant talent on the part of the leader. Creating a context that makes innovation possible involves a great deal of work in transforming the system in a way that values innovation. Every member of the work community brings something to the innovative process. Leadership is required to determine the particular and unique characteristics of individuals, discern the contribution these characteristics can make to the innovation process, and build a community of innovators that balances the skills and talents in a way that makes the innovation process work.

As a group, think of a specific innovation that would improve the life of practice in your department, service, or unit. After identifying a specific innovation, reflect together on the staff that makes up the service. List their unique attributes and characteristics with a mind to what role they would play in innovation. Place this information on a flip chart using a mind-mapping or concept-mapping approach. Think about how each might contribute, the role he or she might play, and the manner in which you might organize the innovation initiative to best make use of member skills and to serve and advance the innovation idea. Once the design is concluded, test it out and see where it takes you.

It is incumbent upon leaders to create a context for creativity and innovation that reflects more horizontal and adult-to-adult relationships among all members of the service and unit. The challenge for effective leaders is to confront existing boundaries of roles that reflect a more parent–child, superior–subordinate, manager–staff, boss–employee set of relationship parameters that result in prescribed perceptions and role interactions. Breaking past these highly vertical patterns of behavior is essential to effective leadership of professionals.

If leaders can effectively translate their role of manager to partner with staff colleagues and clarify expectations of the role in a way that reflects specific accountabilities embedded in that role, a more normative relationship can be generated in a way that supports the requisites of innovation.

> **Key Point**
>
> Leaders of innovation must see staff as partners. This is especially true in the professional organization where knowledge work is the center of the profession's activities. Here, leaders engage the staff as peers, as owners of their practice. Out of this sense of ownership and the obligations associated with it, the professional demonstrates commitment to advancing care and the innovations necessary to make the processes associated with it better, more effective, and more sustainable.

Here, leaders generate a clear understanding of the accountabilities of the role in delineating the frame for those accountabilities in the requisites associated with the management of human, physical, material, support, and system resources. These management definitions and the roles and decisions associated with them need to be as clear to staff partners as they are to managers. Some of the greatest impediments to developing the partnership role between management and staff are the ambiguity around issues of locus of control and the possibility that legitimate locus of control is malleable, personality dependent, and can change at a moment's notice, totally based on the feeling and temperament of the manager at any given time. Clarity around manager role expectations and patterns of behavior creates a level of consistency and trust in the role so that stakeholders have an accurate perception of expectations and actions upon which they can both depend and build real partnership.

Innovation and the Membership Community

Innovation is essentially a collateral process that engages a number of interested stakeholders. Once the foundations of manager consistency and role expectation are well established and clearly performed, the expectations of staff member roles in an innovative organization can be explored and clarified. Sustainable organizational innovation depends on the ability of leaders in the system to create a heightened awareness of the system as a membership community made up of individual relationships and networks of relationships necessary to advance the purposes of the organization (Greenhalgh & Abimbola, 2019). It needs to be understood and embedded in organizational culture such that when a new member comes on board with the organization, the obligations and expectations of membership form the foundation of role value, performance, and behavior.

Just as there can be no ambiguity about the parameters of the manager/leader role, ambiguity about the membership in the organization must also be eliminated. This is especially true in professional and knowledge worker–driven organizations. Managing professional and knowledge workers requires a significantly different leadership frame of reference and capacity (**Exhibit 4-9**). These expectations must be clearly prescribed and described upon an

Innovation and the Membership Community

Exhibit 4-9 Creating a Professional Practice Community

- Membership in the work community is not simply a job. From the outset, membership implies commitment and alignment of personal goals and actions with those of the organization and an agreement to fully participate in advancing them.
- Each individual recognizes the unique skills and talents he or she contributes to the community and can articulate precisely what these are along with a commitment to fully access and use them in the best interest of the community.
- Mechanisms in the organization clearly articulate processes that assess, value, and evaluate the goodness-of-fit between the personal characteristics of the individual and the collective values of the community. Creating goodness-of-fit is the critical first-stage emphasis of developing a value-based relationship between the individual member and the membership community in which members seek to participate.
- Policy and documentation of the system clearly state membership rights and obligations, as well as expectations for participation and engagement in the creative and inventive processes of the innovative organization. These foundations present a clear position for the new member regarding the organization's expectations that members will be creative and fully participate in activities that advance the viability of the system in a constantly changing external environment.
- A full and clear explanation and demonstration of the processes and activities associated with the innovation role of the individual in the system is detailed at the outset of the relationship and incorporated into the fundamental orientation experience of new members.
- Mentorship of new members includes activities associated with the innovation dynamic and the member's participation in it, along with an evaluation and a plan for developing and refining individual member's skills and competencies associated with fully participating in the activities of innovation.

---

individual's entry into the organization in a way that signifies an adult contract between the individual and the organization. Associated with the idea of membership are two elements: rights and obligations. Both must be enumerated clearly. The rights of membership are the personal benefits and recognition that comes with engaging other members in the system in a way that advances the net advantage of each and of all. Obligations are the individual's requisites for contributing to the mission and purposes of the community, the work expectations necessary to obtain outcomes and sustain the community, and the performance and behavioral expectations that reflect the actions of membership and the functions that contribute to it.

The assumption that underpins the context for innovation is that each member of the organization plays a role in the innovative dynamic embedded in the culture of the system (Desveaux et al., 2019). This allays the idea that innovation is a special talent or unique capacity of a very few individuals with distinct personal characteristics. In an organizational culture of innovation, the expectation is that all members of the network are full participants in the organization's processes of innovation and that each member contributes to sustaining the dynamic of innovation embedded in the character of the organization (Porter-O'Grady, 2013). As a result, the following fundamental role expectations are embedded in each member's participation in the innovative life of the organization.

Creating a culture of innovation is purposeful work. Both the infrastructure and the processes of the organization must reflect the characteristics of innovation, and these must be fully embedded in the expectations, operations, and functions of every place in the organizational network. Skill development and innovation attributes are neither obtained by nature nor accident. This deliberate work must be reflected in every level of the network in a way that can be seen from governance to service, from policy to practice, from decision to action, and from person to product. Creating a context for innovation means creating the culture within that innovation is innate—it resides within each person and is a normative behavioral expectation, not the exceptional gift of the relative few (Samet & Smith, 2016).

Obviously, there needs to be an infrastructure and a structural framework for innovation as a discipline in the organization. Building innovation communities of practice and organizational infrastructure that allows consideration of transdisciplinary innovations, protection of intellectual property, business strategies/solutions for product development, marketing, production, sales, and evaluation are all critical to promulgating successful innovations. Leaders demonstrate their awareness of these realities by expanding their knowledge and insight regarding best practices and organizations of preference for structures supporting innovation. While such structural design and construction is beyond the scope of this text, the innovation leader needs to be well versed in the business and structural components that ensure effective and sustainable innovations as a part of the life of the system.

Balancing Innovation with Value

Creating a culture for innovation requires more than simply creating an environment where innovative processes can freely unfold. It is equally important to ensure that the focus on innovation connectivity actually advances the interests of the organization. The organizational network, the actions and coalitions converging around the purposes and goals of the organization, must reflect a consistency of focus and energy directed to truly meeting the interests of the organizational community as a whole. From the strategic imperatives established through the governance process for the focused activities of delivering outcomes directed by those at the point-of-service, each component of the organization must demonstrate the convergence of plans and actions around those priorities that represent significant value for the organization.

Value now has larger implications for healthcare leaders. In health reform, value is a national strategic goal for the delivery of health services. Focus is on the value of creating truly healthy outcomes where the health of the nation is advanced and the cost of ensuring that health is controlled. The move from volume-based to value-driven health care now calls for a major shift in the mental model of care delivery and in the structure of organizations and leadership in ensuring that the health of the nation is advanced. Real value must now be clearly enumerated, defined, delivered, and measured in ways that represent effectiveness, efficiency, efficacy, and good use of available resources. Value implies stewardship of both services and resources in a convergence that ultimately positively affects service, outcome, and national health.

While leaders are creating the infrastructure and conditions that make the creative processes an operational characteristic of the work of the organization, they must discipline this creativity with the value creation process, which is just as essential to the dynamic integrity and sustenance of the organization and to those it serves. Working with individuals to develop creative processes during idea generation and valuing experimentation is important, as is developing good predictive capacity and intuition. Good leaders also need to build processes that move people and systems out of the box, aiding them in implementing innovative group dynamic processes and in translating ideas into action, as these are the critical factors of innovation as a way of life at each and every node and network interface in the organization. Each factor must be valued, developed, and refined as the foundational skill sets of the innovative organization that are truly reflected in the operation of the organization. And value demands that they make a difference.

At the same time, these creative and innovative elements need the discipline of direction. All innovative processes and organizational systems should respond to the organization's relationship with its external communities and the strategic demand of the organization to excel and to thrive (Elrod & Fortenberry, 2017). This means that leadership and staff must be as cognizant of and as fully engaged in the value creation processes that bring form and substance to innovation and the creative frame within which the creative endeavors unfold. Although this is a delicate dance, viability requires insightful balance and continual review of the components of value creation: mission, vision, value, trade-offs, priorities, resources, risks, markets, margins, and outcomes. Leaders, therefore, have the obligation to continually and carefully balance the vagaries of the innovation process against the discipline of organizational direction and goals.

> **Key Point**
>
> Innovation is not merely a process. It is a dynamic and emerges from broad worldviews. Innovation gives new meaning and direction, and challenges the historic, the expected, and the routine. It calls innovators to adopt an attitude that reflects that all work processes and activities are subject to the discipline of constant inquiry and reassessment.

The innovation dynamic should be as much a part of ensuring the integrity and sustainability of the system as it is part of responding to the ever-challenging and changing demands of the external environment. No system can be all things at all times; this is why systems are disciplined by mission and purpose. Although mission and purpose may be altered over time as the organization is reviewed in the context of a changing environment, they do give the organization a sense of self and place, and they call members to more clearly see themselves in that place. Mission and purpose further call leaders to raise the questions of innovation in light of how it advances the integrity and sustainability of the system given its position and role in the greater social, political, and economic contexts. Leaders of innovation remain constantly aware of this strategic balancing act and deal with the ambiguities and vagaries inherent in innovation. This is reflected in the struggle between operations and innovation and the ever-present potential of self-transformation in an ever-changing environment (**Figure 4-8**).

Differentiating Roles in Innovation

Different locations in the organization or system focus on different kinds of innovation. Clearly, leadership does not want administration to undertake activities associated with clinical innovation, and neither does it expect clinical leaders to lead physical plant innovations. Although there must be a point in the organization where a range of innovations undertaken by the system is assessed and determined, specific innovations should reflect the content and character of the innovators who will lead them. At the same time, "setting the table" for specific innovations may necessarily include interdisciplinary and multifocal membership at the table to address the full range of elements associated with a particular innovation. Whatever the case, the infrastructure and construction of models and processes of innovation should be located and reflect the character of the obligation of those to whom the innovation is related.

Figure 4-8 External "Fit" and Role of Mission.

1. External changing environment
- Always changing
- In motion
- Reflecting "users"
- Providing the "new"
- Emerging technology

Good strategic decisions

2. Health system mission, purpose, action
- Good tactical translation
- Effective decision infrastructure
- Good staff engagement
- Action impact

- Informed and active board
- Prepared and proactive C-suite

Exhibit 4-10 Forum for Innovation Priority Management

- Tie innovation initiatives to strategic priorities.
- Represent organizational arenas and stakeholders.
- Create format, structure, process, and evaluation.
- Integrate innovation activities to advance system's viability.
- Assess process, competence, progress, and impact.
- Champion innovation structure, learning, and action.
- Communicate all innovation progress to system.

Providing leadership opportunities in innovation at the places in the organization and with the people located there is a centerpiece of structuring effective innovation.

A part of creating the structure and context for innovation is the development of an interdisciplinary forum whose primary obligation is to act as a clearinghouse for establishing innovation priorities and the linkage of those priorities with the strategic imperatives and direction of the organization. The primary purpose of this group is to help discipline and direct the innovation process in the organization in ways that prevent the organization from dissipating its energy and resources and, instead, help focus resources and processes on those innovations that most likely address the strategic and directional priorities of the system (**Exhibit 4-10**). The infrastructure for this process should be as important and central as any decisional process in place in the organization. Here, the integration of strategic choices and innovation priorities takes place, and the challenges of ambiguity, external driving forces, and internal service demands, as well as the interface of mission, operations, and practice, are deliberated and delineated. Also, this forum serves as a centerpiece for evaluating the various elements of innovation and innovation projects in the system to determine their continuing viability, progress, and efficacy in light of the changing circumstances and conditions that drive the need for innovation in the organization.

Differentiating Roles in Innovation

It is also important that there is a clear delineation of role expectations and work processes with regard to innovation. Although it is the role of governance to establish a firm strategy, that process cannot be successful if it is not appropriately informed. Clearly, the work of being fully and appropriately informed cannot be thoroughly and adequately undertaken unilaterally by the board. The officers of the corporation, those that occupy the C-suite, have a significant role to play in ensuring that the board is appropriately informed regarding the conditions and circumstances that influence decision making around strategy. With regard to the innovation process in the organization, the interdisciplinary forum whose obligation is to coordinate, integrate, and facilitate the various innovation tactics and processes in the organization informs senior leadership and the board. They do this by providing them accurate and up-to-date information about the place, progress, and impact of current innovations. Furthermore, they share information they have garnered about issues of organizational fit with the external environment, potential challenges to organizational integrity, and predictive-adaptive indicators of a shift in the external environment. Finally, they articulate the resource implications and demands affecting innovative choices and the potential for future innovations.

Consistent with these contextual accountabilities are the activities associated with the various innovation projects enumerated in the organization. Incorporated into the innovation process and the activities located in these places are mechanisms that define methodology, decision making, work process, design progress, and the activities associated with successful implementation. Equally important are the evaluations that determine whether particular innovations and the processes associated with them are making progress or are stalled or even blocked. Activities and progress with regard to these local innovation processes need to be reported back to the network innovation forum for review and decision making. The forum needs to indicate their continuing support or a need for altering processes, direction, or goals for the innovation (**Figure 4-9**).

Creating a culture of innovation is both easier and wiser than simply attempting to change culture as a way of responding to external demands. If the infrastructure and the culture of the organization are grounded in innovation, and innovation is a part of the operation and functional mechanics of the system, adaptation to change becomes incorporated into the DNA of the system, its way of doing business. Whereas the processes, mechanics, and techniques of innovation can be found in other textbooks and learning resources, it is important here to

```
┌─────────────────────────────────────────────┐
│ Organizational interdisciplinary/systems forum for │
│  innovation structure, processes, and evaluation   │
└─────────────────────────────────────────────┘
         │
  ┌──────┼──────┬──────────┬──────────┐
  │             │          │          │
┌─────┐    ┌─────────┐ ┌─────────┐ ┌──────────┐
│Board│    │C-suite, │ │Managers │ │Staff     │
│strat│    │scanning,│ │translat-│ │designing,│
│egy  │    │assessing│ │ing and  │ │deciding, │
│and  │    │informing│ │tactical │ │acting,   │
│pred-│    │         │ │formation│ │evaluating│
│iction│   │         │ │         │ │          │
└─────┘    └─────────┘ └─────────┘ └──────────┘
```

Figure 4-9 Role Alignment for Organizational Innovation.

emphasize innovation as an essential constituent of all health systems going forward. If innovation is seen as a role obligation of each member of the network community, it is easier to actualize the processes associated with innovation and to build them into the organization's work processes (Albert, 2018; Conger, 2016).

Leadership and the Will to Innovate

If we've learned anything over the past decades with regard to people at work, it is the centrality of the effectiveness of leadership. If the leader is not willing, neither is the staff. This notion of will and its congruence with the innovative dynamic is critical to the understanding of the contextual demand of a truly innovative organization. Many organizations "miss the boat" because their leaders are operationally and functionally fixed. The real obligation of vision and predictive and adaptive capacity is often simply ignored, the competencies associated with it never developed, and the readiness of the organization lost under the burden of myopia, inert stability, and internal fixation.

Innovation is a dynamic, not simply a process. As such, innovation demands leaders and organizational members to be fully aware of those circumstances and conditions that call each to discern the reality of their work, the challenges associated with doing it, and the changes necessary to sustain it (Boston-Fleischhauer, 2016). Interestingly, though, individuals bring to organizations a whole range of cognitive, behavioral, and perceptive skills that, when appropriately and successfully converged, create the very synergy necessary to respond appropriately to shifting demands that affect person and organization. The issues related to this understanding frequently have to do with the capacity of the leader to engage human diversity, the organization's continuing challenge to respond to an ever-shifting environment, and the competencies necessary to implement processes that effectively address and appropriately respond to the convergence of these forces in a way that ensures individual and community thriving.

Human systems have a natural tendency to stability and rigidity. Human organizations tend to work diligently to control the ambiguities and vagaries of the internal environment as a way of advancing normative and stable work processes, relationships, and organizational routines. Through such mechanisms, people and organizations determine that they can better handle the stressors of permanent "white water" by eliminating all risk associated with it. The problem with this perspective is that the chaos, complexity, and uncertainty of organizational life in the larger context of reality are normatively uncertain. Attempting to eliminate uncertainty and to create stability as the prevailing mechanism for organizational integrity and viability is both inadequate and inappropriate as a strategic, organizational, or operational activity (Thayer et al., 2018).

> **Key Point**
> Innovation is a skill set and a contemporary capacity for the leadership role. Innovation is no longer an option with regard to organizational vitality and the construction of the future. Innovation is now a way of life for organizations that seek to advance and to be sustained. The ability to both understand and express predictive and adaptive capacity has become a subset of leadership competence and can no longer be optional if the role and the organization to which it relates seek to be successful.

Truly innovative organizations fully understand the inability to create any sense of permanent contextual frame for their work and life. These organizations seek to harness these dynamics and create the processes of response to them as the normative vehicle for organizational life. Chaos, complexity, and uncertainty need not be permanently accompanied by stress, reaction, and the feeling of being continuously overwhelmed. Once leaders recognize the constituents of the dynamic context of change, they begin to discern and to articulate the appropriate mechanisms that harness this energy and give insights into the behavioral modalities that best inform the life of the organization and its response to these prevailing circumstances. Once this is understood, the organization becomes imbued with the very life that it represents and incorporates in it the energy that reflects the congruence between its internal life and the external conditions and circumstances to which it must always respond if it seeks to continually thrive.

Leaders seek both to meet this challenge and to address it within structure and role. Leaders at all places in the organizational network seeking to create the innovative dynamic are a part of the construct of the network's operation and pattern of behavior. These leaders seek to align the innovation dynamics with the operational processes of the organization. Here, leaders construct the organizational framework, the operational modalities, and the decision and action processes in a way that reflects creativity and innovation as the normative response to the organization's place in the larger culture. In doing so, leaders heighten the awareness of the organization as a system and its individual members about the fundamental necessity to be fully engaged in the life of the organization and involved in the work process in ways that are inherently innovative and creative (Weatherford et al., 2018). In these organizations, leaders and members are constantly looking for the challenges to historical and current ways of being and doing, seeking to inform organizational action in a way that alerts them early enough in the dynamic to respond to these challenges appropriately. In this way, they avoid the critical reaction that comes from late awareness, inadequate response, and an existing infrastructure that narrows people's focus to function and action rather than to purpose, value, and outcome.

Group Discussion

You are leaders of innovation. As a leadership group, you are charged with developing a program of learning for all of the management leadership in your health system regarding value-driven health care. As a part of its vision and leadership expectation, the health system has committed to constructing a strategic imperative and an infrastructure for innovative value-based care delivery to help transform the organization into a truly health-based, population-designed, and innovative enterprise.

Your group has been charged with helping to develop leaders with the innovative insights and capacity necessary to build a truly patient-centered, value-driven health service enterprise. You are putting together a 12-month education program that will ensure that each level of leadership understands its role and that each leader has the capacity to fully engage and express confidence in the exercise of his or her leadership role in the movement to value-based health care.

Respond to the following questions about how you might structure this innovative value-based care delivery system:

1. Based on this chapter, what are the various role expectations for value-based innovation of board members, C-suite members, managers, and professional staff?
2. What might the content of the program be if emphasis must reflect the construction of policy, principles, protocols, structures, and processes associated with making the organization a patient-centered, value-driven enterprise?
3. In your attempt to be innovative in the design of leadership development for value-based patient care, what innovative learning dynamics and processes might you incorporate into this learning program as a mechanism for more deeply embedding this new innovation into the patterns of leadership in the system?

Conclusion

We are deep into a value-driven age. The question of this age is no longer, "What are you doing?" The real question of the time is, "What difference are you making?" The answers to these questions are as different as the questions themselves. The innovative organization asks the questions related to whether the organization matters, has value and impact, and, indeed, makes a sustainable difference. A system's sustainability and continuing need to make a difference define the relationship and the synergy between the external environment that constantly grows, adapts, and changes and an internal environment that accepts the challenge of change; creates modalities that incorporate change into its way of life; and creates structure, process, and relationships that embrace its own becoming. In this way, both the person and the collective of the organization advance the life of the system, its purposes, and the integrity and synergy between the innovative work of the organization and the creation of its own future.

Chapter Takeaways

1. Our postdigital and postreform age is increasing the demands on organizations and systems to engage and embrace essential structural and technological shifts that lead to innovations in the creation, design, delivery, and evaluation of health delivery in every setting.
2. Creating a culture of innovation requires different structures, infrastructure, strategic leadership, practice, and work constructs and designs that transform the traditional vertical institutional organization into a multilateral, multifunctional, transdisciplinary, user-engaged network of services that positively impact health.
3. The innovative organization is one that engages stakeholders at all places in the organization and recognizes the fundamental truth that innovation is driven from the point-of-service and requires the full investment and engagement of those who do the work of health care supported by those who lead healthcare systems and networks.

4. Organizations now must be structured and aligned in a way that provides a seamless linkage between stakeholders and users, resulting in a network of relationships, interactions, and structures that support engagement, ownership, creativity, and the capacity to innovate and adapt quickly in a way that accommodates emerging knowledge, technology, and practices.
5. Innovation must be balanced with value in a network of strategically aligned and professionally engaged interactions that advance user satisfaction, the fulfillment of specific quality metrics, and the appropriate stewardship of resources reflected in cost-effective service pricing. This triple aim of satisfaction, quality, and price is the driving force for clinical practice for the foreseeable future.

Case Study 4-1

Developing a Culture of Interprofessional Collaboration

As the chief nursing officer (CNO) of a large metropolitan hospital, Jesse has established a strong reputation as a "mover and shaker" in nursing leadership circles. He is greatly admired by his colleagues who are CNOs at other hospitals in the region. For the most part, Jesse is proud of his many accomplishments and very satisfied in his current role at the hospital, but lately he has been feeling restless and is concerned that the entire organization could do a better job of creative thinking to address needed changes to ensure excellence in patient care, excellence in the work environment, and excellence in individual professionalism.

Jesse shares his concerns with his colleagues on the hospital executive team, and they all reassure him that he should simply be satisfied with the hospital's reputation as a premier place to work, receive care, and practice professionally. Despite his colleagues' opinions, Jesse feels that there is an opportunity to make the best even better. He feels that there are a number of age-old issues confronting nursing that never seem to be completely addressed or resolved. The notion of interprofessional practice and collaboration is one example. Jesse realizes that the nursing profession has talked about the importance of interprofessional practice for at least 45 years, and in 2010, interprofessional practice was cited as critical for optimal patient outcomes in the Robert Wood Johnson Foundation's *Future of Nursing* report, the Institute of Healthcare Improvement's report, and the Agency for Healthcare Research and Quality's report.

Jesse realized that the healthcare literature is replete with articles citing the benefits of interprofessional collaboration and its importance in enhancing job satisfaction, organizational commitment, and professionalism and for minimizing job stress and interprofessional conflicts. In spite of all of the evidence and rhetoric about interprofessional collaboration, Jesse realized that the hospital had not achieved interprofessional collaboration or practice. Although the hospital had made great strides in improving the organizational culture by addressing behavioral standards and values that were to be the norm for every employee and every physician affiliated with the hospital, there were many instances when physicians practiced very independently from the nurses caring for their patients.

Both nurses and physicians were frustrated, feeling that they were not valued or respected by the other party for their knowledge and skills in caring for patients and families. Several particular situations triggered Jesse's concern about the subject, and he felt that there was an underlying tension that could be a platform upon which to initiate some creative dialogue and ideas for changing the culture to support and encourage interprofessional collaboration and practice. He realized, however, that it was impossible to motivate others to make a change in their relationships and interactions with others, but he considered his options for developing some internal motivation that would spur individuals to take the lead in championing such a change. Jesse wanted to ensure that there was alignment among nurses and physicians with the hospital's behavioral standards and values, which were widely accepted by employees and physicians throughout the organization. It seemed, however, that some physicians and nurses felt that collaboration was not a part of the accepted values. Jesse wanted to change this perception so that interprofessional collaboration would be a valued behavior among all disciplines and specifically between nurses and physicians.

After much thought Jesse decided to form an interprofessional task force composed of nurses, physicians, and key individuals from other divisions such as radiology, dietary, surgery, and laboratory services. In choosing individuals to be a part of the task force, he invited individuals who were exemplar collaborators and some who were referred to as "problem" individuals. He also identified a group of individuals who could be champion leaders on each of the nursing units from the recommendations of the directors of the respective nursing services. The plan was to roll down the work of the task force to the point-of-service and to bubble up ideas from the point-of-service to the task force.

One of the directors suggested that all newly hired nurses and nurses in the nurse residency program be rotated for a day or more in each of the ancillary departments, which would give the orienting nurses the opportunity to see the internal workings of each of the departments and how they interfaced with the respective nursing units. All directors felt that this was a very worthwhile plan, although there were some front-end investment costs because the on-boarding of new nurses would take at least an extra week. They all believed that this action would create a better understanding of the intersections between nursing and ancillary support departments.

The first meeting of the interprofessional task force was very introductory in nature, and most participants were a bit skeptical about the efficacy of such an initiative. The "problem" physicians and nurses were the most skeptical, and their body language spoke loudly that they did not value this new initiative, nor did they value the notion of collaboration. Some of the more skeptical physicians were of the belief that physicians were the authority for the patient plan of care and that nurses were simply to follow physician orders. A few nurses on the team were quite content simply to follow physician orders and had no need for any further interaction to discuss a patient's condition, needs, or plan of care. On the other hand, a few very progressive physicians and nurses were excited about an initiative to improve communication and collaboration among all team members for the benefit of patients and families. Fortunately, Jesse noticed that these individuals were more vocal in the task force, and he hoped that they would create the context for an innovative strategy to improve point-of-service interprofessional collaboration and provide some peer pressure for the others to follow. Jesse realized that this entire initiative was a cultural change and that it would need time to be formulated, implemented, and solidified in the minds of individuals for collaboration to become a new value and behavior.

The interprofessional task force convened a number of meetings, and the group brought forth many ideas. Part of the process included presentations of studies in both the medical and nursing literature that demonstrated the importance of interprofessional collaboration in ensuring optimal patient outcomes. Most task force participants were very engaged in the process, inquired as to how certain actions might be initiated at the unit level, and asked how they might ensure that nurses and physicians at the unit level could take ownership of the change. Jesse and the rest of the executive team reviewed the progress of the task force and attended many meetings to assure the team that they were supportive of their work. The executive team also brought in an industrial organizational psychologist who was a noted specialist in organizational change to facilitate the team meetings and discussions. The group was quite energized with this external consultant, who brought a new perspective and fresh ideas to the table.

After several months of meetings, the task force was finally ready to roll out an innovative strategy to promote interprofessional collaboration at the unit level. Jesse and the rest of the executive team were amazed at the ownership that the team had taken and how enthusiastic they were to launch the initiative. One physician leader offered to be the physician champion, and the group planned that she would present the initiative and plan at each of the specialty physician meetings and to the medical executive committee. Similarly, a clinical nurse offered to be the spokesperson for nursing because it was hoped that the initiative would quickly be embraced by nurses at the point-of-service if it was presented by a clinical nurse, rather than a line manager or director.

Because competency of the bedside nurse is one of the most important attributes of collaboration, emphasis on knowledge and skill development of all nurses was a component of the initiative. As a part of the nursing competency skill list, communication, conflict management, crucial conversations, and the art of collaboration were added as learning modules that would be included in hospital orientation and annual competency checks. The modules were added to the on-boarding orientation program for physicians as well, and interprofessional collaboration, teamwork, and conflict management topics were added to medical staff education. The hospital elected to add collaboration to its list of values and behavioral standards, and statements related to collaboration were added to every employee's annual performance appraisal form.

Although a number of different initiatives were used to facilitate building the culture of collaboration, there was a belief that nurses and physicians interacting together at hospital-based celebrations, social gatherings, educational venues, and on the unit would build the trust level necessary in collaborative relationships. Clinical nurses and clinical nurse specialists (CNSs) were frequently invited as participants in medical staff education programs to present the nursing perspective on topics. Also, physicians were invited to be speakers at quarterly leadership meetings and other nursing education venues.

Jesse suggested that the director of research conduct a formal study to evaluate nurse and physician perspectives on the level of collaborative behavior existing before and after the roll-out of the task force initiatives. The chief of the medical staff was invited to be a co-investigator and assisted in preparing an institutional review board (IRB) proposal. Post IRB approval, the baseline level of collaborative behavior of nurses and physicians were evaluated. Initial findings were presented by the director of research and chief medical staff together at medical staff and nursing unit level meetings. A year after some task force initiatives were implemented at the unit level, nursing staff and physicians were surveyed again to determine the level of change in perceptions of collaborative behavior. In analysis, they found a small improvement in the level of nurse–physician collaboration. They completed an IRB amendment to make the study longitudinal, and planned to survey nurses and physicians every year as part of the employee opinion survey and the physicians' satisfaction survey.

Approximately 5 years after the first interprofessional task force meeting, Jesse proudly sat in the audience as the director of research and the chief of the medical staff presented 5-year collaboration outcomes. In longitudinal analysis, they learned that perceptions of nurses and physician collaborative behaviors improved over time became highly valued. Nurses and physician engagement during rounding at patient bedsides was cited as one of the most appreciated factors.

While reflecting on the past 5 years in progress toward this cultural change, Jesse realized that he had simply set the stage for the change to occur, chose individuals who were passionate about the topic (both positively and negatively), identified champions who would lead the change process, and was available to provide support as necessary.

Questions

1. How would you consider Jesse's vision for a cultural change to normalize interprofessional collaboration as an expected behavioral standard and personal value as an innovation?
2. How did Jesse and the rest of the executive team create the context for an innovative solution to this age-old problem in health care?
3. In what ways did Jesse and his directors create the context and expectation of new employees and new physicians for collaborative behaviors?
4. How did Jesse and the executive team create alignment with this organizational goal and the overarching behavioral standards in the value statements?
5. What were some of the initiatives that motivated the interprofessional task force to become engaged in the process and to become owners of the solution?
6. How would you have handled the dissenting physicians and nurses who did not recognize the importance of collaborative behavior and who held on to past values of hierarchy, authority, and submissive, task-based nursing?
7. Although all of the initiatives were not described in this case study, if you were Jesse, what might you have done or suggested to set the context for such an important cultural change?
8. Describe what you might do as an innovation leader to ensure point-of-service engagement and ownership in creating a culture of collaboration? How would you ensure the support of other executives who might not be familiar with nor value the benefits of collaborative relationships among healthcare team members?

Case Study 4-2

Creating a Culture of Innovation

Fred is the president of a large multihospital healthcare system that is nationally recognized as one of the most successful vertically integrated healthcare systems in the nation. The organization was recently designated as one of the first providers in a statewide accountable care contract because of its organizational structure, which supports community-wide point-of-service care, holds exemplar quality standards, and is a positive workplace for healthcare providers.

Even though Fred holds a lofty position, he often interacts with individuals at all levels of the organization. He makes a point of visiting each hospital campus and talking with gardeners, nurses, dietary aides, physicians, and, of course, patients and their families. Fred is committed to excellence in patient care and strongly believes that an empowered and engaged workforce is the best way to achieve that goal. Even though the healthcare system is widely recognized for excellence, Fred is uncomfortable simply resting on the status quo. He realizes that the competitive forces in the region and in health care and the sweeping changes in how health care is provided and reimbursed threaten the status quo.

He meets with his senior executive team and tells them, "We can't sit still and wait for the future to happen. We must invent the future and write the script for how we will interact with the forces that can either make or break us as a healthcare system. If we are truthful with ourselves, none of us really thrive in a constantly changing environment, and we often long for stability. Unfortunately, we do not live in a stable environment. We see major changes in healthcare reimbursement, challenges in serving the community as it changes ethnically and economically, threats from a union environment that demands more than our organization can offer, and a constantly deteriorating physical plant that needs replacement or refurbishment. We are compelled to accelerate new and creative thinking to proactively address some of these challenges."

He goes on to tell the team that he is not comfortable with slow, incremental changes, and he challenges them to consider ways that organization leaders can incentivize innovation from the point-of-service all the way to the top of the organization. He informs them that he recently attended a national meeting of presidents of healthcare systems and that innovation was the most discussed and hotly debated topic at the meeting. It seemed as if all healthcare leaders were feeling the need to reinvent their organizations to position them for Accountable Care Organization expectations and the consequences of other national issues, such as the potential for community terrorist acts, natural disasters, growth of diverse immigrant populations, the opioid crisis, and the impact of an aging population with chronic and acute illnesses.

Fred recommends that a comprehensive strategy be developed to create a culture of innovation and instill excitement about developing new and more economical ways to meet patient needs while still supporting the enhancement of professionalism among caregivers. Fred states that this is not a new budget-cutting initiative to meet the financial bottom line, but rather a willingness to invest in new, innovative ideas that can revolutionize how care is provided in primary care settings, hospital settings, and the home environment after discharge. He wants the executive team to consider how the organization's leaders can partner with physician groups, community leaders, the organization's nursing leaders, and clinical directors to instill and incentivize a culture of innovation.

Later, Fred meets with all of the CNOs from the system's hospitals and informs them of his new vision for a culture of innovation. He states that he believes that nursing is a key stakeholder in creating innovations at the bedside and that he is willing to support key innovations in their testing and implementation phases of changes.

The CNOs discuss Fred's vision and the need for innovative thinking. They are convinced that advancing nurses' knowledge and expertise in evidence-based practice will be an important step in creating a culture of excellence and innovation. The CNOs asked the respective leaders in research and professional development to develop a plan to advance evidence-based practice at all hospitals. They also discussed having an annual nursing innovation conference that would recognize nurses who developed innovations in care, education, or leadership and then disseminate new knowledge to the entire healthcare system. They discussed a plan to financially reward the top innovation, which would be chosen by the executive team with clinical nurse representation and evaluated on financial and clinical outcomes and alignment with the healthcare system's mission, vision, values, and behavioral standards. They asked Fred for an innovation development budget that would finance an evidence-based practice institute and an annual innovation conference with financial prizes of $2,500 for the first-place winner, $1,500 for the second-place winner, and $1,000 for the third-place winner.

The evidence-based practice institute would use an established framework for project development and a mentor–mentee format. Research mentors would be CNSs, but it was anticipated that future mentors would be past graduates of the evidence-based practice institute. Mentees would be recommended by their unit managers. Each mentee would be given 8 hours of pay per month to attend the evidence-based practice institute didactic classes and 4 hours to work on their evidence-based innovation projects. The institute would be conducted once a year with an annual evidence-based conference to recognize program graduates and to disseminate findings from completed projects. The cost of the institute would also include expenses to have a nationally known nursing leader as a keynote speaker and to display poster presentations of projects, with podium presentations from those that meet criteria and had the greatest impact on unit changes and patient outcomes.

The CNOs decided to make the annual innovation conference interdisciplinary and invited physicians and other discipline representatives to help plan the next conference. Using the evidence-based practice institute as a model, they invited nationally recognized healthcare leaders to be a keynote speakers on innovation and then the rest of the day was filled with presentations from the healthcare system's employees and physicians who developed innovations to improve workplace environment, patient outcomes, or workflow processes.

The CNOs are excited to present three proposals and prospective budgets to Fred and the senior executive team for consideration, and in addition, a proposal to advance the culture of innovation. The CNOs recommended that their healthcare system partner with major businesses in the region to expose healthcare leaders to research and development (R&D) processes of businesses and to engage business leaders in advancing innovations in health care. Several major healthcare vendors had corporate offices and production plants in the region, and would be perfect partners to design, build, and finance innovations involving the physical plant, medical equipment, information technology systems, workforce planning and resource procurement. Fred and the senior executive team are really interested in the three proposals and the plan to partner with regional businesses to advance innovations. They embraced advancing clinical nurses' knowledge and expertise in evidence-based practice and the healthcare system's leaders in R&D processes of regional businesses. The annual innovation conference was also well received, and the senior executive team committed themselves to support these initiatives and to allocate funding to ensure their success.

Questions

1. How do you think the three initiatives will facilitate the development of a culture of innovation in the healthcare system?
2. What types of incentives do you think would be necessary to encourage and facilitate innovation among clinical nurses or other clinical leaders in the healthcare setting?
3. How effective do you think the initiative to expose the system's leaders in the research and development of regional businesses will be in developing a culture of innovation?

4. What effect will advance nurses' knowledge and competence in evidence-based practice on innovations at the clinical level?
5. What purpose do the annual conferences for the evidence-based practice institute and the innovation conference serve in promoting a culture of innovation?

References

Albert, N. M. (2018). Operationalizing a nursing innovation center within a health care system. *Nursing Administration Quarterly, 42*(1), 43–53.

Bates, D. W., Sheikh, A., & Asch, D. A. (2017). Innovative environments in health care: Where and how new approaches to care are succeeding. *Health Affairs, 36*(3), 400–407.

Batras, D., Duff, C., & Smith, B. J. (2014). Organizational change theory: Implications for health promotion practice. *Health Promotion International, 31*(1), 231–241.

Berry, J., Noles, K., Eberhardt, A. W., & Wingo, N. (2019). Acceleration of clinical innovation: A collaboration between biomedical engineering, nursing and honors undergraduates. *Journal of Biomechanical Engineering, 141*(12), 121003.

Bismark, M. M., & Studdert, D. M. (2014). Governance of quality of care: A qualitative study of health service boards in Victoria, Australia. *BMJ Quality & Safety, 23*(6), 474–482.

Boston-Fleischhauer, C. (2016). Nurse executives wearing two hats as strategic leaders. *Journal of Nursing Administration, 46*(10), 487–489.

Brown, A. (2019). Understanding corporate governance of healthcare quality: A comparative case study of eight Australian public hospitals. *BMC Health Services Research, 19*(1), 725.

Bucknall, T., & Hitch, D. (2018). Connections, communication and collaboration in healthcare's complex adaptive systems comment on "using complexity and network concepts to inform healthcare knowledge translation." *International Journal of Health Policy and Management, 7*(6), 556–559.

Businger, A. C., Fuller, T. E., Schnipper, J. L., Rossetti, S. C., Schnock, K. O., Rozenblum, R., Dalal, A. K., Benneyan, J., Bates, D. W., & Dykes, P. C. (2020). Lessons learned implementing a complex and innovative patient safety learning laboratory project in a large academic medical center. *Journal of the American Medical Informatics Association, 27*(2), 301–307.

Chan, M. C., Bayer, A. M., Zunt, J. R., Blas, M. M., & Garcia, P. J. (2018). Kuskaya: a training program for collaboration and innovation in global health. *Journal of Multidisciplinary Healthcare, 12*, 31–42.

Clavelle, J. T., Porter-O'Grady, T., Weston, M., & Veran, J. (2016). Evolution of structural empowerment: Moving from shared to professional governance. *Journal of Nursing Administration, 46*(6), 308–312.

Cochrane, B. S. (2017). Leaders go first: Creating and sustaining a culture of high performance. *Healthcare Management Forum, 30*(5), 229–232.

Conger, M. D. (2016). Building a healthcare system's innovation program. *Frontiers in Health Services Management, 33*(2), 16–26.

Crow, G., & DeBourgh, G. (2017). Shared governance: The infrastructure for innovation. In S. Davidson, D. Weberg, T. Porter-O'Grady, & K. Malloch (Eds.), *Evidence-based innovation in nursing and health professions* (pp. 401–437). Jones & Bartlett Learning.

Davidson, S., Weberg, D., Porter-O'Grady, T., & Malloch, K. (2017). *Evidence-based innovation in nursing and health professions.* Jones & Bartlett Learning.

Desveaux, L., Soobiah, C., Bhatia, R. S., & Shaw, J. (2019). Identifying and overcoming policy-level barriers to the implementation of digital health innovation: Qualitative study. *Journal of Medical Internet Research, 21*(12), e14994.

Elrod, J. K., & Fortenberry, J. L. Jr. (2017). Peering beyond the walls of healthcare institutions: A catalyst for innovation. *BMC Health Services Research, 17*(Suppl 1), 402.

Fleiszer, A. R., Semenic, S. E., Ritchie, J. A., Richer, M. C., & Denis, J. L. (2016). Nursing unit leaders' influence on the long-term sustainability of evidence-based practice improvements. *Journal of Nursing Management, 24*(3), 309–318.

Franklin, C. M., Bernhardt, J. M., Lopez, R. P., Long-Middleton, E. R., & Davis, S. (2015). Interprofessional teamwork and collaboration between community health workers and healthcare teams: An integrative review. *Health Services Research and Managerial Epidemiology, 16*(2), 2333392815573312.

Garcia-Sierra, R., Fernández-Castro, J., & Martinez-Zsragoza, F. (2016). Work engagement in nursing: An integrative review of the literature. *Journal of Nursing Management, 24*(2), E101–E111.

Greenhalgh, T., & Abimbola, S. (2019). The NASSS framework—A synthesis of multiple theories of technology implementation. *Studies in Health Technology and Informatics, 263*, 193–204.

Hilligoss, B., Song, P. H., & McAlearney, A. S. (2017). Aligning for accountable care: Strategic practices for change in accountable care organizations. *Health Care Management Review, 42*(3), 192–202.

Jones, L., Pomeroy, L., Robert, G., Burnett, S., Anderson, J. E., & Fulop, N. J. (2017). How do hospital boards govern for quality improvement? A mixed methods study of 15 organizations in England. *BMJ Quality & Safety, 26*(12), 978–986.

Keynejad, R. C., Mekonnen, F. D., Qabile, A., Handuleh, J. I. M., Dahir, M. A., Haji Rabi, M. M., Read, C., & Adan Ismail, E. (2018). Gender equality in the global health workplace: Learning from a Somaliland–UK paired institutional partnership. *BMJ Global Health, 3*(6), e001073.

Liu, Y., Aungsuroch, Y., & Yunibhand, J. (2016). Job satisfaction in nursing: A concept analysis study. *International Nursing Review, 63*(1), 84–91.

Lynch, M., & Verner, E. (2013). Building a clinical leadership community to drive improvement: A multi-case educational study to inform 21st century clinical commissioning, professional capability and patient care. *Education for Primary Care, 24*(1), 22–28.

Malik, N., Dhar, R. L., & Handa, S. C. (2016). Authentic leadership and its impact on creativity of nursing staff: A cross sectional questionnaire survey of Indian nurses and their supervisors. *International Journal of Nursing Studies, 63*, 28–36.

Malloch, K., & Porter-O'Grady, T. (2017). Shifting workforce paradigms: From quantity to value-driven staffing using evidence and innovation. In S. Davidson, D. Weberg, T. Porter-O'Grady, & K. Malloch (Eds.), *Evidence-based innovation in nursing and health professions* (pp. 369–400). Jones & Bartlett Learning.

Marciano, P. L., & Wingrove, C. (2014). *SuperTeams using the principles of RESPECTT to unleash explosive business performance.* McGraw-Hill Education.

Mazhindu, D. M., Griffiths, L., Pook, C., Erskine, A., Ellis, R., & Smith, F. (2016). The nurse match investment: Exploring professional nurse identity and professional nursing values for future nurse recruitment. *Nurse Education in Practice, 18*, 36–45.

McCovery, J., & Matusitz, J. (2014). Assessment of collaboration in U.S. health care delivery: A perspective from systems theory. *Social Work in Public Health, 29*(5), 451–461.

McKimm, J. (2015). Clinical leadership effectiveness, change and complexity. *British Journal of Hospital Medicine, 76*(4), 239–243.

Minvielle, E., Waelli, M., Sicotte, C., & Kimberly, J. R. (2014). Managing customization in health care: A framework derived from the services sector literature. *Health Policy, 117*(2), 216–227.

Murray, Z. (2015). Community representation in hospital decision making: A literature review. *Australian Health Review, 39*(3), 323–328.

Pines, J. M., Farmer, S. A., & Akman, J. S. (2014). "Innovation" institutes in academic health centers: Enhancing value through leadership, education, engagement, and scholarship. *Academic Medicine: Journal of the Association of American Medical Colleges, 89*(9), 1204–1206.

Porter-O'Grady, T. (2013). Building the practice community. In M. Bahuth, K. Blum, & S. Simone (Eds.), *Transitioning into hospital-based practice: A guide for nurse practitioners and administrators* (pp. 181–204). Springer.

Porter-O'Grady, T. (2019a). Principles for sustaining shared/professional governance in nursing. *Nursing Management, 50*(1), 36–41.

Porter-O'Grady, T. (2019b). Turning the page: Nursing in the digital age and beyond. *Nursing Management, 50*(9), 40–47.

Porter-O'Grady, T., & Malloch, K. (2016). *The leadership of nursing practice.* Jones & Bartlett Learning.

Read, E. A. (2014). Workplace social capital in nursing: An evolutionary concept analysis. *Journal of Advanced Nursing, 70*(5), 997–1007.

Rounds, K. E., McGrath, B. B., & Walsh, E. (2013). Perspectives on provider behaviors: A qualitative study of sexual and gender minorities regarding quality of care. *Contemporary Nurse.* doi:10.5172/conu.2013.2440

Rubin, G. D., & Abramson, R. G. (2018). Creating value through incremental innovation: Managing culture, structure and process. *Radiology, 288*(2), 330–340.

Rumball-Smith, J., Ross, K., & Bates, D. W. (2020). Late adopters of the electronic health record should move now. *BMJ Quality and Safety, 29*(3), 238–240.

Samet, K. A., & Smith, M. S. (2016). Thinking differently: Catalyzing innovation in healthcare and beyond. *Frontiers in Health Services Management, 33*(2), 3–15.

Sangaleti, C., Schveitzer, M. C., Peduzzi, M., Zoboli, E. L. C. P., & Soares, C. B. (2017). Experiences and shared meaning of teamwork and interprofessional collaboration among health care professionals in primary health care settings: A systematic review. *JBI Database of Systematic Reviews and Implementation Reports, 15*(11), 2723–2788.

Saxěn, S. (2018). Same principles, different worlds: A critical discourse analysis of medical ethics and nursing ethics in Finnish professional texts. *HEC Forum, 30*(1), 31–55.

Schultz, S., Abercrombie, S., Crownover, B., Hoekzema, G., Krug, N., Maxwell, L., Mazzone, M., Mitchell, K., Shaffer, T., & Tuggy, M. (2013). Accountable care organizations: An opportunity for synergy. *Annals of Family Medicine, 11*(3), 283–284.

Setoodegan, E., Gholamzadeh, S., Rakshan, M., & Peiravi, H. (2019). Nurses' lived experiences of professional autonomy in Iran. *International Journal of Nursing Sciences, 23*(6), 315–321.

Thayer, A. L., Petruzzelli, A., & McClurg, C. E. (2018). Addressing the paradox of the team innovation process: A review of practical considerations. *The American Psychologist, 73*(4), 363–375.

Thompson, J., Schwatka, N. V., Tenney, L., & Newman, L. S. (2018). Total worker health: A small business leader perspective. *International Journal of Environmental Research and Public Health, 15*(11), pii. E2416.

Valaitis, R., MacDonald, M., Kothari, A., O'Mara, L., Regan, S., Garcia, J., Murray, N., Manson, H., Peroff-Johnston, N., Bursey, G., & Boyko, J. (2016). Moving towards a new vision: Implementation of public health policy intervention. *BMC Public Health, 16*, 412.

Weatherford, B., Bower, K. A., & Vitello-Cicciu, J. (2018). The CNO and leading innovation. Competencies for the future. *Nursing Administration Quarterly, 42*(1), 76–82.

Wiljer, D., & Hakim, Z. (2019). Developing an artificial intelligence-enabled health care practice: Rewiring health care professions for better care. *Journal of Medical Imaging and Radiation Sciences, 50*(4S2), S8–S14.

Willis, C. D., Saul, J., Bevan, H., Scheirer, M. A., Best, A., Greenhalgh, T., Mannion, R., Cornelissen, E., Howland, D., Jenkins, E., & Bitz, J. (2016). Sustaining organizational culture change in health systems. *Journal of Health Organization and Management, 30*(1), 2–30.

Wong, F. K., Liu, H., Wang, H., Anderson, D., Seib, C., & Molasiotis, A. (2015). Global nursing issues and development: Analysis of World Health Organization documents. *Journal of Nursing Scholarship, 47*(6), 574–583.

Yarbrough, S., Martin, P., Alfred, D., & McNeill, C. (2017). Professional values, job satisfaction, career development, and intent to stay. *Nursing Ethics, 24*(6), 675–685.

Zuber, C. D., & Moody, L. (2018). Creativity and innovation in health care: Tapping into organizational enablers through human-centered design. *Nursing Administration Quarterly, 42*(1), 62–75.

Suggested Readings

Cristiansen, C., Johnson, C., & Horn, M. (2008). *Disrupting class: How disruptive innovation will change the way the world learns*. McGraw-Hill.

Metcalf, M. (2012). *Innovation leadership: Workbook for emerging managers and leaders*. Integral.

Ness, R. (2012). *Innovation generation*. Oxford University Press.

Skarzynski, P., & Gibson, R. (2008). *Innovation to the core*. Harvard Business School Press.

Terwindt, F., Rajan, D., & Soucat, A. (2016). Priority setting for national health policies, strategies and plans. In G. Schmets, D. Rajan, & S. Kadandale (Eds.). *Strategizing national health in the 21st century: A handbook* (Chapter 4). World Health Organization.

Quiz Questions

Select the best answer for each of the following questions.

1. Which of the following best defines *disruptive technologies*?
    a. Normal changes that alter the way things work
    b. Radical changes that result from normal evolution
    c. Significant shifts that alter how we think, act, and behave
    d. The results of changing how an existing product or service looks and works

2. How has medical superiority and decision making, including financial support of nursing services, directly affected the nursing profession?
    a. It created a lack of interdisciplinary collaboration, linkage, and interaction.
    b. It removed practice boundaries that limit nursing scope of practice.
    c. It removed political and legislative limitations to clinical practice opportunities.
    d. It created a desire for nurses to seek evidence-based clinical practices.

3. How does focus on functionalism and process-oriented work affect innovation?
    a. It eliminates responsiveness to innovation-based solutions.
    b. It encourages practical foundations for innovation.
    c. It connects innovation to real work issues.
    d. It maintains a focus on innovation within work.

4. Equity is essential to innovation for which of the following reasons?
   a. Everyone does equal work in the organization.
   b. Equity reflects the value placed on an individual and his or her work.
   c. It is important to acknowledge that not everyone's work has equal value.
   d. Knowing what work contributes to innovation and what work does not is important.

5. The term *professions* differs from the term *employees* in which important way? Professions:
   a. make more money.
   b. are more important to the work of the organization.
   c. are directed by their social mandate for the people they serve.
   d. are not obligated to the members with which they relate.

6. *Worker motivation* can be described as:
   a. an increase in monetary rewards to get better work performance.
   b. internal values that direct and satisfy individuals in their work.
   c. encouraging, directing, and reinforcing workers to be more productive.
   d. helping workers feel better about their work so they want to do more.

7. Why is innovation always driven from the point-of-service?
   a. Investment, engagement, and ownership of the outcomes of work are directly located.
   b. People do more work there, and that is where the money is made.
   c. People are more creative and innovative when they are on the front lines.
   d. People will do new things close to the places where they do the work.

8. Why is partnership among the board, executives, and managers critical to innovation?
   a. The staff are required to do what the board and managers determine.
   b. Executives and managers generally do what the board directs.
   c. Managers are primarily accountable for making sure the organization works.
   d. Each group has a specific role to play in the innovation process to make it successful.

9. Why are first-line managers the most important leader group in the innovation process?
   a. They know more about what is really going on in the organization.
   b. Their proximity to the point-of-service creates a strong partnership with the place where innovation becomes action.
   c. They do what they are told and know how to get the staff "on board."
   d. They can translate change in a way staff can best understand.

10. Which of the following characteristics demonstrates that an organization is innovative?
    a. The board of governors is willing to be ready for the next change.
    b. First-line leaders constantly create new products and ways of doing work.
    c. Members use collaboration and integration to demonstrate their commitment to their organization's vitality in the presence of change.
    d. Leadership staff ensures that their organization can survive and produce new products and ways of working.

11. In the current age the leader must now:
    a. create both a strategic and structural imperative that incorporates new and emerging technologies and innovation as a "way of doing business."
    b. change daily functions and activities to better reflect the requirements of the organization.
    c. adjust current practices so that they better reflect the contemporary demands of daily healthcare practice.
    d. help non-leaders to support the organization's current practices and a changing environment.

12. The primacy of the physician's role has:
    a. been reaffirmed by health reform and now calls physicians to help guide other disciplines into value-based practices.
    b. been redefined so the position now plays a secondary role to policy makers in making decisions about medical practices and healthcare delivery.
    c. been altered in an environment that now requires collaboration and partnership across the disciplines in order to serve patients better in a value-based delivery system.
    d. been redefined by health reform in a way that affects their role and significance in care delivery decisions.

13. Equity is a statement of:
    a. clarity.
    b. economics.
    c. equality.
    d. value.

14. In the contemporary age, building communities of practice and partnership is essential to the future of health care; therefore, it is:
    a. the requirements of each discipline to direct their own work and define their own parameters in advancing quality health care.
    b. the obligation of individual practitioners to demonstrate their specific and unique contribution to the aggregate contribution of all disciplines in advancing health care.
    c. the obligation of all disciplines to work together to define one set of practices with which they will all engage to advance the health of the community.
    d. the responsibility of users of healthcare services to more fully participate in directing healthcare practices in ways that best meet their own needs.

15. One of the first steps necessary to building a context that truly stimulates and sustains innovation is:
    a. more clearly defining the manager's role and positional authority.
    b. more specifically defining the role of the practitioner at the point-of-service.
    c. the reconfiguration of infrastructure to be based on decisional accountability.
    d. a better orientation of the board to the work of the healthcare system and to the priorities that now drive it.

16. Locus of control means that:
    a. managers drive all decisions and take accountability for decisional responses at the point-of-service.
    b. staff assume responsibility for decisions that were traditionally the role of the manager.
    c. organizational leadership must determine the most effective place to take action.
    d. decisions and actions are located at the most legitimate place where they are effectively acted upon.

17. In all living systems and networks, homeostatic mechanisms:
    a. are the essential linkage between smaller and larger system elements to which the interaction and convergence of smaller elements contribute.
    b. are a hierarchy of linked and integrated control mechanisms operating throughout a system.
    c. represent the diversity of mechanisms that represent the unique and individual characteristic of each element in the system.
    d. are the clear compartmentalization of tasks and functions of each element and process.

18. The life of all systems is driven from:
    a. the bottom of a system.
    b. the top of a system.
    c. laterally, from the outside in.
    d. from its center or point-of-service.

19. Alignment, not motivation, is critical to the effective functioning of any system because:
    a. motivation is an externally generated capacity and therefore cannot be managed.
    b. alignment creates the critical context for innovation and action.
    c. alignment eliminates the need for personal motivation and stimulates consistency in action.
    d. motivation requires the use of external resources like pay and benefits to change behavior.

20. It is virtually impossible to undertake the activities of innovation in a "closed" environment with rigid hierarchy, tight control, compartmentalized structure, and narrowly vertical organizational structures.
    a. True
    b. False

21. In work environments predominately composed of professionals (knowledge workers), professional governance structures that ensure that stakeholders are represented and engaged in decision making reduce the opportunity for involvement, creativity, and innovation.
    a. True
    b. False

22. The central tenet of value recognizes that:
    a. all people are committed to collective action.
    b. all work is inherently valuable.
    c. people are involved in personal activity that validates their value in the world.
    d. people will give up personal identity, meaning, and value to advance the meaning of their work.

23. In an innovative organization, the role of the board is to:
    a. support and select strategy and the organizational constructs necessary to advance dynamic innovation.
    b. direct the activities of the organization to ensure that innovation occurs as a part of the work of the organization.
    c. direct and guide management/leadership to undertake innovation in advancing the interests and viability of the organization.
    d. make decisions about the organization's work and function to succeed in a competitive healthcare environment.

24. The primary role of the first-line leader in an innovative organization is to:
    a. create an operating milieu (a context) that supports and interfaces with the action of innovation at the point-of-service.
    b. drive innovation by creating innovative priorities and engaging the staff in fulfilling them.
    c. help staff understand their role in relationship to innovation, provide them the strategy and processes, and support them in implementing innovation.
    d. fulfill the obligations for implementing strategy defined by executive leadership and ensure staff behaviors and practices operate in a way consistent with board requisites.

25. It is incumbent upon the point-of-service leader to create a context for:
    a. employee solidarity with the innovation requisites of the organization.
    b. creativity and innovation that reflects more horizontal and adult-to-adult relationships among all members of the service and unit.
    c. compliance with manager-defined innovation priorities for the unit or service.
    d. unilaterally driven employee creativity and engagement of specific innovations in a way that results in high levels of employee satisfaction.

CHAPTER FIVE

From Evidence to Innovation: Measuring the Foundations of Practice and Value

We cannot deny our connectedness while we build our separateness.
—M. J. Wheatley and M. Kellner-Rogers (1996)[1]

Chapter Objectives

At the completion of this chapter, the reader will be able to:

- List five major drivers for documentation of value-based outcomes.
- Discuss the leadership challenges in selecting metrics for healthcare organization evaluation.
- Describe innovative leadership strategies for measurement in complex social systems.
- Gain an appreciation of the realities and challenges of creating more robust measurement models reflecting the complexity of health care.

There is a great and pressing need to reformulate the way in which health care is valued, measured, and reimbursed. Quantum leaders have experienced both the challenges of linear measurement models and the potential for integration of complexity principles into the healthcare system measurement models. Further, quantum leaders are well positioned to lead initiatives that challenge current measurement assumptions and create models more reflective of the complex nature of healthcare work.

The purpose of this chapter is not to provide a template for measurement, but rather to offer a new lens for healthcare leaders to consider, compile, synthesize, and evaluate the multiple variables of the healthcare experience. Necessarily, each organization must customize its measurement model to include industry standards and facility-specific measures reflective of its mission and vision. Leaders can create revitalized measurement templates specific to their organizational

---

[1] Reprinted with permission of the publisher. From *A simpler way*, copyright © 1996 by Wheatley, M. J., & Kellner-Rogers, M., p. 51. Berrett-Koehler Publishers, Inc., San Francisco, CA. All rights reserved. www.bkconnection.com

context. Also in this chapter, the challenges of measuring health care and suggestions for reconceptualizing healthcare measurement using the characteristics of complexity are presented.

Key Drivers for Change

The need to challenge current assumptions and create more robust models emanates from multiple sources and issues. Five major issues are discussed in this section and serve to stimulate action. The Points to Ponder challenge each of us to think differently and consider new strategies that can be useful to reach effective measurement and valuing of health care in the United States. The Points to Ponder comments include explorative ideas, challenges, and thoughts about the assumptions that currently drive the healthcare system. The first issue, not surprisingly, is the belief that health care is too costly.

Issue: Cost

The general notion is that health care in the United States is too costly and that the quality of outcomes are less than desirable. Total U.S. national health expenditures as a percentage of gross domestic product (GDP) in 2018 was 17.7%, and health spending for hospital care increased at nearly the same rate in 2018 as in 2017 (Centers for Medicare & Medicaid Services, 2019). Further, patient safety did not substantially improve following the release of the landmark 1999 Institute of Medicine (IOM) report. For example, based on data from 2015 to 2017, disease burden was higher in the United States than in other comparable countries; hospital admissions for preventable chronic conditions (worsening heart failure, asthma, and diabetes) were higher in the United States than in other comparable countries; the United States had the highest rates of medical, medication, and laboratory errors compared to other countries; and in nearly all comparable countries, adults had quicker access to a doctor or nurse when they needed care than did adults in the United States (Peterson-KFF, 2019). In addition, the Affordable Care Act requirements to achieve full or nearly full access for Americans continues to present challenges for managing the cost–quality equation (Olsson et al., 2020).

> **Points to Ponder**
>
> If we are spending too much, how much are we willing to spend? And what level of quality are we willing to fund? Is the real issue how much we spend, or is it the quality and consistency of outcomes? Common understanding is that health care is too costly. Should there be a different question, or many different questions, that would inform us what the dollars should achieve and how much the United States is willing to spend? What kind of health care could we have if the expenditures were at 10% of the GDP, or one-half of what is currently spent on health care? What services at what level of quality are we willing to pay for? If the next phase of the Patient Protection and Affordable Care Act healthcare reform efforts were based on a defined amount of expenditure, level of quality, and defined access, would the recommendations be different or more acceptable? Perhaps a new valuation process that integrates the costs and value of innovation should be considered.

Issue: Cost Shifting

The cost of health care is affected not only by the actual services provided and supporting technologies but also by numerous well-intended initiatives designed to control those costs. Regulations, both national and local, are in place to control and monitor costs and quality. Price adjustments and cost shifting serve to "even the playing field" for payers, providers, and patients. Sophisticated mechanisms to control access to care and payment for services further complicate the system. Not surprisingly, there is an unending quest to reduce the disparity between healthcare costs and quality; however, achievement of this admirable goal has eluded the U.S. healthcare system. Shifting costs between payers has become normative (e.g., in patients with irritable bowel diseases, fewer hospitalizations were replaced by dramatically higher pharmacy expenses; Click et al., 2019); however, fairness of cost-shifting practices is seldom fully supported. Incredible attempts are made to level the payment structure in a social system that is multitiered and based on individual values and rights.

Issue: Demand Without Accountability

Citizens of the United States believe that there should be no limits on access to treatment. Healthcare access and available treatment is believed to be an inherent right for every individual. Further, to date, there have been no expectations of boundaries for receiving care, and importantly, no accountability for healthy behaviors as a requirement for receiving healthcare service funding. Funding continues to be provided to individuals, regardless of engagement or disengagement in healthy behaviors or adherence or nonadherence to self-care expectations (including taking prescription medications) that minimize exacerbation of existing conditions. Healthcare funding is based on a one-way model: presence of illness or disease. Healthcare demands are linked to historical and social developments, and accountability is based on many factors, including citizen knowledge and capability; demographic, socioeconomic, and other patient-related factors; comorbidities and current health status; and a national consensus on the definition of optimal health care when healthy and in acute and chronic diseases. Both themes are complex, interwoven, and challenging to healthcare systems.

Issue: Partial Measurement and Avoidance of Ambiguous Evidence

Measuring empirical or observable and easily quantifiable variables has dominated the healthcare system. Traditional finance references identify metrics for returns on investment, ratios for cash management, and allocation percentages for expense categories (**Table 5-1**). The use of mathematical tools such as graphs, charts, and statistical formulas provides important data that are easily understood. Unfortunately, measurement of selected healthcare elements is often used to inform the totality of the system. In general, they are insufficient to capture the complexity of healthcare work. Although mathematical tools have value, they also have limitations when applied to the nonlinear and multidimensional processes of health care. In the current model, reimbursement is provided for selected and discrete clinical interventions or procedures regardless of the surrounding circumstances and patient status or values. Finally, with the explosion of healthcare papers and the emergence of online journals, a lot of evidence is available on healthcare cost and quality themes. A quantum leader must be able to differentiate high-strength and quality papers from those that do not provide generalizable data or that have errors related to metrics selected, data analysis, or implications.

> **Points to Ponder**
>
> In a free and democratic society, will individuals who are more successful or fortunate always need to subsidize individuals who are less fortunate? Is there a better way to support less fortunate individuals? Is a national health plan the only way to eliminate or control cost shifting? In the United States, should health care be a right to all or a privilege to those who can fund health care—that is, those who have resources for payment?

TABLE 5-1 Complexity and Healthcare Measurement Implications

Property Complexity Description	Implication for Healthcare Measurement
Connectivity	• One standard metric is seldom adequate to tell the story. When measuring, ask the question, "Did the results affect any other metrics?" If hours of care were decreased, were the necessary services provided to ensure the desired level of quality?
Interdependence	• Reliance on other elements of the healthcare system is the norm. • There's more to consider than the financial return on investment. Utility, effectiveness, health, quality of life, and functionality must also be considered.
Emergence	• Be available for unpredictable results/outcomes/events. • Unintended and unanticipated consequences often occur after implementation of or correction of another problem, creating the need to consider other information. • Highly structured forecasting and planning may be of limited value. • Identify "anticipatory metrics"—what could happen with this decision? • Examine traditional metrics and at least three additional sequential evolving metrics to increase awareness of the impact of emergence. • When measuring, focus on principles rather than specific goals and targets. • Be open and available to reconsider existing opinions.

Can we really afford one-way health care? Is the best practice to give and give and give without the expectation for healthy behaviors? The failure of fully engaged patient–provider relationships unnecessarily increases the cost of healthcare services. How do we engage patients in the healthcare process to ensure full-circle accountability within the system?

Until the advent of the CAHPS (Consumer Assessment of Healthcare Providers and Systems) family of surveys and the Patient Protection and Affordable Care Act, ambiguous or qualitative information on patient–provider relationships, effectiveness of procedures, patient satisfaction with care and services, and healthy behaviors practiced were not considered in the reimbursement system (**Exhibit 5-1**). Following the Institute of Medicine's development of a definition of "quality health outcomes," many conceptual and theoretical models emerged to guide research and program development. In Fawcett and Ellenbecker's (2015) proposed conceptual model of nursing and population health, upstream factors, population factors, health system factors, and nursing activities were all identified as components influencing population health outcomes of wellness, disease burden, functional status, life expectancy, mortality, and quality of life.

> **Points to Ponder**
>
> Individuals desire to have all health care without personal accountability, and providers have a propensity to "overhelp," rendering the current system disastrously dysfunctional. Why is it so difficult for Americans to say no when not enough resources are available to match demand? Will changing spending behaviors change the state of the U.S. healthcare system? Will changing our expectations become the best first step to reform? Is it possible to change the healthcare expectations of all citizens? Can we work to guarantee a level of basic services? Should U.S. citizens bite the bullet and continue to give more dollars to the healthcare system? Should every available healthcare service be available to every citizen regardless of the cost?

Exhibit 5-1 The HCAHPS Survey

29 items; 22 substantive items that encompass critical aspects of the hospital experience.

Categories
- Communication with doctors
- Communication with nurses
- Responsiveness of hospital staff
- Cleanliness of hospital environment
- Quietness of hospital environment
- Pain management
- Communication about medicines
- Discharge information
- Overall rating of hospital
- Recommendation of hospital
- Understanding care expectations after leaving the hospital

Data from Centers for Medicare & Medicaid Services. (n.d.). CAHPS® hospital survey. https://hcahpsonline.org/

As discussed earlier, there is more to the healthcare experience than net income margins, cost per case, and hours per patient day (HPPD). Every metric has a story connected to interdependent measures of quality and quantity. Historically, ambiguous evidence such as relationship effectiveness, surveillance work, and team collaboration measurement were avoided. The adage that you cannot manage what you do not measure has been used in healthcare quality and measurement discussions, and this idea further challenges us to develop systems that measure and account for what is valued and managed (Colla et al., 2015; Nordin et al., 2017). Documentation and accounting for the relational and qualitative aspects of patient care in the healthcare model need to be identified and connected to the system. To begin, the antecedents, concurrent processes or interventions, and unplanned outcomes need to be identified and linked to each financial metric, and measurement should include low-value, wasteful, and harmful healthcare services as a prerequisite to improving quality and eliminating waste.

Interestingly, healthcare systems are working desperately to improve the quality of health care, manage relationships, consider the impact of the context in which health care occurs, and integrate patient personal values into care processes. Unfortunately, the emphasis is on creating more discrete and isolated measures rather than inclusion of measures reflective of these variables. Formation of relationships, work of clinical surveillance and oversight, engagement of team members and patients, and perceptions of quality and respect are but a few of the important concepts to which it is difficult to assign quantifiable metrics and dollars.

> **Points to Ponder**
>
> Getting an accurate read on situations may be harder than it appears. Information is filtered, unpopular opinions are avoided, emotional entanglements and tensions are purposely circumvented, and partisan views are veiled as objective arguments. The same can be said for getting an accurate accounting on healthcare services. Too often, the challenges in selecting the most appropriate groupings of financial and quality metrics are insurmountable, and leaders settle on financial and volume measures and standardized quality measures because they become the only thing a leadership team can agree on.

Patient satisfaction measures are rigorous for what they measure. What does not occur regularly is documentation of the story they tell—the connections and interdependencies among providers, patient care processes, values, and the context of care. For example, the events and resources required to achieve levels of patient satisfaction are seldom if ever identified and at best are only inferred.

> ## Group Discussion
>
> The foolproof elasticity formula is believed by some to be critical to successful operations and management. For example, if the cost of care for 5 patients is $50,000, then the elasticity formula dictates that the cost of care for 10 patients would be $100,000, and the cost of care for 20 patients would be $200,000 and so on. Unfortunately, the complexity of the processes and resources involved in patient care render this formula invalid and unreliable. In your discussion group, identify a list of variations that occur in patient care and invalidate the elasticity formula.

The pathway to a meaningful measurement system is not found in magical analyses of costs, charges, and profits. Despite the quest for a foolproof elasticity formula (see the Group Discussion), a formula in which changes are predictable based on past experiences is, at best, incomplete. With formulas, there is always a clarification, an exception, or a confounding variable that marginalizes the value of the formulation. At best, formulas are a beginning, not the final word.

As previously noted, avoiding inclusion of the contextual information (environment, resources, etc.) can be disastrous and costly. Single-source financial metrics can lead to decisions that are short-sighted and incomplete. Further, when one entity tries to improve its fitness or position, it may result in a worsening condition for others. Each "improvement" in one entity therefore may impose associated costs on other entities, either within the same system or on other related systems.

> **Key Point**
> **The following are tips for unravelling ambiguous evidence:**
> 1. Scrutinize and unravel preconceptions.
> 2. Let high-strength, high-quality evidence be your guide.
> 3. Focus on the source (point-of-care or intersection between patient and caregiver) not the second- or third-hand interpretation. Minimize filters of information or interpretations by those removed from the actual situation (use direct evidence from source authors).
> 4. Look around the event. Examine and integrate the connections, antecedents, and subsequent events of healthcare work.
> 5. Tell the story using measurement language and concepts.

Issue: Using Evidence Is Optional

Evidentiary information is inconsistently identified and applied in patient care (Melnyk et al., 2018). The source of the inconsistency is widespread and ranges from lack of knowledge or access to current evidence to personal practice preferences. In national studies, authors documented the significance of evidence-based practice and its relationship to higher quality of care, improved patient outcomes, decreased geographic variations in the delivery of care, reduced healthcare costs, and greater job satisfaction (Durante et al., 2019; Krans et al., 2019; Theofanidis & Gibbon, 2016; Yun & Choi, 2019). The current adoption rates for the provision of care based on evidence, caregiver expertise, and patient values is unconscionably slow.

Perhaps greater accountability and ownership of health care should be placed on providers and caregivers in addition to organizational leadership. Given the clearly defined scopes of practice, licensing regulations, and independent practice models, it would seem that more emphasis should be placed on the source of the practice. This is not to minimize the role of the organization and leadership in creating the appropriate context for evidence-based practice, rather it is shifting the accountability to the locus of practice. It is about shifting from being rule or policy driven to principle driven. The principle of patient safety that is adopted by every employee should negate the need for innumerable policies and procedures telling individuals how to be safe!

> **Key Point**
> Focus on principles versus specific actions or rules. It may feel comfortable to develop an annual quality plan with sharply defined strategies and targets, but a better approach is to outline general goals and boundaries for improvement through which the organization moves toward the desired emergence.

The six major issues of high cost, low quality, cost shifting, demand without accountability, partial measurement, and the inconsistent use of evidence provide significant incentives for us to consider the healthcare system in a different way. Given the current state of disarray and dysfunction in our system, continuing with the same practices and valuation model can only perpetuate more of the same. A measurement system that reflects the complexity of health care is desperately needed, one that provides evidence to assist individuals to address these issues and improve the allocation of healthcare resources more effectively.

A Very Complex System

Other healthcare challenges could be added to the list; however, the six issues that have been raised describe the major problems emanating from the complexity of the healthcare system and serve as the foundation for the creation of a contemporary healthcare valuation model. In this section, a discussion of the phenomena of complex systems—connectedness, interdependence, emergence, and uncertainty—is provided to further inform the new valuation model.

Complexity science rejects the belief that systems and processes are like machines with parts that can be separated, analyzed, and modified or replaced. All healthcare organizations are complex and evolving social systems with innumerable behaviors, not mechanical assembly-line models. The realities of complexity are evident in nearly every aspect of the healthcare system and

> **Points to Ponder**
> Using available evidence seems so logical. The increasing availability of computerized systems and availability of the internet to most providers and patients strongly support the use of evidence in practice. Such strategies as linking the use of federal or state funds to evidence-based practice and penalties for failure to use state-of-the-art practices deserve careful consideration. The IOM goal to have 90% of clinical decisions based on evidence by 2020 is ambitious and requires all leaders to embrace it and clearly link it to organizational productivity and quality metrics.

> **Key Point**
>
> An example of selecting and analyzing an isolated component is the root cause analysis model. Organizations have typically approached complex problems from the angle of ferreting out and eliminating specific factors (root causes) thought to be responsible for undesired results. In fact, targeting precise improvement strategies toward singular root causes may result in the unpleasant and unexpected emergence of new problem-laden systems. The key to mastering desired change begins with a focus on holistic systems and the relationships among components in those systems.

can better inform how healthcare value can be determined and documented more effectively. What is not evident or understandable is the continuing reliance on mechanistic models of thinking and measurement; thus, these principles are discussed as impetus to rethink the current model.

Connectivity and Interdependence

In complex systems, all things intersect and interact with each other and necessarily provide the energy to sustain and enhance the life of the system. No person, event, or process is ever fully isolated or immune from influences of other persons, events, or processes. Intuitively and intellectually, leaders recognize this reality, yet they operate on the premise that events and individuals are isolated and processes are linear. Table 5-1 includes a description of complexity principles and the implications for healthcare measurement.

The implications for the healthcare system are significant. Connectivity means that a decision or action by any individual (group, organization, institution, or human system) affects other individuals and systems. That effect may not have equal or uniform impact and will vary with the "state" of each related individual and system at the time. The connections or relationships between events provide the essential information to create an accurate representation of what needs to be considered for valuation. Documenting and determining value in an organization necessarily include valuing of the relationships and interdependencies among components in a system and the impact of those relationships as an essential part of the value statement. For example, the trajectory of communication is seldom linear or unidirectional. Communication may emanate from one individual and ultimately connect to numerous other individuals. The interactions and interdependencies in the worlds of patients, families, visitors, and healthcare professionals result in innumerable communication pathways and variables.

Beyond simple connectivity of elements of a system, relationships and dependence among elements quickly emerge as entities collaborate and support each other (**Figure 5-1**). Interdependence occurs among individuals within a system and between systems. Individual components in a process or system are not independent of other factors of the environment, technology, or political influence. Interdependence assumes mutual reliance on individuals and entities of a system. Behaviors and systems in which health care occurs are multidimensional, with multiple dimensions interacting and influencing each other. The social, cultural, technical, economic, and global dimensions continually interact and intertwine in the creation of healthcare outcomes.

Emergence and Uncertainty

In a complex and highly interconnected system, the future is rarely known and only somewhat predictable. Beyond our connections and interdependencies, systems offer us the possibility of becoming something different: the possibility to emerge into entirely new ways of being.

Emergence and Uncertainty

Figure 5-1 Diagram of Interconnectedness.
©VLADGRIN/Shutterstock

Group Discussion

Emergence and the electronic health record
From the implementation of the electronic medical record, new challenges and opportunities emerge. Brainstorm with your team members a list of positive emergent events and negative emergent events.

- Were these events anticipated?
- What is the cost of the events?
- Finally, create a mind map of all of the emergent events that occurred to further illuminate the concepts of connectivity and interdependence.

Emergence of virtual reality in nursing orientation/education
As new methodologies are used to educate hospital-based clinical nurses in critical thinking, new challenges and opportunities emerge. Brainstorm with your team members a list of positive emergent events and negative emergent events. What is the likelihood that these events will occur? Explain.

> **Key Point**
>
> We witness emergence any time individuals come together and accomplish more than what was thought possible. The collective wisdom and creativity of individuals seldom disappoint us.

> **Key Point**
>
> No metric, such as hours per patient day or salary expense, should ever stand alone. Each metric has an important and essential story that cannot be isolated and considered as a complete representation of the work.

Emergence, or the evolution of new behaviors, relationships, processes, and products is the result of our interdependencies. This reality requires recognition of these phenomena and accounting for the management of the uncertainty or essential course corrections that must continually occur. Emergence is evident in the basic nature of patient care. To illustrate further, patient care is often guided by standards of care and algorithms for evidence-driven practices; however, despite the best map for care, the actual care is determined when all of the information and conditions connect. In essence, patient care is *underdetermined* until the situation is at hand and the caregiver and patient are engaged. The time of day, presence of family, mental and emotional status of the patient, and level of pain all converge to determine what and how care will actually happen.

Although glaringly obvious, these fundamental characteristics of our healthcare systems are not central to mainstream business management and leadership, where the focus is largely on measuring and controlling certain system components, discrete financial indicators, and specific performance goals.

The driving assumptions for a new model focus on addressing current issues and recognizing the complexity of the work and expectations for ongoing evolution and course corrections as the future unfolds. Quantum leaders can now guide their organizations in the development of more robust models for the valuation of health care. The goal is to measure the reality as completely and accurately as possible. A new model for healthcare valuation must necessarily serve to document traditional financial data as well as the value of teamwork, patient–provider engagement, and the degree of evidence integration.

New Healthcare Valuation Model

Given the complex nature of the healthcare experience, traditional metrics viewed in isolation are limiting and short-sighted for effective decision making in health care. Financial metrics should be the beginning and not the end for measurement of healthcare effectiveness. Evaluation should occur in light of multiple, interconnected variables rather than a single traditional financial metric. Multiple metrics and information are needed specific to the achievement of goals and patient experiences as well as financial resources in the determination of healthcare value (Valentijn et al., 2016). No metric should ever stand alone for decision making without a supporting story. The following strategies are presented to begin the value transformation.

Strategy 1: Document the Story

A healthcare system driven by cure of disease, promotion of health, and prevention of disease is not sustainable if the context is not considered in every step of the process and evaluation. It should never be assumed that practices that work well in one place can simply be transplanted elsewhere. Replication of practices in another environment or patient population ignores the notion that systems that appear analogous often have underlying differences. This is not to say that healthcare quality's current emphasis on transplanting best practices is ill-placed but rather that common sense, flexibility, and a smattering of creativity must accompany the introduction of any new practice into an organization. Using patient-centered care approaches, such as listening to patients explain their diagnoses, helps clinicians understand complex situations and also helps patients understand the interdependencies affecting their health (Khan et al., 2018). Insightful leaders encourage their organization to consider how the organization's unique norms, histories, values, and processes may impede or facilitate adoption of guidelines, recommendations, and other improvement strategies.

Group Discussion

Create a story or narrative that identifies connections, interdependencies, accountability, evidence, and evolving conditions. Describe both the realized past scenario and the desired future(s). Narratives include the individuals, their roles and motives, relationships between the individuals, the activities, and the potential outcomes. The narrative of what actually occurred serves to document the connections, interdependencies, and emerging events. The desired narrative serves to document how patient needs are evolving, which new provider services are being offered, and the challenges occurring in the environment.

Consider the ever-present expectation to increase profitability (see **Exhibit 5-2**). A long-held assumption is that the profit margin can be controlled by clearly defined and discrete actions or individuals. Mandating a change in financial processes or expenditures is believed to be the requisite for success. The reality is that the profit margin is affected by many unknown and evolving influences and is connected to and intertwined with nearly every variable within the healthcare system. The traditional model with its well-intentioned steps to cut expenses at believed intervention points requires serious reconsideration. Consider the following two scenarios in which two approaches were used: (1) the traditional mandate for expense reductions (Story A) and (2) the more contemporary shared leadership approach to increasing revenues (Story B). The process focus begins with decreasing expenses by selected percentages. However, the trajectory and interdependence of the impact of this action are seldom articulated. A decrease in labor hours affects far more than the individual whose hours are reduced.

The outcomes from Exhibit 5-2 of Story A and Story B are successful from the perspective of the target goal; however, the connecting variables were affected quite differently. In Story A, the effect on staff and patient satisfaction was decidedly negative. Patient safety and quality were also negatively affected, as was long-term caregiver turnover. The results in Story B are quite different. This approach sought to engage caregivers and support staff in addressing the challenge to increase the profit margin. Not only did the revenues increase with minimal increases in expenses, but the approach also increased caregiver satisfaction and long-term tenure. No negative impacts on patient satisfaction were identified.

Exhibit 5-2 Profitability of Two Healthcare System Facilities: Story A and B

A 15% increase in profitability was the target for two facilities in a large healthcare system. Both facilities achieved their goal.

Story A
To achieve this increase in profitability, the facility implemented an initiative to decrease expenses, beginning with labor hours. All staff hours were decreased by 20% to achieve the desired increase in profitability. To achieve the decrease in labor hours, nurses increased the number of patients cared for, decreased hourly rounds to twice a shift, and decreased discussion of medications with patients during medication administration. As a result, patient satisfaction decreased specific to response time to call lights, understanding of medications decreased, and the number of falls with injury increased. Further, nurse turnover increased and job satisfaction decreased.

Story B
To achieve the increase in profitability, the facility engaged the shared leadership councils to develop innovative ways to increase revenue. Three creative online projects were developed to package the facility's unique clinical standards and practices for clinical simulation, technology adoption, and transplant services to other organizations. Marketing staff assisted with both national and international advertising for Asia, Japan, and Australia. A total of 160 staff hours were required to create the new revenue center and begin generating revenue. Specific metrics that were affected include caregiver satisfaction, labor hours for creation of the new center, and internet support for the service.

Measurement Category	Story A	Story B
Revenue	Unchanged	↑3%
Expenses	↓15%	↑0.5%
Labor hours	↓15%	↑0.5%
Nurse-to-patient ratio	↑25%	Unchanged
Patient satisfaction with response for call light	↓10%	Unchanged
Patient satisfaction with education regarding medications	↓15%	Unchanged
Patient falls	↑15% (2 falls with injury)	Unchanged
Caregiver satisfaction and perceptions of quality patient care	↓20%	↑5%
Caregiver perceptions of involvement in decision making	↓15%	↓10%
Caregiver turnover	↑7%	↑5%

The challenges of measuring health care are the result of the limitations of traditional analyses and measurement tools as well as many firmly entrenched practices believed acceptable. Rarely, if ever, can a single metric such as net income or profit margin reflect the totality and reality of the situation, namely, an effective healthcare system. A profitable enterprise may in fact have delivered substandard care, alienated caregivers, and created negative relationships within the community. Traditional measurement approaches, though vital, do not hold all the answers. Most measures are limiting and may be deceptive because of the hidden variables contributing to the single metric. Antecedent and concurrent events affect outcomes in multiple ways.

> ## Group Discussion
>
> Very specific information from caregivers can be obtained at the end of the shift. In light of the increasing computerization resources associated with time and attendance systems, discuss the value of a quick yes/no survey from every caregiver at the time of clock out. The questions, limited to three or four, could be:
>
> 1. I provided quality patient care today.
> 2. My team worked well together.
> 3. I had the supplies I needed to do my work well and in a timely manner.

Strategy 2: Extend Traditional Tools to Manage and Oversee Complexity

In light of the limitations of traditional financial measurement methodologies, quantum leaders need to explore and develop new tools to illuminate connectedness, interdependence, and emergence as the means to better understand system complexities and nuances. Often, leaders wonder if new roles or support staff are needed to advance this measurement and data analysis work. Some organizations have created chief data officer (CDO) positions to assist with this work. What is especially important is for leaders to focus on the work to be done rather than the title of a position. Managing and analyzing large datasets is an emerging discipline and requires high-level analytical competencies (Mehta & Pandit, 2018; Sanchez-Pinto et al., 2018; Schaeffer et al., 2017). Information from large datasets provides access to great numbers of experiences and outcomes that are useful to improve outcomes and reduce costs. Further, the digitization of data supports the analysis and filtering of the available data that were previously in disparate files. Large datasets now make it more likely for the evaluation of multiple variables rather than that of just a few select variables once challenges are overcome.

> **Key Point**
>
> "Big data" in health care refers to digital data that are generated in high volume and that create datasets that are too large for traditional data-processing systems (Sanchez-Pinto et al., 2018).

Moving beyond the emphasis on the selection of appropriate quantitative variables for value determination such as net profit, revenues, expenses, and return on investment is the beginning. This is not to say that these metrics are not important; rather, they are incomplete when disconnected from the totality of the variables representing the healthcare situation. Complex quality problems within complex systems rarely have one root cause or a single solution. Tools and methods that identify multiple aspects and relationships are needed for complex valuation. Although it is impossible to predict the unpredictable and to design solutions for every potential scenario, three contemporary tools provide new insight into valuation: mind maps, geographical information system (GIS) models, and scenario planning.

> ## Group Discussion
>
> Consider the persistent and unresolved issue of patient medication errors. An organization may monitor medication error data over time, using measurement tools such as run charts and control charts. Unfortunately, these tools do not include the antecedents and concurrent events that influence the outcomes on the run or control chart. Use a mind map to describe and display the same situation. What are the advantages and disadvantages of each tool?

> ## Key Point
> Measurement missteps:
>
> - *Measuring against yourself*. Both internal and external benchmarks are important to recognize available resources and the potential for increasing patient quality and safety.
> - *Looking backward*. Historical performance occurred under a different set of circumstances, for example, patient types, caregiver skills, physical settings, regulations.
> - *Putting your faith in numbers*. Return on investment is only one of the variables for evaluation; cost-effectiveness and cost utility add information to the analysis. Further, the story associated with the numbers is of equal importance.
> - *Gaming your metrics*. Some metrics result in users "manipulating" numbers to meet targets. Moving expenses to different categories to avoid inclusion defeats the purpose.
> - *Sticking to your numbers too long*. Metrics can lose their essence as the business evolves. The use of hours per patient day has long been seen as an incomplete metric given that the associated costs of support staff, education/quality/research time, and patient engagement are not included in this metric.
> - *Not enough metrics*. Single-minded metrics can lead to focusing on the wrong priorities.
> - *Focusing on inputs over outcomes*. Although the processes and inputs of work are important, the results or outcomes are the real measure of organizational success.
>
> Modified from Anthony, S. D., Johnson, M. W., Sinfield, J. V., & Altman, E. J. (2008). *Innovator's guide to growth: Putting disruptive innovation to work*. Harvard Business Press.

Mind Mapping

The mind map tool has become a powerful vehicle for collecting, organizing, and synthesizing large amounts of information, and for increasing understanding of complex phenomena. The use of diagrams, shapes, and colors provides individuals with the means to expand and explore ideas, creating linkages between elements while maintaining focus on the central theme.

The mind map is a very useful tool for documenting connectivity, interdependencies, and emerging phenomena in health care. When a particular healthcare scenario is mapped, the identified elements, linkages, and pathways become the essential elements for consideration in valuing health care more accurately and completely.

GIS Models

GIS models integrate hardware, software, and data as the means to capture, manage, analyze, and display multiple forms of geographic reference information (Shaw & McGuire, 2017). The unique feature of GIS models is their ability to display multidimensional, multilayered aspects of complex situations. GIS models provide for unique views of complex situations as the means to question, interpret, and better understand the phenomenon of interest. In addition, they provide a means to solve problems by looking at data in a way that is quickly understood. The utility of GIS models in healthcare analyses is that perspectives from point-of-care, local communities, regional areas, and national impact can be viewed and analyzed quickly and expertly.

Scenario Planning

Scenario planning is the third tool that provides a unique way to capture the essential elements for valuing healthcare situations. Scenario planning is especially useful in creating capacity for the unknown future. Participants in a workgroup are challenged to think more broadly and more creatively in addressing an unknown or extremely outrageous problem. The purpose is to move out of traditional thinking patterns and develop creative solutions not previously considered. This information now becomes available to teams as they confront uncertainty and embark on course corrections. The outrageous scenarios provide background ideas and potential solutions for consideration.

Strategy 3: Quantify the Value of Teamwork

It is no secret that expertly functioning teams are more likely to achieve excellent results and have minimal or no errors as a result of their effective collaboration. The financial value of expert teamwork and the cost of poorly functioning teams are not traditionally integrated into value formulations. Teamwork across disciplines is critical and at the same time very difficult to monitor and quantify. The increasingly complex nature of health care and the complex issues that caregivers face require a unique balance of responsibility and freedom to do the right work. The conditions for teamwork where issues are complex—namely, an environment that supports involvement in decision making, professional autonomy, and creativity in ensuring achievement of patient goals—are supporting variables that are linked to positive patient outcomes. **Exhibit 5-3** provides eight behavioral processes of teamwork. In addition, respect, social support, and psychological safety are affective components of teamwork, and understanding role responsibility and shared objectives are cognitive components of teamwork (Valentine et al., 2015).

Measurement strategies to identify levels or degrees of teamwork contributing to patient care processes and outcomes begin with qualitative assessments, quantification of the specific cost of labor hours associated with the identified work, and examination of outcomes. The unit of analysis best begins with the shift of work or the patient event. **Exhibit 5-4** presents the group of metrics that integrate expert functioning teamwork. Once the variables are identified, comparisons can be made to identify best practices among optimally functioning teams.

Exhibit 5-3 Eight Behavioral Dimensions of Teamwork

Core Dimensions

1. *Communication*: Is communication frequent, informative, direct, and open?
2. *Coordination*: Are individual efforts well-structured and synchronized with the team? Is there mutual adjustment, when needed? Team synergy? Use of resources?
3. *Balance of member contributions*: Does the team make use of all contributors' expertise?

Other Dimensions

4. *Shared decision making*: Does everyone participate in decision making?
5. *Collaboration*: Does the team self-report performance and satisfaction when working with another department?
6. *Mutual support (shared workload)*: Do team members help and support each other in carrying out their tasks?
7. *Effort*: Do team members exert all efforts to the team's tasks?
8. *Cohesion*: Are team members motivated to maintain the team? Is there team spirit? Is there active conflict management?

Data from Valentine, M. A., Nembhard, I. M., & Edmondson, A. C. (2015). Measuring teamwork in health care settings: A review of survey instruments. *Medical Care, 53*(4), e16–e30.

Exhibit 5-4 Measures of Teamwork Outcomes

1. Hours of work
2. Skill mix
3. Levels of education of members
4. Years of experience of members
5. Overtime hours and/or missed lunches
6. Patient complaints
7. Patient satisfaction (global and specific in relation to noise, responsiveness, and others)
8. Caregiver feedback
9. Negative patient outcomes

Strategy 4: Focus on Engagement of Providers and Patients

The need for full engagement of patient and provider has never been more important as the resources for health care become scarcer. Creating and supporting accountability for evidence-driven interventions and healthy patient behaviors that support healing and maintenance of health can be cost-effective and important to achieving desired health goals (Riegel et al., 2019). Collaborative care planning that fully engages patients and their families to commit to healthy behaviors requires skilled dialogue that creates both accountability for progress and sharing of information when plans are not working. The relationship between patients and caregivers is best supported with integrated, computerized electronic record keeping that can be accessed by both patient and caregivers. It is no longer acceptable for records to be provider controlled and not accessible by patients.

Engagement of providers and patients also involves a shared decision-making model. Shared decision making includes creating choice awareness of treatment options using standardized or tailored information. The goal is to assist with mutual decision making; however, there is no one unified view, currently. In some models, the process is stopped after providers describe treatment options. Shared decision making involves learning about the patient and creating choice awareness (Bomhof-Roordink et al., 2019). Quantum leaders need to consider the mental and behavioral complexities surrounding provider–patient decision making given the many factors that influence implementation of shared decision making and also the dyad responsiveness to the model. For example, consider poor quality information due to an intervention's novelty or a patient's emotional state. In this situation, dyad relationships related to who has power and insufficient time for discussion are important barriers. Factors that facilitate shared decision making with patients are used in low-stake decisions, when provider–patient trust and respect are high, when tools are available that aid discussions, and when providers demonstrate skill in using the model (Boland et al., 2019).

Group Discussion

System components depend on each other for their success. For example, a nurse depends on the presence of patients to provide care, a place to provide that care, supplies, medication, and support staff. For the care of your assigned patients for one shift, create a mind map that identifies the components required for patient care, the sequence of events, and the factors affecting patient outcomes.

- How many relationships did you identify?
- Which elements are working well together?
- Are there areas of congestion or dysfunction that are not working?
- How often during the shift was shared decision making an appropriate component of care?

Group Discussion

When organizations are attempting to empower staff at the point-of-service, getting caregivers engaged is usually not the hard part. Often, senior leaders are scared, and it is usually the senior leaders who pull the rug out based on the belief that point-of-care–driven work is disturbing the system, not directing it. The lack of clear knowledge of expected outcomes is unacceptable and a threat to patient safety. To prevent a premature death of point-of-care creativity and innovation work, it is important to communicate regularly, understand the complexity system mental model, and realize the need for continuing growth.

Consider a unit in your organization that has many opportunities for improvement. Design a plan to empower staff to identify issues, prioritize challenges, select tools of innovation to address issues, communicate progress to key stakeholders, and evaluate progress.

Strategy 5: Begin Locally with Change

Changing a long-standing culture of single financial measurements requires courage, persistence, and a plan that begins at the point-of-service, not in the boardroom. Given the challenges at the unit level specific to medication administration accuracy, safe environments, teamwork, nurse–physician collaboration, time spent in direct patient contact, work distractions (false alarms), and retention of competent staff, opportunities are available for unit-driven activities to begin the processes working from the inside out.

The work of leadership is not to direct change; rather, it is to be a committed leader who understands the importance of a receptive unit culture, achieving a shared vision by thinking differently and having protected time, and who empowers staff at the point-of-care to be aware of challenges and to use tools of innovation to create better processes and outcomes. In addition to protected time, leaders need to provide the infrastructure-specific role expectations and resources to test new models. Senior leaders need to learn to let go; to empower direct caregivers to operate within loose boundaries and be creative in finding better solutions. Indeed, local change is reflective of the transformation of cultures from a controlling, mechanical model to a shared leadership model that embraces the complex nature of human systems.

Strategy 6: Plan and Budget for Course Correction Work

In light of the reality of complex systems interactions and uncertainty, the work of course corrections must become recognized as normative and part of the work of adapting and growing; thus, mechanisms and measures for this work need to be included in the budgeting process. Specifically, it is important to at least determine a percentage of resources that will be needed for course correction. Developing expertise in quantifying course correction resources requires creativity and persistence. Assessment begins with comparisons of planned work and actual work through pre- and postanalyses of events or variance data as objective information that can facilitate more accurate resource planning. To be sure, no leader ever believes that 100% of work will be perfect. It is expected that revisions or modifications are part of the process to achieve goals. The work for each organization is to determine a percentage of resources that needs to be allocated for course corrections.

Strategy 7: Create the Business Case for the Healthcare Story and Course Corrections

Building the business case for new work is essential. Although leaders cannot use experience or history as a guide, there is an expectation for achievement of certain processes and outcomes, and an expectation of new work value once diffused into practice, consistent with the definition of innovation (Kelly & Young, 2017). Thus, process and outcome information and the stated value of new work/ideas needs to be systematically collected and integrated into a plan or road map that serves as a method to manage new ideas.

The following steps are essential components of the innovation business case:

1. Create the narrative for the product or service.
2. Identify the goal or purpose of the product or service. Include the relationship to mission-driven and financial goals, patient care quality, and patient safety.
3. Determine projected costs, course correction costs, and excluded costs. Include the rationale for each category, namely, why costs were included or excluded.

4. State predicted project benefits. Examples include meeting quality and safety goals, increasing profitability, and enhancing teamwork or the organization's reputation.
5. Target levels of performance goals. Ideally, the goals should be 100% satisfaction and zero errors.
6. Anticipate profit or loss.
7. Determine expected nonfinancial benefits, which may include information related to ambiguous evidence or evidence that has not traditionally been quantified, such as the degree of patient–caregiver engagement or the effect of reputation or brand strength on recruitment potential.
8. Determine key stakeholders, namely, those individuals who have a significant influence on success of this work.
9. Anticipate risks and plan to mediate risks or unexpected results.
10. Create an overall summary of long-term and short-term value to the organization and community.

The following exemplar is provided to demonstrate the creation of a business case for the healthcare story. Each leader and organization has different experiences and information that can further enhance this important work. A story from a very satisfied patient serves as the foundation for determination of value.

1. The healthcare story: *My neighbor's mother died recently and left this story in her will with directions to donate a specified amount to the healthcare system.*

    My last year of life has been blessed with incredible support from the healthcare system for my aging body and the realities of the end of life. During this time, my hypertension, diabetes, and irregular heart rhythm required routine monitoring and evaluation. My chronic constipation has been a problem for years; however, I am willing to live with it with the occasional oral remedies to manage it. I never felt like I was overtreated or asked to have tests or studies that I did not understand or for which there was an expectation that a positive change could be made. My healthcare providers and coaches, Dr. Karen (physician), Dr. Michael (nurse practitioner), and Mary (office receptionist), consistently assured me that my records were complete and shared appropriately with other providers as needed. Getting an appointment with my providers was handled efficiently and effectively—I never waited when I thought I needed to be seen—or at least got a call from Karen or Michael to discuss my questions and concerns.

    One short episode in the hospital was incredible—my blood sugars were out of control and the members of the healthcare team quickly reviewed my records and worked diligently to stabilize me. There was very little paperwork and interviewing—the only questions were about updates and new events in my life. I felt like I was one very special person and recovered quickly and went home within 2 days. I am now able to read again, watch TV, and walk to the mailbox. I am thrilled to be able to do these things without shortness of breath or anxiety.

    Charges, billing, and payment for my care were always clear. Before I left the office or hospital, my bill was presented and the exact amount Medicare would cover was identified as well as the amount I would need to pay. I never received bills for things I had not been advised about.

    I know this is special health care because my neighbor didn't have the same experiences that I did. She, too, had many illnesses associated with aging. She was seldom able to get an appointment with her provider in less than a month. She went to the emergency department several times last year for things that she was waiting to see the provider about. In addition, she had two colonoscopies in the last 2 years—she didn't know why but thought it had something to do with her constipation.

The metrics or measures for this story offer the beginnings of a new mental model for health care: begin with a successful story and identify the associated metrics to support similar care. In this story, metrics are extracted to identify the meaningful variables that are not often identified with traditional measurement approaches. These metrics contribute to the business case for complex patient care and provide for a more complete measurement picture of the healthcare experience.

Within this story, there is an incredible amount of information that can serve to illuminate new strategies for healthcare measurement. Multiple categories of value that reflect traditional metrics and those reflecting the complexities of health care are embedded in the story. The following can be learned from this story:

- *Patients can be realistic and do not want every symptom managed aggressively.* Living with chronic constipation, although uncomfortable, is tolerable for many individuals. They are not looking for the miracle cure (or multiple colonoscopies) to a chronic problem.
- *Understand and integrate the patient's values; age does matter.*
- *A complete and integrated patient medical record reduces redundancy and the chance for errors.*
- *Access to care providers in a timely manner is important because it can avoid unnecessary stress for the patient and unneeded visits to the emergency department.*
- *Teamwork and communication make a positive difference.*
- *Clarity and communication of charges and patient accountability for copays are essential parts of the service of health care that needs to be addressed along with the service rather than months after the event.*
- *Single-source billing is possible.* It's like a Visa bill: all charges on one simple statement.

2. Goals and purpose of this story: The expectations from this story are multifocal and relate to the patient, the caregivers, and the organization. Examples of expectations are as follows:
   - *Integrated and accessible medical records available 24/7 to enable communication among providers and caregivers specific to patient's multiple diagnoses of hypertension, diabetes, and heart disease.*
   - *No redundancy of services or requests for information already provided.*
   - *Access to providers and feedback within 24 hours.* Providers are accessible for unanticipated needs as well as every 3 months for monitoring of diabetes and hypertension. No visits to the emergency room.
   - *Respectful and meaningful relationships with providers.* Patient is elderly, hard of hearing, and has some vision impairment. Decisions for care are made by the patient with full information from providers and supporting evidence. Patient does not want unnecessary diagnostic testing or medications unless they will support or enhance current quality of life (shared decision making).
   - *Personal level of independence and functionality includes limited ambulation with a cane and limited driving to church, bank, and grocery story.*

- *Payment and billing of healthcare services are fully understood at the time of treatment.* At the time of service, all charges and costs to the patient are known and discussed. There are no unanticipated charges to the payer or the patient.
3. Cost of care is identified as office visits, medications, blood glucose monitoring equipment, and +10% allocations for course corrections should the patient need to visit the emergency room.
4. The benefits of this coordinated and respectful plan of care include sustained quality of life for the patient, a high degree of patient satisfaction, and a positive community reputation for the healthcare system.
5. Anticipated levels of performance are 100% patient satisfaction and zero medical errors. Also, zero visits to the emergency room are the goal.
6. The anticipated profit for these services is 2%.
7. The stakeholders include the patient, providers, office staff, and the local pharmacy.
8. The anticipated risks in this plan are the potential emergency room visits for unexpected emergencies or unavailability of office staff.
9. The short-term and long-term benefits of this model of patient care include health maintenance and functionality for the patient, financial viability of the organization, and a positive community reputation for the organization as a resource for quality healthcare services.

Conclusion

In summary, this healthcare valuation model is innovative and requires courage to be tested and implemented. What is most important for healthcare leaders is recognition of unresolved issues in the current system, adoption of healthcare reform, and an understanding of the ever-increasing complexity of healthcare systems. To be sure, the system will not improve with waiting and thinking; action is required to begin remodeling and testing new ideas that reflect the complexity of the healthcare system.

Chapter Takeaways

1. Documenting value requires variables reflecting connectivity, interdependencies, and emergence of the process or product being assessed.
2. Metrics for value can include costs, profits, perception, clinical improvements, goal achievement, and negative or unanticipated events/outcomes.
3. Strategies to document healthcare value include documenting the story, extending traditional measurement tools to assess complexity, quantifying the value of teamwork, and assessing the engagement of providers and patients.
4. Healthcare success stories are useful to create a list of metrics associated with the patient's positive experience.
5. Effective teamwork is a foundational requirement in creating healthcare value that can be learned and quantified.

Case Study 5-1
Are We a System or a Confederation of Hospitals?

Pacific Grove Healthcare System comprises six community hospitals located in a 100-mile radius, two major integrated physician organizations (IPOs), a healthcare plan, a hospice and home health service, and a freestanding rehabilitation center. The corporate executives recently hired a chief nursing executive (CNE) to simplify the reporting structure for all of the CNOs at each hospital and IPO. The new CNE has a PhD in nursing and is nationally recognized for his success in developing integrated systems for health care. The new CNE has just completed a 10-year engagement at another large healthcare system that made dramatic changes in nursing services resulting in a system-wide Magnet designation by the American Nurses Credentialing Center (ANCC). The CNE published many papers and spoke at national conferences about the challenges and successes of integrating nursing services across a multi-hospital system.

One of the first changes that the CNE made was to develop a new structure for nursing services that included several system-wide councils for (1) operations, (2) research and innovation, (3) professional development and scholarship, and (4) clinical excellence. The CNE announced that the intent and purpose of these system-wide councils were to facilitate planning, implementation of programs and services, and evaluation of the effectiveness of nursing services across the system. The CNE emphasized the importance and value of creating the system-wide councils and the need to lead the system effort and let go of the traditional unilateral decision making by inviting others in the organization to participate in decisions that affected patient care and nursing practice.

At first the CNOs at each hospital resisted reporting to the system CNE and participating in the expansion of membership on the various system councils to individuals other than the CNOs. They viewed this structure change as marginalization of their roles and power structure. The CNE met with them individually and as a group in a planning retreat to address their concerns and shared stories and case studies from his previous organization that illustrated the benefits and outcomes of integrating nursing across the system. As a group they developed a list of attributes that they believed essential for a fully functioning system and the strategic actions that would need to take place before nursing in the system could be completely integrated. They also discussed the benefits and barriers to system work. The CNE led them through a mind-mapping experience to expand their thinking about the challenges and opportunities in leading system work. From the mind-map bubbles, the CNOs explored scenarios that would illustrate some of the situations that they might be facing in the future. The group discussed possible leaders and the membership for each of the councils and decided to invite some of the top leaders from each hospital's Magnet council structure to participate in the system-wide councils.

To facilitate the effectiveness of this change, the CNE also engaged the services of an academic partner from one of the local universities to facilitate a professional development curriculum focused on leading group meetings, building consensus, managing conflict, managing change, financial planning and management, and system integration. Once the membership was decided and the leadership selected for each of the system-wide councils, each of the members was invited to participate in the learning experiences to build their skills and competencies in system work.

Case Study 5-1

The CNE invited all of the system council members and CNOs to participate in a retreat where he presented his vision for an integrated nursing service line across all system entities. He shared that "success" would have many definitions, but one measure of success would be system-wide Magnet designation. He presented the characteristics of a high-performing system with examples of cost savings, financial gains, and program and service expansions from other system organizations that had achieved integration of patient care and nursing services across their systems. He outlined several measures that would guide the evaluation of their work, including financial, quality, satisfaction, work environment, and patient-outcome metrics. He indicated that each hospital would continue to report their individual progress on these metrics, but the aggregate of all of the system entities was a better measure of system performance. Each of them would also be evaluated on system metrics in addition to their individual entity goals. Each of the councils would include clinical nurses who were active in their unit practice councils and their entity's collaborative governance councils.

Bolstering his vision for integrated patient care and nursing services, the CNE mentioned several business partners whose companies were interested in funding and involvement in the Research and Innovation Council, which was a tremendous opportunity to expand patient care and nursing research efforts. Academic partners representing the local colleges would also participate in the Professional Development and Scholarship Council in an effort to provide additional opportunities and resources to advance the education level and leadership skills of clinical nurses and frontline managers. It was also suggested that patient representatives be selected to participate in the Clinical Excellence Council to ensure that the "voice of the customer" was heard as a focus area for planning. Clinical nurses and interprofessional partners would be invited to participate on the Operations Council to integrate efforts of nursing and other professional providers.

At the end of the planning retreats, the CNOs and others who had participated were excited but a bit overwhelmed at the layers of change that were planned for each of their entities and for the entire system for patient care and nursing services. Some had doubts about the value of such a change, but most trusted that the new CNE would be able to direct and facilitate such a change because of his experience and reputation for accomplishing a similar process in another organization. Most were eager and pleased to be empowered to participate in such a lofty goal of integrating nursing services across the entire organization.

Questions
1. What is your impression of the new CNE's plans for a layered change process to integrate patient care and nursing services across the healthcare system?
2. What barriers do you think will challenge the efforts toward system integration?
3. How do you think that the CNE can ensure accountability of his CNOs to support such change and promote systemness in their own organization as opposed to promoting their own entity's interests?
4. What other metrics or measures would you recommend to assess the success of the integration process?
5. Describe the attributes that you think would be essential for a fully integrated nursing system.
6. To achieve the attributes that you outlined in question 5, what developmental elements would be needed to achieve an integrated nursing system?

Case Study 5-2

It's That Time of the Year Again!

"Good grief, it's that time of year again!" This seemed to be the mantra of the entire group of nurse directors at St. Thomas Hospital as budget season approached. There seemed to be a spirit of quiet anticipation and resignation to the fact that each of them would be spending the next 6 weeks reviewing operational and financial data, planning unit budgets, negotiating for changes in financial and productivity targets based on last year's information, and presenting the final budget to their direct reports once they were approved by the finance department. There never seemed to be enough financial resources to support all of the proposed initiatives, planned volume for the future, and changes that seemed essential, causing great conflict among the various layers of management in the organization as they competed for a greater "piece of the pie" for their respective departments. The finance department disseminated the budget forms and the operational and productivity data trended over the past 3 years.

Irene, one of the department directors commented, "It's like planning the future looking in the rearview mirror!" Irene was particularly sensitive to using the past data for staffing projections because her department had experienced significant changes affecting staffing, productivity, and expenses. The entire department had moved into a new building with a completely different configuration of the nursing units, all private rooms, and centralized nursing station that increased distances that nurses had to walk when providing patient care and retrieving supplies and equipment. The new unit configuration completely changed the way that nurses practiced, making the past 3 years of data ineffective for planning the future. Irene realized that she would have difficulty convincing the chief financial officer (CFO) of this fact because the goal of the hospital was to have a budget-neutral plan for the next year to accommodate major changes in reimbursement methodologies proposed by the new Affordable Care Act. It had been clearly announced that none of the departments would receive more money for staffing than they had been allocated in the past, making Irene a bit nervous about how she would justify the need for additional dollars needed because of the unit configuration change in the new building.

To prepare her case for presentation to the CFO, Irene benchmarked her units with other hospitals of similar size, complexity, and configuration. She had asked the architectural firm that designed the new unit for names of other hospitals so that she could interface with their nursing directors. She had many questions about how they allocated staffing in the new configuration and particularly with a remote centralized nursing station. Irene had hoped for a design that would allow for a documentation area between every two private rooms, locating the nurses closer to the patients, but space constraints prevented the achievement of this design; at least this is what Irene had been told by the architects and the hospital's executive team. Now Irene was accountable to staff the unit with the same resources that had been used in a more compact semiprivate configuration with the same number of patient beds. Therefore, Irene felt that it was essential that she gather evidence from directors at other hospitals who had also made the change to a new unit configuration.

Irene also needed to add additional money for cross training the staff to the new computerized documentation and medication administration systems, and these expenses would not have been realized in the budget snapshots for the past 3 years. It seemed that all of these changes not only affected the budgetary expenses but also the staff morale on the unit because they were becoming "change fatigued." Irene was certain that any budgetary restraints on staffing levels would tip the staff into becoming more negative about the organization. She did all possible to make her staff aware that she was advocating for their needs and included some of the clinical nurses in the budget-planning meetings so that they could share information from a clinical perspective and provide input to their colleagues as well. Irene included representation from pharmacy, dietary, and the therapies because their workload had also changed with the new unit configuration. Irene's intent was to develop a comprehensive proposal making the business case for her additional needs with the input of her interprofessional partners. Together they created a narrative that would support the new budget and developed two separate budgets that would illustrate how the unit configuration changed the resource needs for each of their respective departments. One of the proposals reflected the resource needs that would have been budgeted for the previous unit configuration and compared that with a second budget developed for the new unit configuration, which demonstrated the incremental increases resultant from changes in the physical design. Irene realized this was an important step in presenting her case to the CFO because patient type, acuity, and volume did not change appreciably over the past 3 years but rather the physical design affected nursing care hours needed for the same projected volume and acuity.

Questions

1. If you were Irene, how would you present your business case to the CFO requesting additional nursing care hours and staffing dollars for the new budget?
2. What are the benefits of an interprofessional approach in supporting Irene's proposal to the CFO?
3. What evidence does Irene need to acquire to support her budget proposal?

References

Anthony, S. D., Johnson, M. W., Sinfield, J. V., & Altman, E. J. (2008). *Innovator's guide to growth: Putting disruptive innovation to work*. Harvard Business Press.

Boland, L., Graham, I. D., Légaré, F., Lewis, K., Jull, J., Shepard, A., Lawson, M. L., Davis, A., Yameogo, A., & Stacey, D. (2019). Barriers and facilitators of pediatric shared decision making: A systematic review. *Implementation Science, 14*(1), 7.

Bomhof-Roordink, H., Gärtner, F. R., Stiggelbout, A. M., & Pieterse, A. H. (2019). Key components of shared decision making models: A systematic review. *BMJ Open, 9*(12), e031763.

Centers for Medicare & Medicaid Services. (n.d.). CAHPS® hospital survey. https://hcahpsonline.org/

Centers for Medicare and Medicaid Services. (2019, December 22). National health expenditures 2018 highlights. https://www.cms.gov/files/document/highlights.pdf

Click, B., Lopez, R., Arrigain, S., Schold, J., Reguero, M., & Rizk, M. (2020). Shifting cost-drivers of health care expenditures in inflammatory bowel diseases. *Inflammatory Bowel Diseases, 26*(8), 1268–1275.

Colla, C. H., Morden, N. E., Sequist, T. D., Schpero, W. L., & Rosenthal, M. B. (2015). Choosing wisely: Prevalence and correlates of low-value health care services in the United States. *Journal of General Internal Medicine, 30*(2), 221–228.

Durante, A., Paturzo, M., Mottloa, A., Alvaro, R., Vaughan Dickson, V., & Vellone, E. (2019). Caregiver contribution to self-care in patients with heart failure: A qualitative descriptive study. *Journal of Cardiovascular Nursing, 34*(2), E28–E35.

Fawcett, J., & Ellenbecker, C. H. (2015). A proposed conceptual model of nursing and population health. *Nursing Outlook, 63*(3), 288–298.

Institute of Medicine (IOM). (2000). *To err is human: Building a safer health system*. The National Academies Press.

Kelly, C. J., & Young, A. J. (2017). Promoting innovation in healthcare. *Future Healthcare Journal, 4*(2), 121–125.

Khan, S., Vandermorris, A., Shaperd, J., Begun, J. W., Lanham, H. J., Uhl-Bien, M., & Berta, W. (2018). Embracing uncertainty, managing complexity: Applying complexity thinking principles to transformation efforts in healthcare systems. *BMC Health Services Research, 18*(1), 192.

Krans, E. E., Campopiano, M., Cleveland, L. M., Goodman, D., Kilday, D., Kendig, S., Leffert, L. R., Main, E. K., Mitchell, K. T., O'Gurek, D. T., D'Oria, R., McDaniel, D., & Terplan, M. (2019). National partnership for maternal safety: Consensus bundle on obstetric care for women with opioid use disorder. *Obstetrics and Gynecology, 134*(2), 365–375.

Mehta, N., & Pandit, A. (2018). Concurrence of big data analytics and healthcare: A systematic review. *International Journal of Medical Informatics, 114*, 57–65.

Melnyk, B. M., Gallagher-Ford, L., Zellefrow, C., Tucker, S., Thomas, B., Sinnott, L. T., & Tan, A. (2018). The first U.S. study on nurses' evidence-based practice competencies indicates major deficits that threaten healthcare quality, safety, and patient outcomes. *Worldviews on Evidence-Based Nursing, 15*(1), 16–25.

Nordin, P., Kork, A. A., & Koskela, I. (2017). Value-based healthcare measurement as a context for organizational learning. *Leadership in Health Services, 30*(2), 159–170.

Olsson, M., Bajpai, R., Yew, Y. W., Koh, M. J. A., Thng, S., Car, J., & Järbrink, K. (2020). Associations between health-related quality of life and health care costs among children with atopic dermatitis and their caregivers: A cross-sectional study. *Pediatric Dermatology, 37*(2), 284–293.

Peterson-KFF. (2019, March 28). Health system tracker. https://www.healthsystemtracker.org/chart-collection/quality-u-s-healthcare-system-compare-countries/#item-start

Riegel, B., Jaarsma, T., Lee, C. S., & Strömberg, A. (2019). Integrating symptoms into the middle-range theory of self-care of chronic illness. *Advances in Nursing Science, 43*(3), 206–215.

Sanchez-Pinto, L. N., Luo, Y., & Churpek, M. M. (2018). Big data and data science in critical care. *Chest, 154*(5), 1239–1248.

Schaeffer, C., Booton, L., Halleck, J., Studeny, J., & Coustasse, A. (2017). Big data management in US hospitals: Benefits and barriers. *The Health Care Manager, 36*(1), 87–95.

Shaw, N., & McGuire, S. (2017). Understanding the use of geographical information systems (GIS) in health informatics research: A review. *Journal of Innovation in Health Informatics, 24*(2), 940.

Theofanidis, D., & Gibbon, B. (2016). Nursing interventions in stroke delivery: An evidence-based clinical review. *Journal of Vascular Nursing, 34*(4), 144–151.

Valentijn, P. P., Biermann, C., & Bruijnzeels, M. A. (2016). Value-based integrated (renal) care: Setting a development agenda for research and implementation strategies. *BMC Health Services Research, 16*, 330.

Valentine, M. A., Nembhard, I. M., & Edmondson, A. C. (2015). Measuring teamwork in health care settings: A review of survey instruments. *Medical Care, 53*(4), e16–e30.

Wheatley, M. J., & Kellner-Rogers, M. (1996). *A simpler way*. Berrett-Koehler.

Yun, D., & Choi, J. (2019). Person-centered rehabilitation care and outcomes: A systematic literature review. *International Journal of Nursing Studies, 93*, 74–83.

Suggested Readings

Anthony, S. D., Johnson, M. W., Sinfield, J. V., & Altman, E. J. (2008). *Innovator's guide to growth: Putting disruptive innovation to work*. Harvard Business Press.

Christensen, C., Kaufman, S. P., & Shih, W. C. (2008). Innovation killers: How financial tools destroy your capacity to do new things. *Harvard Business Review, 87*(1), 98–105, 137.

Davis, P. D., & Marshall, D. R. (2014). Teamwork: An essential for leading and launching innovation. *Nursing Administration Quarterly, 38*(3), 221–229.

Jena, A. B., & Philipson, T. J. (2008). Cost-effectiveness analysis and innovation. *Journal of Health Economics, 27*(5), 1224–1236.

Kinch, M. S., & Moore, R. (2016). Innovator organizations in new drug development: Assessing the sustainability of the biopharmaceutical industry. *Cell Chemical Biology, 23*(6), 644–653.

Li, J., Talari, P., Kelly, A., Latham, B., Dotson, S., Manning, K., Thornsberry, L., Swartz, C., & Williams, M. V. (2018). Interprofessional teamwork innovation model (ITIM) to promote communication and patient-centred, coordinated care. *BMJ Quality & Safety, 27*(9), 700–709.

Likierman, A. (2009). The five traps of performance measurement. *Harvard Business Review, 87*(10), 96–101, 141.

Roberts, J. P., Fisher, T. R., Trowbridge, M. J., & Bent, C. (2016). A design thinking framework for healthcare management and innovation. *Healthcare, 4*(1), 11–14.

Quiz Questions

Select the best answer for each of the following questions.

1. Which of the following statements characterizes customizing measurement in health care?
    a. Customization creates a need for leaders to ensure that local facility resources are identified to create optimal measurement.
    b. Customization is frowned upon as it makes it difficult to compare healthcare practices across the country.
    c. Customization is irresponsible given the need to develop safe and reliable systems that can be replicated.
    d. Customization allows leaders to include industry standards and facility-specific measures that match mission and goals.

2. Why does cost continue to be an issue in health care?
    a. Healthcare reform is too costly.
    b. Cost shifting prevents improvements.
    c. The overall system is fragmented and inconsistent.
    d. Most citizens "expect" healthcare services as a right.

3. Which of the following statements characterizes cost savings in health care?
    a. Cost savings are possible if patient accountability for provider instructions is required.
    b. Cost savings are difficult to determine in light of system complexity and current inefficiencies.
    c. Cost savings are possible if adults would practice healthy behaviors and lifestyles.
    d. Cost savings are most likely if the private sector assumed control of the healthcare system.

4. Which of the following statements characterizes personal patient accountability?
    a. It is only a minor influence in the cost of health care.
    b. It significantly affects the demand for health services and medications/treatments.
    c. It is an untapped component of the healthcare equation for rational spending and allocation of resources.
    d. It is a violation of individual rights and should not be considered in the healthcare model.

5. Which of the following is true of complexity theory?
   a. It illuminates the challenges of valuation in the healthcare system.
   b. It introduces unnecessary information into the system.
   c. It limits the applicability of shared decision making.
   d. It is an outdated paradigm that further complicates healthcare issues.

6. Which of the following statements best characterizes ambiguous evidence?
   a. Ambiguous evidence is a reality that should not be considered in healthcare valuation because of its subjectivity.
   b. Ambiguous evidence provides an opportunity for manipulation of the reimbursement system.
   c. Ambiguous evidence is a reality of the healthcare experience and system complexity that needs to be considered.
   d. Ambiguous evidence should be discounted in financial analyses.

7. What does emergence, a reality of human relationships, require of leaders?
   a. Planning for eventual conflict between providers and patients
   b. Ensuring there is a well-planned patient care plan
   c. Identifying the budgeting implications for unanticipated changes
   d. Recognizing the need for course corrections when planning

8. Which of the following statements characterizes documenting the story?
   a. Documenting the story is interesting, but it is nearly impossible to integrate it into a measurement system.
   b. Documenting the story requires skilled clinicians to interpret subjective information.
   c. Documenting the story is not accepted by financial experts because of subjectivity in reporting.
   d. Documenting the story is a robust method to illicit as much information as possible about the patient care experience.

9. Which of the following statements characterizes traditional measurement tools?
   a. They are tried-and-true measures that meet the complexities of most healthcare centers.
   b. They require supplementation with more comprehensive models of healthcare measurement.
   c. They should be minimized as hospital measures to decrease the complexity and cost of care.
   d. They have limitations; however, they are accepted by legislators and financial experts.

10. What is the business case for the healthcare story?
    a. It is another iteration of a strategic plan, but with a personal touch.
    b. It requires additional resources and does not provide additional information.
    c. It integrates the healthcare situation, comprehensive information, and challenges of valuing new models.
    d. It is an excellent model that can be widely replicated to support national healthcare reform.

11. The drivers for healthcare change are multifaceted and interconnected. Which response reflects emergence from a complexity perspective?
    a. The cost of care now is now regulated by the Affordable Care Act.
    b. Evidence-based hospital and ambulatory practices result in improved care.
    c. Partial measurement has led to incomplete recognition of total costs of services.
    d. The amount of cost shifting is unanticipated and metrics to create equity are not available.

12. HCAHPS (Hospital Consumer Assessment of Healthcare Providers and Systems) surveys resulted in which of the following?
    a. Standardized assessments of patients' perceptions of care, providers, and information received while hospitalized
    b. Standardized assessments of patients' perceptions of care, providers, and information received during any healthcare visit or hospitalization
    c. Duplication of existing surveys used by hospitals to understand patient satisfaction needs
    d. An approach to measurement that does not support value-driven health care

13. The concept of interdependence from a complexity perspective recognizes all of the following, *except*:
    a. physicians' need for nurses to provide care to support patient recovery.
    b. the healthcare organization's need for providers and patients.
    c. patients' need for reimbursement resources.
    d. fully functioning equipment that does not require service.

14. Medication administration often results in unexpected outcomes. Which response does *not* reflect the complexity phenomenon of emergence?
    a. All patient medications are accurately prepared and labeled.
    b. The patient experiences an unexpected allergic response.
    c. All medications result in the desired outcome.
    d. The patient refuses all prepared medications.

15. Documenting the story about successful or unsuccessful care is a strategy to:
    a. learn more psychosocial information about the patient and family.
    b. uncover unknown areas of influence on outcomes.
    c. limit the amount of data collection about traditional metrics.
    d. confirm the current measurement process used for quality assessment.

16. Mind mapping is a useful tool to explore a situation because it reflects all of the following, *except*:
    a. interconnectedness.
    b. relationships.
    c. outcomes.
    d. quality of available research.

17. Teamwork quantification has been difficult to achieve due to the:
    a. cost of care providers compared to the average length of stay.
    b. satisfaction scores of team members and patients.
    c. combination of costs of labor, communication assessments, and team outcomes.
    d. skill mix of team members, team member education levels, patient complaints, and the attendance records of team members.

18. Great new ideas for health care are discovered at conferences, in the literature, and on the internet. Beginning locally or at the unit level with a pilot study is appropriate in all of the following situations, *except*:
    a. implementing a new needleless system.
    b. using 3D printers for patient education.
    c. implementing legislative mandates for drug restrictions.
    d. implementing a new self-scheduling process.

CHAPTER FIVE   From Evidence to Innovation: Measuring the Foundations of Practice and Value

19. Budgeting for course correction is seldom considered. Which of the following should be quantified on an annual basis?
    a. Labor time and supply costs to change two to three practices that did not succeed
    b. Communication costs of policy changes
    c. Labor time for strategic plan review and revisions
    d. 5% of the total unit budget

20. The comparison of Story A and Story B used quantifiable metrics to determine the value of each scenario. What were the significant differences in each scenario?
    a. Story A used a traditional approach; Story B used an innovative approach.
    b. Story A focused on increasing revenue; Story B focused on decreasing costs.
    c. Story A had engaged caregivers; Story B created caregiver turnover.
    d. The impact on patient satisfaction in Story A was positive; Story B was neutral.

21. High-quality teamwork in healthcare is increasingly important to achieve patient engagement and desired outcomes. Teamwork efforts:
    a. result in little collaboration.
    b. prompt individuals to work in groups doing their own individual work.
    c. lead to frustration, because teamwork requires consistent team members.
    d. are not considered a unique competency and one that must be learned and practiced.

22. Creating a business case for healthcare/nursing work is:
    a. not always possible due to patient requests.
    b. essential when implementing new programs and services.
    c. essential to determine the value to the patient and cost to the organization.
    d. essential for the finance and cost-accounting services to document for regulatory reviews.

23. In the chapter story, the authors note that some patients do not want every symptom managed.
    a. It is acceptable because it respects the patient's values and preferences.
    b. It is unacceptable and unethical not to treat identified symptoms.
    c. It is unacceptable to ration healthcare services and treatments.
    d. It is acceptable, because it eliminates non-value-added services.

24. Making decisions with adequate information that reflects the whole story is often challenging, because:
    a. the amount of time to select and gather the needed information is limited.
    b. partial measurement is more effective than trying to quantify ambiguous evidence.
    c. decisions can be made with one data point that has been tested.
    d. reimbursement allocations are the bottom line and the only issue that matters.

25. When an innovation does not succeed as planned, leaders often use a root cause analysis to guide course corrections. When is it appropriate to use the root cause analysis method?
    a. When the individual source of error or failure has been identified.
    b. When the specific organizational factors influencing the error/failure have been identified.
    c. When ineffective relationships among team members have been identified.
    d. When all of the organizational factors and individuals involved in the error/failure have been identified.

CHAPTER SIX

Diversity and Difference: Managing Conflict in a Transdisciplinary Network

Cooperation is the thorough conviction that nobody can get there unless everybody gets there.

—*Virginia Burden*[1]

Chapter Objectives

At the completion of this chapter, the reader will be able to:

- Recognize the key principles of conflict resolution in dealing with a wide variety of conflict-based issues.
- Apply conflict management principles and processes in the everyday work of leadership.
- Distinguish between normal conflict management and the management of differences.
- Formulate personal insights regarding how to apply conflict management skill sets as part of the leadership role.
- Distinguish between identity- and interest-based conflicts and describe the best approach to dealing with each type.

Conflict is central to all human interaction. Conflict simply codifies the deep and abiding understanding of the fundamental diversity of the human experience. Managing conflict is the vehicle through which we negotiate our differences and work to find passage to common ground. As a metaphor for difference, normative conflict represents the foundational aspect of human interaction and communication. The challenge presented by individual, interpersonal, or organizational (workplace) conflict is that it is often rife with pain and violence. The frequency of occurrence of these two features is evidence of our inability to see conflict as normal and to develop mechanisms for managing it well. Because it is so much a part of the human

---

[1] *The Process of Intuition* by Virginia Burden Tower, Theosophical Publishing House, Wheaton, Illinois, 1987. Reprinted by permission.

experience, we would do better to learn the dynamics of conflict and incorporate its management into our human skill set. This chapter treats conflict as normal and offers a range of techniques and methodologies for managing it in such a way as to ultimately achieve purposeful action and improved relationships. The emphasis is on developing skills for facilitating the use of conflict as a tool for promoting good interaction and advancing relationships. The chapter also outlines the difference between interest- and identity-based conflicts and describes the processes used to address each.

Conflict is normal. It is present in every human relationship and represents diversity in action. Conflict is the dynamic content of diversity. Managing human conflict requires an understanding that diversity needs to be valued and negotiated to facilitate effective community relationships.

Conflict should never be avoided or suppressed. Instead, it should be embraced as a fundamental part of every human interaction. Conflict is the most frequently occurring dynamic in human relationships. And yet it is the most misunderstood and misused element in the whole arena of communication and interaction.

Embracing conflict is easier said than done! A particular instance of conflict can involve a significant emotional overlay that adds stress to the interaction. The emotional component can take the conflict to a level of intensity that is uncomfortable and potentially destructive. At higher levels of intensity, the process of being in opposition becomes its own end, and the purpose and product of the conflict disappear in the dust raised by living in opposition. The emotional component creates so much unpredictable and untenable content that most people simply back away from the conflict, unable to figure out how to deal with it or cope with its pain.

In making conflict normative, leaders create a frame for conflict that turns it from an event into a process. The more conflict is looked at as a normal occurrence, one that reflects the usual vagaries of human interaction, the more likely it can be handled appropriately. This notion of normative conflict is a relatively recent understanding of the role conflict plays in organizational dynamics. Good leaders recognize that the tensions associated with normative human conflict simply represent the usual and ordinary differences that exist between people at all levels of the human community. Conflict itself is never a problem.

> **Key Point**
> Conflict is normal. The challenge is to know what it is when it happens and what to do about it when it is recognized for what it is.

However, *unresolved* conflict continues on a growth trajectory that becomes increasingly problematic to the extent that it is ignored or unaddressed. Wise leaders, therefore, never ignore conflict; in fact, they search for it in the human community and, always finding it, address it in an appropriate and timely fashion.

Good leaders recognize that conflict cannot be avoided. In fact, good leaders do everything *not* to avoid conflict. Rather, leaders create an environment that provides a safe space to identify and express conflict. Good leaders recognize that conflict management is a fundamental obligation of the leadership role. Knowing that conflict cannot be ignored, good leaders embrace it. The best way for leaders to deal with work conflict is to create an environment (culture) that makes it comfortable and safe to engage conflict and build a culture where conflict is accepted as part the interaction of the human community. More important, good leaders recognize that opening interactions to the noise, ambiguity, and challenge of expressing differences creates a safe milieu for the expression of differences, even though it can often be especially demanding for leaders to manage.

Good leaders are responsible for creating a positive context for the work of others. Leaders continually attempt to provide a framework for work that is positive, encouraging, and growth oriented. A good part of leaders' work in creating a positive context is building relationships that facilitate a high level of partnership, openness, and trust. Leaders must consider conflict management to be a regular part of their responsibilities; they must confront conflict directly so that it becomes a part of effectively expressing their role. A willingness to explore conflict rather than denying its presence will allow leaders to recognize that fear of confrontation is a significant impediment to resolving interpersonal and relationship-based conflicts.

The best time to address conflict is early in its expression. Seeing a conflict situation emerge is a forewarning that it is likely to blossom. Leaders need to know that conflict does not go away of its own volition. Because it is normal for almost all human interactions, when left unaddressed, conflict simply changes its form and emerges somewhere else in a kind of "wolf in sheep's clothing." The longer conflict simmers, the more difficult it is to resolve. Conflict is never a static process that just sits there, failing to gather energy. It is common for unresolved conflict to grow in intensity as it lies just below the surface, collecting energy and building toward a cataclysmic eruption. Unresolved conflict always intensifies. Good leaders have an intuitive sense of the potential for conflict. They know that every interaction is rife with the seeds for conflict. Human differences drive its continual unfolding. If not recognized early, individual, interpersonal, or organizational conflicts will continue to gather potential and grow in possibility until their more volatile expression becomes likely. Leaders must do three things in the presence of the potential for conflict: understand the factors that make up healthcare conflict (individual, interpersonal, or organizational), address it early, and address it appropriately.

Conflict management takes into account that people differ in a whole range of ways and that factors as broad as culture, race, gender, social status, and income group and as specific as personal beliefs, family position, mental health, intelligence, and emotional maturity all can influence the onset and process of a particular conflict. Many factors are associated with conflict, and the consequences are often rooted in the source and factor(s) (Kim et al., 2017). Further, the best interventions to manage conflict may be related to the source (Almost et al., 2016). **Exhibit 6-1** provides nonexclusive examples of factors that can produce healthcare conflict, based on their source.

Leaders need to recognize that early engagement of conflict means recognizing it soon enough to address it without noise and/or overwhelming personal emotion. In the earliest moments of an interpersonal conflict, the beginning signs of the impending conflict are always present. An attitude of disrespect, an unkind word from one person to another, an offhand remark, discourteous or bullying actions, disrespectful wording, or an inappropriate phrase can be early signs of the gathering storm of a conflict. Good leaders let no remark or behavior that represents anger, misunderstanding, incivility, or personal apprehension go unaddressed. Each of these communication breakdowns or actions is an indicator of an underlying set of concerns that begs to be addressed. Interrupting the course of a conflict in these early stages gets the real issues out in the open and raises the chance that addressing them will allay further opportunity for the conflict to accelerate.

In the earliest stages of conflict, leaders should look to determine if people are creating positions and taking sides. Indeed, in the earliest stages, a conflict-driven individual creates boundaries and limits to a view or position as a way of emphasizing differences. People

Exhibit 6-1 Factors of Healthcare Conflict

Individual Sources	Interpersonal Sources	Organizational Sources
• Ego or concept of self is threatened • Personality • Identity • Intimate relationships • Misperceptions of others' beliefs, worldviews, or abilities • Perspectives • Education • Position and role • Race, culture, nationality • Religion • Politics • Economics, class, society • Resources • Low psychological capital related to hope, resilience, or optimism	• Communication breakdown • Absence of timely or specific feedback • Unclear expectations around task completion or information sharing • Power differentials in positions, roles, or expertise • Stereotyping • Stigmatizing • Treated disrespectfully • Lack of support • Lack of trust • Lack of fairness • Reporting to multiple managers • Leader's management style	• Workflow complexity • Task-based, related to procedures, policies, standards • Processes tied to perceptions of team members • Task assignments are demeaning, unfair, or insulting to capabilities or reputation compared to what others receive • Job environment, including time pressures, job stress, overtime, and staffing and scheduling • Accountability and decision-making process • Role ambiguity

creating conflict often become exclusionary or exclusive to perceptions or notions that represent their chosen position. Ownership and expression of the position and extreme defense of it creates the initial conditions and circumstances upon which further conflict can build.

Fear, conflict avoidance, ignorance or lack of insight about issues that generate conflict, and lack of use of the legitimate processes of conflict management are the primary causes of the ensuing problems that arise when conflict occurs. When people become embroiled in a conflict, many feelings rush to the surface and begin to be expressed in one form or another, until eventually, people are dealing with feelings rather than the conflict that generated them. As a result, the original reason for the conflict can get lost in the interaction and may even be forgotten, replaced by another reason. In this scenario, ending the conflict amicably does not resolve the underlying problem, which has the potential to bring about another skirmish. The cycle can continue indefinitely, building layer upon layer over the underlying problem and making it ever harder to discern and resolve.

Growth and Transformation

All conflict provides a dynamic opportunity for growth and transformation, and leaders should treat conflict as simply another tool of good leadership. Leadership involves addressing human behavior issues. Good leadership involves facilitating optimal communication and therapeutic interpersonal relations and fostering mutual respect among healthcare teams. Good leaders understand that conflict management is unavoidable and that it is an important aspect of their roles (McKibben, 2017).

The secret of good conflict management is simple, but the process is not. The secret is to get the parties in conflict to discern the root issues and mutually agree on actions to be taken. Actually building an effective process to accomplish this goal is a complex task. In addition to understanding the source and factors associated with conflict, leaders must take into account that typically the parties involved in conflict are unequal in some way; that is, one party may have a substantial advantage over the other (e.g., the lion's share of power). Conflict management must involve interventions that closely reflect the source, character, and content/context elements of the conflict and moves it toward a mutually agreed upon resolution. If a satisfactory outcome is to be obtained, the conflict management process must create equity. The conflict management process must address power equations so that any unevenness can be accommodated and the process can unfold in a balanced and fair way.

> **Point to Ponder**
>
> About 90% of the average leader's responsibilities involve dealing with human behavior and human interaction. Given that this is true, why do leaders spend so little time learning how to resolve the issues that arise out of human dynamics?

Much of the structural inequity alludes to individual and collective issues generated out of personal insecurity and inequality. In health care, there is an overwhelming and almost suffocating lack of scholarship and dialogue around issues of gender, power, and role inequity. Although frequently alluded to, formal structures and processes specifically directed to resolving conflicts related to inequity are few. The traditional masculine and medical caste structure of the health system represents a serious relational disequilibrium and generates a set of values related to power, importance, significance, and value that subordinates roles and creates structural barriers to equity. As value-driven healthcare reforms unfold with increasing intensity over the next decade, issues of collateral relationships, interaction, value, and mutual contribution will come to the fore and require formal processes that help construct more effective and collateral relationships among healthcare disciplines. Even though the competencies and skill sets of multidisciplinary or multicultural practitioners or those of asymmetric power dynamics bring a unique set of talents to the continuum of care, there could be unintended consequences and a need to ensure that their collaborations are collateral, partnered, and equity based (Janss et al., 2012; Lewicki et al., 2015).

Nurses have a unique set of concerns regarding conflicts and their resolution. In some ways, the history of nursing parallels the history of the women's movement, including the subordination and powerlessness experienced by both women and nurses (most of whom have been women). Education of nurses and other health professionals has promoted intellectual and role equity, but long-standing medical practices and legal constraints on the scope of practice makes many health professionals, including nurses, uncertain of the agendas of physicians and administrators and skeptical of the processes that have been used to resolve conflicts. For many nurses, relationships with physicians and administrators were historically one-sided and biased against them, and their sense of being ignored or even silenced did not create a good foundation for building equitable relationships and resolving conflicts. Conflicting interests were also created when pseudo-teams (e.g., a nurse and physician) had independent objectives (e.g., a physician wants to schedule surgery when the nurse perceives the patient is at the end of life and should receive palliative care) (Kim et al., 2017). Even as nursing practice has expanded to meet critical needs for advanced practice, pejorative enumerations and identification of the role by other disciplines such as "midlevel practitioners" or "physician-extenders"

> ## Group Discussion
>
> It has been said that health care is both risk adverse and conflict adverse. Discuss this claim. First, consider whether it is indeed true that health professionals avoid conflict to an unusually high degree. To reach a conclusion, it may be helpful to consider the following questions:
>
> - Does the structure of healthcare services create clear lines of demarcation between people?
> - Does the hierarchical nature of healthcare services promote or prevent conflict?
> - Are there fewer, more, or similar personality issues in healthcare settings than in other settings?
> - How does the physician's role and position affect the incidence of conflict?

characterize advanced practice practitioners in subordinate and comparatively subservient roles compared to that of the historically predominantly superior role of physicians.

As a result, out of frustration, nurses are sometimes inclined to engage in passive-aggressive, hostile, uncooperative, or avoidance behavior, even if the consequences are damaging to themselves (Johansen & Cadmus, 2016). One explanation is that they have not always been able to avail themselves of the maturity that comes with development, dialogue, conflict resolution processes, and any aggregated measure of success. Another explanation may be that the practice and service delivery models in use generally do not require nurses to interact at a high level outside of their own discipline or with other disciplines. Most nursing work is designed to be performed by interdependent nurses or nursing teams assigned to defined groups of patients acting inside of the nursing community. Nurses primarily speak with each other regarding the specifics of nursing practice and the processes and values of nursing-driven decisions and actions. Nursing teamwork involves little interdisciplinary interface and sharing and keeps nurses from the vital multilateral interactions that would develop their broader relational skills. Conflicts among nurses and between nurses and other health professionals fall into the category of identity-based conflicts, and their ultimate resolution requires, among other things, reconstructing the relationship between nursing and the other professions (Maung et al., 2015).

Leaders, to do their job well, must acquire basic conflict management skills. Most lack these skills or have failed to master them, and as a result, in many organizations, a whole range of conflicts festers and grows. Avoidance of conflict is one of the greatest sources of human relationship and interactional problems in the workplace. The possession of well-honed conflict management skills has become even more important because of the increasingly interdisciplinary nature of the workplace and because questioning or attempting to change these historically uneven relationships can easily raise the potential for conflict.

Avoiding Unnecessary Conflict

Because conflict is an essential component of human interaction, trying to create conditions in which conflict is completely absent is a pointless exercise. There is generally a prevailing sense that conflict is negative. Nothing could be further from the truth. Conflict is simply the indication of the presence of differences. Ignoring essential differences provides solid ground for encouraging unnecessary conflict. It is not good use of leaders' skills or time to try to prevent inevitable conflict. Instead, leaders should devote themselves to managing conflict, which also includes preventing unnecessary conflict. Some of the conditions that help prevent unnecessary conflict are described in the following sections (Dignath et al., 2015).

An Environment of Open Communication

It goes without saying that creating a climate of openness and trust is an excellent way to facilitate work and relationships. However, some leaders believe that tightly controlling work creates the fewest problems and that a "tight ship is the best run ship." This is not true for the normal activities of work. Leaders must realize that the relationship between the members of the work team is the most critical factor influencing the extent to which any conflict situation becomes a way of life. A sense that there is nothing that cannot be dealt with, that there are no "undiscussables," is essential to avoiding unnecessary conflicts.

> **Key Point**
> An environment that abounds with "undiscussables" is an environment that breeds mistrust and unnecessary conflict.

The senior-level leaders of an organization have enormous influence over the organization's culture. The leaders' style of relating to and communicating with others sets the tone for the workplace, and it does not take long for others in the organization to discern what is acceptable to leaders and what is not. Leader behavior toward staff and their responses to the stressors and challenges of work create the model of acceptable conduct and act as the framework for which topics can be approached and which behaviors are appropriate.

Groups become very skilled at seeing and noting the permissible and the political. Group members know the workarounds needed to get things done. What cannot be dealt with openly and directly is addressed secretively and behind closed doors. It is when open communication is absent that the infrastructure of conflict begins to take form and processes leading to irresolvable differences begin to emerge.

Congruence Between Organizational and Professional Work Goals

A good way to prevent conflict is to ensure that the goals of individual workers and the goals of the organization support each other. It is commonly understood that complementary goals prevent conflict and competitive goals generate conflict. The history of work in America is rife with instances where organizational goals and processes were at odds with the goals and expectations of those doing the work and where inherent conflict sprang up as a result.

When there is goal congruence, people are more open, cooperative, engaged, and supportive and less angry and frustrated. When everyone is clear about expectations and processes and there is a supporting structure that contributes to meeting expectations, less conflict is generated (Zavotsky & Chan, 2016).

Of course, congruence between goals is not always possible. Therefore, people must be given the opportunity to disclose differences in goals and how they are affected by differences. If the reasons for the differences and the character of the differences

> **Key Point**
> Facilitators must understand that the conflicts they attempt to resolve never belong to them. A conflict is owned by those who experience it, and transferring the locus of control is not good for the parties or the process.

can be made clear, people find them easier to accommodate or accept. In addition, they find goal differences easier to accommodate or accept if they understand that all issues and situations are transitional (subject to inevitable change) and all relationships operate within the context of the constantly shifting human and relational journey (**Figures 6-1** through **6-5**).

Managing Conflict Productively

Leaders should devote resources to the tasks of recognizing sources of conflict soon enough to handle disputes in the right way and at the right time, rather than devoting resources to avoiding conflict. Following are some rules for handling conflict appropriately and productively.

Time and place can play a role in diffusing or inflaming a conflict. For example, if a conflict arises in public, wise leaders act to remove the parties to a private place where the issues can be dealt with directly and freely. In many cases, a conflict first reveals itself at a critical or stressful moment, fooling participants into believing that the situation is the source of the conflict rather than simply an occasion for its expression. In such a case, trying to deal with the conflict within the context of the situation will likely escalate the conflict, and so it is better to put the participants into a different environment or deal with the conflict at a later time when everyone can focus the dialogue on the issues, not the event.

Figure 6-1 Structural Conflicts.

Figure 6-2 Value Conflicts.

Avoiding Unnecessary Conflict

Figure 6-3 Information Conflicts.

- Insight
- Skill
- Facilitation

- Availability
- Specificity
- Relevance

What can be changed: Different information; Different data, assessment, and interpretation; Geography Demography Environment

Figure 6-4 Interaction Conflicts.

- Insight
- Skill
- Facilitation

- Capacity
- Expression/passion
- Maturity/ego

What can be changed: Perceptions of others; Communication and language; Geography Demography Environment

Professional standards

Figure 6-5 Interest Conflicts.

- Insight
- Skill
- Facilitation

- Wants
- Approaches
- Breadth

What can be changed: Competition and position; Politics and processes; Geography Demography Environment

225

CHAPTER SIX   Diversity and Difference: Managing Conflict in a Transdisciplinary Network

The implications of appreciative leadership are important as an underpinning to appropriate conflict management behaviors and strategies. The capacity of leaders to see creative potential as a consistent undercurrent to all positive behavior is important to a productive view of the work of conflict management (du Plessis, 2016). Understanding that conflict is simply a metaphor for human differences and that conflict management is essentially "difference management" is important. Leaders must have a productive and positive mental model that reflects on their capacity to appreciate the value of every individual, their ownership for their own action and lives, and the requisite that they simply act to enable individual ownership and action. In this difference management framework, a positive search for what is best in the organization and among individuals, undertaking of positive narratives with all stakeholders, the generative focus of all conversations, and centrality of relationship-building in every human interaction are the driving characteristics for positive conflict management (Bleich & Hessler, 2016). The leader's pursuit of a deeper understanding of the appreciative characteristics of human interaction and communication is an essential foundation to the critical and successful development of a personal leadership capacity in understanding and handling conflict. Although outside of the scope of this text, it is advised that leaders broaden and deepen their understanding of appreciative approaches and incorporate patterns of leadership behavior and interaction into the management of all of their relationships with those they lead (Butani & Plant, 2016).

Remember, conflict is primarily about behavior, not about people (although see the section titled "Identity-Based Conflict," which follows). In dealing with conflicts, leaders need to be clued into the behavioral patterns and concerns and their impact on the parties' relationships because the ultimate goal is to sustain effective relationships (Morreim, 2016). Leaders should look to accommodate behaviors that are needed to develop a working relationship that matches the values and commitment necessary to complete the work of conflict management and sustain optimal relationships. In addition, the goal is to fix the problem, not to affix blame. No conflict is unilaterally driven—there is always enough fault to go around (thus, faultfinding is a waste of time). Wasting time and resources on trying to affix blame invariably delays long-term resolution of the conflict.

Resolution of a conflict depends on achievement of some level of agreement about change in the parties' behaviors or responses. Agreement in a change in behaviors or responses to differences must be clearly articulated and understood by all parties. Further, at some point the parties must formally or publicly define their common ground in joint communication (written or in a meeting).

If a conflict is to be resolved, the parties involved must have a sense of ownership over their own feelings and the resolution agenda. Leaders must ensure that the parties own their feelings and do not cast them onto the shoulders of others. Leaders should never interpret what others mean without confirming that their interpretation is correct. The use of "I" approaches is critical to the dialogue. By making certain that each party's insights, feelings, and views are expressed from the party's own perspective and in their individual (own) language, leaders keep both parties away from "us versus them" and "you" statements. Leaders can also help maintain the focus and flow of the dialogue by making certain it stays within the limits of self-directed communication and personal ownership of the dialogue.

A white board, flip chart, sticky notes, or other visual tools can be used to get the conflict elements out in front of the parties in a two-dimensional way. The use of visual tools can overcome some of the obstacles likely to be raised by poorly chosen language. Visual tools place the ideas of all the parties before their eyes in a way that automatically creates equity. Visual tools also help balance the dialogue and move issues closer to real resolution by expanding the foundation of understanding between the parties.

Vagueness must be constantly fought. Although a certain amount of ambiguity is unavoidable as people sort out their issues, continued vagueness obscures the issues and stops the dialogue. Leaders involved in the conflict must work to facilitate clarity around every issue of concern. By naming names, identifying events, describing situations, and illustrating behaviors, leaders seek to get down to basics. The goal is to ensure that the real issues and processes are laid out on the table in clear enough terms that all the players can see them plainly.

In the conflict, each person (party) with a similar view is looking for something, and unless this something is obtained or willingly given up for something else, the conflict will not end. First, each party must articulate what they want in a way that all can understand and agree to. Second, each party must leave the conflict with a sense that they each obtained something valuable; and, each must feel good about the other party's resolution as well. In other words, each party must view the resolution as equitable. This does not mean that what everyone gets is equal. It means that the resolution dispensed to each party is enough to satisfy that party, regardless of the level of importance to the other parties.

Advice on how to manage conflict is not all-inclusive. For instance, leaders must take into account both situational/organizational and individual (e.g., cultural) factors when trying to facilitate resolution of conflicts. Leaders must demonstrate flexibility in incorporating contextual factors in discussions as part of the conflict management skill set.

> **Point to Ponder**
>
> The team, not the individual, is the basic unit of work. Individuals must always be seen in the context of their relationships with others. Because work is the aggregation of the efforts of many people, for work to result in sustainable outcomes efforts must be coordinated and integrated. The task of team leaders is to synthesize the efforts of team members and take advantage of the resulting synergy to achieve team goals efficiently and effectively.

Team-Based Conflict Issues

Working together to provide healthcare services can be intense and difficult and can easily lead to conflict. To reduce the chance of unnecessary conflict, leaders must pay attention to relationship issues and create and keep an open and honest context for the work. Still, even in the best circumstances the behaviors and characteristics of people can lead to conflict (Hamblin et al., 2016).

Different personalities deal with conflict in different ways. Some people are naturally generators of conflict, whereas others are skilled avoiders of it. Most adults fall somewhere in between the two extremes. Because different interests and personalities are present in the workplace, there is always opportunity for conflict to emerge.

Leaders of a healthcare organization should always be on the lookout for the potential for conflict. Because conflict eventually arises in any human environment, its potential is always present, at least to some degree. Further, when a conflict is detected in its very early stages, it can be addressed soon enough to keep it from becoming critical and requiring extensive intervention. In general, the amount of effort needed to resolve a conflict is directly related to how early in the conflict's development the issues are dealt with.

Leaders must be aware of the multiple factors that lead to team-based conflict. If team members believe they are on the receiving end of unfair or inequitable treatment, they will descend Maslow's hierarchy of needs (organizational source of conflict). Conflict and acting out inevitably occur unless everyone is given an equal opportunity to provide input and have an impact. One source of inequity surrounds the tendency of people to use each other or the team for their own agendas or advancement. All team members must try to be just and fair in their dealings with each other to ensure the playing field is level and even and everyone is treated impartially.

Everyone does not need to know everything, but there must not be a lack of essential information, especially the information people need to do their work and to function and relate efficiently. Team members must have a common understanding of information and be able to see it within the correct context. It is common for people to believe they have the information they need, only to discover upon further investigation that each individual has a different understanding of it. Team leaders must make sure that everyone shares a common understanding. At the end of an interaction, session, or meeting, it is always wise for leaders to poll the group regarding their level of mutual understanding of what has been deliberated and decided on prior to anyone undertaking action. Further, team members need to share their knowledge, insights, and experience in a way that can influence the team and what it does. Expressing what they know and believe is critical to their own sense of value and place on the team and is likewise critical to the viability of the team.

Game playing always leads to conflict. Team leaders must be certain that members are singing off the same song sheet. The rules that govern the team's activities should be clarified to and by the team members at the outset and often along the way. Members also need to be reminded that they will be held accountable for respecting the rules. Although any team must be able to accommodate different personalities, the interaction of team members must keep within certain boundaries. Processes that impede good interaction and communication between members ultimately lead to conflict.

Not acknowledging everyone's unique contribution can be a source of trouble. Every person approaches his or her work differently, has a different array of talents and skills, and has a different background and set of experiences. Team leaders must not only recognize the differences between team members, but must use them to advance the work of the team. For instance, some members are more reflective, and others are more active. Leaders usually do not need to prompt the more active members to make themselves heard—they are usually the first to initiate dialogue or action—but leaders may have to ask more reflective members for their views. Because the reflective members often have excellent insights and thoughtful opinions, their contributions must be considered in the team process to ensure that the team's work is fully effective. Thus, leaders must recognize that the presence of personality and role differences can actually enhance the team's effectiveness, and that getting the full range of contributions from members avoids conflict because no one feels unjustly neglected.

Behavior based on hidden agendas is a prevalent source of team conflict and is extremely difficult to address (individual source of conflict). Almost every team has members who are not "on board" because they are pursuing their own agendas. Members with hidden agendas attempt to realize their goals by manipulating others and preventing others from attaining their objectives. They tend to see the world solely from their own position and treat others simply as a means of advancing their own interests. Whether they keep the team from growing or move the team in the direction of their choosing, they damage the integrity of the team and its sense of purpose. Team leaders must try to detect patterns of behavior reflecting hidden agendas early in the team process and correct them before they do serious harm. If members are allowed to pursue their own agendas with impunity or for a long period of time, they reduce the team's effectiveness and eventually cause the team to descend into a state of chaos and conflict.

Lack of mutual appreciation among team members impairs team integrity. Old adages that reflect this theme are "I can only be me through your eyes" and "we are only as strong as the weakest link." Who people are and the gifts that they bring are sacred and important. All team members should believe they have value and are there because they have a unique contribution to make. They should know what it is they offer and be acknowledged for it by other members. Members should be aware of the character and role of any other member and understand how to advance and honor their own role. By clearly articulating the gifts that everyone brings to the table and the value of those gifts, team leaders keep all team members mindful of everyone's importance and thus diminish the potential for conflict and breakdown.

Power issues are a common source of conflict. How power is dispersed and used has a great influence on the occurrence and intensity of conflict within a team. In particular, conflict inevitably occurs if the expression of power is not seen as competent or balanced, or if the location of power is not seen as appropriate. A team operates like a community, and team leaders have the responsibility to maintain a sense of community among members. Leaders are always looking for breaks and potential problems in the relationship between members as a way of anticipating conflict and dealing with it before it develops into a major crisis requiring substantial time and resources (Almost et al., 2016).

Getting ahead of conflicts that emerge is the best possible method for diffusing them and mitigating their consequences. Team leaders should set up their team's structure and processes to make conflict a normal part of interactions and relationships among members. Leaders should not ignore conflict but instead implement strategies to expose the essential differences between members early enough to resolve the inevitable episodes of conflict as quickly as possible. By valuing and validating differences among team members and accommodating them, leaders reduce the number of conflicts and at the same time decrease the chance that any of them will become crippling.

> **Key Point**
>
> Power is a sensitive issue in health care. For example, the word *power* is rarely used by health professionals, as if they do not really believe it operates in their relationships with each other. Of course, it always does. It is vital that the issues of power and authority be open for discussion because they are critical elements in the interaction of team members at every level of the system.

Identity-Based Conflicts

Conflicts generally fall into two categories: interest-based conflicts and identity-based conflicts. Interest-based conflicts arise from circumstances or interactions and often can be resolved quickly; in contrast, identity-based conflicts go much deeper and last longer. Rothman (2018), in laying some foundations, suggested that identity-based conflicts are rooted in threats to people's need for dignity, recognition, safety, control, purpose, and efficacy. For identity-based conflicts to be adequately addressed, their origin and their meaning to the opposed parties must be adequately appreciated. In general, identity-based conflicts have the following characteristics:

- Reflect the parties' culture and beliefs
- Involve questions of identity and sense of self
- Arise out of the parties' commitment to their values
- Are of long duration
- Are the most difficult conflicts to resolve
- Can be passed on from one generation to next

Sources of identity-based conflicts include:

- Values
- Religion
- Language
- Heritage
- Culture
- Family
- Community
- Country

Each person has a unique background and set of life experiences and brings a personal and a cultural framework to any dialogue or deliberation with others. Further, because each person is unique, relationships and interactions exhibit a dynamic pattern and identity-based conflicts are possible. Differences between people create life's mosaic—its fabric. The richness of human experience is driven by the broad diversity that is characteristic of human life and that forms the foundation for human interaction. It is no surprise that for conflict resolution activities to be successful they must be based on an understanding of the ingrained differences between the parties and must encompass a respect for and appreciation of these differences.

Conflict is a normal part of all human affairs, from marriage to politics. Recognizing this fact encourages us not to ignore conflict, downplay it, or leave it unaddressed. The best strategy is to accept that conflict is inevitable and to acquire the skills and methods for safely and

Group Discussion

Look around the room at other occupants and write down as many differences as you can in a few minutes. After listing all the differences on a flip chart, discuss how each might lead to a conflict. Also discuss how the resulting conflicts might affect relationships, interactions, and the work environment. Then, identify how different types of conflict are related to each other and consider the possibility that together they could result in an irresolvable state of conflict. Finally, discuss how the conflicts identified could escalate, and then describe the impact such escalation could have on patient care.

effectively dealing with it, including paying attention to what it means and the positive direction it is trying to move us toward.

Identity-based conflicts are very difficult to either define or resolve. Because they are rooted in historical, psychological, cultural, and experiential factors, their boundaries and content are hard to determine. Because they are deeply embedded in personal sentiments, contending parties are less willing to compromise. Therefore, people with identity-based conflicts demand a deep and creative engagement.

Protracted religious, ethnic, tribal, regional, and national conflicts are the best examples of the persistence of identity-based conflicts. Long-term, persisting "enemy images" create a permanent "other" that influences notions of equality, equity, value, and identity. Enemy images that are believed to be valid and that are stereotypic are embedded in a group's set of beliefs, hypotheses, or theories about another group. Over time these images become normative and set up intransigent images that reinforce the stereotype and hostility toward it. Group consensus around beliefs and stereotypes reinforces acceptable enemy characterizations and socially entrenched opposition behaviors as normative parts of the sentiments toward the "enemy group." These behaviors, in fact, become a way of life such that not having them would be inconceivable. Because the idea exists over a sufficiently long time, the "enemy other" often becomes inherently inequitable, less than, innately subordinate, and is often subject to the grossest maligning, objectification, and the worst levels of inhuman violence. Such hostility reinforces hostility, generates more intensive hostility, and sustains hostility over generations. Like all conflicts, the longer it remains unresolved, the more entrenched it becomes, and the more difficult it is to resolve.

> **Point to Ponder**
>
> Although conflict is normal, unresolved conflict is dysfunctional. Further, a particular conflict will remain unresolved if it remains unnamed or undiscussed.

Giving the Parties a Voice

When confronted with an identity-based conflict between two or more parties, a "third-party" leader must facilitate resolution of the conflict. Acting as facilitator, the leader's first job is to give the parties a voice and listen to their essential insights and their perceptions of the conflict. They must be allowed to express where they are located in the conflict and what their feelings are about the conflict. Note that their perceptions do not have to be correct, right or wrong, because the main goal is to simply lay out what each party has experienced from inside the experience. The stated perceptions of the parties constitute a personal expression of their experiences of the conflict and are bound to be different from the stated perceptions of the other party. In some cases, the parties' perceptions are so different that an objective third person may wonder if each is describing the same situation, condition, or scenario.

> **Key Point**
>
> Difference is a cause of conflict and, as a prerequisite of dialogue, part of the solution to conflict. In fact, both difference and dialogue are necessary for good and sustainable human interaction.

Getting the parties to give expression to their perceptions of the conflict is an essential first step in understanding and resolving the conflict. The way the perceptions are formulated should reflect the feelings and sentiments of those who have the perceptions. This stage, when the parties give voice to their sentiments and perceptions, is not the time for structured clarification and process. The facilitator needs to allow the expression of perceptions to be natural and unconstrained. The result is sometimes uncomfortable because the emotion can be intense and raw. Yet intensity of feeling indicates to the parties how critical the process is and just what the stakes are.

Perceptions of the conflict are accompanied by sentiments and emotions that are largely not grounded in sound facts or occurrences. Historical perceptions of a wrong or fault have often been embellished by story and mythology over the long term to the extent that it becomes difficult to separate the myth from the real, fiction from fact. As has often been done in emerging nations where ethnic groups have played enemy roles for generations, grievances have been acknowledged and accepted as true by all stakeholders, recognized as undeniable, and simply acknowledged as a part of history. Such processes are always followed by significant national or ethnic symbols of forgiveness and separation so that a new foundation or demarcation can be laid, upon which a fresh and emergent pattern of social compatibility can be structured between former divergent groups ("enemies"), representing a level of mutuality and agreement about the future that all parties can agree to.

For there to be movement toward resolution and/or acceptance, the facilitator must make sure that all the issues and all facets of the issues believed by the parties to be critical are laid out in detail, including issues related to dignity, recognition, value, and meaning. Nothing is more threatening to the process of resolution than for a party to believe that his or her story was not told, the story has not been fully heard, or the origin of the conflict has not been fully appreciated and, as a result, that the process is skewed and therefore flawed.

Identity-based conflicts are rooted in the parties' need to protect their value and identity (**Exhibit 6-2**). People with identity-based conflicts believe there is a threat to who they are—a threat to the very foundation of their being—and they often respond by going on the attack. For example, conflicts between nurses and physicians over practice are rooted in their notions of who they are as professionals and their sense that their value and even survival are threatened by the other professional group. Some physicians believe that advanced practice nurses jeopardize their independence as practitioners and their economic well-being, and some advanced practice nurses believe that physicians obstruct their ability to practice, grow, thrive, and contribute as professionals at the top of their license. In fact, each group views the other group as a major threat to its own interests, predisposing members of both groups to let their negative perceptions of the conflict inform every interaction they have on issues of practice and service.

Interest-based conflicts, if left unresolved long enough, can and often do become identity-based conflicts, but the latter, no matter what their origin, require strategies different

---

Exhibit 6-2 Identity Characteristics

- Needs
- Self-image
- Insight
- Knowledge
- Skills
- Balance
- Clarity
- Investment
- Breadth
- Ownership

from those used to resolve conflicts that are simply interest based. For instance, legal and negotiation-oriented strategies tend to alienate the parties to an identity-based conflict. These strategies limit the amount and types of dialogue that occur, preventing the parties from establishing the kind of relationship they need to deal with the issues affecting them. Using resolution strategies aimed at getting to an early agreement can poison the conversation and keep the parties from finding common ground and some points of mutual value and shared identity. People are not willing to compromise those things that they believe are fundamental to their own identity and survival. For them, some issues simply are not subject to negotiation.

> **Key Point**
>
> Identity-based conflicts take longer to resolve than do interest-based conflicts. They arise out of people's identity—who people are as opposed to what they do—and often have substantial historical content. In an identity-based conflict, to reach a resolution the two parties must come to appreciate each other's value and respect each other's uniqueness—a very challenging task given the passionate attachment of each party to his or her own identity.

Time and Patience

In trying to resolve an identity-based conflict, it is a mistake to begin by pushing the parties to compromise, often the strategy of choice for interest-based conflicts. Another mistake is to try to get the parties to separate their feelings from the so-called facts of the conflict because their feelings, especially their sense of identity, are at the root of the conflict. Using a strategy that threatens their identity makes the parties more suspicious of each other and of the conflict resolution process.

The resolution of identity-based conflicts takes a great deal of time, especially the first stages of the process. However, these stages are the most crucial and warrant the extra time and patience. Naming and certifying issues, feelings, and positions clearly at the outset establishes a firm foundation on which to construct a process that moves effectively to a successful outcome.

In a traditional negotiation process, the parties try, through compromise, to arrive at a place where they can essentially split the difference. This process works best when the issues are clear, the goals are well defined, and the parties are reasonably clear on what the common ground looks like. Unfortunately, the underlying issues in an identity-based conflict are blurred, and the parties feel especially vulnerable because the stakes are seen as consequential. The parties therefore are hesitant to compromise early in the process, and moving too quickly toward a resolution could threaten the process itself and prevent the parties from dealing with the underlying issues, in which case these issues would ultimately give rise to another episode of discord.

> **Point to Ponder**
>
> Conflicts love to hide in ambiguity. If a conflict remains unclear or undefined, it also remains elusive and hard to eradicate. The parties, only able to deal with the symptoms, almost certainly will allow the conflict to have an impact on all their joint activities, leading to negativity and uncertainty far beyond the boundaries of the conflict itself.

Building Trust

Much of the early work in the resolution process is directed toward getting the parties to change the way they think about each other and agree on a process and method for interacting.

Chapter Six Diversity and Difference: Managing Conflict in a Transdisciplinary Network

The parties are essentially suspicious of each other. Their suspicion is itself a great source of conflict, and getting to a place where the rules of engagement are clear and can be used as the vehicle for dialogue increases the probability that the parties can work out their differences.

In an interest-based conflict, the root issues are not always put on the table, and the negotiation strategies are typically as important as the issues. In contrast, in an identity-based conflict, posturing and positioning are generally ineffective because the parties need to disclose their powerfully held sentiments and beliefs—those things that reveal who they are and what they do. To build a proper foundation for resolving the conflict, they must fully understand these sentiments and beliefs—their own and those of the other party—and identify whatever common ground exists.

Because of the high stakes involved in an identity-based conflict, the facilitator should move the parties toward negotiations slowly, after a trusting foundation has been established. Often, using informal familiar and familial interaction and relationship development humanizes the participants, makes them real to each other, and gives them an opportunity to witness common frames of references related to children, family, and community. These informal opportunities at relationship help to humanize those who have lost their humanity through enemy metaphors of prejudice, objectification, humiliation, and subordination. In the initial stages of dialogue, the facilitator should encourage the parties to set practical goals, such as arriving at a common view of the conflict and agreeing to a description of the issues in a common language. By achieving these goals, the parties are more inclined to accept that resolution of the conflict is a real possibility and can feel comfortable with the resolution process. In short, the parties must develop a sense of relationship with each other before moving further along toward resolution.

The facilitator must realize that building a trusting atmosphere and getting the parties to recognize they each have a substantial stake in resolving the conflict are both essential steps. By showing the parties their relationship in the larger context, the facilitator helps them see where their common values lie and what a resolution equitable to everyone might be.

The facilitator is likely to find that one or both parties exhibit a currently prevailing pattern of behavior characterized by deviousness, secretiveness, manipulation, and a sense of "us against the world." This pattern provokes a response of unilateral defensiveness that is hard to break through. To fight against it, the facilitator must try to nurture cooperative inquiry, establish credibility, and engage in relationship building. A good part of the resolution process must be devoted to creating a common identity around the issues in a way that allows all the parties to believe they are mutually contributing to a justifiable end of the conflict.

The parties must arrive at a place where they can honestly say what they value and believe. Getting them to this place may not be easy because the parties may have strong emotional blocks that prevent them from articulating their real issues. Sometimes the parties believe they are articulating the issues by stating how they feel, but in doing this they are focusing on the results of the issues, not on the issues themselves. The facilitator must get them to focus on what caused these feelings—the conflicts that lie at the heart of their emotions.

The long-term work involves helping the parties reconceptualize the conflict, perceive their relationship in a new way, change the language they use to describe the conflict, and even change the nature of the conflict altogether. The conflict may be rooted in a lack of clarity, and one or both parties may say things that are inconsistent with what they do. Both parties need to achieve a good understanding of their own motives and desires before attempting to move toward an end to the conflict. Otherwise, each will be unable to hear the other and understand where the other is coming from.

Finding Differences

As mentioned earlier, each person is a unique blend of differences, and these differences are what make people exciting and intriguing to each other. We celebrate our differences and honor diversity in culture and personality. Yet differences can become an impediment to understanding a relationship, and given enough time, any human relationship will give rise to some level of conflict. When it does, those in the relationship must understand that it is not the conflict that is problematic but its nonresolution.

> ## Group Discussion
>
> In any organization, unresolved conflict eventually creates a culture of conflict, increasing the incidence of conflict at every level (Almost et al., 2016). After identifying personally experienced unresolved conflicts in the workplace, discuss the impact that each conflict had on relationships in the workgroup. In talking about this issue, consider the following questions:
>
> - What kinds of factions formed?
> - Did the one conflict lead to others?
> - Did the group leader take any action to ensure that the conflict would be resolved? That it would not be resolved?
> - What was the long-term impact of the unresolved conflict?
> - Was the conflict ever resolved? How?

To figure out just what caused a conflict, the parties to the conflict must frame the issue in a way that gives it focus. One method is for each party to ask, what do I want here? To answer this question, each must be clear on how he or she stands on the differences between the two parties. Framing their notion of the conflict or of their position in relationship to it gives the parties a foundation on which to take a position. To get there, they need to ask themselves some specific questions.

Do the parties remember the period before the conflict existed? Looking at the before and after can help the parties give the conflict a time and a frame of reference, allowing them to identify its elements in a way that makes it real. Furthermore, the parties, in reviewing the period before the conflict, give the facilitator an opportunity to see how each perceives the beginning of the conflict and to detect any differences in their perceptions.

What antagonisms emerged? What did they look like? How did they feel? Here, the focus is on perceptions of the moment of conflict. The issues of resentment, behavior change, and cultural and personality differences get expressed in the unique language of each party. Both parties begin to express their special insights about the feelings and animosities that emerged and grew as a result of their differences, and the individual flavor of the conflict starts to become clear. The parties now get a chance to express not only how they felt but why and what it meant to them at the time, allowing the circumstances to be reflected through the lens of personal experience. This process disciplines their insight and forces them to focus on the conditions and circumstances that give form to their sense of the conflict.

Who is to blame and what is he or she to be blamed for? Answering this question is a good way to get to the dynamics of the conflict. A strong element of blame lies at the heart of almost every conflict. The parties need to get some idea of what the blame is, where it resides, and what form it takes. Not only is it important to uncover the blame, the facilitator must push each party to describe the content of the blame it points at the other party and explain why it is justified. The explanation is likely to make reference to stress, pain, or anguish experienced by the party doing the blaming and indicates how the other party was responsible for it.

These questions get at the fundamental antagonisms causing the conflict. The parties' perceptions and feelings need to be articulated at the beginning of the resolution process for two reasons. First, both parties must see and say where they are in relation to their notion of the conflict. Second, the facilitator must get some sense of where the parties are at the start of the resolution process. The agenda for building the process and achieving reconciliation is constructed at the very beginning of the process. By getting the parties to delineate the differences in their perceptions and positions, the facilitator gains information about the work yet to be undertaken.

To get information about party differences, it is best to talk with each party independently. The facilitator should keep the meetings informal and focused on gathering information and helping the parties get ready for their work within the process. These meetings also offer a good opportunity to discuss the rules of engagement that will be used when all the parties are at the table. Note, however, that the rules of engagement must be finally deliberated and agreed to when both parties are present.

Who Wants What?

People in conflict generally know what it is they believe they want. When individuals or groups are at the point of conflict, they generally have reached the stage of holding black-and-white positions—positions that are mutually exclusive and sit at some distance from each other.

> **Key Point**
>
> Parties to a conflict must be allowed to express their feelings, even their passionate feelings. If not expressed, these feelings become intensified and move deeply inward, poisoning every interaction and preventing a resolution from being achieved. Therefore, facilitators must create a safe space for the parties to get their feelings out.

To bring the positions closer, the facilitator must be steeped in the resolution process and look for every opportunity to foster congruence, strengthen trust, and improve the interface between the parties as their relationship begins to grow. As noted previously, the parties to an identity-based conflict must establish a relationship and not simply obtain a resolution of their issues. The facilitator helps them do this by knowing them as well as possible and being familiar enough with their issues and positions so as not to miss opportunities for bridging differences and constructing common ground because such opportunities rarely are presented twice. The facilitator's knowledge is his or her main tool for advancing the process and moving the relationship through the tough times.

ARIA Conflict Engagement Theory

In his seminal work on identity-based conflicts, Rothman (2018) suggested a format for the resolution process. The stages of the format, which he called ARIA Conflict Engagement Theory, are antagonism, resonance, invention, and action. They are outlined in the following subsections.

Antagonism

In this first stage the facilitator pushes the parties to express their antagonism, which, besides helping the facilitator move the process along, helps the parties lay out their raw emotions in plain view and, in so doing, diffuses them, thereby reducing the temperature of the conflict. Given the proper context, this initial expression of antagonism also provides extra motivation to do something about the conflict and the negative feelings that it generates—to end the pain and discord and move to a better place, where there is more peace and stability and opportunity.

In addition, it can reveal to the parties their own limitations and constraints. They are able to see how their own intensity of emotion polarizes their views and positions. Although unlikely at this point to be able to make substantial changes, they can at least get a picture of what their positions look like and how strongly they hold their views, possibly opening a window to understanding. Indeed, expressing their antagonism and hearing it reflected back in the language of the facilitator may surprise them and finally make them realize just how fixed, strident, or polarized they have become. After all, the flames of antagonism are fanned by a wide range of emotions that, regardless of their legitimacy, are strongly felt and often just as strongly expressed.

Blame helps the parties avoid focusing on their part in the conflict. By concentrating on why it is the other party's fault, each party evades having to reflect on the role he or she has played. The parties never have to consider how they might have acted differently, experience the pain of admitting their own contribution to the conflict, or engage in the work of reaching a resolution. Indeed, blame suggests that a resolution to the conflict is not possible.

Blame helps keep the conflict external—safe and free of personal content. It puts the responsibility for resolving the conflict in the other party's court and suggests that if the other party would make certain changes or act differently, the issues and the conflict would simply disappear.

Blame never has any real inherent or intrinsic value. The facilitator's best strategy is to pursue naming the feelings of each party and their intensities. Even when restating accusations of blame, the facilitator does not spend time in the blame. Discussing the blame that has been leveled merely helps the facilitator figure out (1) where the parties are in relation to each other and to the issues at the root of the conflict and (2) how to move the parties toward reconciliation.

Blame also generalizes feelings and perceptions and keeps the parties from being specific and reaching clarity. The facilitator's role is to get the parties into and through the blame and on to focus on the particulars and delineate their own positions.

> **Point to Ponder**
>
> Blame keeps the parties from owning their part of the conflict—from naming their own issues and identifying them as causes of the conflict—and thus keeps them from achieving a resolution. In pointing a finger, each party focuses exclusively on the other party's actions, whereas each should instead attempt to see clearly and admit to his or her role in the conflict dynamic.
>
> In a typical conflict, one or both parties blame the other side to strengthen their own position, at least in their own eyes. Blame serves to escalate the conflict and give it a justification. It creates an "us and them" position, locates the enemy, and defines the terms of opposition. It puts the other party at fault and provides a reason to be angry at and in conflict with the other party. The natural tendency to place blame is best exemplified by the common childhood claim, "He hit me first."

> ## Group Discussion
>
> Greg Shue, the manager of a hospital department, was angry with the head of critical care. She had beaten him out of a part of the budget he needed to make programmatic changes in his own department. He occasionally referred to her in derogatory terms and seemed unable to get past his anger, which was beginning to have a serious effect on the relationship between Greg and the other department head and on the entire organization. You are the conflict mediator in this case. How would you begin the conflict resolution process? What would you do to get Greg to own his anger? What would you do to induce Greg to move beyond his feelings and begin dealing with the real issues?

Posturing and positioning commonly act as intensifiers of conflict. They support the culture of justification and rights and lead to rationalizations of the polarization that typically occur in a conflict. The parties give reasons for the polarization and construct a whole logic to support it. In other words, they "circle the wagons" and make the war their cause, rather than the issue at the root of the war. They then devote more time and energy to conducting the war than they ever did in pursuing the underlying issue.

At this stage, the conflict has taken on a life of its own. Nothing the other party does with regard to the issue is right or appropriate. Further, because each party is acting out of his or her own identity, the other party not only does the wrong thing but becomes wrong. The next step is to describe the other party as bad and to conclude that he or she must be opposed. If the one party did not oppose the bad party, the former would be bad, too, and in the same way. This would be untenable. Thus, each side builds the polarization between the parties and raises the intensity of the conflict.

Also, as the characterization of each party by the other grows increasingly negative, the less necessary each believes it is to resolve the conflict. Who would want to resolve a conflict if it meant giving up a justifiable fight against what is bad, perhaps even evil? In the mind of each party, what needs to happen is for the other party to stop being bad, and, if that occurred, the conflict would automatically end.

The facilitator must realize that each party has a selective memory. Each vividly remembers events that led to the conflict and for which blame could be laid on the other party. On the other hand, both parties tend to forget contributing events for which they were responsible, not to mention their own dishonorable motives.

When the negatives run high, each party's desire to resolve the underlying issue wanes. Their energy is instead devoted to building a culture of opposition and to placing themselves in the right. They act to strengthen their position and have it validated by prospective allies. Correspondingly little energy is devoted to pursuing strategies that might lead to a resolution of the conflict.

As time goes on, each party becomes increasingly critical and disapproving of the behaviors, practices, and even culture of the other party. Words and actions become opportunities for the one party to challenge, skewer, or demean the other and further validate continuation of the conflict.

Projection is commonly used by parties in a conflict to strengthen their positions. Projection involves attributing to others problematic behaviors we engage in or embarrassing characteristics we possess. It is universally understood as a defense mechanism for avoiding responsibility for such behaviors and characteristics. In a conflict, one party, in addition to viewing the other party as fundamentally different, might project, for example, unacceptable motives onto the other party, and thus avoid confronting their own motives.

If failure to confront motives occurs, the facilitator's goal of getting the parties to see what they share in common becomes even harder. Each party resists admitting that the other could in any way be similar because doing so might involve acknowledging parallel objectionable behaviors. Though daunting, the facilitator's task at the outset is to achieve as much clarity about the antagonism as possible, and his or her initial activities largely are spent on getting the parties past this part of the conflict so that they can pursue resolution strategies.

> ## Group Discussion
>
> The parties to a conflict each possess values and beliefs. If the conflict is identity based, their ownership of their values and beliefs and their sense of who they are unavoidably have an impact on their interactions with each other. Assume you are assigned the job of facilitating the end of an identity-based conflict between two people. How do you break through the identity issues to get the parties to talk with each other? What should you explore and settle with the parties separately before you bring them together? Break the discussion group into two and give each subgroup the role of acting as one party in an identity-based conflict (a conflict arising out of a difference in nationality, ethnicity, religion, or politics). List the elements of conflict as they come up during the ensuing dialogue.

Resonance

Resonance is the process of moving away from antagonism and toward the identification of common ground. Through *reflexive reframing* the parties begin to articulate their values and concerns and seek commonalities on which to build dialogue.

In the preceding phase, the focus of each party is on the behavior of the other. Each party's view is outward and other oriented. Reflexive reframing refocuses the gaze of the parties back to themselves so that they can clarify who they are and what they want before trying to fashion a resolution.

An identity-based conflict is likely to involve intangible and subjective issues. The facilitator might have a hard time believing the two parties are talking about the same concerns. In point of fact, they may not be. The two parties are likely to have different cultural and experiential backgrounds, have different perceptions of the conflict, and use different language to express their perceptions. The notion of objective truth is irrelevant because each party cannot help seeing the conflict through his or her own eyes and treating his or her own perceptions as true.

However, by expressing their deepest feelings and values, the two parties start to fashion a common frame of reference. Each begins to sense that the other shares certain sentiments and each develops a fuller picture of the other. By going deeper into their own experiences, the parties build the foundation for future dialogue. They discover that their initial views and positions—those expressed during the first stage—are inadequate and cannot be supported.

The personal and "why" questions they ask help turn the conversation into a vehicle for learning about each other's different perspectives and values.

Reflexes come in two varieties, the automatic reflex to external stimuli and the reflective response based on study and assessment. The latter type is characteristic of good conflict management. It requires the ability to step back and look at issues and concerns from a far enough distance to see the whole landscape related to the conflict. The goal of the facilitator is to get the parties to take the necessary step back. Ideally, they would see each other's pictures of the conflict, understand the circumstances and variables placing them in the conflict, and understand how all of that stands in relationship to everything else. Ultimately, the facilitator wants to create a double-loop experience for the parties. Once each has articulated his or her experience and completed the circle of experience, the two parties would link their experiences in a way that exposes their similarities and intersections. Common elements and frames of reference begin to emerge as a result, and the relatedness of the elements become clear to the parties and form a foundation for further dialogue.

The two parties also need to see clearly that they both have the same fears, uncertainties, meanings, and values, and to recognize that they could find themselves saying the same things. When one party says, "I am concerned," "I am afraid," or "I am angry," the other should be able to admit honestly that he or she could easily utter the same statement. Furthermore, through the "I" form of the expression, the individual ownership of thoughts and feelings ultimately becomes mutual. It is precisely because of the deep ownership each party has of his or her own insights and feelings that mutuality can begin to emerge without causing the threats of challenge, accusation, or alienation. It is hard to reject in another what you just affirmed in yourself.

Identity-based conflicts can exhibit elements of reaction. Each party's sense of self may actually be formed in opposition to the other party's sense of self. The parties' discernment of who they are not can sometimes be as important as their definition of who they are. For instance, they might see themselves as not having characteristics that they attribute to the other party, possibly just because they perceive the other party as having them. They are likely to view themselves not just as possessing different interests, but as *being* fundamentally different. Religious, cultural, ethnic, national, and sexual differences often serve as the basis of identity-based conflicts. After all, there is nothing any of us can do about our gender, nationality, ethnicity, or religion, and so these are seen as defining us and differentiating us from the "other."

> **Key Point**
>
> Fear keeps people from disclosing how they really feel and focusing on resolving the issues at the root of a conflict. Therefore, early in the conflict resolution process, the facilitator must give the parties a strong sense of safety so that they can confront their anxieties and talk openly and honestly.

In health care, discipline, role, function, and license can similarly act to divide people in fundamental ways and create a priori positions that are hard and sometimes impossible to get around. For example, "I am the doctor; the buck stops with me" or "I am the nurse; I manage the processes of care" or "I am the caregiver; I do the work of health care." Each of these statements is partially true, but by holding to them the parties can become polarized and entrenched. Moving them from their positions is a challenging task, but it can be done by persuading them that no role is the most special, important, critical, powerful, or viable, and that no person can do what needs to be done if the other parties fail to meet their responsibilities.

The fact is that "I am because you are." That is, we are all interdependent, and indeed the clearer I am as to how I stand in relation to you, the clearer I am as to who I am and who I can become. It is essential that the parties understand the interdependence of their roles so that they can reach a sustainable resolution of their differences.

The parties to an identity-based conflict are faced with a fundamental choice: they can continue to maintain an isolated identity against the world, or they can search for and uncover their common roots and frames of reference and find their mutuality. To get them to do the latter, the facilitator should help them move

- from blaming to articulating their sense of self,
- from antagonism toward the other to identification with the other,
- from the attribution of negatives to understanding,
- from projection to ownership,
- from anger to acceptance, and
- from fear to a sense of safety.

As the parties move through these initial stages of the conflict resolution process, they clarify the conflict, obtain ownership of the process, and explain to each other what is most present in themselves, thereby deepening their self-understanding and establishing a foundation for the later stages.

Invention

During this stage, the parties begin to see some payoff for the work they have done. The focus is on inventing solutions that can take the parties to a place where they can live in peace and engagement. In short, they begin the work of resolution.

Their main task is to look at solutions through a larger lens or use a greater frame of reference—in other words, to think outside the box. They should try to develop new ways of looking at the conflict and come up with new solutions. As noted, in identity-based conflicts negotiating a compromise is fraught with difficulty because the parties would view compromising as giving up something of who they are, not simply something they have, and would thus find it unacceptable.

Instead of seeking compromise, the facilitator must challenge the parties to apply a broader framework and see the situation in a new way. They both have a stake in the outcome and stand to gain from a solution. They must therefore reconceptualize the conflict, which is the purpose of the invention process. This process is about developing whole new ways of seeing the issues and working through them. It demands a focus on the practical and the real, and by going through the process the parties should be able to develop a different vision of their concerns and a different image of each other. In particular, they should recognize that they are interdependent and need each other, and that the resolution of the conflict requires everyone to get on board.

> **Point to Ponder**
>
> In trying to resolve an identity-based conflict, the facilitator should help the parties differentiate themselves and develop a clearer sense of who they are and what they bring to the table.

The first step is to develop and agree on statements of objectives. These are derived from statements of the issues. They help the parties see and say what they want to get from the process, especially it as relates to their fundamental needs for safety, security, value, dignity, and so on. They also inform the more detailed discourse the parties will engage in regarding the steps and processes intended to move the parties to where they would like to be.

This step includes components that allow the parties to educate each other on what they need and to explain their reasons why. The education expands on what has already been shared but with a new focus on safety, security, values, and so on. Because the issues at the root of the conflict are identity issues, the parties must try to explain how what they are asking for advances or protects their identity.

Working out the details is critical. Watching negotiations, uninformed observers often believe that the haggling that occurs over the smallest detail is disingenuous and foolish. In an identity-based conflict, each detail has implications for the identities of the parties after the resolution, and thus each one counts.

Note that there is a significant difference between interests and needs. Interests generally play a central role in resource- or interest-based conflicts but a subsidiary role in identity-based conflicts, where needs are primary. Consequently, in an identity-based conflict the most critical task is to get parties to express their needs and then to reach an understanding of their interests based on their needs. For example, as they see it, nurses in a healthcare organization need to give care to patients unconstrained by financial considerations. On the other hand, managers, as they see it, need to ensure the financial health of the organization. Both needs—the nurses' need to give good care and managers' need to ensure financial viability—relate to a common interest, ensuring the existence of enough financial resources to render good service to the public. If the two groups understand that because of their needs they share an interest, they are more likely to reach a resolution of their conflict.

Of course, achieving a resolution does not mean that the parties get everything they desire. At best, they can negotiate a method for meeting their needs—a method that may involve working together, such as one of those described next.

Sometimes differentiating between the parties more clearly—that is, accentuating and enumerating their differences—can lead to a more suitable resolution for each. Although their needs may differ, clarifying them and seeking alternative ways to satisfy them through common action can help move the parties to a new place. For example, imagine that a respiratory therapy union is seeking greater recognition for its members and a stronger role for its leaders, whereas the management wants a reduction in complaints and grievances instituted by the union. Both groups agree to apply a different method of problem solving, one in which the

Group Discussion

Nina Conners really did not want to settle the issues she had with Frank Kliener. They had been feuding for 3 years. Both she and Frank used their conflict as a way of getting more for their own departments and keeping their staff energized and competitive. However, the organization has been paying the price, and its goals are sometimes held hostage to the war between the two departments. Discuss how a mediator would begin to resolve this conflict. What are the apparent issues? What might be the real issue? How would the mediator structure the resolution process? As part of the exercise, create a resolution plan that contains steps for addressing the issues and resolving the conflict.

union leadership plays a more direct role. The result is less use of the grievance procedure. Here, the different needs of the two groups provide a basis for resolving their conflict creatively.

A second technique involves expanding the playing field so that the parties can each get more of the resources they need. For example, nurses may request more staffing, and management may want to save more money. The two groups may agree that if the nurses meet set productivity targets, then management will use part of the savings to hire more nurses. By consenting to work together to expand the organization's resources, they each help meet their own needs and those of the other party. The result is a win–win resolution of their conflict. To reach a mutually beneficial resolution, the parties usually have to identify joint activities that move them past the issues that prevented them from ending their conflict in the past.

If the parties find that their needs are seemingly irreconcilable, the solution may lie in offering compensation for not meeting a certain need by bestowing something different of equal value. If one party is asking for money that the other party cannot afford to give, it may agree to accept something it views as equally valuable, such as more vacation time. The two parties must engage in clear and creative dialogue to ensure that the substitute is truly viewed and explicitly accepted as equivalent; otherwise, the issue of just compensation will likely arise later and cause problems and further conflict.

The facilitator must look for signs of enough movement and energy to take the parties to the next step—or provide the necessary energy. There is nothing like a small success now and again for maintaining the momentum. Once successes begin to occur, they serve to spur the process and move it in ways that nothing else could. The process, energized by the successes already achieved, begins to change the dynamic, the emotions, and the relationship of the two parties without any further intervention. Through good timing and careful pushing, the facilitator can get the parties to work on the more difficult issues in the midst of good momentum, increasing the chance that they will be finally settled.

The inventing stage is when the parties' interaction changes from being oppositional to being collaborative. It is an essential stage on the journey to a resolution, and the techniques of differentiation, expansion, compensation, and momentum all have the potential of increasing the probability that the parties will achieve an end to the conflict.

> **Key Point**
>
> Conflict resolution is a process with its own timing and techniques. It requires training and experience. Leaders should develop the necessary skills and practice using them until they are adept at bringing parties in conflict step by step through the process to a sustainable settlement of their differences.

Action

The final stage is devoted to crafting a plan of action. There is nothing more disheartening than to get through the touchy issues and concerns, establish a strong commitment to pursue possible solutions, build an effective relationship, and then have the process fall apart because an action plan either could not be constructed or was not detailed enough to guide the parties to a final resolution.

As the process progresses toward action, the parties need to reaffirm where they have come from and where they believe they are in relation to their own needs and their interaction with each other. The mutual understanding that results serves as the ground for the subsequent focus on action. In the action phase, the new questions are what to do, who is to do it, why is it being done, and how to do it.

The first step is to set the agenda for action. What are the priorities of the agreements reached? Where do the parties start? What are the items that must be translated into substantive work, enabling the agreed way of relating and behaving to be realized? These questions serve as the basis for the next level of critical dialogue. Here again patience and attention to detail are required from both parties and from the facilitator.

Setting the agenda includes deciding the priority of actions, their timing, their criticalness, and what other actions must be done in preparation. It also includes reaching an agreement on who is to be accountable for the actions.

New kinds of structures and institutions may have to be constructed as vehicles for implementing conflict resolution actions. If built early on, structures provide a framework for implementing actions and evaluating their progress. They also help ensure that issues important to the parties are addressed as expected and that any problems or concerns that arise are defined precisely (Ramsbotham et al., 2016).

Once problems are defined, they need to be solved, which means building problem-solving mechanisms into the implementation process. Unaddressed problems have the potential to negatively affect the relationship between the parties and eliminate the progress made to date.

Parties need to clarify immediate and long-term goals and priorities based on the critical elements identified during the reflexive reframing process (which occurs in the second stage of ARIA). Parties also need to ensure that the principal, pivotal, and relational items are handled first during the implementation.

> **Point to Ponder**
>
> A conflict resolution facilitator must keep the parties centered by reminding them what is at stake and which issues need to be addressed. The facilitator must also remind the parties of the expectations agreed upon so that these can be reaffirmed or altered as the process moves forward.

The facilitator must try not to upset the delicate balance achieved between the parties. The facilitator's tasks include determining the specific needs each party wants to satisfy as a result of the implementation process and devising an evaluation schedule so that progress can be assessed at critical points. Evaluating the process regularly keeps the parties on board and ensures the process remains in line with their expectations.

Equally critical is the assignment of accountability for specific outcomes. Who does what should be a practical rather than a political issue, yet at this stage politics often take precedence in a way they never should, typically because the skills, talents, and roles of participants have not been discussed in advance of the assignment. Participant skills, talents, and roles must be ascertained before the point of assigning accountability if political machinations are to be kept at a minimum.

Content (goals) must always be placed before process (methods). Once the parties set their goals, they need to choose methods for achieving them. In thinking about methods, the parties need to anticipate potential impediments and select those methods that are most likely to succeed. Each party will judge the other by their actions because their actions are the visible evidence of that party's commitment to the agreement. Actions represent what the one party has done on the other's behalf. Therefore, the parties' actions require as much attention as any of the other components of the resolution process.

The facilitator must always keep the parties focused on what is at stake and how important it is. The parties must have the sense that they are a part of a meaningful effort that is larger than their own contributions and that will lead them to a better place.

In any conflict resolution process, no matter whether the conflict is interest or identity based, the facilitator must establish his or her neutrality at the outset. If that cannot be done, the facilitator should consider relinquishing his or her role. Facilitators who are seen as too close to the issue or unable to act in a neutral manner are more of a hindrance than a help.

Facilitators must be as committed to the process as to the parties. Facilitators have an important position of trust and are responsible for moving the dynamic in critical ways. If not careful and skillful, facilitators will cease to be credible to the parties and will lose their confidence, thereby crippling the process and ensuring that further problems will arise.

Facilitators must make it clear at the outset that they are working for the whole, not one side or the other, regardless of how they got there. Further, the parties must agree to the notion that facilitators are neutral or the process simply will not progress. If one side or the other is paying for facilitator services or the facilitator holds a specific role in the organization, accommodation may have to be made at the outset of the process to ensure that the parties trust and support the facilitator equally.

Although identity-based conflicts are the most difficult of all conflicts to deal with, they can be resolved using the processes and mechanisms outlined here. Many conflicts are allowed to continue because leaders have no idea that these tools even exist and mistakenly try to use approaches suitable only for interest-based conflicts.

In the current world of health care, the potential for conflict is greater than ever. Various disciplines and workgroups must revise their relationships and their boundaries—or even establish them for the first time. Team-based and continuum-driven approaches to service place a great emphasis on who people are rather than simply what they do (Caspers & Pickard, 2013; Eisler & Garrick, 2018). Thus, a vital part of the leadership role in the new age of health care involves working through the differences between professionals and building mutuality as a basis for preventing unnecessary conflict and resolving unavoidable conflict when it arises.

Interest-Based Conflicts

Interest-based conflicts are situations that present the potential to affect or compromise the impartiality of a person or an issue because the situation involves an individual's self-interest, diverging interpersonal interests, organizational/professional interest, or public interest. In legal terms, one representation of interest-based conflicts is a situation where an individual party's responsibility to a second party limits the first party's ability to discharge its responsibility to a third party because of interest conflicts. In negotiating interest-based conflicts, the substantive assumption is that parties in conflict are much more amenable to reach mutually satisfying decisions when their respective interests are honored and met in a way that suggests mutual advantage or satisfaction.

Most interest-based conflicts involve questions related to the distribution of interest among the disputants, often related to money, property, personal benefit, or obligations. With these sources of conflict, questions relate more to a symbolic "pie" and just how equitable the pieces of that pie can be distributed among the stakeholders that have some investment or interest in all or some parts of the pie. Interest-based negotiation depends much more strongly on win–win processes, and many of the elements of interest-based dialogue and negotiation are directed toward achieving that kind of outcome.

Types of Interest-Based Conflicts

Like any other human dynamic, conflict has content, particular elements, and specific processes. Conflict generally falls into relationship-based, values-based, structural-based, and data-based categories. Each has its own characteristics and elements that mark it as unique. The leader becomes skilled at identifying the kinds and characteristics of conflict being dealt with and the responses that best address them.

Because the leader is always looking for specific conflicts, it is wise to become skilled in identifying the particular characteristics of conflict that most often appear within the culture of the service or department. Each setting is unique with regard to the makeup of the staff and the stressors on them and the work that they do. Good leaders perform a conflict-potential assessment as part of delineating which strategies are going to be most helpful in dealing with conflict. In this assessment, leaders attempt to get a handle on those specific potentials for conflict that will most often be a concern in the ordinary management of the service.

Leaders look at the staff makeup, demographics (both cultural and age related), breadth of the work, and skill level. Embedded within these factors is the potential for specific kinds of conflict that may recur. In this manner, leaders make the potential for conflict a normal and usual part of their organizational and resource planning. Good leaders know that the greater the awareness of the circumstances and characteristics of conflict, the earlier it can be addressed appropriately.

Relationship-Based (Interpersonal) Conflicts

In any work environment, there are a number of personalities and situations whose vagaries create conditions that can lead to conflict. Differences between people always provide a source for a variety of relationship-driven crises or conflicts. Differences in personality create problems in interaction and communication and often lead to misunderstandings. Interpersonal differences can frequently lead to specific altercations reflecting emotional involvement and personal animosity. Left unaddressed, differences can escalate and create real polarization between the involved parties and those who relate to them. Relationship conflict is the most frequently experienced conflict in most organizations. Communication irregularities emerge and miscommunication becomes common. Negative behavior becomes repetitive and, if not resolved, becomes a way to sabotage and offend the opposing party, which can affect the work, workers, and those they serve.

Good leaders recognize the potential for relational conflicts early. Unkind words, snide comments, asides, negative comments to others, and avoiding behaviors are the early signs that a relational conflict is present. Because leaders understand that some level of relational conflict exists in the workplace, they are able to see signs and begin to take action right away.

First, leaders must get at the originating source of the conflict. Confronting both parties separately with regard to the behaviors expressed is the critical path to getting at the root problem underlying the behaviors. Beginning the questioning with an open-ended approach is best. The leader might say one of the following:

"I'm noticing that . . ."
"Can you tell me . . ."
"I'm wondering if I'm seeing . . ."
"Help me see if I'm perceiving this right . . ."

At this stage, leaders are just trying to get a level of understanding about the existence of a problem and the basic perceptions of what the problem might be through the words of each party. Through this process, leaders are simply validating whether a problem exists and the underlying nature of the concern. Leaders are also ascertaining the degree of perceptive agreement that exists between the parties regarding their issues. Leaders initially respond to emotions and feelings. It is impossible to get at the problem without first going through the emotional content of each party's issues. In relationship conflict, the parties are reacting to their own feelings and impressions of what has happened to them and how they are feeling about it rather than to the real issue that may be the causative factor.

If leaders try to get to the causative issues too soon, the parties may block and refuse to move there because they have not had an appropriate opportunity to work through the emotional content related to the issue. Sometimes leaders might need to carefully move individuals through their feelings by validating and supporting the person while clarifying the underlying issues along the way. Leaders attempt to get the individual to a more reality-oriented place from which some rational work might be done as the individual moves through the conflict. At some point, the parties must be in the same place to move the conflict closer to resolution. Leaders attempt to prepare each party to understand where the other party is in relation to feelings and content. Leaders, acting as neutral parties, seek to have each conflicted party express their feelings with a language that accurately expresses feelings without further polarization, energizing a new level of emotional intensity.

As the process moves toward engagement, leaders seek to focus on expression and rules of engagement as well as to remind each party of the expectations regarding communication and conflict management in the service or the department. Having created an appropriate milieu for conflict management, leaders want to ensure that the parties are aware of the expectations and need to resolve issues that impede the ability of the staff to communicate and deal with differences. Leaders identify the conflict resolution process as one of the mechanisms that exemplifies the components of communication within which the unit operates. It is only at this point that leaders begin to bring the parties together to a dialogue and to work through their differences.

Values-Based Conflicts

Perhaps one of the most difficult classes of conflict to resolve are those that represent differences in values. Conflicts of these types are often categorized within the context of identity-based conflicts discussed earlier in this chapter. Every person brings different experiences and beliefs to the expression of their human journey. Cultural, social, religious, moral, and personal values are all part of what defines an individual. In a multicultural society such as that reflected in the American experience, cultural and personal differences are common. Yet with the richness of these differences comes the inevitable conflicts that arise when individual values come in conflict with the values of others. Leaders create a culture of acceptance and openness to differences and to the vagaries of response they reflect. In anticipation of the potential for conflict, leaders see to it that cultural and value awareness is inculcated into the educational and developmental activities of the service. Everyone should be expected to participate in activities that teach them about the value and practice of acceptance and about the negative behaviors that are unacceptable between and among different ethnic, cultural, national, and religious groups.

Like identity-based conflict, values-based conflict is very difficult to resolve late in the cycle of conflict management; it is wise to confront it at the earliest possible moment. A breach in the code of conduct or expectations of behavior should be addressed as soon as it happens. The absolute unacceptability of such patterns of behavior should be clear to everyone at the outset. Refusal to conform one's personal behavior to these rules of good relationship should be grounds for the strongest disciplinary action. Ethnic discrimination has no room for dialogue or debate. Any discrimination based on color or disparaging remarks that reflect on ethnic origins have no legitimacy. In a world of many colors and ethnic backgrounds reflecting the broadest array of human beings, any conflict based on this has no room for negotiation and misunderstanding. In the human experience, there are some a priori considerations that operate beyond question. Race and ethnicity are two of them. The only room for conflict in this arena is where a misunderstanding or misrepresentation of one's remarks or behavior has occurred and needs clarification and restating between the parties. Cultural or language difficulties or misrepresentations can create a perception that simply may not have been intended. The process of continuous cultural and values education for staff should keep such misunderstandings to a minimum.

Religious and values differences can create significant problems. A number of problems can arise from religious differences related to beliefs, practices, and accommodation. Special considerations to religious and values practices can create negative feelings in others who do not hold the same beliefs. Resentment and feelings of preference can emerge, creating conflict. Here again, being clear in advance about what the expectations are regarding the presence of staff with different practices and the impact of those on the staff relationship is a critical obligation of the leader. Adjustments required in the schedule and even assignments and role adjustments need to be clear to all staff members with attention paid to how equity is maintained between and among staff members. Achieving equity between and among staff members with different religious beliefs or values is challenging for leaders and staff. Dialogue and negotiation regarding these adjustments must be delineated up front with the staff. This approach keeps the issue before the staff, makes it a part of their ongoing work experience, and creates an expectation that such accommodations are always a part of the work environment.

When accommodations to the expression of particular religious practices are especially difficult for staff to accept or verge on creating resentment, the leader must reanimate dialogue around the differences in light of reinvigorating acceptance. Leaders and staff can find creative ways of addressing the related issues and resolving the conflicts these issues generate. If leaders have been successful in the aggressive creation of an environment of acceptance and openness, the expectation is that conflicts can be dealt with and ultimately resolved.

In cases where there is intractable religious-based conflict, it is often wise for the leader to expand the dialogue and include experts from outside the service to guide the discussion and advance resolution. It is often helpful to involve pastoral assistance from representatives from the religious traditions at issue and have them help the participants find some common ground and define areas of resolution or accommodation. Leaders always acts as a resource purveyor when conflicts require an alternative mechanism for resolution.

In values-based conflicts, it is also helpful for leaders to expand the dialogue to values that can be shared by all participants. Values that operate in the broader human context and reflect common human needs and interests can help refocus the issue to one that engages human experience, regardless of value tradition or expression. Attempting to find common areas of value (such as family, home, nation, loyalty, sentiment, children) can change the emotional and relational content of the conflict and create a common frame of reference for its resolution that might not have originally been anticipated.

Finally, it is important for leaders to know that it is sometimes necessary to allow people to agree to disagree. Values are sacred to the individual who holds them; they cannot easily be surrendered to others. Leaders may have to get the parties to determine how they will live with their differences and make the necessary accommodations to those differences as a part of their relationship. Respect is critical to effectiveness of this process. If each can respect the position of the other, common ground can be found and progress can be made with regard to the quality of the work relationship.

Structure-Driven Conflicts

Structure-driven conflicts recognize inequities inherent in the system or structure of work. These can be classified as inadequate or unfair policies, processes, rules, behaviors, and practices, as well as contextual and organizational factors that inhibit cooperative relationships.

Leaders recognize that no workplace is free of structural and operational challenges to the capacity to do work and to build relationships in the system. Differences in pay grades, benefits policies, reward systems, and job and role status all contribute to perceptions of structural inequity. Even if there is a rational basis for these practices, the inherent inequity needs to be addressed as a possible source of unresolved conflict.

Leaders recognize that there must be openness with regard to people's specific concerns about any particular structural inequity. Leaders acknowledge its presence and clearly enumerate the logic behind the apparent inequity. Understanding the value of implementing a particular advantage by one group in relationship to others is a valuable first step. In those places where the inequity established is sufficiently egregious, mechanisms and efforts at self-correction must address the structural element. Where such inequities can be changed or struck down in the organization, they should be, as soon as possible, with a solution that can actually be implemented.

There is a perceived inequity and imbalance at the professional level in a number of organizations. These perceived imbalances generally indicate that one profession or work group is preferred or treated favorably compared with another profession or work group. This perceived inequity often creates much internal conflict in the organization that may not always be directly expressed. Hidden conflict operates as an organizational subtext or frequently lies just below the surface. In this specific set of circumstances, the leader must recognize the foundations of the perceived inequity early and clearly. If it is status inequity evidenced by differentiation of role or reward, the justifications and support for these differentiations must be clear enough to make sense to the group that feels disadvantaged. Although these inequities cannot always be changed, they can be understood—and the role of leaders is to generate understanding.

Where there are more challenges in justifying the inequity and it does not appear to be legitimate or functional, leaders must support individuals in undertaking a process in which the inequity can be actively addressed and pursued further. In such circumstances, advocacy for a particular approach or solution, communication with the appropriate leadership individuals, or structural or organizational approaches to finding solutions must be determined by the stakeholders in the conflict. Without the leader advocating for a specific process for problem resolution, the structural problem will continue to frustrate and challenge the effectiveness and integrity of the work group.

Additional structural challenges that can generate conflict relate to the environmental or the architectural construct within which work unfolds. In many clinical organizations, the structures of the organization impede the effectiveness of the work. Where the structures can be altered, they should be. Where the architectural and structural elements of work cannot be altered or adjusted, those affected by the structural impediments can explore mechanisms and methods for accommodation or modification. In addition, continuing leadership attention and focus must be centered on challenging and addressing structural barriers in a way that ultimately removes the issues. By addressing structural barriers, leaders show that they are committed to supporting clinical work of the organization. Whether the architectural modifications or structural adjustments can be undertaken is not as important as the commitment of leaders to continuous support of the staff by challenging organizational leadership to modify structural impediments.

Data-Based Conflicts

Conflicts related to data are generally driven by either limited access to information or lack of information. Information is critical to the effectiveness of organizations in today's clinical workplace. Without appropriate information in a useful configuration, clinical work cannot be successfully undertaken. In fact, the complexity of information necessary to do work now makes clinical (and non-clinical) work completely information dependent. Information is critical to the ability of all disciplines to fulfill their obligations in rendering clinical service throughout the healthcare system. Furthermore, business, clinical, support, and material information must interface to create a sufficient data foundation upon which high-quality, effective clinical choices can be made. Information must be seamless with work and reflect a portability and mobility that links the provider in real time with data essential to work quality and effectiveness. The growing intensity of the generation and interface of information creates some of the most difficult and intractable contemporary problems and conflicts.

Information is resource intensive. As a result, there is wide variability related to the distribution and quality of hardware and software across the healthcare system. Emphasis has historically been placed on building a business infrastructure and information system, and much business sophistication has emerged as a result. In the growing accountable care environment, clinical information infrastructures are just now being expanded, perfected, and linked to business and clinical infrastructure in ways that can have an impact on resource use and clinical decision making. However, information priorities, mechanisms for generating information, tools for using data, distribution of resources in building information infrastructures, and the quality and kind of information generated all have an impact on organizational effectiveness and integrity. Therein lies the source for the emergence of conflict. Each of these issues can generate its own internally fixed sources of conflict from access, availability, accuracy, quality, efficacy, and utility of information.

Leaders must recognize that a fit between resource allocation and information usefulness is necessary. Because there are intersecting groups, all requiring various components of the information complex, some level of agreement must be achieved as to what information is necessary, important, and vital to clinical decision making. Organization-established priorities and clinically useful data processes and information must be interfaced in a way that is wise and reflects service utility. In addition, leaders must ensure that there are structural and process formats within which information priorities are understood. Format elements should reflect the useful and common set of criteria to which all stakeholders have contributed.

Leaders' roles are to reduce the structural opportunities for conflict by ensuring that appropriate processes and interfacing regarding information collection, management, and generation have been delineated and structured in the organization. Leaders make sure that the right stakeholders are present so that deliberations include those whom decisions will affect. When issues have been overlooked or forgotten, leaders, recognizing that the process is fluid, bring the stakeholders together again to deliberate and reassess, with the intent of establishing a process that works successfully. There may be challengers to the skill set and ability of stakeholders. Leaders ensure that appropriate experts and expertise are available to guide the team to correctly delineate needs and create resolutions or information management solutions. Through this complex of activities and systems approaches to handling the information infrastructure, leaders create an ongoing mechanism that embeds conflict resolution in the information system utilization process.

In each of the arenas of interest-based conflicts are specific and unique activities related to resolving conflict. Although this chapter certainly introduces some of the steps leaders can take to address conflict, it is not comprehensive. Leaders must recognize that conflict management is a significant skill set, and they must obtain as much development and education as necessary to build conflict management skills. Facility in conflict management comes with discipline, practice, and time. Leaders, recognizing how important conflict management is to successful group interchange and group dynamics, therefore commit considerable time and energy to understanding and developing their skills.

In dealing with interest-based conflicts, leaders act essentially as mediators, a neutral third party who helps the parties resolve their issues and bring closure to the conflict. Interest-based conflict requires much more negotiation and give-and-take than the resolution process for identity-based conflict. Offers are made and countered as the parties try to work out an agreement consistent with their interests.

The mediator typically undertakes two kinds of intervention: contingent and noncontingent. The noncontingent interventions focus on the processes necessary to any mediation. Contingent interventions are implemented in response to specific circumstances arising from the process itself. Problems, emotions, issues, and other contingencies can individually or collectively have an impact on the mediation process (**Figure 6-6**), and the mediator occasionally has to respond by adjusting the process accordingly.

Isolating Interest-Based Conflicts

As with all conflicts, as we have emphasized in this chapter, leaders must recognize that early engagement of an interest-based conflict is important. Here, leaders recognize as early as possible the need to address the "noise" related to an emerging conflict between parties. From the earliest stirrings of conflict between persons, signs of the impending conflict are present. If leaders are aware, they notice an attitude of disrespect, unkind words from one person to another, offhand remarks, an inappropriate phrase, or an emerging situation that has in it the potential for later conflict. Good leaders do not let a remark, behavior, or potential issue that has any embedded elements of anger, misunderstanding, or personal apprehension go unaddressed. Conflict is often evidenced in early emotional language and demonstrated in particular patterns of behavior. Such early expressions are indicators of underlying or emerging concerns that beg to be addressed. These are early characteristics of interest-based conflicts that, when interrupted in an early stage, point to substantive issues at the foundation of the conflict, moving them into the open and increasing the opportunity that addressing them can allay acceleration of conflict.

Personal elements	Process	Results
Interests	Negotiable	Outcomes
Wants	Possible	Deliverables
Needs	Related	Agreed to
Desires	Obtainable	Required
Initiation	Progress	Resolution

Figure 6-6 The Interest-Based Conflict Resolution Process.

In these earliest stages of conflict, the leader continually looks for individuals creating positions or taking sides on issues. In fact, in the very earliest stages, individuals begin to drive conflict, construct boundaries and limits for strongly held positions, or demarcate differences in a way that represents a strong unilateral position that is exclusionary or exclusive. The individual ownership, expression, and defense of such positions create conditions and circumstances upon which further conflict can be built and interest positions can be taken.

Through constant awareness and careful listening, leaders prepare to address conflict at the earliest possible moment using appropriate tools. It is vital for leaders to identify the key elements of the impending conflict situation as quickly as possible. What most often appears are signposts to real issues that are deeply buried and of which the emerging conflict is symbolic. The ability of leaders to dig deeper to find the source of conflicts is critical for problem solving (double-loop problem solving). Often, the conflict-laden language represents feelings, not circumstances. These feelings generally mask the true roots of the conflict.

In interest-based conflict resolution, leaders need to enumerate feelings and sentiments, allowing them a language and expression, with the intent of finding the underlying issues that are driving the conflict expression. There are often triggers, remarks that serve to indicate the intensity of feeling and perception, which leaders will need to sort through and get past to enumerate the conflict. Often leaders hear feelings and response triggers similar to the following:

"She always does this to me."
"He is forever dumping this on me."
"She never stops criticizing me."
"He always makes me so angry."
"What she says or does just wants to make me scream."
"He is mean to me all the time."
"She doesn't trust me."

These comments are filled with reactive emotional content. These sentiments represent feelings and powerful emotions that reflect a sense of impotence and helplessness. Sometimes these feelings are even accompanied by related behaviors; at times, they are merely feelings.

Either way, these feelings are powerful indicators of an impending and a potentially irresolvable conflict if they are not addressed.

Of course, not all conflict can be addressed by a leader on the spot. Good conflict resolution may require that the conflict temporarily goes into the leader's "parking lot" of responses until it can be more reasonably and fully addressed. Even so, when the leader hears comments from an aggressor in the conflict or from the offended individual, it is important that an immediate response be offered while noting the potential for longer-term follow-up action. Short, yet key, immediate responses from the leader to the individual are advisable. Some sample responses are the following:

> "I'm concerned about what I'm hearing; I'll need to talk with you about it after we finish this task (work, procedure, meeting, etc.)."
> "I hear what you're saying, and I think we need to talk about it after we're done here."
> "I'm very unclear about what you are saying, and I think we need to talk about it right after we're done here."

To the offended person, the leader might respond:

> "I need to know more; let's talk when we're done here."
> "I'm concerned about how you're feeling right now. Let's talk when this task (meeting, procedure, work, etc.) is finished."

Note that leaders address the fact that there is an issue but postpone focusing on the issue to a more appropriate time. Also, note that leaders do not address all parties to the conflict immediately. Leaders need to establish clarity around individual perceptions and reactions to the conflict before purposeful collective resolution activities begin. At the outset, simply getting notions, perceptions, and facts related to individual responses to the conflict is a critical element in the initial data-gathering process that informs the later resolution processes.

Perhaps the most important aspect of straightening out the underpinnings of conflict is found in gathering all pieces of the information related to the conflict. Good conflict leaders pay attention to what is being said and what is being felt. Getting to the facts of the conflict requires travel through an emotional landscape, dealing with perceptions and feelings first because these lead ultimately to a deeper understanding of the situation, a clear contextual framework for the conflict, and opportunities for the parties to be fully heard and to express sentiments early in the process. What happens most often is that the leader seeks to resolve the conflict too early in the process, hoping that by doing so the conflict and its emotional content can be short-circuited, and thus kept from escalating. However, the opposite occurs. In moving too quickly the leader fails to address strongly felt personal sentiments, emotions, and feelings that, left unaddressed, cloud and slow the movement to meaningfully addressing the facts of the conflict.

Ten Steps to Resolving an Interest-Based Conflict

The resolution of an interest-based conflict typically includes 10 steps (**Figure 6-7**). Each step requires a different amount of time and a different approach. By keeping track of each step of the process, the mediator can discipline the parties and keep the process moving steadily in the right direction.

CHAPTER SIX   Diversity and Difference: Managing Conflict in a Transdisciplinary Network

Step 1 Establishing the initial relationship
- Contact the parties
- Build credibility
- Rules of engagement
- Contract to proceed

Step 2 Developing strategies to guide the process
- Assess approaches
- Select approaches
- Coordinate approaches
- Develop plans

Step 3 Constructing the initial database
- Analyze relevant data
- Get to substance of conflict
- Verify data accuracy
- Sort out inaccurate data

Step 4 Organizing the plan for mediation
- Develop strategy plan
- Define techniques
- Define the right moves
- Accommodate contingencies

Step 5 Building trust and communication
- Deal with feelings directly
- Create a safe space
- Name the right issues
- Develop effective communication

Step 6 Beginning the resolution process
- Define expectations
- Apply an approach
- Devise structure and flow
- Ensure parties are heard

Step 7 Defining concerns and setting priorities
- Ensure correct understanding of issues
- Ensure mutuality of the issues
- Agree on the issues
- Develop tactics to move beyond the issues

Step 8 Looking for the unseen
- Find the real issues
- Pull out hidden information
- Name hidden agendas
- Determine personal agendas

Step 9 Naming values and options
- Move to agreement
- Choose options
- Name places of consensus
- Affirm understanding and choices

Step 10 Concluding the conflict process
- Converge around options
- Agree to proceed
- Contract for performance
- Develop an action plan

Figure 6-7 The 10 Steps of the Conflict Resolution Process.

Step 1: Establishing the Initial Relationship
The mediator's first task is to establish credibility with the parties and introduce them to the process. A conflict resolution process has components and rules that the parties must understand and agree to if the process is to result in a resolution.

Step 2: Developing Strategies to Guide the Process
The mediator should discuss approaches and processes and the rules of engagement with the parties up front to strengthen the relationship between all participants. In addition, it helps the parties learn about the process and select those activities they determine will best assist them in moving effectively toward resolution.

Step 3: Constructing the Initial Database
The mediator needs to become familiar with the parties and the issues as soon as possible. Thus, early in the process the mediator should ask the parties about their histories and experiences and for their insights to build a foundation for establishing priorities and deciding on an approach. Verifying the accuracy of the collected information and the central issues of concern is part of the data-gathering process. After the gathering stage, participants should spend time reflecting on the content of the conflict and its implications for the resolution approach and process. Here again, they get to know each other better. In particular, the mediator obtains a view of the personal processes and behaviors of the parties within the context of the mediation process and can adjust the approach accordingly.

Step 4: Organizing the Plan for Mediation
In this stage, the mediator considers the approach and structures to use for the mediation. The goal is to develop a plan of approach that fits the situation and the parties, accounting for the contingent factors discernible thus far. The mediator designs the noncontingent structures, considers process elements that could move the parties closer to agreement, and constructs a framework for guiding the process. The plan is simply contingent; it is not cast in stone. The participants need to be flexible and adjust the process in response to the inevitable emergence of new information and unexpected factors.

Step 5: Building Trust and Communication
It is essential to build trust between the parties and to strengthen the parties' trust in the mediator. The challenge is obvious: the parties have entered the mediation process precisely because they are in conflict and have negative feelings toward each other. The mediator's job is to get the parties at least to trust the process enough to get from it what it has to offer. Through exploring the emotional component of their perceptions of each other and of the process, the participants can lay a firm foundation for the subsequent work they will do.

The first five steps of the conflict resolution process set up the parties for everything that is to follow. The mediator clearly lays out rules of engagement at the beginning, ensuring that the parties understand what to expect and how to proceed. Rules include guidelines for meeting together and for expressing feelings. The mediator also clarifies the areas of focus and the mechanisms used to proceed and apprises the parties of the opportunities they have to be heard, have their issues considered, and be included in deliberations.

Step 6: Beginning the Resolution Process
Familiarizing everyone with the structure of the process is essential because that increases the participants' flexibility. Flexibility is especially important for mediators because they must

respond appropriately to what emerges along the way and take advantage of any opportunity to bring the parties to agreement.

Step 7: Defining Concerns and Setting Priorities
Here, doing one's homework pays off. The mediator, having come to understand the beginning issues, gives the parties an opportunity to explain their individual perceptions and how they formed their related expectations. The mediator also gets agreement from the parties on their understanding of the issues. Participants discuss the substantive points and positions until they are clear to everyone, work out the flow of events, and express their expectations of the methods for dealing with the issues.

Step 8: Looking for Hidden Information, Agendas, and Interests
The mediator constantly focuses on what the real issues are and on finding clues that could direct the parties toward sustainable solutions. During this stage, many issues, concerns, and problems are likely to emerge, and the mediator must be on the lookout for opportunities to get the parties to work them out. The seeds of solution are to be found in the parties' dialogue. The parties are engaged in a great amount of detailed work, sometimes together and sometimes apart or one on one with the mediator.

Step 9: Finding Potential Solutions and Determining Their Value to the Parties
As the parties move closer to an agreement, the mediator concentrates on getting them to understand where they appear to be in accord. The mediator's main task is to help the parties work out and state in detail any points of agreement between them, assess the applicability of potential solutions to the issues, determine their acceptability, and do whatever else is necessary to bring closure to the issues. As part of this process, the participants figure out the expected benefits and costs of meeting the obligations of the solutions.

Step 10: Formalizing the Agreement
Once all the issues in the dispute have been dealt with and the parties understand what they have agreed to and find it acceptable, the mediator and the parties fashion an official agreement that is both clear and acceptable to the parties. Depending on the breadth and complexity of the agreement, different levels of documentation may be necessary. The parties must make certain they all have the same understanding of what they have agreed to. In this final stage, the mediator prepares the documentation that formalizes the agreement and forms the foundation for carrying out the solutions. The parties, once they are satisfied there is a mechanism for implementing the agreement, formally accept it.

Keeping the Process on Track
The conflict resolution process summarized here is influenced by the issues, behaviors, personalities, and circumstances of the parties to the conflict. Some of these are unanticipated and move the process in directions not initially imagined by the mediator. However, the mediator, by paying attention to the dynamics of dialogue and remaining flexible, can guide the process in a way that ultimately gets the parties to an agreement and/or an end to the conflict.

The mediator uses many techniques to get the parties unstuck and moving toward a workable consensus. Taking the parties aside and working with them individually (commonly called *caucusing*) helps each deal with the issues in a way that is impossible when they are all in the same room. Getting more information, expanding the options, introducing new considerations, moving horizontally on the issues, pressing the parties to consider other factors, and expanding the parties' perceptions, among other strategies, are all tools in the mediator's tool box.

The mediator attempts to move the parties toward a negotiated settlement by means of a joint problem-solving process in which the parties work out the solutions themselves. The mediator is not invested in any particular outcome. The parties must be satisfied. They own the issues and the solutions. The mediator simply provides them with tools and a structure within which the resolution can be more assuredly achieved. The mediator stays neutral, not favoring either party and moving both toward a state of mutual satisfaction.

> **Key Point**
> Mediating any dispute involves helping the parties remain "unstuck," which is often a time-consuming task. It is all too easy for the parties to retreat to known territory, pushing for their own advantages and sustaining the polarization that has occurred. The best strategy is to stay focused on the larger picture and on the mutual benefits to be gained from a resolution.

The mediator is also constantly aware of the need to maintain a balance of power between the parties. In any dispute, issues of power are embedded in the process, and each party is tempted to pursue his or her own advantage to the exclusion of the other party's interests. Aware that jockeying over power occurs, the mediator does everything possible to make sure that the balance of power remains constant so that no party is disadvantaged as a result of the process. The mediator must not become an advocate for one party and must not act in a way that creates a perception of favoritism. The best strategy for dealing with issues of power is to be as public as possible about maintaining a balance, making it clear to the parties that this is a necessary feature of mediation.

Conflicts come in all shapes and sizes and levels of complexity, but in any conflict the mediator's role is to guide the process of problem solving and solution seeking for people who have been unable to get through this process by themselves. Although the details of the mediator's role are subject to debate, the mediator must recognize that the issues and their solutions belong to the parties. The mediator can bring his or her insights and skills, as well as sophisticated techniques and new concepts, to the process, yet the parties essentially own it. Whatever solutions are obtained are chosen by the parties and implemented by them. This is not to deny that sometimes the parties might want the mediator to control more of the process or take over responsibilities that properly belong to them, either because they view the responsibilities as too difficult or because they see the mediator as better placed to handle them.

The mediator must keep in mind that the process lends itself to tricks and stratagems that can slyly or inexplicably change the character or context of the interaction between the parties with such subtlety that it happens unnoticed. To avoid such shifts from occurring, the mediator needs to remain constantly focused on the process and its dynamics, evaluating its viability and efficacy and working to ensure that it is unfolding as it should.

People and Behavior

In conflict situations, stress levels are high and not everyone is at their best. Further, because of the history of conflict and people's general attitude toward it, people in conflict are not disposed to engage in relationship building and problem solving.

Parties to a conflict generally take the position that someone must win and someone must lose. The role of the mediator is to see that this outcome does not occur. It should be clear that only a mutually satisfying solution is likely to end the conflict permanently.

In the effort to "win," either party might try one or more tactics to unbalance the situation. The mediator needs to be on the lookout for these tactics and counter them through good techniques and a good process. In addition, the mediator needs to be aware of other factors that often influence the outcome of a conflict resolution process, such as those discussed next.

Communication Technique

The mediator must always be listening. And not just listening but listening actively, which means continually restating points in a way that is understandable to all the parties and that gets the issues out in the open. Almost any conflict is rife with emotional energy, and the mediator must manage and diffuse as much of it as possible through being clear and understandable and by translating every nuance and every embedded message into an explicit assertion. The parties are more likely to come to an agreement if they fully comprehend all the issues and each other's positions.

Meeting Setting and Schedule

The meeting place should be comfortable and not favor any particular party. The room should exhibit balance, the table should be round instead of rectangular, the seating arrangement should be comfortable and informal, and the lighting should be conducive to dialogue and therefore not bright or irritating. It is important to schedule the meetings at a time of the day when the parties are alert and invested instead of tired and worn out. By being sensitive to the possible influence of the environment on the resolution process, the mediator can ensure that the meeting place is pleasing and congenial and supports the process rather than working against it.

Demeanor

Mediators come from all kinds of backgrounds and have all kinds of personalities. Personality is always a consideration in mediation, and there must be a good fit between the mediator and the parties. If there is not a good fit, the mediator will have difficulty moving the process forward, possibly to such an extent that the process comes to a dead halt. The mediator must exhibit confidence and competence and present him- or herself as someone the parties can depend on in the times of challenge. The mediator is responsible for the process and its culture and dynamics, and by showing a proper demeanor and gaining the respect of the parties, the mediator can do much to create a suitable culture and stimulate movement toward resolution. When the fit between the mediator and the participants is not aligned, mediators must recuse themselves from the mediation process and make room for a neutral mediator who can create a better fit and help facilitate moving the resolution process to success. Mediators should not be offended by their lack of congruence. In many aspects of the human interaction, relationships do not always work as anticipated. Recognizing this and moving on are often critical moments in successful problem solving.

Information Exchange

During a conflict resolution process, lots of information is laid out. The mediator must facilitate the transmission of correct information. The more accurate the information exchanged between the parties, the more likely the process will move along smoothly. There is always a danger of having more information than is necessary for good decision making. Having lots of information is not the same as having the right information. The mediator tries to ensure that the parties have the information they need and can differentiate between desired data and needed data (needed data are data they can use to fashion an agreement).

Use of Experts

The mediator tries to provide the parties with access to whatever will help them resolve their conflict. Because no mediator can be an expert in all the elements and processes associated with every kind of conflict, others may need to be involved in the process. There are no rules limiting access to what or who is needed to resolve issues. Planning for and scheduling the use of experts or other resources and determining the focus of their use are among the critical responsibilities of the mediator.

Conclusion

Resolving conflicts is a fundamental part of managing human relationships. All relationships have the potential for conflict embedded deep within them, especially in our increasingly diverse healthcare system, where professionals with widely different backgrounds and roles are required to work together. As they sort through their unique contributions, they face many opportunities for conflict and are almost guaranteed to fall into disputes and disagreements (Kim et al., 2017). Healthcare leaders are responsible for supervising the relationships between the disciplines, and as the roles of the disciplines change and their relationships become more complex, the leaders have the critical task of helping all who work in the health field to respond to the changes and build stronger, more positive relationships.

The kind of intense interdisciplinary interaction characteristic of continuum-based teams is new to health care. Historically, there were only a very few types of professionals, and each type performed a wide variety of tasks. With the advances in technology that have occurred, more types of professionals exist, but the activities of each type are more narrowly focused. As a consequence, more people will be negotiating the clinical practice landscape, and, to complicate matters, these people will have more divergent roles and views. Working through their differences to find common ground will be essential to creating a more aligned and integrated healthcare system. Leaders have an important role to play in bringing this kind of system into existence by assisting others in solving problems and resolving conflicts.

Dealing with conflict is a normal part of the leadership role as it currently exists, and therefore leaders must understand the basic elements and learn the essential skills of conflict management. The implications for the role will only accelerate in the emerging and growing interdisciplinary work environment. Finding common ground among the disciplines and achieving true relational equity will imply the management and resolutions of many heretofore unaddressed relational and interactional conflicts. Like any skill, conflict management leadership requires continuous development. Leaders must recognize this and persevere in their learning efforts. The payoff is that these skills serve any leader well in dealing with the increasingly complex set of relationships in the delivery of health services. To the extent that a leader develops the necessary skills and takes on the role of conflict resolution facilitator, he or she will strengthen the relationships between health professionals and, most important, increase the effectiveness of health care.

CHAPTER SIX   Diversity and Difference: Managing Conflict in a Transdisciplinary Network

Chapter Takeaways

1. All conflict is normative and represents the key and fundamental characteristic of differences in human communication and interaction. For leaders, managing conflict is simply a vehicle through which people negotiate their differences and work to advance the journey to finding common ground.
2. Conflict operates on a continuum. If not engaged early at the very elemental stages of conflict, the process grows in intensity, veracity, and difficulty. Left unaddressed, all conflict ultimately leads to emotional, intellectual, physical, relational, or social death.
3. Conflict can be positively addressed by recognizing that conflict management is a leadership process and by utilizing appreciative approaches. The primary role of leaders is to develop an understanding of the systematic approach (process) to effective conflict management and with patience and perseverance develop skills with the good use of a disciplined process.
4. The five categories of conflict are structural (organizational), value, information, interaction, and interest conflicts. Each category requires an understanding of the root of conflict and a unique approach. Appropriately diagnosing the foundation and category of conflict helps inform the leader with regard to the choices related to the approach, the use of an effective conflict method, and the strategy for effectively addressing and moving the conflict toward resolution.
5. Leaders generally assume a neutral role in managing organizational and interpersonal conflict at work. This means that leaders focus on an equity-based approach, use of a good process, management of the interests and needs of the parties, and movement toward a mutually beneficial outcome.

Case Study 6-1

Managing an Unhealthy Work Environment

Isabella is new to the management role and has been the nurse manager of the Mother Infant Care (MIC) unit for 6 months. She recently graduated with her master of science degree with an emphasis on leadership in micro healthcare systems. She was excited to be chosen from a candidate pool of five more experienced nurses, and she was eager to apply what she had learned in graduate school in shaping the culture of the MIC unit. After getting to know the staff and assistant nurse managers, Isabella made some changes to put structure and processes in place that would facilitate staff involvement in decisions related to patient care and their practice of nursing. She encouraged the assistant managers to change from developing the staff schedule to allowing self-scheduling based on a few rules and principles that the staff had part in developing. It was decided that the more senior staff would have first choice in their schedule, followed by the part-time, and finally the per diem staff. Requests for time off were to be submitted to the assistant managers prior to the new schedule being posted so that the unit would be staffed appropriately.

All seemed to be going fairly well with the self-scheduling system for the first 4 months, but with the holiday season approaching, Isabella was receiving feedback that some of the staff were extremely unhappy with the system. There had been some arguments among staff in the nursing lounge, and Isabella was informed that one of the staff members left work in tears. Apparently, some of the more senior staff were being unreasonable with the less tenured full-time staff and refused to cover personal requests. The assistant managers informed Isabella that a powerful clique had formed with a few senior staff who were bullying some of the new nurses and refusing to assist them in patient care activities or to answer any of their questions. It seemed as if the situation was becoming quite unsettling, and two of the newly hired nurses had put in a request to be transferred to another unit.

When Isabella interviewed the nurses who had resigned or were transferring to another unit, she was surprised to hear their stories of verbal abuse, the "silent treatment" with no communication, or refusal to cover for them during required break times. She was also told that several of the more senior nurses refused to assist in turning patients and often withheld information that was important to patient care. Although Isabella was not able to convince the nurses to stay on the unit, she realized that the culture of the unit had to be changed.

Isabella called all of the assistant managers together and told them that they needed to work as a team to change the culture on the unit. She listened to their perspectives on what was happening and quickly identified that some of the assistant managers may have contributed to the problem because they had refused to become involved in managing the situation on their shift. It seemed to Isabella that the assistant managers may have been afraid of some of the staff members, and therefore were not comfortable confronting them about their inappropriate behaviors in the workplace. The small group of senior staff seemed to have control over staff members as well as the assistant managers. Some ethnic clashes also contributed to the problem.

Isabella decided to meet with the human resources specialist for her area and her director to apprise them of the situation and to ask for assistance in developing a strategy to resolve the conflicts. After discussing the situation and identifying potential options for resolution, they decided that the problem needed to be discussed openly at staff meetings and that performance and clarification of expectations would be discussed with offending staff individually and all staff collectively. A series of short presentations by a clinical psychologist on workplace bullying was planned with follow-up discussions with the staff.

New group norms for professional behavior and consequences for unprofessional conduct were presented and discussed with the staff. Each staff member was asked to sign an agreement outlining his or her knowledge of and acceptance of the new behavioral standards. This process allowed Isabella to meet with each staff member with the individual's assistant manager to reinforce the importance of acceptable behaviors in the workplace. Isabella and the human resources specialist helped the assistant managers give disciplinary warnings to the more offending staff members, and Isabella reiterated her expectation to these staff members that if they could not accept the new behavior standards or demonstrate the necessary changes, she would assist them in "making other career choices."

Finally, Isabella announced a zero-tolerance policy for workplace bullying and unprofessional conduct. She told the staff, "Everyone has a right to feel safe, respected, and valued when at work. How we feel at work affects our ability to provide the best possible care to our patients." She told the staff that each of them could expect to be treated fairly and that she wanted them to feel safe in expressing their feelings in a professional and positive manner. She listened to their views on how to improve the self-scheduling process to ensure fairness for all. Isabella also arranged for every staff member to attend educational sessions that included discussions on cultural, gender, and age diversity in the workplace. Every staff meeting included open discussion on progress that was being made on each shift toward resolving the conflicts and creating a healthier work environment for all of the staff. She encouraged the staff to meet with her if they had any concerns about conflicts on the unit, and she made frequent rounds to speak with individuals and to make her presence visible among the staff.

Isabella also worked with her assistant managers to increase their leadership competencies in facing conflict and developing strategies to resolve the conflict rather than choosing to ignore the situation. She reminded them of their responsibility as leaders to face conflicts early, before they became unmanageable. She discussed the need for improved teamwork among the assistant managers to ensure support for one another during these times of crisis. She reassured them that she would be available to each of them to support them through any difficult situation, and that she would secure any resources needed to create a healthy work environment for them and for the staff.

Questions

1. What were some of the sources and possible causes of the conflict that emerged on the unit?
2. What were some of the signs that the conflict had escalated to an unacceptable level?
3. What leadership roles did Isabella assume in managing the conflict process?
4. How did the assistant managers' actions affect the level of conflict and the resolution of the conflict?
5. If you were Isabella, how would you have handled the conflict and mediated the situation?

Case Study 6-2

He Said, She Said, and No One Is Listening!

It started out a good day, and Mike reviewed the long list of items that he needed to accomplish that day. He had planned to meet with his managers to discuss the operational budget goals for the department and to initiate discussion about needed capital equipment that had to be projected for the upcoming year. Mike was the director of Medical Surgical Services and had six direct reports who were nurse managers over the following units: Oncology, General-Medical, Postoperative Surgical, Bariatric, Orthopedics, and Observational (short stay). In addition to the six nurse managers, the medical director for Internal Medicine and the medical director for Surgical Services also reported to Mike. The management team was an eclectic group with very different levels of education and experience, which made for lively discussions in their team meetings.

Each nurse manager brought a list of capital needs to the meeting. It quickly became apparent that there was more need than there was allocated budget, because Mike's service line was only one of four for the entire hospital. As the nurse managers began to present their proposed capital needs, the group dynamics began to change from friendly to conflicting and competitive. The Orthopedics department had the longest capital need list with the biggest dollar amount. As the other managers began to defend their list of needs, the nurse manager of the Orthopedics department mentioned that his service line also contributed the greatest amount of revenue as compared to the other departments. He used that fact as a rationale for why his department should receive a larger piece of the allocated budget. Other nurse managers argued fiercely about their contribution to the hospital's bottom line and the value that their department brought to the organization. When the discussions became heated, Mike suggested that they take a recess as a "cooling off period." They agreed to meet again the next day to finalize the capital budget plan.

The next day the nurse managers came prepared to defend their units' needs, and they had formed a coalition against the nurse manager of Orthopedics. They had met outside of the meeting and agreed that they might have more power in the discussion if they presented their needs collectively rather than individually.

The nurse manager of Orthopedics also had a strategy. He had met with the chief of the Orthopedics service line and the medical director of Surgical Services. He asked them to join him in the meeting and indicate how important it was for Orthopedics to receive the requested capital budget items. He also presented information about the threat to the hospital's market share if the Orthopedics department did not keep up with state-of-the-art equipment.

Not long after the meeting started, it was clear to Mike that the cooling-off period had not worked but rather had served as an opportunity to strengthen the conflict. As each of the nurse managers stated their case and rationale for their requests, tempers began to flare, and accusations were made on both sides. Mike realized that further discussion was not going to be helpful in resolving the conflict. Although the capital budget for his department was due in 2 days, Mike decided to stop the meeting once again. He informed the group that he would meet with two representatives from the coalition group and two representatives from the Orthopedics group. Although the others were not happy about this plan, they were also not happy with the group's inability to negotiate a fair and equitable capital budget plan within the overall allocated amount.

The next day Mike met with the four representatives in a quiet, subdued setting that he felt would facilitate the mediation process and create a favorable environment for open dialogue, negotiation, and resolution. His opening remarks addressed the need for the four representatives to make decisions for the entire team that would be appropriate within the budget limitations. Mike had reviewed in his head the steps of the negotiation process and reminded himself not to take sides or contribute to the discussion until both sides were able to find common ground and begin to develop some realistic solutions.

Mike led them through a meeting norming process with the participants agreeing to "rules" for the meeting. They agreed that they would (1) respect the person speaking, and only one person would speak at a time without interruption; (2) focus on the common good in contrast to their individual units' needs; (3) create a list of the top 10 priorities for the entire department, and then negotiate the list down to the allocated budget amount; and (4) vote on items until consensus was reached. Needless to say, it was not easy in the beginning, and Mike had to continually remind them that there was a finite amount of money that could be allocated and that they needed to make decisions for the whole based on the allocated budget amounts. With this constant reminder and norming process, the four began to work together using the strategic plan for the department as a foundation for their decision making. They also developed rationale for each of their decisions that could be presented to the whole group. It took a full two days of meetings to finally have a proposed budget that could be presented to the rest of the group.

Mike called the entire group together and informed them of the decision-making process that led to the proposed budget. Two of the representatives prepared a presentation for the entire group and provided handouts of the proposed budget with a rationale for each item suggested. As it turned out, Orthopedics did receive a greater allocation than the other units, but there was clear justification using the strategic goals for the department as a foundation. Not everyone in the group was happy with the proposed budget, but they did agree that the rationale was sound. After discussion, the group finally decided to adopt the new proposed capital budget and to develop proposals for the hospital's foundation to fund some of the other items that they felt were important to their units.

Mike submitted his final capital budget on time, but he recognized that there was still some discontent among some managers within the group. He realized that he could not please everyone, but the method that he used to resolve the open conflict resulted in a budget that was supportive of the department's strategic initiatives even though some capital items were not approved, as some had hoped.

Questions

1. Identify the potential causes for the conflict among the managers.
2. If you were in Mike's position, what might you have done differently to manage and resolve the conflict?
3. What are your thoughts about why the splintering among the group occurred when they began to form a coalition and bring other team members into the process?
4. How did Mike help or hinder the negotiation process?
5. Although the capital budget has been submitted, what work does Mike need to focus on to improve the group dynamics?
6. Describe the power imbalances that existed within the group, and discuss how these imbalances affected the group dynamics.
7. How were the 10 steps to conflict resolution used in developing the final solution to the capital budget plan?

References

Almost, J., Wolff, A. C., Stewart-Pyne, A., McCormick, L. G., Strachan, D., & D'Souza, C. (2016). Managing and mitigating conflict in healthcare teams: An integrative review. *Journal of Advanced Nursing, 72*(7), 1490–1505.

Bleich, M. R., & Hessler, C. (2016). Appreciative inquiry and implementation science in leadership development. *Journal of Continuing Education in Nursing, 47*(5), 207–209.

Butani, L., & Plant, J. (2016). Building connections with role models using an appreciative inquiry approach. *Academic Pediatrics, 16*(4), 411–412.

Caspers, B. A., & Pickard, B. (2013). Value-based resource management: A model for best value nursing care. *Nursing Administration Quarterly, 37*(2), 95–104.

Dignath, D., Kiesel, A., & Eder, A. B. (2015). Flexible conflict management: Conflict avoidance and conflict adjustment in reactive cognitive control. *Journal of Experimental Psychology. Learning Memory and Cognition, 41*(4), 975–988.

du Plessis, E. (2016). Caring presence in practice: Facilitating an appreciative discourse in nursing. *International Nursing Review, 63*(3), 377–380.

Eisler, R., & Garrick, L. (2018). *Leading the shift from a dominator to a partnership culture.* The Systems Thinker. https://thesystemsthinker.com/leading-the-shift-from-a-dominator-to-a-partnership-culture/

Hamblin, L. E., Essenmacher, L., Ager, J., Upfal, M., Luborsky, M., Russell, J., & Ametz, J. (2016). Worker-to-worker violence in hospitals: Perpetrator characteristics and common dyads. *Workplace Health & Safety, 64*(2), 51–56.

Janss, R., Rispens, S., Segers, M., & Jehn, K. A. (2012). What is happening under the surface? Power, conflict and the performance of medical teams. *Medical Education*, 46(9), 838–849.

Johansen, M. L., & Cadmus, E. (2016). Conflict management style, supportive work environments and the experience of work stress in emergency nurses. *Journal of Nursing Management*, 24(2), 211–218.

Kim, S., Bochatay, N., Relyea-Chew, A., Buttrick, E., Amdahl, C., Kim, L., Frans, E., Mossanen, M., Khandekar, A., Fehr, R., & Lee, Y. (2017). Individual, interpersonal, and organizational factors of healthcare conflict: A scoping review. *Journal of Interprofessional Care*, 32(3), 282–290.

Lewicki, R. J., Saunders, D. M., & Barry, B. (2015). *Negotiation*. McGraw-Hill Education.

Maung, A. A., Toevs, C. C., Kayser, J. B., & Kaplan, L. J. (2015). Conflict management teams in the intensive care unit: A concise definitive review. *Journal of Trauma and Acute Care Surgery*, 79(2), 314–320.

McKibben, L. (2017). Conflict management: Importance and implications. *British Journal of Nursing*, 26(2), 100–103.

Morreim, H. (2016). Story of a mediation in the clinical setting. *Journal of Clinical Ethics*, 27(1), 43–50.

Ramsbotham, O., Woodhouse, T., & Miall, H. (2016). *Contemporary conflict resolution* (4th ed.). Polity Press.

Rothman, J. (2018). *The "ARIA" approach to conflict resolution*. The Systems Thinker. https://thesystemsthinker.com/the-aria-approach-to-conflict-resolution/

Zavotsky, K. E., & Chan, G. K. (2016). Exploring the relationship among moral distress, coping, and the practice environment in emergency department nurses. *Advanced Emergency Nursing Journal*, 38(2), 133–146.

Suggested Readings

Brown, J., Lewis, L., Ellis, K., Stewart, M., Freeman, T. R., & Kasperski, M. J. (2011). Conflict on interprofessional primary health care teams—Can it be resolved? *Journal of Interprofessional Care*, 25(1), 4–10.

Busch, M., & Hostetter, C. (2009). Examining organizational learning for application and human service organizations. *Administration and Social Work*, 33(3), 297–318.

Cahn, D., & Abigail, R. (2013). *Managing conflict through communication*. Pearson.

Cheung, F., & Tang, C. (2009). The influence of emotional intelligence and affectivity on emotional labor strategies that work. *Journal of Individual Differences*, 30(2), 75–86.

Deutch, M., Coleman, P., & Marcus, E. (2006). *The handbook of conflict resolution: Theory and practice*. Jossey-Bass.

Malloch, K., & Porter-O'Grady, T. (2009). *The quantum leader: Applications for the new world of work*. Jones & Bartlett Learning.

McKibben, L. (2017). Conflict management: Importance and implications. *British Journal of Nursing*, 26(2), 100–103.

Peterson, M. B., & Laustsen, L. (2019). Dominant leaders and the political psychology of followership. *Current Opinion in Psychology*, 33, 136–141.

Quiz Questions

Select the best answer for each of the following questions.

1. Conflict in everyday relationships is:
    a. to be avoided.
    b. unacceptable.
    c. normal.
    d. destructive.

2. Conflict resolution facilitators must recognize the value of:
   a. uniformity.
   b. diversity.
   c. anxiety.
   d. humanity.

3. When is conflict destructive?
   a. When it is not resolved
   b. When it is accompanied by anger
   c. When it is secretive
   d. When it becomes physical

4. The perceived imbalance of power can occur during a conflict. Power should be:
   a. viewed as a necessary evil that enhances positive outcomes.
   b. placed in the hands of managers and mediators.
   c. placed in the hands of staff not involved in conflict.
   d. balanced by both conflicting parties.

5. What do two parties in conflict generally know?
   a. Each party's position
   b. Why they are angry
   c. What they want
   d. What they dislike

6. Which of the following is a true statement about conflict?
   a. Interest-based conflict concerns how the parties view themselves.
   b. Identity-based conflict concerns how the parties view themselves.
   c. Identity-based conflict involves tangible issues.
   d. Interest-based conflict is harder to resolve.

7. What is the primary role of a conflict resolution facilitator?
   a. To bring the conflict to an end
   b. To establish a good resolution process
   c. To keep the parties moving through the process
   d. To help both parties get what they want

8. What must a conflict resolution facilitator never do?
   a. Move through negotiations slowly
   b. Encourage expressions of antagonism
   c. Push to uncover who/what is at blame/being blamed
   d. Get invested in a particular outcome

9. To reach a successful completion of the 10-step conflict resolution process, the mediator must ensure which of the following?
   a. That the interaction between the parties is friendly and their dialogue is courteous
   b. That the parties use effective techniques for communicating and exchanging information
   c. That the parties meet with the mediator together, not one on one
   d. That the parties receive as much information that the mediator acquires

Quiz Questions

10. The attribution by each party of negative motives and qualities to the other party usually indicates which of the following?
    a. That both parties have identity-related conflicts
    b. That each party has relational conflicts
    c. That the parties hold similar organizational-related conflict
    d. That each party wants to sabotage conflict resolution

11. In making conflict normative, the leader creates a frame for conflict that turns it from:
    a. a dynamic into a situation.
    b. a process into an event.
    c. an event into a process.
    d. the situation into an event.

12. A good leader does everything possible to avoid conflict.
    a. True
    b. False

13. When left unaddressed, conflict simply changes:
    a. its form.
    b. its substance.
    c. its content.
    d. its intensity.

14. When conflicts occur, problems that arise are usually generated from:
    a. emotional maturity and position.
    b. anger and aggression.
    c. hurt and pain.
    d. fear and avoidance.

15. Nurses have a unique set of concerns regarding conflicts and their resolution because of:
    a. lack of education in conflict management.
    b. history of subordination and organizational powerlessness.
    c. aggressive physician workplace behaviors.
    d. a lack of medical knowledge that supports a clinical situation.

16. Game playing _____ lead(s) to conflict.
    a. can sometimes
    b. usually
    c. rarely
    d. always

17. Which of the following are sources of identity-based conflict?
    a. Personality, relatives, coworkers
    b. Religion, heritage, culture
    c. Policy, rules, roles
    d. Leaders, professionals, personalities

18. Acting as a facilitator, the leader's first job is to:
    a. give the parties a voice and listen to their essential insights and perceptions.
    b. identify an apparent conflict and its source.
    c. plan potential solutions and strategies related to the identified elements of the conflict.
    d. gather the stakeholders to the problem in one place and begin exploring their problems.

19. For there to be movement toward resolution and/or acceptance, the facilitator must:
    a. make sure conflict processes are interrupted so that their negative impact does not continue.
    b. protect the organization and leadership against the negative impact and aspects of the conflict.
    c. ensure that all the issues and facets of the issue held by the parties are laid out in detail.
    d. communicate with the staff about the conflict and its potential impact on their work.

20. In conflict management, *resonance* is the:
    a. intangible and subjective assessment of issues within interpersonal relationships.
    b. process of moving away from antagonism and toward identification of common ground.
    c. articulation of values and concerns that indicate strong differences affecting dialogue.
    d. identification of common concerns that have very similar elements.

21. During the early stages of the conflict resolution/mediation process, one of the first steps is to:
    a. agree on solutions to be sought.
    b. advance the movement from problem identification to solution process.
    c. help all parties understand their disagreements with respect and inclusion.
    d. develop and agree on mutual statements of objectives.

22. The final stage of a conflict resolution/mediation process is:
    a. crafting a plan of action.
    b. determining individual behaviors following the mediation.
    c. listing the agreed-upon conflicts clearly and precisely.
    d. sorting out the details of the remaining differences.

23. A step that may help parties get unstuck and move toward a workable solution is to have the mediator:
    a. develop a solution based on the single most important locus of responsibility for the original conflict.
    b. assign accountability for specific outcomes to different party members.
    c. take the parties aside (individually) to help each deal with previously unresolvable issues.
    d. ensure that one of the rules put in place is to consider corrective action when needed.

24. Part of being a successful mediator is the mediator's capacity to:
    a. exhibit confidence and competence in addressing the conflict.
    b. ensure that blame and responsibility remain with the parties, not the mediator.
    c. identify the elements and characteristics of the conflict to clearly identify conflict problems.
    d. manage the communication of each party to remove the emotional and behavioral impact.

25. The conflict management leader should use experts in resolving the conflict:
    a. in a very limited fashion, so as not to shift the focus of resolution from the participants to the expert.
    b. to transfer the locus of control to the parties and the processes in motion.
    c. as frequently as needed to help parties resolve the conflict.
    d. only when there is a particular problem that needs an expert to prevent stalling of problem resolution.

CHAPTER SEVEN

Leading Constant Movement: Transforming Chaos and Crisis

For the past 33 years I have looked into the mirror every morning and asked myself: "If today were the last day of my life, would I want to do what I am about to do today?" And if the answer were "no" for too many days in a row, I know I need to change something.
—*Steve Jobs*

Chapter Objectives

At the completion of this chapter, the reader will be able to:

- Define *crisis* and expand on the essential elements of crisis within a leadership context.
- Enumerate the complexity of systems and the role crisis plays in moving them to change.
- Explain the role of crisis in the change process and identify the characteristics of crisis in the process of change.
- Understand and apply the concepts of predictive and adaptive capacity in the role of the leader.
- Use a systems model for crisis management as a way of systematically confronting and addressing crisis as a normative part of the change process.

This is a time of great transformation for healthcare systems. And great challenges. Cultural, social, and global political shifts and challenges create a milieu for increasing risk and uncertainty across societies and within organizations. There is an increased focus on patient-centered, value-based, and coordinated care, and digitalization of health services (accessibility, accountability, and finding the right provider) and its related data. Transformations also include major initiatives related to continuing national health reform, the growing technical transformation of therapeutics and service delivery, and management of patients and communities with or at risk for novel viruses. All of these transformations converge to create the perfect storm of chaos and complexity throughout the health system. Leaders increasingly understand the vagaries of complexity and chaos and the implications of unplanned events. Leaders also increasingly understand the connectivity of the business of healthcare in that if there is a crisis in a foreign country that is the leading manufacturer of essential healthcare equipment and supplies, there is a ripple effect thousands of miles away in the United States.

In fact, the unexpected has become the norm. Increasingly, unplanned events and broad-based crises are all part of doing business and of natural occurrences in the cycle of human experience. No amount of planning and all of the anticipation that accompanies planning can change the contingencies that are a constant and that require leadership responses.

Crises have always been with us. Since the dawn of time, natural and human events have combined to create conditions and circumstances that have raised the intensity of human life and even threatened its very existence. From natural disasters and environmental shifts to human-made war to outbreaks of new strains of viruses or diseases without antidotes or treatments to conflict and social and cultural change, crises have accompanied human beings on the human journey. Only in the last couple of decades have we begun to study crisis and to sort through its characteristics, elements, and all aspects that operate to affect the "critical" human experience. Through studying crisis and understanding its vagaries and variables, humans can anticipate, perhaps even predict, crises in a way to help us better manage the impact on our social and individual experiences (Stephens et al., 2016; St.Pierre et al., 2016).

Normative and Nonnormative Crisis

Crises are not always stimulated by cataclysmic events. Sometimes, a crisis can be stimulated by simple occurrences. An accidental moment of invention, turning down the wrong street, a casual conversation with another individual, and the choice of where to spend one's vacation all represent simple decisions and actions that might result in significant and important challenges and shifts in events and experiences. These kinds of critical events and unanticipated situations can be the end product of a convergence of forces unknown at a given time, yet operating inexorably to create an impact or cause a result that was fully unanticipated. Violent acts emerging out of severe mental illness, terrorism, significant natural calamities, and human errors can occur at a moment's notice and interrupt the norms and routines of human action and throw us individually and collectively into the throes of chaos.

> **Point to Ponder**
>
> Crisis is a fundamental component of the human journey; it accompanies change.

Although unplanned events are normal parts of human existence, people do not like crises and significant change events. Individuals demonstrate the most discomfort when normal patterns of human experience are interrupted with a radical or immediate shift in reality or conditions. An apparent contradiction exists between the normality of unplanned events and people's unwillingness to accommodate them that creates the foundation for much of the conflict, stress, and anxiety related to confronting and addressing normative crisis. If crisis could be seen as a routine and fundamental element of everyone's personal experience and life process, perhaps more attention would be paid to developing adaptation, anticipation, and coping mechanisms to help people accommodate and deal with the crises that inevitably occur in their lives.

Early Warning

Crises very rarely occur without some level of early warning (VanVactor, 2015; Zhuravsky, 2015). The critical factor in early engagement of crisis is the development and presence of tools and mechanisms that enable leadership to become aware of the potential for crisis in advance of crises actually occurring. The first step of any early warning system is the leaders' understanding and acceptance that the occurrence of crisis is a normative part of the human experience and that crises are to be anticipated. Understanding the inevitability and normative circumstances related to the potential of the onset of a crisis helps to condition organizational leaders to create a programmatic and systematic approach to confronting crisis. In short, a systematic framework—a model—needs to be incorporated into the operational and structural characteristics of the organization as a way of ensuring that well-planned mechanisms for addressing the onset of crisis events are in place long before crisis actually arises.

Hospitals and health systems are very good at anticipating clinical crises as well as community and natural disasters. Their capacity for disaster planning is unparalleled. However, these crises tend to be the least common occurrences affecting the viability and stability of the hospital or health system. Usually, other major significant crises place the hospital or health system at greater risk than do natural or clinical disasters. Crises related to readiness for health reform, finance, management, market, competition, environment, and operations create more significant risks for the organization than do natural or clinical disasters.

Much of the reason for the impact of this kind of risk is the lack of systems that predict and anticipate changes in current conditions and the challenges that threaten the traditional work patterns of the status quo (Mather et al., 2018). For all leaders, the ability to develop these skills requires a deep understanding of social and organizational complexity and the processes associated with facilitating human dynamics within the context of complex systems. The ability to comprehend the action of complexity and the human response to immediate and dramatic change is an important leadership skill that is required as a basic foundation for the expression of leadership competencies related to the management of crisis. And it is now a leadership competency that must be considered as essential in the operation of healthcare agencies and facilities that respond to the potential and realities associated with environmental, social, political, and behavioral crises. Complexity theory and science have provided leaders with major new insights regarding predictive and adaptive capacity and the need to incorporate particular dynamics and applications into the ordinary and usual management practices of organizations (Storkholm et al., 2019).

The ability to understand both the complexities of and applications essential to a positive response to crisis demands an understanding of the cybernetic nature of all action and human experience. Leaders must recognize the cyclical nature of all action, including human action, and the inevitability and eventuality of major and dramatic shifts in both experience and reality (Goralnick et al., 2015). Because of this inevitability, all human organizations must reflect a strong capacity for adaptation and change. Because change is the only constant in the universe, structuring organizations to be continuously adaptive and mobile is a critical requisite for long-term viability. The need for an organization to continue to thrive calls for its leadership to be ever-vigilant with regard to the continuous and unrelenting risks embedded in change dynamics operating both internally and externally and having both negative and positive implications for the organization's health and existence (Graves & Nikpay, 2017).

The Leader's Perception of Crisis

Contemporary leaders must recognize the importance of adaptive and predictive skills related to managing crises. The contemporary leader must understand that crisis management is as important a part of the process of management as the normative operational considerations

> **Key Point**
>
> If leaders are unable to accommodate the critical variables embedded in the crisis of change, followers will be no more successful in confronting the demand to change.

of day-to-day function. At the same time, crisis is not always appropriate in the work environment. Leaders must be able to separate crisis management as a functional activity from crisis leadership as a strategic imperative. Leaders who continually manage within a crisis mode create the conditions and circumstances that ultimately blind people to the legitimate and normative crises that confront their lives and work from time to time. At this level of intensity, crisis management both prevents people from dealing effectively with the crisis and creates a set of circumstances that makes them uniquely unprepared to adequately address a legitimate crisis.

Often, leaders who manage in a crisis mode like the intense feeling of the "high" that comes from living at an accelerated level of energy. For these people, everything has a serious potential for implications beyond what normally can be expected in a given situation. Raising this level of crisis and applying it to routine and ritual functions and activities ultimately causes people to burn out and become immune to responding appropriately to situations that might be potentially significant or dangerous. This kind of leadership is neither effective nor valuable; in fact, it is destructive. Wise leaders recognize the value of conflict and crisis, understand its appropriate context, and prepare for it without living it.

Understanding Crisis

Crisis comes in all forms, from natural disasters to human-caused crises such as war, terrorism, novel viruses with high morbidity and mortality, national disasters, and economic meltdowns. In human organizations, the more complex the system, the more likely the onset of crisis. Human development has resulted in a burgeoning of technologies and systems that create increasingly more complex infrastructures. The more complex the infrastructure, the more interdependent the elements that make it up become, and the more likely it is subject to the vagaries of external and internal forces causing the crisis. Technologies themselves increase the intensity through magnification of processes, elements, and experiences in ways that advance the human experience and the opportunity for a wide variety of human expressions. Technologies may be identified in the instruments of creativity and in the products of human ingenuity. From medicines to new products, from ideas to new insights regarding the technology itself, the impact of human ingenuity is increasingly vital to everyday human activity (Meskó et al., 2017; Sturmberg & Bircher, 2019).

Technology further refines the human experience. In the presence of technology, the quality of human life is advanced and improved such that illnesses can be healed, diseases prevented, discomfort alleviated, and enjoyment and comfort in the human experience advanced. Technology becomes the means for fulfilling every human desire and expectation. Through the use of technology, the human experience can be expanded, deepened, and broadened. A part of the impact of technology, however, is the complexity that it brings to human experience.

> **Point to Ponder**
>
> Technology is accompanied by crisis. Destructive technologies always radically change our lives.

Complexity and Technology

Human beings have lived in organizations of every level of complexity. We depend on the well-being and functioning of complex human systems in small and large aggregates of human interaction and relationship. Organizational and relational issues are highest on the priority list of human interest and exploration. As the human culture has grown in diversity, breadth, and complexity, it has become increasingly complex and challenging to both understand and manage (Therrien et al., 2017).

Human beings shape the form of their organization through cultural, social, political, and relational interactions. The impact of each of these has led to highly complex and successful societies emerging from the earliest experiences of human history. From Greek societies and Chinese culture, to the Roman Empire, to the development of European and Asian powers, to the emergence of North American cultures and the political and social influence of the West, social and political aggregations of human organizations have continually made an impact on the human experience and the dynamics of change.

Our world has become more complex and diverse. In this diversity, it has also become more prone to the conflicts that difference creates. Crises that result from conflicts usually demonstrate problems with the regulation of human organizations, the ability to control function and interaction, and the inability or unwillingness of various cultural organizations and groupings to deal effectively and peacefully with others (Grady, 2016; van Rossum et al., 2016).

> ### Group Discussion
>
> Identify a recent global or national social shift (like health reform) or a national tragedy (like the COVID-19 pandemic) and the unknown and unanticipated elements of the event. List the ways in which people were unprepared, and identify how being unprepared contributed to the crisis. What elements of the crisis drove people into chaos and uncertainty? What role did the lack of technology play in exacerbating the crisis? How do human beings behave in the absolute absence of technology? What role does technology play in anticipating and managing crisis? In this scenario, is technology a means or an end?

Conflict in the Human Community

Many crises can be traced to problems within and between the organizational infrastructures of human communities (Curt & Tacnet, 2018). As a result of infrastructure inadequacies and conflict, various pathologies emerge that represent inadequacies within and between groups when dealing with issues that negatively affect other groups. Various systems technologies have been developed within societies, organizations, and large groupings. Systems approaches deal with the complex interactions of variables that affect the quality of the human experience. From the development of economics, sociology, politics, psychodynamics, engineering and architecture, and other innovative and creative technologies, social groups find ways to optimize their collective and individual experiences and to create opportunities to advance their organizational infrastructure, even at the risk of challenging current organizational configurations. Entire fields of science have been developed within the context of emerging complexities of human societies and organizations for researchers to find ways to solve problems associated with large, complex human communities. Out of these sciences have emerged intellectual, theoretical, and practical processes directed to managing and creating ways to advance the social experience; ensure that societies live in harmony, peace, and comfort; and reduce the potential for war (Laapotti & Mikkola, 2016).

In the past 2 decades, scientific endeavors have led to a deeper understanding of the complexity of systems and the elements of complexity as applied to human dynamics and human organization (Podgorski et al., 2016; Turchin et al., 2018). This examination attempts to move past assumptions and serendipitous models of human process into understanding more complex systems and creating an increasingly adaptive and broad-based field of inquiry with regard to systems and human organizations. A variety of systems theory and cybernetics has emerged that recognizes the unfolding of a growing language for complex human organizations. A wide breadth of variables affect human relationships and the ability of societies and organizations to work and thrive in increasingly complex circumstances. Out of these systems approaches, a new synergistic understanding of human systems and organizations and the processes of human dynamics, interaction, innovation, and complexity has emerged, recognizing a complexity of processes and utilizing the insights and skills of a wide variety of disciplines.

Understanding complexity in systems requires understanding the integration, coordination, and facilitation of complex human groups (Kelders et al., 2016). Understanding complexity in organizations enables leaders to control the variables affecting human interaction, decision making, innovation, technology, and direction. Leadership skills are critical to the sustenance and advancement of both societies and organizations. Complexity science requires an effective conceptual foundation for successful social systems management. This brings to mind the need to manage the dynamic cybernetic capacity of human experience that lies embedded within this complexity, with all the related organizational and human challenges that implies. The cybernetics of organizational human life (cycles of unrelenting change) and the application of complexity science related to explicating it and communicating complexity become a management skill of translating understanding of human dynamics and social enterprise. Leaders' capacity to do this helps to better articulate human interaction, autonomy, behavior and values, and significance in the application of work and issues related to advancing the human experience and achieving self-actualization.

> **Key Point**
> Complexity sciences now form the foundation for thinking about existence, organization, and human functioning.

Complexity and Organizations

Human organizations, especially those organized for work, are exemplars of both a broad and a narrow aggregation of human activity. However, to thrive and grow cybernetic and life-generating intelligent organizations require a systematic integration of a number of forces.

Human organizations must adapt quickly to changing circumstances. Adaptation is a critical factor in an organization's ability to continue to thrive and succeed. Adaptation is a fundamental predictor of continuing existence and requires a clear conceptualization of the elements and processes necessary to ensure thriving. Thriving means building a goodness-of-fit in the intersection between an organization's external and internal rela-

> **Point to Ponder**
>
> Adaptation is central to survival. Those who do not adapt die!

tionships and circumstances in the broader world. As the world continues to shift as a result of improving conditions, changing technology, environmental transformation, or political and social change, organizations must reflect those changes within the context of their own operations. Nothing remains constant. Organizations must expect that the ever-transitioning environment will be challenging, perhaps even threatening, because the transforming social conditions and circumstances affect what the organization does and its place in the world (van Wietmarschen et al., 2018).

Effectively managing change means leaders create an internally and externally adaptive environment that has the capacity to anticipate, even predict, the impact of changes, internal and external, that affect its ability to continue to function. The management of change is a constant, rather than an exception, and is a critical leadership skill in complex systems. Because change is ever-present and continuously affects the organization, leaders must recognize in their own roles an adaptive capacity that helps the organization and its people shift and adjust practices, processes, and behaviors in the face of a shifting demand for them.

Adaptive Capacity and Change

Several factors need to be addressed for an organization to adapt to its changing realities. First, of course, senior management needs to be fully invested and committed to the change dynamic (Lal, 2019; Velthuis et al., 2018). This level of leadership requires that the strategic frame for the organization incorporates change as a normative part of the operating decision-making infrastructure. Strong executive leadership requires that a strategic focus and a well-planned process related to contingent and disruptive conditions be incorporated into the normative planning activities of the organization (Jeffs et al., 2019). Senior leadership's commitment, skill, investment, and ability to organize and plan systematically around the potential for crisis are strong indicators of effectiveness in the face of constant change.

Second, there must be organizational commitment both in the design of the infrastructure of the organization related to its work and in the processes associated with undertaking work. Change never occurs when expected. Although predictive processes in the organization can look for the signals and triggers that indicate imminent change, these shifts often cannot be anticipated at a particular or given time in the organization's history. However, through the incorporation of a broad-based organizational construct for crisis, change, and contingency and an organized response to the possibility of a change event, the potential for crisis can be incorporated into the ongoing expectations of all in the workplace. In this way, successful organizations can demonstrate clear and specific goals for all the issues at every level of the organization that are affected by the potential change event.

> **Key Point**
>
> Adaptive capacity is the ability to identify the key responses necessary to thrive in a change situation and to build new and related responses.

Third, there is a need to understand elements of the change process and a coherent organized response to the dynamics of change. Change is neither difficult to understand nor difficult to incorporate into the operating realities of an organization. Addiction to historical rituals and routines, often present in clinical environments, can impede or block adaptation to change. Leaders must articulate the vagaries and characteristics of change, incorporate that understanding into the work processes of all workers, and show by their own behaviors a willingness to adapt and change to the new realities brought on by critical events (Chaffin & Gunderson, 2016). In addition, the communication system in the organization must adapt and adjust to the various emerging demands that arise at any given moment. Communications systems require a multifocal, multichannel approach to information generation and the management of communication around specific change events. The communication of particular signals indicates an impending shift in the way of doing business and links those signals to the trigger events initiating the organizational action stage. This operates in response to the external and internal signals that anticipate a need for a change in a way of doing business. Also, the communication channels must not impede patient service and clinical activities in a way that interrupts the viability and effectiveness of the services. Although change may occur in a number of different forms, from payment changes to environmental and contextual changes, and even clinical and technological changes, the patient experience should never be threatened or undermined as the organization responds to the demand for change.

The many challenges of healthcare reform create both context and content to which most of the tool sets identified in this chapter are applicable. Significant whole-systems reconceptualization, redesign, and recalibration are the fundamental work of change agents across the healthcare system. Moving from a volume-driven to a value-based approach to delivering service and paying for it calls for fundamentally rethinking at the environmental, systems, tactical, operational, and point-of-service arenas of increasingly complex health systems. As health service and system regional mergers and integration accelerate along the current trajectory to improved accountable care and broad-based population service models, the structural and contextual framework identified in this chapter is increasingly relevant and critical to ensuring that full-scale system-wide approaches are well led and sustainable. Failing to adequately and thoroughly address the demands of each stage of change, component of response, and network action limits the development of an adequately supporting infrastructure and the sustainable processes that advance health system viability and success.

Of course, it would be inadequate not to also include brief discussion on the unplanned and serendipitous events related to terrorism and the expression of human evil. While the focus in this text is not related to the exploration of such forces, increasingly healthcare systems must accommodate in their operational construction the occurrence of disasters related to human-caused social, political, and personal crises. Increasingly, these scenarios are rising at points across the globe in response to the social, religious, cultural, ethnic, and racial conflicts emerging out of issues of increased globalization and related population and personal disasters. However, the discipline of crisis management and the ability to respond appropriately still holds true in these scenarios as in any other arena of crises. The studied, cautious, informed, and disciplined format for incorporating crisis management into the normative aspects of operating health systems is just as relevant in these arenas of crisis as in any other. Leaders are advised that the mechanisms addressed in this chapter apply to crisis regardless of its origin or nature. The issue for leaders is their capacity and their willingness to create a framework and format for operationalizing the discipline of crisis response in a way that demonstrates an understanding of its elements and create a detailed analysis of appropriate responses in the careful implementation of plans that were developed in response to the need for good crisis management (Corrigan et al., 2016).

The Human Resources Focus

Good human resources management systems are critical to the organization's ability to adjust and adapt personal behaviors and work processes to critical change events. Human resources focuses on the value and processes associated with normative change. These responses should be included in the ongoing education and development of all workers. This means incorporating the understanding of change elements and the management of change into every level of educational development within the organization. Clinical education, as well as organizational and management leadership education, should incorporate the elements, characteristics, and stages of crisis. Increasingly of concern is the alignment between clinical resource demand and the disposition of adequate human resources that meets the numbers, kind, and quality necessary for specific population and service demands in the emerging accountable care environment. The complex relationship between these factors must be considered if related problems are to be appropriately resolved. For example, addressing the need for better-educated nurses prepared in advanced practice for the growing primary care infrastructure of health reform is impossible without addressing the aging and diminishing numbers of competent faculty necessary to prepare them.

Effective human resources models should include cybernetics and change management as fundamental parts of the role expectations of leaders and the professional staff. Many organizations suffer in the face of inevitable change because their human resources have not been educated in the processes and activities of complexity and change management and the impact of inevitable change on clinical and service processes and response. In an era of service innovation, evidence-based practice, and accountable care, it becomes even more important to incorporate adaptive skills into the professional skill set of every clinical leader in the organization.

Group Discussion

Identify a particularly rancorous change process in your organization (health reform provides many such opportunities) or one that was psychologically stressful (change processes associated with the COVID-19 pandemic). Discuss and then list the particular elements that made this specific change event difficult. Also include in your discussion the personal and emotional reactions that occurred in the center of the change event. What were the particular elements of this change that created problems? What were people's attitudes toward the need for this change? How were people prepared and incorporated in determining the need for this change? How was engagement of the stakeholders in this change incorporated into determining how best to respond to it? How would you do it differently, if it were to be done correctly?

A crisis critical-planning process should be incorporated into the operating activities of the leadership of the organization. All healthcare facilities have disaster plans and plans for specific critical events. These focus on the occurrence of particular crises that are environment or disaster related. Disaster, however, no longer is the only driver of crisis. Broad-based immediate social, political, and economic shifts create their own level of crisis, shortening response time and intensifying the degree of risk related to effective immediate, incremental, and sustainable responses.

Response planning should also encompass those normative strategic and alignment changes that affect the ability of an organization to continue its work. Because of the growing digital infrastructure and its ability to compress data, time, and response, traditional Industrial Age response mechanisms are no longer sufficient. Often, the introduction of a new technology or new regulations regarding payment policy or patient safety can create as much impact as a critical environmental event or community disaster. Recognizing that ongoing operational and planning activities should relate as much to normative change as to exceptional change is a vital leadership capacity for the 21st century. Incorporating these elements of the organization's critical-planning processes and the activities associated with adapting to environmental and contextual changes ensures that the organization remains constantly vigilant as it reviews signals and trigger events that may lead to a change in the conditions and circumstances within which clinical practitioners work. Leaders must always be aware of the need for and the processes associated with deliberation of the critical action steps to organizational, contextual, and strategic shifts affecting the viability of the organization. These effects are as significant to the organization's success as any environmental or disaster-related critical event.

Adaptive Capacity in Human Organizations

Traditionally, organizational activity and learning have been considered continuous and dynamic processes that reflect inclusion of the organization's adjustments and adaptations to internal and external individual and collective contingencies that affect individuals' ability to learn and adapt. Resulting from this process are practices and routines that reflect the normal life and activity of the organization in response to strategic, market, and process demands. Each individual, when joined with the collective effort, contributes to these organizational values and routines in a way that reflects consistent and viable performance, reliability, and the achievement of expectations and outcomes. In this way, the organization maintains a continuum of rituals and routines that, when uninterrupted, comprises the usual and ordinary processes of work and contributes to achieving desirable outcomes.

At the same time, people and organizations live in a larger context. The dynamics of internal and external vagaries and variability have a direct impact on the life and activities of individuals and organizations. The influence of these random factors frequently creates a level of organizational and individual uncertainty and ensures an embedded ambiguity. This condition, called noise, creates a level of personal and organizational interference with the continuum of normative work and the sustenance of the rituals and routines associated with it. The organization's availability and adaptability to these vagaries give form to its

> **Point to Ponder**
>
> Organizations are dynamic living organisms. They operate less like a machine and more like an organism. Leaders must now see them as ever-changing dynamics with no permanent form.

general adaptive capacity. The ability of an organization to accommodate these uncontrolled factors, making adjustments in work processes and individual behavior, reflects the level of flexibility and fluidity built into the organization's work processes that ensure its continuance.

Still, uncontrollable variances create instability in the mind of workers and the processes of the workplace. Often, learning processes and programs in most workplaces employ process learning and apply it in a way that assumes a normative continuum of activities and stable, uninterrupted work processes. Rarely are the influence and force of constant, uninterrupted change embedded in the processes of organizational and individual learning. In many ways, it is assumed that these interruptive patterns of behavior are nonnormative and exceptional, and are therefore not to be included in the usual processes of learning. Yet every worker is reminded that "change is constant" and that they must be willing to accommodate it. What often fails to be communicated is the notion that "change is the norm" and that stability, ritual, routine, and process activities are, themselves, nonnormative. Contemporary and adaptive organizations recognize this reality and must now begin to incorporate into their operating framework the continuous and unrelenting demands of external and internal adaptation.

Organizational learning theory was based on a mechanistic notion of organizational life. Contemporary organizational learning approaches shift away from that foundation and now reflect the belief that organizations are not so much like machines but more like organisms. This biodynamic approach indicates that organizations and individuals can learn and adapt to external change and stressors through behaviorally oriented cognitive and adaptive processes. Adaptive approaches in human organizations enable the organization to adapt through learning processes that incorporate those realities.

> **Point to Ponder**
>
> Leaders frame adaptation by looking carefully for the intersections and interaction between seemingly unrelated systems and processes and dynamically managing these connections.

Chaos, Complexity, and Crisis

Contemporary chaos and complexity theory characterizes complex human systems and organizations as spontaneous and self-organizing (Chandler et al., 2016). This approach recognizes behavior as nonlinear, understanding that small changes and shifts in behavior can have significantly large implications. Complexity theory goes beyond simply defining the impact of randomness and universal disorder. Furthermore, the theory recognizes that order can be found deeply within the seemingly random complexities. In addition, chaos theory reflects the constant contest between stability and chaos where the activities of creativity unfold. Chaos approaches attempt to understand the impact of change on systems; complexity theory attempts to understand how organizations and environments adapt to changing circumstances over time (Tsai et al., 2017).

> **Point to Ponder**
>
> The potential for crisis is constantly present. Understanding this concept of potential is critical to the exercise of good leadership. The wise leader is always living in this potential.

The interaction between seemingly unrelated systems and processes creates the frame for adaptation. The notion of emergent order is consistent with adaptation. In complexity theory, emergence suggests that a fundamental and inherent order exists within an apparent disorderly and chaotic condition. Adaptation contains within it a certain amount of spontaneity and self-order that results from awareness of the connections and intersections to which the organization reacts or responds. Imbedded in the adaptation process are all the necessary elements: goodness-of-fit, feedback loops, and organizationally responsive strategies.

This borderland on the edge of chaos at the intersections between systems represents the conflict between stability and chaos. It is here that innovation, adaptation, creativity, and flexibility all thrive. In essence, these elements create a dance of interaction, the confluence of which results in the conditions, circumstances, and forces that require human and organizational response and adaptation. In this place creativity and learning, adjustment and adaptation, flexibility and fluidity combine to encourage new patterns of behavior, action, and organizational response. However, this set of circumstances also creates the conditions for crisis.

Crises are embedded in the juncture between contemporary and normative organizational activities and occur at the critical moment when the external and internal forces converge to force a change in the organization's circumstances (Montgomery et al., 2017). Often, crisis is not easily anticipated, but it can always be expected. For the leader, anticipating crisis is a state of mind; responding to its inevitability is an organizational construct. The potential for crisis is consistently present regardless of the stability apparent within any current state. By understanding this potential, leaders can see that through the constant movement across time, the opportunity for the impact of change is ever-present. One of the most significant leadership skills is the leader's ability to recognize the constant potential of crisis and identify the signs of convergence of factors and forces leading to a paradigm shift for the organization and its people.

Strategic Crisis Management

The key to thriving in the context of crisis conditions is a strategic ability to anticipate, identify, and respond. Organizational leadership should focus on developing the resources, both financial and human, that create a frame of reference to ensure that the organization adapts to crisis and does not simply react to it. Because there will always be unanticipated surprises that can negatively affect the organization, the more strategic tools, supporting infrastructure, and planned approaches available to the leader, the better likelihood of sound response and recovery. Whenever models exist, they must be dynamic and represent the organization's continuous effort to anticipate and identify those internal and external factors affecting the work of the organization. This process must be inculcated into the operating structure of the organization and become a part of the life and work expectations at every level of the organization. The ability to read signals and to anticipate challenge can be generated at any place in the organization where the indicators and signs of impending impact can be diagnosed. From the front lines to the executive office, points of intersection within the system, between systems, or with externally generated variables can be anticipated and responded to regardless of position or role.

Leadership must enroll practicing professionals and managers by structuring and framing work activities so that workers can quickly assess and respond to crisis influence and impact. Furthermore, the cybernetic process, which is any action in a system that generates a change in its larger environment and cycles back to further "trigger" a system's change of whatever dynamic mechanism is built, must make it possible—indeed desirable—for workers at all levels of the organization to own the obligation of identifying and responding to shifting realities that affect their ability to address the purposes of the organization and undertake their own work. A systematic and organized response to building the infrastructure that makes such fluidity and flexibility the frame for doing business and undertaking action is a critical variable that results in either negative impact or positive response.

The model for addressing critical variants needs to contain several elements. First, it must address team activities and relationships in the course of doing business and the activities of the organization in everyday rituals and routines. Every member in the organization must be aware of his or her connection to the strategy, mission, and purposes of the organization and how individual and collective work contribute. All the work elements of the model must tie the individual and collective action of the work team to fulfilling the goals of the organization. The work must also meet the needs of the various constituencies and customers, ultimately resulting in advancing the health of individuals and the community. In contemporary, value-driven care, evidence of the impact of such a model is witnessed in the seamlessness of service connections, supply chain supports, the clinical continuum, and the continuous highest level of healthy functioning of patients, populations, and communities.

Second, the model must assist the organization and its players, and every point in the system, in anticipating and predicting the impact of external and internal forces and how their convergence affects the work of the organization. Local and global influences affect the organization's viability and responsiveness to changes in its contextual circumstances. Influences often can be identified at the clinical sites as changes in practice, technology, therapeutics, or clinical evidence. Identification of the signals, such as health reform legislation and policy formation that indicate a convergence of forces and triggers of change that will impact the organization, should occur wherever they can be first anticipated. There is a need to inculcate the value at every level of the organization of the role of all players in sharing the identification, prediction, and adaptation of the organization to realities that affect its continuing viability.

Third, crisis planning must not simply be isolated to particular dramatic and critical events, as often associated with disaster planning. The model should encompass the inherent but less clearly visible crises embedded in contextual and external social, political, and economic changes, which are not so easy to respond to because of the organization's focus on current-stage work. Crisis planning should include the construction of an organizational frame within which predictive and anticipatory transformations and changes can be incorporated in the ordinary course of doing business. Developing these planning components for the normative trajectory of transformative crisis helps to normalize the notion of critical change and inculcates into the lives and activities of workers in every part of the organization the processes associated with predictive and adaptive capacity.

Group Discussion

An organized and systematic response is necessary to building a good infrastructure that supports constant change. Particular elements of this infrastructure are necessary for it to be effective, such as addressing team activities and relationships. What are some of the other elements that are necessary in creating an effective adaptive model (think of the necessary adjustments and changes embedded in responding to the demands of health reform)? What would you do to incorporate this model into your way of doing work? How would it affect the expression of leadership? And what would be the role of workers in making the model work effectively?

Dynamic Cybernetic Team Model (DCTM)

Teams are the fundamental unit of work in the contemporary workplace. If an organization is to fully engage the full range of activities to respond to both process and critical events and seek to be successful, it will do it through teams. Therefore, any model that focuses on predictive and adaptive organizational response to external and internal variances requires full engagement of teams. As previously identified, the ability to isolate environmental signals and triggers that indicate organizational impact may occur anywhere in the organization. Effective and adaptive organizations access insight and response from wherever in the system the indicators of change or crisis first appear.

Most important to the organization is the formalization and construction of rational and sequential approaches to team action (**Figure 7-1**). These responses should be tied to such action and to the purpose, mission, and goals of organization. This operationalizes the work of teams, such that team processes are strongly linked with all the major system characteristics and processes that can make the team ready and available to do its part in anticipating, predicting, and responding to critical indicators.

A DCTM is an evidence-building, organized systematic cybernetic feedback crisis response that uses an interdisciplinary approach and emphasizes cognitive processes that engage teams to act in a reflexive, integrated, competent, broad-based, cross-system manner to appropriately and meaningfully respond to crisis and change. Not only are team outcomes achieved, team competence is continuously impacted because knowledge gained is continually incorporated into the framework of team work/process quality and outcomes performance (Porter-O'Grady et al., 2006). The DCTM promotes team communication and decision making in dynamic, complex, or uncertain situations by controlling and reducing the element of uncertainty as much as possible and keeping a focus on team dynamics (participants) and on the change vision (leaders).

Figure 7-1 Dynamic Cybernetic Team Adaptation Model.

The team's participation in engaging the challenges to organizations cannot occur effectively unless a frame or discipline is available to give form to the team's work. This framework must be structured enough to provide direction and context, yet fluid enough to respond nimbly to whatever vagaries and variances might confront the organization. Critical to this format is evidence of synthesis of the various flow components of the team's action and the systems framework that gives form to the team's work. The DCTM is discussed in the following sections.

Macro Considerations for Organizational Crisis

Although crises can and do occur within organizations, most crises are caused by external conditions or circumstances outside the unilateral control of an organization. As COVID-19 clearly reminded humanity, crises can and will arise at any moment and have an unlimited potential for challenge and harm. In complex adaptive systems, leaders recognize the potential reality of external conditions and the inherent connection between and among all elements affecting the life and activity of a human organization and its relationship to its external environment. Effective leaders are always scanning the influencing forces and dynamics of the external environment as a part of predictive work in an effort to both anticipate and adapt to this existential reality.

A number of convergences must occur in order to ensure appropriate responses to an unanticipated crisis. Preparedness for crisis within systems is always a reflection of the fundamental awareness that, by definition, the actual occurrence of a crisis is consistently a surprise to those who experience it. Crisis preparedness includes a clear measurement of risk and the establishment of a priority plan for the highest crisis risks to the system. There is always variability in risk readiness. The degree of readiness is dependent on the level of crisis priority and concomitant risk status.

Five key external influencers affect readiness and response to risk for the healthcare organization: command structure, supply chain, local support systems, clinical engagement, and infrastructure. Leaders must be aware of the status of each influencer and the degree of accommodation that must be made to adapt to their influence and impact on system response (**Figure 7-2**). As with all complex adaptive systems and the complex responsive processes associated with them, leaders need to be available to compensate for inadequacies in any one or more of the five influencers. In addition, leaders must be able to segue to other actions and resources when there is brokenness in any one of the influencers or within or between several of them. One of the key characteristics of adaptation is innovation and creativity to the immediate circumstances or given situation while plans are being formulated to address longer-term adaptations or correct deficiencies.

Command Structure

Every organization has the duty and obligation during a crisis to have the right accountability/decision models and structures at every stage of the command structure in the society and the system. The integrity of command operations along the public and private chain of command depends on the participation of all parties in the construction, regular testing, and periodic adjustments of command structures. Problems or flaws that emerge in the response to crises can often be identified and addressed through testing of command structures and through mock decision/action authority related to any element of the chain of the external and internal models and structures. Brokenness or ineffectiveness in command locus of control for decisions and actions will always have a deleterious effect on every one of the influencers in any crisis.

Figure 7-2 Key External Influencers That Affect Readiness and Response to Risk.

Supply Chain

The ability to access needed resources in a timely fashion is critical to the effectiveness of response. Of course, supply chain configuration and utility is dependent upon the nature of the crisis and the facility for response. The capacity of the supply chain and its efficacy is dependent on the nature of the crisis (e.g., a flood requires a different set of specifics than a pandemic). Issues should be included in the macro and micro planning for priority crises along every critical stage in the supply chain. Also, leaders need to be keyed into unique and creative supply sources that can provide innovative opportunities to meet immediate demand. There is nothing more frustrating and devastating to those on the front lines of a crisis than not having sufficient amounts of the right tools to respond to the demands that emerge at key stages of crisis management.

Local Support Systems

In every aspect of a crisis, leaders will have limited success if they attempt to address it alone. Within complex adaptive principles, a key tenet is that all parts of any human system will ultimately be impacted by what happens to any one member in the system. The common statement that "we're all in it together" is not so far-fetched from the principle to which it alludes. In fact, behaving in a unilateral way to one's specific advantage will, at some point, negatively impact all responses, including that of the unilateral respondent. The network of connections in the human community call for a confluence of effort on the part of all in a way that negotiates the intersections and ensures the convergence of community effort to address and remediate the crisis for one and for all. Relationships and interactions are affected by crisis, including that of the community, and relationship dynamics will instruct the crisis plan with which the appropriate players have been engaged. And, as with the command structure, local support systems need to be regularly tested and updated as realities and resources change.

Clinical Engagement

In every healthcare network, key personnel at every point-of-service are the service providers who do the work of the enterprise. Critical key personnel in health care are nurses, doctors, and other clinical service providers that make up the service team impacting the delivery of health care. In any effective complex adaptive system, key personnel must be included in the planning, design, and engagement of service accommodation and adaptation for any crisis. Furthermore, key stakeholder leaders will be involved in any command structure and in the decision/action continuum related to operations, supply, clinical partnerships, and clinical policy and practices within the system.

Infrastructure

We have come to learn in the past decade that formative structure is either an enabler of positive behavior or a barrier to it. Structure directly informs human behavior. With this in mind, the conscious effort of leaders should be to eliminate as many barriers as possible to healthy and effective organizational behavior. The effective medium of the clinical work environment of health care should reflect the essential and key values of the health of the community and the individuals who make it up. Again, in complex adaptive systems, leaders should consider the principle that in a network (system) there should be only as much structure as necessary to support its function. Excess structure becomes an impediment to the efficiency and efficacy of the system and those who work within it. Leaders need to carefully assess and review the infrastructure of the workplace with an eye to addressing the potential or emergence of anything that is not directly related to "lean" effectiveness of the existing infrastructures that directly supports the work of the system. If this critical work is not done, any crisis will be burdened with unnecessary layers of human and systems structures that will demand resources and servicing that draw strength of effort away from the pressures of the moment.

Synthesizing External and Internal Factors

Creating a predictive awareness of the potential of critical events to affect the work of the team requires the team to maintain a broad focus on issues that influence its actions. One of the most significant problems with clinical teams is their disciplinary isolation, hyper focus on the issues of the day, and lack of awareness of the influences and circumstances affecting team viability occurring outside the immediate locus of the team's action. Environmental and contextual changes in health policy, finances, market, clinical and service characteristics, technology, social structure, priorities, and organizational goals all have a direct impact on the viability and vitality of the team's work.

> **Point to Ponder**
>
> The team is the centerpiece of all work. It is important that the team be involved in the change process from first identification of the need for change to final implementation of the processes of change.

However, team member efforts often are diluted by the team's focus on function and action. There is a belief that the quality of a team's activity is sufficient to ensure its effectiveness, when, instead, external realities have a greater impact on the team's viability than its own actions do.

From a broad view, it is frightening to note how often teams are surprised by shifts in the prevailing reality that affect their ability to succeed in their work. Most teams have a complete lack of awareness of contextual, business, social, and relational changes that affect their work. Even more concerning is leaders' lack of insight regarding how important this level of contextual awareness is to successful action and interaction of team members with the system and with those they serve. Whatever model is created to systematically address team operation and its predictive and adaptive capacity to anticipate and respond to crisis, it must be formalized and become a fundamental part of the discipline in the expression of the role of the leader. This model must be fluid enough to alter priority and practices, yet sufficiently structured to ensure the necessary continuum of actions that attempt to focus the work on reaching goals and achieving outcomes.

Strategic Core

Any systematic activity associated with the team's work must reflect how closely aligned the activity is with the strategic priorities of the organization. In this arena most healthcare organizations reflect the greatest dissonance. Clinical teams often see their focus unilaterally as how well they serve particular patient needs. What they often do not recognize is a broader strategic obligation to which they must contribute. This broader obligation operates at a level of complexity that requires teams at every level of the organization to frame their activities within the context of contribution to the strategic, financial, operational, and service goals of the organization. Simply providing adequate work performance to meet individual patient needs may actually be an impediment to advancing the strategic priorities of the health organization. Failing to make a difference in the health of the community, lack of evidence of the relationship between clinical activity and positive patient outcomes, and a level of resource use intensity that outstrips the financial viability of the organization are examples of how the team's unilateral focus on patient-related activities and functions actually limits or impedes its ability to adequately address the strategic imperative to create a healthy community.

Leaders can demonstrate focus on critical factors by encouraging team members to align patient-related activities with strategic priorities in the conscious application of team thinking and team members' work. Continuous awareness of the alignment of purpose, mission, and professionals' motivation and competence enables leaders and staff to focus on the constant need for goodness-of-fit between the organization's strategic core and the functional priorities and actions of its clinical providers. Partnership between each team member's personal effort as aggregated in the team's work and the strategic priorities of the organization represents the continuous, seamless thread of collective commitment to ensuring the organization's vitality.

A part of the flexibility of strategic direction is the fluidity and adaptability of that strategy when external and internal (externalization/internalization) forces and factors create a need to reconceptualize and reconfigure direction and goals. The tremendous external obligation to create more strongly aligned models of accountable care and the partnerships that sustain it is just one such example. Once a strategy has been redefined to reflect the changing parameters influencing the team's work, the leader must inform the team and inculcate the new factors on the template of the team's mental model and work processes to incorporate changing expectations into team action (socialization/internalization/combination) (**Figure 7-3**). Addressing adaptive processes is a critical component of the leader's role. Leaders at all levels of the organization are required to contribute to the fluidity and flexibility of the organization's strategy in responding to the continuously changing circumstances that affect the system priorities and the team's work (McHugh et al., 2020).

> **Key Point**
> Once a strategy has been redefined, the leader must always inform the team and engage it with regard to how the change will affect the way the team does its work.

Socialization externalization
Team core:
Purpose/mission
Meaning/motivation
Commitment/competence
Work = learning
Internalization combination

Figure 7-3 Strategy Core.

Team Performance

Essential to a team's capacity to respond to change and critical events is its basic internal, structural, social, and relational integrity. For a team to function well, it must be clear about the goodness-of-fit among team members in terms of relationship, competence, and work capacity. The degree of integration, efficacy of interaction, and intersection among team members is critical to smooth and effective functioning of the team. Leaders who do not spend sufficient time constructing effective teams pay a price for this failure at the time of a team's encounter with crisis or conflict.

Teams are themselves small systems, reflecting the same level of complexity as other levels of systemness do. Effectiveness with regard to work styles, communication, and clinical skills and an individual's ability to think critically, express competently, work well with others, accommodate differences, and approach work activities with a high level of flexibility are all requisites for successful team membership (**Figure 7-4**). By failing to balance the essential elements when creating team membership, leaders are challenged when the team members attempt to work together. Although each member of the team can develop each of the team performance capacities, these skill sets must be present at the outset if effective team synthesis is to be ensured.

To ensure long-term team effectiveness, it is important for leaders to ensure a good level of synthesis between and among team members. Leaders must establish corollaries with regard to basic clinical competence, conceptual skills, social skills, personal attributes, and the balance of skills between and among team members because these are priorities that influence team effectiveness. Wise leaders create competency grids related to the clinical, social, personal, and collective parameters necessary to create a frame for defining an effective team within the specific clinical and service characteristics of the department. This "setting the table" for subsequent team interaction and action is perhaps one of the most critical elements of effective team construction.

Once the individual characteristics of team members are combined to create a team's "personality," it is important for leaders to focus on making clear the performance and work expectations that define the functional elements of the team's activities. Here, leaders establish the link between performance and strategy such that the work efforts of team members are tightly aligned with the purpose and goals of the organization as represented in the focus and activities of the specific clinical service. Leaders begin to match the characteristics of the team with

Team performance:
- Member roles
- Empowered members
- Individual competence
- Team skills
- Accommodating variance
- Work effort
- Outcomes focused

Figure 7-4 Team Performance.

performance expectations and activities represented in the team's work. In an evidence-based approach to structuring team effectiveness, leaders make sure that team members are aware of expectations, goals, and the specific outcomes to which good performance must ultimately lead.

Once the basic elements of team construction have been configured appropriately, leaders must determine the team's adaptability to changing circumstances and address how vagaries embedded in their work life can be addressed appropriately through team action. Although it is important for teams to work effectively and undertake their day-to-day routines with care and consideration, the forces of change are always working inexorably on the periphery of organizational life. Forces of change operate sometimes directly and other times discursively to create a shift in conditions and circumstances that affect the viability and sustenance of work. Sometimes forces of change can be predicted and anticipated, but often they cannot.

However clearly change can be anticipated, group adaptation and adjustments to the realities and impact of a given change must be part of the work construct of the team. Here, leaders must ensure that team members receive appropriate education and development in their role of identifying and adapting to change events, to facilitate team effectiveness. To ensure that the team responds appropriately to critical events, leaders must help team members understand that events are normative, and that when they appear they will directly affect the ability of the team to undertake its work processes. Ultimately, the team must demonstrate its ability to incorporate the demand for adaptation and change into team routines and rituals and, indeed, approach these changes as a normatively interruptive reality.

This critical and adaptive capacity must be present in all levels of team effort in the organization. From the board and executive team focusing on strategy and goal development throughout the organization to include administrative and financial support teams, organizational and clinical support, and clinical services, each makes a contribution to synthesizing and incorporating the demand for change into the collective and individual work processes that result in sustainable outcomes and the ability of the organization to thrive.

Team Outcomes

Teams have no purpose or meaning if purpose and meaning are not driving their work. Contemporary focus on outcomes ties the notion of strategic imperative and work process to the achievement of goals and sustaining work outcomes (**Figure 7-5**). A focus on outcome requires the team to have clearly delineated deliverables against which its performance can be measured. However, all too often in the clinical environment the clinical team's work becomes an end in itself such that

Outcomes:
- Precise
- Timely
- Quality based
- Excellent
- Satisfied customer

Figure 7-5 Team Outcomes.

the process becomes the outcome where clearly articulated deliverables are never really expressed. In an evidence-driven and value-grounded world, a process-as-an-outcome circumstance is not acceptable. As digitization of clinical practice and communication, accountable care, and value-based health practices increasingly become the norm, the expectation for the team is that some evidence of impact, of a difference being made, must be incorporated into the performance expectations of team members, just as it is the expectation of the organization.

> **Key Point**
> A leader must always make the team aware of the realities affecting advanced planning, which demonstrates commitment to the normative construct and dynamic of change. In this case, adaption is even more important than anticipation.

Value-based practice requires that the team's work activity is viewed from the perspective of the difference it makes, the impact it has, and the health it produces rather than simply from the view of the quality of the work processes. Teams might work well and with a high degree of commitment and precision and still not make a difference or achieve specific health objectives. This has been the Achilles' heel of most clinical teams in the past. Incremental and unilateral patient impact has historically remained unconnected or unlinked to other similar patient efforts such that an aggregate body of knowledge regarding specific and definitive clinical activities related to defined clinical outcomes has yet to be achieved. The potential for clinical standardization has created the fear that somehow a "cookbook" approach to clinical practice might emerge, robbing practices of responsiveness and spontaneity and creating a clinical format that may be disconnected and unfeeling. The fear of standardization has kept clinical professions from developing a broad-based standard of clinical performance that can be effectively compared and contrasted and out of which would emerge clear notions of what worked best and what did not (value-driven, evidence-based practice). Now, with the ability to aggregate information across a broad frame, creation of foundations for practice is real and increases demand on the clinical team to align its work with a broader body of knowledge.

Standardization can now be seen as simply a mechanism for establishing the "floor" of practice, the norms of clinical decision making and action understood by every practitioner and forming the platform upon which any improvement or advancement occurs. Value-based efforts at finding points of excellence at the "ceiling" of practice demand increasing levels of clinical and service customization made possible by increasingly sophisticated levels of digital utility and applicability. In this dynamic, neither standardization nor customization remains a static notion. When they are continuously informed by increasingly discrete and sophisticated data, clinical practices simply reflect appropriate and timely reactions. On this dynamic trajectory, practice changes are the normative response to evidence that both informs and provides the impetus for continuous practice change.

User Expectations

Use of digital tools allows teams to be more objective and definitive with regard to clinical action. Teams can measure performance against national, regional, or local aggregated databases to determine effectiveness and efficacy. As part of evaluating and delineating the most effective clinical processes likely to achieve defined expectations and outcomes, teams must adapt strategies that integrate their unilateral action with the action of other similar teams. In generic terminology, outcome value must also include customer (patient) satisfaction, but only if that satisfaction is based on clearly enumerated, legitimate user (patient) expectations. Team members must ensure that providers and patients (users) have a clearly understood set of expectations with regard to what is legitimate to achieve under the circumstances.

In achieving sustainable outcomes, one of the performance expectations of team members is reeducation of the user, shifting expectations and roles as the parameters and conditions of service change in response to new technologies, therapeutics, and interventions. The constant enhancement of clinical activities over increasingly shorter periods of time requires that user reeducation be a constant activity of the clinical team in relationship to those they serve. Also, outcome expectation includes more clearly defining the performance roles of users (consumers or patients) in managing that part of the clinical journey for which they are primarily accountable. As healing increasingly occurs in settings other than the clinical institution, user accountability in undertaking activities and roles related to the individual's healing process is now a fundamental work expectation of the clinical team. Indeed, this is one of the centerpieces of value-driven health reform.

Notions of excellence and value with regard to outcomes must also include how clearly specific clinical and performance outcomes have fulfilled the overall strategic purpose and goals of the organization. The clinical team must always maintain a two-pronged focus on outcomes. First, it must meet the individual clinical needs of the population it serves as those are defined from the perspective of the user (patient/consumer). Second, the overall organizational goals, which include community impact, overall health status, reduction in process risks, and any other specific clinical performance goals, must also be included in the performance expectations of team members. Making the connection between individual consumer impact and aggregated organizational effectiveness becomes the frame for delineating outcome value at the point-of-service and within the context of the work of all teams, regardless of where they are located in the system.

Here again, crisis and critical events are constantly lurking at the boundaries of the organization's intersection with the larger community and the team's intersection with the organization and consumers (patients). Inherent in all team action is the team's continuing awareness of and preparedness for environmental, financial, technological, social, and market changes that dynamically intersect with current operations and occasionally converge to create a demand for change in strategy, operations, and clinical practice. At best, in the course of doing business, teams can adjust to predicted and anticipated changes with sufficient time and resources. However, just as likely, other critical events, disasters, and unanticipated and unplanned events will require teams to change

> **Point to Ponder**
>
> Excellence in performance is no longer optional. Therefore, teams must focus on value and outcomes, not just processes. What the patient receives—not just what the provider gives—is important. For providers, there must be strong goodness-of-fit between process and outcome to achieve and sustain value.

behaviors and practices immediately, demonstrating their inherent flexibility and fluidity as well as the applicability of their crisis planning model.

The Partnership Team Process Factors

The best methodology available for confronting crisis events is an infrastructure that builds on the normality of good process. Building a good process infrastructure creates a frame for response to any particular work activities and, further, provides a construct within which critical events can be addressed through good form, format, and structure.

Process factors break down the framework for work activities into a series of steps that relate specifically to the work itself and the staged activities that represent particular points of reference in relationship to the work (**Figure 7-6**). In addition, process factors tie each stage of the work process to the goals and purposes that give direction and meaning to individual work. Process factors structure the work activities so that they best relate to the goals and objectives to which those work activities are directed. In the midst of a crisis or critical event, dependence on the stability that comes from process factors provides a solid frame of reference. What often happens in the midst of critical process is the loss of the routine and ritual embedded in process factors. Through this loss, organizations become chaotic and directionless and fail to incorporate the critical process into a ritualized series of activities that can ensure all issues affected by the crisis are addressed appropriately.

Process factors can be broken down into five types: goals, competence, resources, work demands, and results. There is a sixth factor that follows the successful flow of the five process factors, and that factor is the outcome, evaluation. This factor is separate from the other process factors because evaluation depends on their successful implementation and action related to them. The elements that identify and explicate outcomes are clearly enumerated in the first five process factors.

Process factor 3
Resources:
Support the work
Reward sufficient
Outcome appropriate

Process factor 2
Competence:
Work specific
Task appropriate
Skill mix/fit
Learning needs

Process factor 4
Work demands:
Sufficient time
Design/work processes
Outcome appropriate

Process factor 1
Goals:
Clear
Specific
Understood

Process factor 5
Results:
As defined (goals)
Customer driven
Quality values

Figure 7-6 Process Factors.

> **Process factor 1**
> Goals:
> Clear
> Specific
> Understood

Figure 7-7 Process Factor 1: Goals.

Process Factor 1: Goals

In moments of crisis or in the midst of critical events, organizations lose their bearing, their sense of directedness, and as a result become reactive and focused on the short term. They can be "eaten up" by the immediate issue or situation, often at the expense of other important factors. The purpose of goals is certainly clear during the normal processes of the organization in the absence of critical events (**Figure 7-7**). However, critical events do not change the need for goals; if anything, they advance them. An important and appropriate role of leadership during a critical event is refocusing the organization on its goals and purposes so that, in responding to the critical event, the organization does not wander away from its key purposes and directional priorities. Goals serve as a point of demarcation even in the most critical change event, such that when a change occurs, a clear delineation of the impact of the change can be better made when compared to the originating goal.

> **Point to Ponder**
>
> Competence is not simply what people know. Competence is what people do with what they know and how well that makes a difference for others.

Leaders help the organization in crisis by bringing leader and staff attention to the fundamental purposes and values of the organization as it confronts its crisis and attempts to continue to thrive. This notion of thriving is important in the midst of crisis. Often, during crises organizations move to survival mode. Although some of the immediate actions may focus on precise and definitive responses to the crisis, the organization should not forget its fundamental drive to achieve its goals and fulfill its purpose in a way that both acknowledges and accepts the impact of a change on originating goal content. Failing to do so maintains a crisis format for the organization and keeps it from returning to a focus that represents its core values and goal priorities.

Goal clarity and specificity are the two most important elements of goal setting. Goals must be defined in such a way that the purpose and mission of the organization are made transparent to all members and can be clearly articulated by individuals and workgroups whose activity ostensibly fulfills the purposes of the organization. The ability to clearly enumerate particular goals and priorities helps the organization keep focus on the purposes of work and the long-term values to which even critical responses must ultimately be directed. Furthermore, it keeps workers grounded and promulgates the particular values that relate to the organization thriving and the activities necessary to ensure that happens.

Process Factor 2: Competence

Ensuring competence at every level of the organization is never so important as during a critical period of events. Lapses in identifying and managing issues of competence become especially

> **Process factor 2**
> Competence:
> Work specific
> Task appropriate
> Skill mix/fit
> Learning needs

Figure 7-8 Process Factor 2: Competence.

risky when critical events intervene. At these times, the organization needs to depend on the ability and skills of those who do its work (**Figure 7-8**). If the critical competence factors necessary to ensure effective work processes are missing, the price that is paid during a critical event is additionally burdensome to the organization. Assurance that every level of work operates at a specific level of competence becomes very important in positioning organizations to address the inevitable noise and crises that come with unplanned occurrences. Individuals need to act independently and interdependently at a number of critical levels in the midst of a crisis event. This expectation that the organization can count on the skills and talents of its workforce is an important factor in the organization's preparedness and readiness for crisis events.

Competence includes not only the skills, abilities, and capacity of performing job assignments, but also workers' ability to take focused action. The focus is on individual competence as well as on team response. Teams are the basic unit of all work. The ability of teams to respond appropriately and with efficiency to crisis depends on team members' ability to act in concert with each other, in direct response to the crisis as it affects the team's work, and in relationship with other teams with specified roles in responding to the critical event. The notion of the centrality of teams to respond and act is especially critical in the development and refinement of models of accountable care where transdisciplinary partnerships, interactions, and relationships are central to obtaining high-level and sustainable clinical outcomes and advancing community health.

Competence in crisis also means the ability to adapt to additional challenges and activities necessary to ensure the organization's appropriate action in the face of crisis. Sometimes a crisis broadens role expectations beyond the usual and ordinary course of an individual's or a team's working over time. Critical events may change the mix of work expectations and demands, requiring workers to shift roles, performance, and expectations. Competence means the flexibility, fluidity, and adaptability necessary to meet the challenges and shifting demands that frequently arise in moments of crisis.

Incorporated in the notion of competence is the commitment of the organization, teams, and individuals to continuing education and development in preparation for or anticipation of inevitable crises or critical events. Continuing education and development of individuals and teams to respond to potential crises are important parts of the organization's development program. Although every kind of crisis cannot be anticipated, the demands of crisis are often generic and can be incorporated into the learning curriculum of employee development. Incorporating the elements of crisis, characteristics of crisis response, and individual and collective roles in reacting and adapting to crisis and addressing issues of flexibility and fluidity in the presence of crisis are all important learning elements that can advance the competence of leaders and teams in the face of inevitable critical events.

Process Factor 3: Resources

It is surprising how few organizations manage their fiscal distribution and operational budgets in a way that includes the anticipation of critical events and crisis situations. A certain amount of the organization's capital resources should be directed to addressing inevitable critical events. Often organizations that have failed to adequately create resource reserves find themselves in serious financial trouble too late in the crisis cycle to adequately respond and to return to thriving (**Figure 7-9**). In fact, this set of circumstances most often permanently cripples organizations in the face of crisis, ending in serious decline or corporate failure.

Appropriate resource allocation means that the organization has set aside sufficient financial, material, and human resources to respond immediately and effectively to crises that affect the normative operations of the organization. The ability of the organization to adapt specific job functions, roles, and fiscal commitments to address crisis plays a major part in ensuring the organization can quickly recover from critical events and move forward into normal operations. Taking additional time and resources to adjust the normal flow of business to respond to the crisis, if not carefully managed, can be a formula for failure. Quickly responding to critical events and creating a goodness-of-fit between the response and the demand of the event indicate a good allocation of appropriate resources and an ability to adapt the focus of the organization to the issues immediately affecting it. This ability to reallocate and shift the distribution of capital and resources creates the level of flexibility and fluidity necessary to respond appropriately to crisis. Furthermore, flexibility reflects the organization's understanding that the social milieu for all organized human activity in the current digital social reality is to remain continuously portable and mobile in every endeavor. All levels of the organization should consider their individual and collective ability to shift focus and resource capacity to adequately address critical events without endangering the long-term viability and service provision of the organization.

One can imagine the secondary crisis created in an organization where staffing and financial resources are already tightly configured. The introduction of critical events often places additional demand on existing work infrastructure, making it virtually impossible for resources to meet the demands of the crisis and the routine and usual expectations for work (Langan et al., 2017; Veenema et al., 2017). Not adequately accessing additional resources or adjusting the focus of existing resources in a timely fashion creates a double demand on staff, further burdening them with additional work, increasing levels of emotional stress, and decreasing their ability to focus and respond to immediate issues of concern. And yet it is common for just such secondary crisis events to occur in many organizations in the midst of crisis. The staff's inability to respond and the narrowly allocated resources with no financial

Process factor 3
Resources:
Support the work
Reward sufficient
Outcome appropriate

Figure 7-9 Process Factor 3: Resources.

flexibility create a serious constraint on the organization's ability to respond to crisis. This is a far more common set of circumstances than is often perceived. A critical leadership requisite is balancing long-term operational resource needs with the resources required for inevitable crisis occurrences.

Process Factor 4: Work Demands

The configuration of the elements of work and workload become important considerations in critical events. Most organizations operate as efficiently as they can, recognizing the need for appropriate productivity and maintaining a tight relationship between work demands and workload. Although this is certainly an appropriate measure of performance in organizations under normal conditions, planning must include flexibility related to specific work objectives when crisis arises (**Figure 7-10**).

The design of work must include options related to responding to critical events and changes in the normal course and routine of work. In clinical organizations, different levels of census create shifting demands and require flexible staffing and resource use plans. Insight into and need for staffing and resources during critical events are heightened. If a disaster or an unplanned event changes the normal routine, a different resource use plan that accelerates or shifts human resources allocation must be accessible. The crisis planning process team should develop such a plan. Staffing and scheduling programs routinely need to be addressed in light of shifting demand and accelerating changes that affect work distribution and workload. Incorporating flexibility and fluidity into the human resources staffing plan increases the likelihood that the organization can adapt to particular crisis events.

Consider some of the challenges associated with health reform. An emphasis on late-stage, bed-based services is shifting quickly to a focus on earlier engagement of services along the continuum of care and new service configurations that reduce the dependency on bed-related services. Those persons staffing bed-related services are therefore poorly positioned to thrive. Quickly shifting human resources to new care models and retraining them for different roles are critical to hospitals' ability to accommodate changing care and service requirements and practices.

Many organizations build contingency staffing plans based on changing customer demand or productivity and workload issues. Contingency plans help the

> **Point to Ponder**
>
> Almost all crises are unplanned for. Understanding that, leaders always make sure that there is a system for crises, an infrastructure that makes it possible to anticipate and respond to unplanned-for crises.

Process factor 4
Work demands:
Sufficient time
Design/work processes
Outcome appropriate

Figure 7-10 Process Factor 4: Work Demands.

organization respond to shifting work demands that include a different service mix or accelerated product or service demand cycle. Flexibility within plans also can serve an organization well in the midst of planned and unplanned events. Having variability in resource demand and staffing helps the organization adjust resources based on the nature of the crisis and the skills of and demands on the workers.

Continuing education and specific role development with regard to unplanned and critical events are important corollaries to the routine education and development of teams and workers. As in the process factor related to worker competence, it is important that the ability to act in a complex or crisis situation is also expected and incorporated into the role and routines of specific workers in the organization. Here again, many crises are unplanned, yet the nature of crisis often requires timely and effective response. The talent and ability to anticipate and respond in crisis can be likened to volunteer fire departments and voluntary medical emergency units: the focus is on skill development of individuals whose primary work activity is focused in another arena. Using this dynamic in corporate crisis response helps prepare key workers to play specific roles in unplanned or critical events and ensures a heightened level of preparedness of the organization.

Process Factor 5: Results/Impact

Results normally validate the achievements of goals to which the team and individual work has been directed. Clearly, the goodness-of-fit between the goals and the achieved results is an indicator of the level of success of the organization and its members. In critical situations, the notion of focus on results is as important as in the normative and routine operations of the organization. A significant difference between the two is that results orientation of normal work processes is long term and continuing, whereas the results orientation of critical events has a much shorter cycle of productivity and performance. Critical events lead to redefining and reconfiguring goals and results based on the immediate activities and actions that must be undertaken to return the organization to thrive status. Results in a critical situation must be defined early so that work processes can be focused specifically on achieving corrective short-term objectives in an efficient and effective manner (**Figure 7-11**).

Short-term goal orientation related to crises should still at some level be evaluated against the long-term operational goals of the organization. Critical intervention intends to return the organization to its normative level of operation. To create normalcy, leaders must continually assess critical goals directed at stabilizing and renewing the organization in the context of the longer-term functional goals that supply the drive and purpose to its work. Matching critical goals helps create a process that fits with the return to normalization necessary to stabilize the

Process factor 5
Results:
As defined (goals)
Customer driven
Quality values

Figure 7-11 Process Factor 5: Results Focus.

organization and ensure its long-term viability. Leaders at every level of the organization must be aware of this need to address both the normative long-term goals and the short-term and immediate goals necessary to normalize organization activities.

Impact on Outcomes

Focusing on the orientation to outcome during a critical event becomes important when considered from the perspective of the customer/user. Critical events have an impact on the will of the organization to serve its users and meet their needs. This orientation to user sensitivity is vital during crisis experiences. Users must be aware of the shift in emphasis, adjustment of resources, and impact on the service or product. The immediate inclusion of the user in consideration of crisis response helps reduce the impact of the crisis, the stress of responding to the crisis, and the negative impact on the user or plan needs. Often, when the focus of a crisis takes emphasis away from meeting the needs of the client or user and when the client or user can be incorporated into the dynamic of solutions seeking or problem solving, the stress and critical nature of the crisis can be significantly reduced. In addition, the client or user can participate in finding alternatives and changing his or her own demand in relationship to pressure on the organization during a critical time frame. Through partnership with the client or user, the organization in crisis can often better identify and address appropriate responses and solutions and return to long-term normative operations.

Certainly, these process factors play a significant role in an organization's response to crisis. The more committed the organization is to systematically and effectively organizing around its specific process factors, the better the tool set the organization has to respond to unplanned events and crises. The discipline with which a company or clinical organization follows its process plan is an important factor in determining that organization's ability to respond well to a crisis. Although, clearly, subsequent processes and dynamics need to be in place to ensure appropriate response to a crisis, the foundations laid by an appropriate team-based process action plan incorporated into the clinical and operating framework is valuable for successfully responding to critical events. In addition, because this is a cybernetic process the impact and value of process factors in a normative work environment are continuous, dynamic, and cyclical in nature. The adaptation of these factors to a critical environment indicates the same level of dynamic, only on a shorter and more heightened cycle. The ability of the leader to apply

Group Discussion

In hospitals and service organizations, crisis has a special impact on patients and people. In planning for and building infrastructure for managing crisis, how does the leader incorporate the patient or the public in responding appropriately to the crisis? What roles do the patient (the user) and significant others play in responding to a clinical or an organizational crisis (such as that indicated by implementation of the various elements of health reform)? Should they be involved in constructing plans for a systematic response to crisis? How are they involved? What processes of communication are necessary in the system to make sure patients (users) are aware and informed of their participation?

CHAPTER SEVEN   Leading Constant Movement: Transforming Chaos and Crisis

> **Key Point**
>
> The model that is created for responding to crisis is cybernetic; that is, a cybernetic system includes processes that are continuous, dynamic (flexible), and cyclical (continuously fluid) in nature and mobile.

process factors to the cycle of crisis intervention as a foundation for evaluating progress and successful intervention is an important indicator of effective crisis management.

Cybernetic and Interacting Environmental Scanning Process

The ability of an organization to respond well to crisis directly relates to the organization's ability to anticipate it. Anticipating and predicting crisis are important parts of the role of leadership throughout the organization. Leaders must recognize the fundamental obligation of leadership; that is, ensuring that the environmental influences that have an impact on the organization's ability to do its work have been considered, and that any change in them has been noted, especially with regard to a shift in the organization. The work of the organization is affected by a number of internal and external forces. These forces continuously interact, and the leader, recognizing this level of interaction, realizes that a change in response may be indicated by a shift in conditions and circumstances.

Organizations are dynamic and living entities. As such, they must achieve a goodness-of-fit and interaction with the prevailing environment and the context within which they function (**Figure 7-12**). Because living organizations exist in a field of continuous and dynamic change,

Figure 7-12 Cybernetic and Interacting Environmental Scanning Detail of DCTM.

the circumstances and conditions within which an organization functions are constantly shifting and adjusting, frequently representing an ever-emerging set of factors that alter the organization's reality and change its operation and action.

Wherever the external environment of the organization comes into contact with the internal mechanisms of the organization, the urge and intersection for change occur. Leaders, recognizing that these intersections are indicators of the potential for critical events or unplanned circumstances, constantly survey the landscape for elements and contents of conditions or circumstances and the potential they have for shifting and adjusting organizational reality (Jadhav et al., 2015).

Internalization and Externalization

Human organizations do not function in isolation. There is a convergence of interactions and intersections within which organizations operate in a continuously dynamic yet cybernetic environment. The external forces at work on organizations relate to social, political, economic, market, and human conditions and circumstances that constantly bombard the organization with different influences. For the most part, these forces can be anticipated and visualized early enough for the organization to respond appropriately. Occasionally, however, these forces converge in an unplanned or unanticipated way and create conditions that force the organization to respond immediately. For example, health reform can be planned for; an unanticipated number of respondents to the state insurance exchanges cannot be so easily accommodated. If the organization is not prepared for the eventuality and possibility of critical impact, reaction is the organization's response to the condition or circumstance. However, if the organization's adaptive and predictive capacities are refined sufficiently to deal with unanticipated change, the organization can actually use the change event as an opportunity to expand or extend its viability and its potential for thriving.

External Forces

The ability of the organization to recognize external forces and to see them in the context of the organization's lived experience in the broader context is a critical mechanism for guaranteeing the organization's ability to respond to immediate change in a positive fashion. Leadership must incorporate the capacity to recognize critical change into the organization's scanning mechanisms. These mechanisms continuously scan for external forces and broadly translate those forces in a way that has meaning and value for the organization and its members.

> **Point to Ponder**
>
> External and internal forces lend equal weight to the process of change. Wise leaders can incorporate both external and internal dynamics in assessing the need for change, and in building a systematic and organized response to it.

The ability of a hospital, for example, to anticipate the impact of changing technology in its cardiac services can be a strong indicator of the adaptability of the organization and its ability to shift its internal environment to meet the radical change in the external technological forces. The movement from coronary artery bypass grafts to drug-eluding stents and/or emerging pharmacological responses is a classic example of the need for an organization to quickly shift its infrastructure, clinical dynamics, and payment processes to address an important new technology. In addition, a healthcare system's move to refining an electronic medical record documentation system is a radical shift in the mechanisms of information management and documentation such that skills, ability, systems, adaptation, and clinical process are all affected by the improvement. Anticipating the increasing demand at the policy and payment levels and with regard to utilization of resources and workload reorganization, the organization must adapt critically and appropriately to this shift in clinical process. Both are examples of external forces having a dramatic and direct impact on internal mechanisms, causing an organization to shift its resources and activities to respond to a new demand, not necessarily a part of its existing infrastructure.

Internal Forces

Internal forces, too, have a strong impact on an organization's ability to respond to changing circumstances and demands that affect its ability to thrive. Structural and operational forces work together to create a context for organizational activities. Unless internal forces are adequately configured to support the organization's ability to address changes and challenges that affect work goals, processes, and outcomes, the ability of the organization to thrive may be compromised. A traditionally satisfactory response to address prevailing or emerging demands may no longer be adequate and, as a result, can actually impede the organization's ability to engage and change.

Internal support structures, work processes, management systems, supply chain, and communication processes may work individually or collectively to create conditions that limit the organization's ability to address real-time issues and concerns. There is a real need for leaders to ensure a true goodness-of-fit between the internal work structures and processes so that when emerging demands, both external and internal, operate to create a change in the mechanisms of work, the organization can respond quickly and effectively (**Figure 7-13**).

> **Point to Ponder**
>
> The internal environment must respond to crisis and change in a fluid and flexible manner because there is now no long-term recovery time between components of the change process.

Figure 7-13 Externalization/Internalization.

This notion of nimbleness is a critical element in the leader's understanding of contemporary work dynamics. There is not a significantly long period of time for adjustment and adaptation. Leaders must adapt and reframe work dynamics in a relatively short time and in a way that ensures appropriate linkage between work processes and changing demand (fluid and flexible). Examples of new medication administration systems, materials management supply chain systems, pharmacy distribution/control/monitoring systems, and an intranet communication infrastructure all represent the internal arena of work structures and processes. They must represent a commitment to reconfiguration and synthesis of changing technologies and processes in the internal work dynamics of the organization.

Ensuring a Strong Service Core

In hospitals and health systems, it is easy to see how leaders can be co-opted by business opportunities, fads, and new ventures in a way that causes them to lose sight of their core work (**Figure 7-14**). Exciting and innovative options can lead an organization down new paths. However, unless these options are disciplined by consistency with mission and purpose, they can also draw the life out of an organization. Leaders must understand that a change in any one part of the structure creates pressures and demands on other parts of the system, leading either to collective sustenance or to failure. To moderate this situation, new ventures and directions should be consistent with the vision, mission, and purposes of the organization.

> **Point to Ponder**
>
> Mission and purpose are fulfilled through an organization's work. Therefore, workers must understand the relationship between their own work efforts and the fulfillment of the mission and purpose of the organization through the commitment of their own effort.

When a mission reflects the vision and values of the organization, it must be inculcated into every person and activity in the organization. For workers, either clinical or support, the meaning and value of their work can become unilateral and nonaligned if it is not both informed and disciplined by purpose and clearly delineated work objectives. Successful organizations require that all stakeholders at any place in the organization be fully committed to living and working consistently with the mission and purposes of the organization. Affirming this ensures that the mission is inculcated in the fabric of the organization and that the work activities of every participant create a core around which all strategic and operational activities can unfold. When this connection is not delineated for everyone in the system, employees often substitute sectional and unilateral purposes and goals and begin to fulfill their own purposes instead.

A strong focus on mission and purpose leads to ensuring that all workers in the system are motivated and committed to achieving positive organizational purposes and, it goes

> Business core:
> Purpose/mission
> Meaning/motivation
> Commitment/competence
> Work = learning

Figure 7-14 Business Core.

without saying, the success of the organization. Individuals are fully aware of how much their ability to thrive depends on organizational success. Building a membership community around this core of understanding and continually reinforcing it establish a firm and continuous foundation on which every work activity can build. In addition, leaders make sure that all activities related to knowledge generation, learning, experimentation, and innovation are evaluated against the mission and purpose. At every level of the organization, the direction, conversation, performance requisites, and work outcomes of all employees should reflect how every participant in the organization fulfills mission and purpose.

At the point-of-service, leaders must translate the usually esoteric language of strategy and mission into a language that can be understood. Clinical practitioners, service providers, and support persons collectively need to be assured that their individual contributions are valued within the context of advancing the mission and purposes of the organization. The language of leadership must reflect the requisites of embracing the mission, identifying how individual work effort contributes to it, and ensuring that work outcomes advance the organization's mission and purpose. This series of activities, linkages, and integration, facilitated by the leader's commitment and effort, ensures the strong point of reference in the midst of intense change. In evaluating critical events or intense moments of change and unplanned crises or challenges, mission and purpose serve as the lens through which leaders can more accurately and appropriately determine specific response. The organization's place in the world is viewed through this lens, which creates both the frame and the discipline for leaders to evaluate crisis and select the most successful responses to it.

Crisis and Environmental Scanning

Wise leaders are always aware of the constancy of change. Change comes in many forms and can emerge at almost any point in the life cycle of an organization. Constancy of change is the only true context, and it has a universal impact on all life processes. Skilled leaders recognize this dynamic is part of the constancy of work and relationship. Leaders are ever-vigilant to the internal and external conditions and circumstances that indicate a significant organizational impact (Nelson-Brantley & Ford, 2017).

> **Key Point**
>
> Unit or departmental leaders see their role from the perspective of the whole system. They do not just lead departments or units; they lead the whole system from the perspective of the department or units where they are located.

In times of great change, such as our current work environment, a talent for environmental scanning becomes vital (**Figure 7-15**). Mobility and the constant transformation of human work and communication systems create the conditions that call leaders to a broader and deeper understanding of the influences and circumstances affecting the organization and the work of its people. Through the development and refinement of strong environmental scanning skills, at every level of management meaningful change can be sorted from fad and superficiality, and appropriate shifts in strategy and work can be more clearly articulated. Effective leaders at every level of the organization understand the internal work dynamics and relationships within the organization with a high level of proficiency. These leaders know the value and contribution the individual

Figure 7-15 Environmental Scanning.

departments or units of the work system make to the whole organization. The reverse is also true: capable department and unit leaders are aware of the impact of the larger system (both external and internal) on the ability of the individual department or unit to function and thrive. This awareness should raise the value of synthesis in the perception of all leaders and emphasize the need for consistency and integration in every level of system decision making and action.

Effective leaders assess information and resources that lead to understanding the convergence of dynamics that create the conditions that influence or affect current operations or work. The strategic decision to implement a high-portability electronic medical record system or paperless processes throughout the clinical organization is a strong indicator of a significant change in information management, documentation, technology, and work applications. Seeing the significance of these forces early in the strategic process provides a response framework for the leader that raises questions related to impact on work design, clinical roles, new learning, support systems, communication, and worker behavior. Once the strategic implications are fully understood, issues of timeline, planning, education, orientation, experimentation, and application can be better defined.

Systematizing this strategic environmental scanning process and formalizing it provide leadership at every level of the health system with both the tools and the processes necessary to anticipate and even predict essential change. Reinforcing in the leader the requisites to read broadly, to stay current with clinical and systems innovations, to remain invested and involved in strategic discussions, and to synthesize information from diverse sources is invaluable in developing effective environmental scanning skills. Leaders at every level of the organization must be free to honestly and openly recognize incongruence between current work conditions, circumstances, and processes and prevailing or emerging realities that challenge or threaten them. These variances create the context for new thinking and raise the challenge for developing innovative approaches. Leaders recognize that in response to shifting realities, work processes never remain the same and must always shift to accommodate new technical or process realities. Here again, leaders create this cultural frame, this context, if you will, within which worker attitude, behavior, responsiveness, and action can demonstrate a willingness and competence to respond in a timely fashion and to act appropriately.

Emerging conditions and forces often can be seen far ahead of their direct impact on organizations and people. Often, leaders suggest how they saw and recognized the coming change but never believed it would have the powerful impact it subsequently did. Anticipating constant change and incorporating it into the discussion related to strategy and response are strong indicators of organizational predictive competence. Also, using alignment strategies that create connections and linkages among emerging technical and work conditions and forces, social and political influences, dramatic economic shifts, and even destructive technologies is useful in determining the specificity and degree of the impact the future change may have on the organization and its people (Lewis & Oyserman, 2015).

Signals

Leaders are constantly alert for major indicators or signals of impending change that are strongly predictive of an impact on the organization and its work (**Figure 7-16**). Changes in therapeutic modalities—for example, movement from mitral and aortic valve replacement surgeries to transcatheter valve replacement procedures—indicate a major shift in cardiac surgical procedures that affect hospital length of stay, supplies and equipment used, operating room space and time, and other factors. Advances in technology and pharmacotherapeutics that shift provider and patient experiences create intense conditional and process challenges that cause hospitals, diagnostic services, key stakeholders that supply and use therapies, finance systems, and support systems to alter their infrastructure and work approaches. Because of the "noise" involved in dramatic shifts, organizations often avoid the upfront conversations and interactions necessary to appropriately anticipate the significance of therapeutic changes and to directly confront the

Signals (examples)
-Global trends
-Potentials
-Critical conditions
-Market fluctuations

Figure 7-16 Signals.

requisites of organizational and personal adjustment. The potential for conflict in not anticipating significant experiential shifts and up- and downstream effects, or undertaking a planned strategic review of important signals, ultimately creates reactive noise and team challenges and slows appropriate adaptation. Without adaptation, conflicts between cardiac surgeons, anesthesiologists, and therapeutic cardiologists are accelerated, and marketing and payment planning and strategies related to novel therapeutic transformations, as well as service and operational adjustments, are severely challenged.

> **Point to Ponder**
>
> Leaders must help those they lead to understand the impact of external trends and changes and how they alter the conception of the work, the way the work is done, and the activities of all workers related to undertaking change in their own way of doing work.

Leaders must regularly scan broad information sources and evidenced-based documentation related to health care or particular health services, identify the signals obtained from scanning activities, share results with key stakeholders, and undertake dialogue with regard to appropriate responses. Leaders must help their stakeholders assess global trends, clinical potentials, critical changes in environmental and work conditions, significant shifts in the market, and new technology if they are to ensure sufficiency in adaptation, prediction, and response.

Triggers

Recognizing significant events or indicators demonstrates the leader's ability to read signals and to draw inferences from them with regard to their potential impact on their organization and service. Eventually, however, all signals converge with external or internal conditions and circumstances to create critical moments. Critical moments serve as trigger events for organizations and people with regard to the dire, immediate, or direct impact of crisis, change, or transformation on the organization and its people (**Figure 7-17**). Still, at this level of intensity trigger events can be missed. When overlooked, the organization diverts to reactive strategies, away from proactive anticipation and response, causing a spiraling down of leadership and staff response toward reactive patterns of behavior; recidivism; poor decisions; market, business, and service losses; and negative human dynamics.

Organizational intelligence is best represented in the effectiveness and success of a system's ability to adapt in a cybernetic way to the vagaries of change that affect it. Sound environmental scanning processes help the organization anticipate strategic, operating, clinical, and technical potential for problems. Trigger events ultimately address any one or all of these in

Triggers (examples)
- Environmental crisis
- Market losses
- Resource losses
- Poor decisions
- Political/legal/socio shifts
- Competition successes

Figure 7-17 Triggers.

any given moment in time. These triggers can be anticipated if appropriately and properly identified through enumerating the signals that, upon convergence, create them. The ability of leaders at every level of the organization to identify signals and respond to trigger events precisely and quickly indicates the degree of adaptation really present in an organization.

Trigger events are the organization's last line of defense against an impending or inevitable shift or change. Triggers indicate that the change impact is "at the door" and now directly influences the strategy and work dynamics of the organization. Ignoring trigger events generally leads to a higher level of organizational crisis and ultimately extends to influencing the viability of the entire system. Leaders who effectively hone environmental scanning skills, formalize methodologies in the organization for identifying signal indicators and processes, and anticipate trigger events aid in the system adapting and thriving.

Crisis Preparedness

Although environmental scanning is an essential skill, it is not, by itself, sufficient for addressing potential and inevitable crises or critical events. The organization's ability to predict and anticipate the potential for critical processes in today's world requires solid strategic planning. Any contemporary organization must have an operating format or infrastructure that specifically incorporates into its management processes adaptive and predictive strategies and crisis preparedness.

> **Key Point**
>
> Crisis preparedness should be incorporated into the organization's strategic processes. Critical events should not be seen as external and not be planned for in advance. The ability to predict and adapt to inevitable crisis and build it into the infrastructure of strategy helps ensure the organization's ability to thrive.

Hospitals and health systems are excellent at developing a variety of community disaster plans. These plans have proven to be excellent templates for healthcare organization responses to crisis and disaster. However, few hospitals and health systems have crisis preparedness plans that are directed to helping them identify and respond to strategic, operational, and service crises and critical changes that directly affect the hospital or health system. In a time of fast-paced technological and therapeutic change, it is no longer optional for hospitals and health systems to anticipate and prepare for significant critical events that affect their very viability and sustenance. Crisis preparedness planning needs to include the hospital's or health system's strategic, operating, human, and technical problem types that invariably result from the impact of a whole host of critical events.

Effective planning for critical events requires that each problem type have specific crisis preparedness planning processes that enumerate the organization's response to a crisis. In addition, the crisis preparedness plan needs to sufficiently address individual or particular threats: environmental, technical/mechanical, and human threats that have the potential to affect the clinical organization through one or all of its problem types.

Planning

A good crisis preparedness plan that focuses on the life of the hospital or health system addresses particular functional priorities of the organization in each of its problem areas (**Figure 7-18**). Effective planning includes specific engagement and anticipation of leadership response in

Planning

Environmental scanning system
-Internal/external variance
-Emerging conditions/forces
-Socio/political/economic shifts
-Destructive technologies

Crisis preparedness plan
-Senior management engagement
-Crisis plan group
-Risk assessment
-Operating priorities
-Data collection
-Written plan
-Plan testing

Hazard plans for threats:
-Environmental
-Technical
-Mechanical
-Human activity

Recovery/salvage
-Damage assessment
-Environmental stabilization
-Activate recovery process
-Restore functions

Rational and objective systems

Problem types
-Strategic
-Operating
-Human
-Technical

Signals (examples)
-Global trends
-Potentials
-Critical conditions
-Market fluctuations

Triggers (examples)
-Environmental crisis
-Market losses
-Resource losses
-Poor decisions
-Political/legal/socio shifts
-Competition successes

Systems evaluation
-Adaptive ability
-Adaptive capacity
-Contingency impact
-Human agency and social structure
-Structural components
-Multiplexity (intra- and interorganizational)
-Redundancy
-Linkage of system elements
-Reformat the plan

Aimless vagaries/variances

Figure 7-18 DCTM Details of Components for Assessing Adaptive Effectiveness.

implementing designated activities in response to signal or trigger events. In crisis preparedness planning, a crisis plan group should be identified and each member should have specific tasks and responsibilities. Members of this group should come from the various forums and levels of the organization representing the breadth of its service and support structures. This DCTM group ties crisis planning to the environmental scanning system and anticipates the potential for specific responses. This requires a well-refined mechanism of assessing risk potential and anticipating risk impact on the organization. Effective crisis planning identifies and defines particular risk-specific operating priorities that can potentially best respond to an impending crisis. The group clarifies these operating priorities and details responses from the involved departments, services, and people in the organization. The group can use environmental scanning processes and data from potential signals and likely trigger events to develop a database that informs particular critical response stages or steps.

The crisis preparedness plan should address the following issues:

1. Describe the various levels and activities associated with leadership engagement and the roles various leaders will play in response to specific categories of crisis.
2. Form the crisis plan group, whose role is to coordinate the activities associated with crisis plan development and application.
3. Identify and determine specific arenas of sensitivity or potential external and internal risk factors that may be associated with the cause of crisis.

Crisis preparedness plan
- Senior management engagement
- Crisis plan group
- Risk assessment
- Operating priorities
- Data collection
- Written plan
- Plan testing

Environmental scanning system
- Internal/external variance
- Emerging conditions/forces
- Socio/political/economic shifts
- Destructive technologies

Recovery/salvage
- Damage assessment
- Environmental stabilization
- Activate recovery process
- Restore functions

Systems evaluation
- Adaptive ability
- Adaptive capacity
- Contingency impact
- Human agency and social structure
- Structural component
- Multiplexity (intra- and interorganizational)
- Redundancy
- Linkage of system elements
- Reformat the plan

Aimless vagaries/variances

Figure 7-19 Crisis Preparedness Plan and Environmental Scanning System.

4. Describe the design, form, format, structure, and process activities associated with operating priorities at a time when trigger events impinge on the usual work cycles.
5. Describe the structure, methodology, technology, and processes associated with data gathering and analysis as a part of the predictive and adaptive data mechanisms.
6. Clearly enumerate and specifically design the written crisis preparedness plan and make it available to all the pertinent leaders and departments of the organization.
7. Implement a regularly scheduled mechanism for testing the veracity and effectiveness of the crisis preparedness plan (**Figure 7-19**).

A written crisis preparedness plan should include all elements and be detailed and clear enough such that it can be understood by all stakeholders and effectively implemented in response to a critical event. In addition, a mechanism for regular testing (6 months to 1 year) should also be included to evaluate the components and the effectiveness of the crisis planning process.

Recovery/Salvage Stage

As a part of the cycle of crisis preparedness, hospital and health system leaders must also recognize the need for quick and immediate response to prevailing factors that affect their clinical work and effectiveness. Crisis preparedness activities assume that, given sufficient time,

Recovery/Salvage Stage

Crisis preparedness plan
- Senior management engagement
- Crisis plan group
- Risk assessment
- Operating priorities
- Data collection
- Written plan
- Plan testing

Environmental scanning system
- Internal/external variance
- Emerging conditions/forces
- Socio/political/economic shifts
- Destructive technologies

Recovery/salvage
- Damage assessment
- Environmental stabilization
- Activate recovery process
- Restore functions

Systems evaluation
- Adaptive ability
- Adaptive capacity
- Contingency impact
- Human agency and social structure
- Structural component
- Multiplexity (intra- and interorganizational)
- Redundancy
- Linkage of system elements
- Reformat the plan

Aimless vagaries/variances

Figure 7-20 Recovery/Salvage.

normative crisis invariably occurs. Immediate crisis response activities and teams should be able to identify specific responses and activities necessary to address both short- and long-term issues in a way that configures the organization's response to a specific critical event (**Figure 7-20**). This intense focus on critical intervention requires attention on the part of involved leaders and staff. This frequently requires suspension of emphasis on normal activities to ensure a timely and correct adaptive response to the critical event.

In this recovery stage, the effectiveness of the critical response enumerated by the crisis preparedness plan can best be demonstrated. Quick damage assessment and immediate corrective action processes enable the organization to establish a short-term investment in critical response, ensuring that the broader normative activities can be resumed as quickly as possible. Whether the critical event is a competing hospital's new cardiac accountable care program that is drawing away an important population of patients or the complete shutdown of an electronic medical record system that requires immediate manual documentation, the crisis preparedness activities should focus on a response strategy in a short period of time. Through this dynamic, specific recovery activities and the necessary reconceptualization or reconfiguration of specific responses should be facilitated. Leaders should recognize that temporary refocusing of resources and efforts may be required in the short term as a necessary part of redesigning and structuring an appropriate response to the crisis.

Adaptive Effectiveness

In any organizational disruption, whether technical, operational, or human, the strategic activities of the organization are directly affected. Any process associated with a hospital's or health system's ability to adapt must also be linked to its environmental scanning processes. In the three-part model provided in this chapter, the interface between multilateral health team effectiveness, environmental scanning, and critical response or crisis preparedness provides a dynamic and cybernetic approach of continuous adaptation and adjustment as an organization responds to the implications and vagaries of change in a highly transforming environment.

> **Key Point**
>
> The relationship among external forces, the leadership's ability to scan the environment, and the organization's preparedness for crisis is a strong indicator of whether an infrastructure for sustainability exists in the system.

In an effort to mitigate strategic challenges and disruptions, the organization's adaptive capacity and response must address immediate needs in a timely fashion. The organization's response must stay one step ahead of the negative forces embedded in a change event. Strategic and operational responses need to be flexible enough to adapt to both the predictable and the unpredictable variances that accompany a significant change event (Cartwright, Hall, & Lee, 2017).

The adaptive capacity of an organization must be exemplified in its ability to resume normative activities consistent with its mission and purposes as soon as possible. Executive leadership needs to be clear about the adjustments related to the interface between strategic, operational, and clinical services. Although a critical event may occur in any one of these arenas, ultimately each one is affected by the other. Leadership must recognize this interface of influencing forces and acknowledge that an issue arising out of one element (strategic, operational, or clinical) ultimately affects the others. Leadership synthesis and demonstration of an integrated response to a critical event are important indicators that the organization has successfully accommodated the crisis and can return to normal operations.

Systems Evaluation

No predictive and adaptive system or approach can succeed unless it is continually monitored, adjusted, and adapted to emerging conditions and circumstances. Predictive and adaptive systems need continuous monitoring to ensure sufficient response capacity and a real goodness-of-fit between the organization's environmental scanning system (which includes its crisis preparedness plan) and the prevailing emerging external and internal realities, which are constantly in a state of flux and affect the organization's continuing viability. The content and character of any crisis represent the environmental conditions or circumstances that initiated it. As timing and technology work to create a different contextual framework, crisis planning and intervention processes must shift to reflect these changes. Close attention must be paid to the content of the crisis preparedness plan that addresses the external and internal contextual challenges that are constantly influencing the organization and its work.

A systems evaluation focuses on the application interface of each component in the process in the system's adaptation to a real-time crisis (**Figure 7-21**). The interface between the cybernetic elements of team process, environmental scanning, and crisis preparedness is indicative of a whole systems approach to ensuring the effectiveness of the strategic

Crisis preparedness plan
- Senior management engagement
- Crisis plan group
- Risk assessment
- Operating priorities
- Data collection
- Written plan
- Plan testing

Environmental scanning system
- Internal/external variance
- Emerging conditions/forces
- Socio/political/economic shifts
- Destructive technologies

Recovery/salvage
- Damage assessment
- Environmental stabilization
- Activate recovery process
- Restore functions

Systems evaluation
- Adaptive ability
- Adaptive capacity
- Contingency impact
- Human agency and social structure
- Structural component
- Multiplexity (intra- and interorganizational)
- Redundancy
- Linkage of system elements
- Reformat the plan

Aimless vagaries/variances

Figure 7-21 Systems Evaluation.

operational and clinical activities of a hospital or health system. The ability of systems leaders to see a cybernetic process such as this as an integrated model and to demonstrate their own skills of synthesis and fluidity in its application is the strongest determinant of a successful model.

Appropriate systems evaluation should include the elements related to the organizational and human response to broad-based change and to critical events. Leaders must demonstrate that the system is effective in its ability, first, to anticipate and predict potential change and, second, to adequately respond in the presence of critical events and unplanned occurrences. Structuring this as a part of the organizational framework ensures that the system and its people can better anticipate, predict, and respond in the presence of a critical change and can consistently reproduce the necessary work and social processes to achieve operational normality within the context of a new change.

> **Point to Ponder**
>
> Evaluation must always be included in the design of the system's response to crisis. Evaluation of the plan must represent as much patient impact and change as are part of the character and content of the crisis. Leaders must always use the insights they gain from evaluation of past appropriate responses to inform how they will manage future crises.

Accountability and authority in the implementation of a systematic approach when creating an operational infrastructure for environmental scanning and crisis planning demand a level of clarity across the organization. Individuals located at various points in the organizational structure must know they have access to and can communicate with key individuals, who can respond in a timely and appropriate way to broad signals and to external and internal triggers that suggest a need for an immediate response. At the same time, the system must have sufficient integrity to avoid a consciousness of crisis and to maintain as normal an operating milieu as possible.

Good systems evaluation should include an assessment of successful approaches that represent the organization's adaptive ability and capacity to respond to the need for immediate change. The impact of the change on the organization's operating environment and the responsiveness of staff to that change give leaders some sense of the contingency impact of the immediate changes created in the organizational system. The ability of individuals and groups to respond and adapt quickly to the demand for a change in context or content of work is a strong indicator of the ability of the organization's social structures to quickly adjust to new ways of working and shifting outcome demands. Systems effectiveness is based on an evidence-driven frame and uses previous experiences, best practices, and innovative approaches to ensure the organization's response to changing environmental conditions or crisis is both consistent with the demand of the crisis and creates the foundation for sustainable normal operations.

Strong systems evaluation includes reviewing the impact of multiplexity (layers of change), of the diversity of interactions and relationships that operate between different elements of the organizational networks, and of redundancy. This review ensures that there is sufficient slack (open time) in the organizational system to anticipate, assess, plan, and adjust human response to a significant change or critical event. Making this time available is especially problematic in health systems and hospitals. The unrelenting focus on time-based productivity at every level of the organization has eliminated sufficient slack in the role of leaders and staff, virtually guaranteeing the organization's lack of preparedness with regard to immediate environmental, operational, and clinical crises.

Assessing the system's responsiveness to critical events requires leaders to synthesize all the components of the system and structures of the organization. Understanding the nature of flow of work processes, external and internal events, and the character of response strategies at the conceptual center of the system creates the proper frame for effective systems evaluation. The ability to see this linkage of multifocal team activity, environmental scanning and influence, and critical response provides the frame for ensuring systems competence and capability with regard to general adaptation.

The three major components of the cybernetic process—team-based synthesis, environmental scanning, and adaptive effectiveness (crisis planning)—each play their part in meeting the demands of the whole-system approach to critical management in response to change. As in all systems approaches, each component must generalize to support the whole, and the whole must converge to ensure consistent and appropriate response to change, resulting in effective adaptation and successful outcomes. In a performance-based, evidence-driven, accountability-based, and outcomes-oriented health system driven by increasingly sophisticated clinical, service, and support technology, leaders must demonstrate systems skills, a capacity for innovation, and a high degree of adaptation. Leader skills are especially important as health systems work to adapt to the demands of health reform and value-driven models of service. Comparable effectiveness between health systems in their service, quality, and price commitment to those they serve will be a transparent witness to the degree of an organization's effectiveness. The future of health care depends on the ability of clinical systems to interface well and work together across the disciplines and the organization, to adjust to increasingly complex technology applications, to operate in a high-mobility accountable care arena, and to ensure that the health needs of individuals are met and the health of our communities is advanced.

Conclusion

Clearly, it is vital that health leaders understand the requirement to be prepared to confront the unexpected. In today's environment, with the complexity of changes that are occurring at a quantum rate, it is no longer optional for leaders to have the capacity to respond to immediate and dramatic change events. The ability to respond to the dynamics of crisis and critical change is not only an inherent leadership skill, it must now be inculcated within the very fabric of the organization and its operation. From the development of strategy through operational efficiency and effectiveness, leadership behavior, and work practices, every element of the system must reflect an ability to both predict and adapt to the drama of crisis and change (Porter-O'Grady, 2013). Developing a systematic and integrated approach that is evident at both the behavioral and operational levels of the system is the critical variable that ensures adaptation and the ability to thrive over the long term.

Chapter Takeaways

1. Crisis is a normative part of the human experience. Crises are not always stimulated or accompanied by cataclysmic events. Most often crises are generated by simple occurrences to create a dramatic shift in the environment. These critical events and unanticipated situations are generally the end product of the convergence of forces unknown at any given time, yet operating inexorably, out of consciousness, causing a result that could not be fully anticipated.
2. A fundamental and basic role of leaders in complex systems is the recognition of the importance of adaptive and predictive skills. This role is essential to successfully anticipate, predict, and adapt to a wide variety of crises. Leaders who adapt to crises fully understand the management of crises as an important part of the process of leadership and as a normative operational consideration of day-to-day function.
3. Well-thought-out and well-planned human resource management systems are critical to any organization's ability to adjust and adapt personnel behaviors and work processes to address critical change events. Such skills must be seen as normative elements of any organizational participant's role and should be a part of the ongoing education, development, and expectation of all workers in the healthcare environment.
4. Strategic crisis management and leadership is a particular discipline within the exercise of leadership. It requires an organized and systematic structure, process, and response cycle with key characteristics and elements, which enumerate it as a way of organizing a systematic response and preserving and advancing the interests of the system and its people for the long term.
5. The DCTM is an organized systematic cybernetic feedback crisis response model that fully engages team action in an integrated, broad-based, cross-system mechanism that ensures an appropriate and meaningful response to crisis and change. Understanding it and applying it is a critical indicator of the system's capacity to successfully manage through complex crisis and change.

Case Study 7-1
Building a High-Performing Rapid Response Team

The chief nursing officer (CNO) at Pine Valley Medical Center has received a written proposal and business plan from the directors of the emergency department and medical surgical services for a new rapid response team (RRT). The two directors recently attended a national conference outlining the benefits of an RRT in improving patient outcomes and preventing cardiac arrest in unstable patients. Their proposal and business plan present a compelling case for the benefits of an RRT and outline the costs and benefits of the new program. The directors discussed how clinical nurses can perceive the deteriorating condition of a patient as a major crisis as they attempt to assess and intervene with the patient while also juggling the needs of other patients and their assignments. It was proposed that an RRT could provide a valuable service in assisting the less experienced nurses in assessing the status of patients and prevent untoward events from occurring from missed observations or interventions. The CNO and the other executives agreed to allow the two directors to develop and pilot the program for 6 months, and then evaluate the program for its success or to identify any changes that might be needed.

Frank, the director of the emergency department, and James, the director of medical surgical services, identified individuals they believed were important stakeholders for the development of an RRT and invited these individuals to the initial planning meeting. James reviewed the past year's data for cardiac arrest in the emergency department and throughout the hospital, patient transfers from medical surgical services to critical care, and other statistics. He shared evidence from the literature and speakers at the national conference who presented data demonstrating how an RRT improved patient outcomes by preventing deterioration of the patients' conditions. Another major benefit noted was the nurses' and medical staff's positive response to an RRT program because it was recognized as an important resource to improve patient outcomes.

James led the group through a process to identify the vision, mission, and purpose of an RRT for Pine Valley Medical Center. The group seemed to be very engaged in the process and quickly embraced the vision for the RRT. Although the group had interprofessional representatives, John and Frank invited members to identify others who might add value to the planning process.

At the second meeting the group identified the critical attributes of a high-performing RRT, including (1) competence of the individual members, (2) team competence, (3) resources for staffing the RRT, (4) metrics to measure outcomes, (5) team roles for each interprofessional team partner, (6) group norms for reviewing performance of the team, and (7) patient scenario practice drills for the team. It was decided that several teams would be needed to cover the hospital 24/7. The initial planning group adopted the name of RRT Steering Committee and agreed that they would organize the initial teams and be the quality review team to review individual and team performance and recommend changes for continued improvement. The steering committee also identified a number of learning modules that would be beneficial to the new RRTs to enhance their understanding of team formation and development, interprofessional communication and collaboration, and assessment and monitoring results.

As the new RRTs developed over the next 6 months, an *esprit de corps* developed among the team members, who were considered as "the elite" and most competent nurses, physicians, pharmacists, and others who supported the effort. The individual teams practiced various patient scenarios, always looking for ways to improve their response and performance. They also held postevent reviews to critique themselves as a team and identify ways to improve their performance individually and as a team. At the end of 6 months, the CNO and other executives reviewed patient outcomes and staff and physician responses to the RRT, and the program was fully adopted with funding appropriated in the annual budget.

Questions

1. How does the DCTM described in this chapter provide a framework for the organizing efforts of the RRT Steering Committee?
2. What might be some of the external and internal forces that could trigger recognition of the need to develop an RRT in a hospital?
3. Describe your perceptions of the process using the DCTM that the steering committee put in place to identify their respective individual and team roles and practice these roles in various patient scenarios.
4. Describe how an RRT fits the description of a complex, adaptive, self-regulating system, as described in this chapter.
5. How could you apply the DCTM to other crisis teams?

Case Study 7-2

No One Could Have Prepared Me for This Experience

Sierra Mountain Hospital was well known for its stellar reputation for nursing and medical excellence, great leadership, and fantastic work environment. The new chief operating officer and her team had done wonders in totally transforming the organizational culture over the past 5 years and dramatically improving the patient, operational, and financial outcomes for the hospital. The executive team had recruited and hired top medical and surgical specialists and talented nursing leaders to create centers of excellence that were second to none for tertiary-level community hospitals. Sierra Mountain Hospital sat at the base of the Sierra National Forest and was surrounded by beautiful, well-established pine and sequoia trees. The hospital had recently been recognized in the national press as one of the top 50 hospitals in the nation for excellence in patient outcomes and patient, physician, and employee satisfaction.

Sierra Mountain Hospital had the usual policies and procedures and annual competency reviews for various crisis situations, particularly disaster planning. The procedures outlined roles and responsibilities of the command post leaders and participants and sites for the safe location of patients for any type of disaster. Every employee in the organization was required to review the disaster policies and procedures annually and to demonstrate their knowledge and competence in carrying out their specific individual roles and team roles in case of a disaster.

In extreme weather conditions with winds recorded at 90 miles per hour, an electrical transformer was blown over and started a fire in dry timber conditions. With the high winds, the fire spread rapidly to the surrounding areas, and embers were blown about as if they were laser darts. As the fire encroached on homes in the community, local fire brigades were dispatched to evacuate residents who were in the fire's expected path. Within hours the state National Guard and other fire brigades were en route to provide assistance in containing the rapidly spreading fire. Per protocol, the leadership of Sierra Mountain Hospital assumed their roles in the command post to assess resources needed, identify patients who could be discharged or immediately moved, identify patients who would need assistance, and determine the level of danger from the fire situation. The nurse director was in radio contact with the police and fire departments and was informed that she would be contacted should patient evacuation be necessary, but it was not expected.

As the command post leader began calling in staff, she realized that the expected number of staff from the callback might not meet expectations because many were actively involved in protecting their own homes and families. Some of the staff indicated that they would come in only if they could bring their young children and pets because they were afraid to leave them behind with other family members who were engaged in trying to protect their homes. The command post leader, knowing that she would need additional help to relieve staff who needed to return to their homes, told the callback staff that they could bring their children and animals to the hospital in this crisis situation. Immediately, the command post leader contacted the facility director and asked for a space to be designated for the care of young children and a space for animals. This situation was certainly one that no one had anticipated when practicing various disaster scenarios.

Within a few hours the nurse director called the police and fire captains for more information about the encroaching fire. It was obvious that they had become so involved in their work that they did not inform the nurse director that the fire was spreading rapidly and in the direction of Sierra Mountain Hospital. It's never an easy decision to make the call for evacuation of all patients, but the nurse director felt that it was in the best interest of the patients and her staff. Evacuation procedures were clearly outlined in the disaster protocol, so the nurse director implemented those procedures and called for the immediate removal of all mobile patients to a safe area in the community's high school on the other end of town. She asked the police department for assistance to use school buses to transport the more mobile patients. Higher acuity patients would be transferred by any available ambulance, and the nurse director mobilized all of her leaders to set up temporary critical care units in the school's gymnasium for the more critical patients who would be transferred with as much equipment and supplies as possible. She made calls to neighboring community hospitals to send ambulances and staff to help. The hospital had several trucks that were used to transport medical supplies and equipment, and these were mobilized to transport the sicker patients in their beds and with their equipment.

The next day authorities determined that it was safe for patients to be returned to Sierra Mountain Hospital, so the staff began the process of moving patients back. After the disaster was over, the nurse director, the command post leader, and others reviewed the situation and how the various unit and department disaster teams performed using the policies, procedures, and practiced roles. Although they were pleased that none of the patients were compromised in the process of protecting them and transferring them to a safe location, the team realized that there were several issues that needed to be addressed to prepare for future disasters. A list of potential changes was identified for implementation. The nurse director and others realized that staff who were called in were reluctant to leave their children and pets. Therefore, it was decided that the hospital would purchase a number of portable pet crates of various sizes and temporary fencing for the containment of animals on the grounds and in large storage areas. Cots and bedding would also be purchased for use when staff needed to bring their children to the hospital during disasters. The role of child caretakers was created and staff were identified for this purpose. Because of the knowledge gained from the review of the fire disaster, Sierra Mountain Hospital led efforts in the community to identify various safe locations for patients and storage areas for cots and other supplies should patients need to be evacuated again in the future.

Questions

1. Using the DCTM as a framework, how would you assess Sierra Mountain Hospital's disaster preparedness?
2. From your own knowledge and experience, what other steps could the leadership of Sierra Mountain Hospital have taken to prepare for this or any other disaster?
3. Describe your perceptions of the review process after the disaster was over in planning for changes that would prepare them for future disaster response.
4. Describe how disaster response teams fit the description of a complex, adaptive, self-regulating system as described in this chapter.

References

Cartwright, C., Hall, M., & Lee, A. C. K. (2017). The changing health priorities of earthquake response and implications for preparedness: A scoping review. *Public Health, 150*, 60–70.

Chaffin, B. C., & Gunderson, L. H. (2016). Emergence, institutionalization and renewal: Rhythms of adaptive governance in complex social–ecological systems. *Journal of Environmental Management, 165*, 81–87.

Chandler, J., Rycroft-Malone, J., Hawkes, C., & Noyes, J. (2016). Application of simplified Complexity Theory concepts for healthcare social systems to explain the implementation of evidence into practice. *Journal of Advanced Nursing, 72*(2), 461–480.

Corrigan, Z., Winslow, W., Miramonti, C., & Stephens, T. (2016). Value-based emergency management. *Disaster Medicine and Public Health Preparedness, 10*(1), 158–160.

Curt, C., & Tacnet, J. M. (2018). Resilience of critical infrastructures: Review and analysis of current approaches. *Risk Analysis, 38*(11), 2441–2458.

Goralnick, E., Halpern, P., Loo, S., Gates, J., Biddinger, P., Fisher, J., Velmahos, G., Chung, S., Mooney, D., Brown, C., Barnewolt, B., Burke, P., Gupta, A., Ulrich, A., Hojman, H., McNulty, E., Dorn, B., Marcus, L., & Peleg, K. (2015). Leadership during the Boston Marathon bombings: A qualitative after-action review. *Disaster Medicine and Public Health Preparedness, 9*(5), 489–495.

Grady, C. M. (2016). Can complexity science inform physician leadership development? *Leadership in Health Service* (Bradford England), *29*(3), 251–263.

Graves, J. A., & Nikpay, S. S. (2017). The changing dynamics of US health insurance and implications for the future of the Affordable Care Act. *Health Affairs, 36*(2), 297–305.

Jadhav, E. D., Holsinger, J. W. Jr., & Fardo, D. W. (2015). Openness to change: Experiential and demographic components of change in local department health leaders. *Frontiers in Public Health, 3*, 209.

Jeffs, L., Merkley, J., Sinno, M., Thomson, N., Peladeau, N., & Richardson, S. (2019). Engaging stakeholders to co-design an academic practice strategic plan in an integrated health system: The key roles of the nurse executive and planning team. *Nursing Administration Quarterly, 43*(2), 186–192.

Kelders, S. M., Oinas-Kukkonen, H., Oorni, A., & van Gemert-Pijnen, J. E. (2016). Health behavior change support systems as a research discipline; a viewpoint. *International Journal of Medical Informatics, 96*, 3–10.

Laapotti, T., & Mikkola, L. (2016). Social interaction in management group meetings: A case study of Finnish hospital. *Journal of Health Organization and Management, 30*(4), 613–629.

Lal, M. M. (2019). Leading effectively through change. *Journal of Nursing Administration, 49*(12), 575–576.

Langan, J. C., Lavin, R., Wolgast, K. A., & Veenema, T. G. (2017). Education for developing and sustaining a health care workforce for disaster readiness. *Nursing Administration Quarterly, 41*(2), 118–127.

Lewis, N. A. Jr., & Oyserman, D. (2015). When does the future begin? Time metrics matter, connecting present and future selves. *Psychological Science, 26*(6), 816–825.

Mather, C. A., Cummings, E. A., & Gale, F. (2018). Advancing mobile learning in Australian healthcare environments: Nursing profession organization perspectives and leadership challenges. *BMC Nursing, 17,* 44.

McHugh, J. P., Zinn, J., Shield, R. R., Tyler, D. A., Gadbois, E. A., Soni, S., & Mor, V. (2020). Strategy and risk sharing in hospital-postacute care integration. *Health Care Management Review, 45*(1), 73–82.

Meskó, B., Drobni, Z., Bėnyei, Ė., Gergely, B., & Györffy, Z. (2017). Digital health is a cultural transformation of traditional healthcare. *mHealth, 3,* 38.

Montgomery, H. E., Haines, A., Marlow, N., Pearson, G., Mythen, M. G., Grocott, M. P. W., & Swanton, C. (2017). The future of UK healthcare: Problems and potential solutions to a system in crisis. *Annals of Oncology, 28*(8), 1751–1755.

Nelson-Brantley, H. V., & Ford, D. J. (2017). Leading change: A concept analysis. *Journal of Advanced Nursing, 73*(4), 834–846.

Podgorski, D., Majchrzycka, K., Dabrowska, A., Gralewicz, G., & Okrasa, M. (2016). Towards a conceptual framework of OSH risk management in Smart Working Environments based on smart PPE, Ambient Intelligence and the Internet of Things technologies. *International Journal of Occupational Safety and Ergonomics, 23*(1), 1–20.

Porter-O'Grady, T. (2013). A new context for service: Healthcare for the 21st century. *American Journal of Maternal Child Nursing, 38*(5), 313–318.

Porter-O'Grady, T., Alexander, D. R., Blaylock, J., Minkara, N., & Surel, D. (2006). Constructing a team model. Creating a foundation for evidence-based teams. *Nursing Administration Quarterly, 30*(3), 211–230.

Stephens, T., Hunningher, A., Mills, H., & Freeth, D. (2016). An interprofessional training course in crises and human factors for perioperative teams. *Journal of Interprofessional Care, 30*(5), 685–688.

Storkholm, M. H., Mazzocato, P., & Savage, C. (2019). Make it complicated: A qualitative study utilizing a complexity framework to explain improvement in health care. *BMC Health Services Research, 19*(1), 842.

St.Pierre, M., Hofinger, G., & Simon, R. (2016). *Crisis management in acute care settings* (3rd ed.). Springer International.

Sturmberg, J. P., & Bircher, J. (2019). Better and fulfilling healthcare at lower costs: The need to manage health systems as complex adaptive systems. *F1000Research, 8,* 789.

Therrien, M. C., Normandin, J. M., & Denis, J. L. (2017). Bridging complexity theory and resilience to develop surge capacity in health systems. *Journal of Health Organization and Management, 31*(1), 96–109.

Tsai, M. H., Sanford, J. A., Black, I. H., Boggs, S. D., & Urman, R. D. (2017). Operating room management at the edge of order and chaos. *The Journal of Medical Practice Management, 32*(4), 250–255.

Turchin, P., Curriec, T. E., Whitehoused, H., François, P., Feeneyg, K., Mullins, D., Hoyer, D., Collins, C., Grohmannd, S., Savaged, P., Mendel-Gleason, G., Turner, E., Dupeyron, A., Cioni, E., Reddish, J., Levine, J., Jordan, G., Brandli, E., Williams, A., . . . Spencer, C. (2018). Quantitative historical analysis uncovers a single dimension of complexity that structures global variation in human social organization. *Proceedings of the National Academy of Sciences of the United States of America, 115*(2), E144–E151.

van Rossum, T. R., Scheele, F., Scherpbier, A. J., Sluiter, H. E., & Heyligers, I. C. (2016). Dealing with the complex dynamics of teaching hospitals. *BMC Medical Education, 16,* 104.

van Wietmarschen, H. H., Wortelboer, H. M., & van der Greef, J. (2018). Grip on health: A complex systems approach to transform health care. *Journal of Evaluation in Clinical Practice, 24*(1), 269–277.

VanVactor, J. D. (Ed.). (2015). *Crisis management. A leadership perspective.* Nova.

Veenema, T. G., Deruggiero, K., Losinski, S., & Barnett, D. (2017). Hospital administration and nursing leadership in disasters: An exploratory study using concept mapping. *Nursing Administration Quarterly, 41*(2), 151–163.

Velthuis, F., Varpio, L., Helmich, E., Dekker, H., & Jaarsma, A. D. C. (2018). Navigating the complexities of undergraduate medical curriculum change: Change leaders' perspectives. *Academic Medicine, 93*(10), 1503–1510.

Zhuravsky, L. (2015). Crisis leadership in an acute clinical setting: Christchurch hospital, New Zealand ICU experience following the February 2011 earthquake. *Prehospital and Disaster Medicine, 30*(2), 131–136.

Suggested Readings

Berstein, J. (2011). *Manager's guide to crisis management.* McGraw-Hill.

Campbell, J. G. (2019). Hospital emergency management: A programming and profession assessment. *Journal of Emergency Management, 17*(5), 349–357.

Chacko, S., Randolph, R., & Morsch, G. (2019). Disaster medicine: Public health preparedness for natural disasters. *FP Essentials, 487*, 17–22.

Crandall, W., Parnell, J., & Spillan, J. (2009). *Crisis management in the new strategy landscape.* Sage.

Fink, S. (2013). *Crisis communications: The definitive guide to managing the message.* McGraw-Hill.

Mitchell, M. (2009). *Complexity: A guided tour.* Oxford University Press.

Sheikhbardsiri, H., Raeisi, A. R., Nekoei-Moghadam, M., & Rezaei, F. (2017). Surge capacity of hospitals in emergencies and disasters with a preparedness approach: A systematic review. *Disaster Medicine and Public Health Preparedness, 11*(5), 612–620.

Wang, B., & Downing, N. L. (2019). A crisis within an epidemic: Critical opioid shortage in US hospitals. *Postgraduate Medicine Journal, 95*(1127), 515–516.

Watkins, M. (2013). *The first 90 days: Proven strategies for getting up to speed faster and smarter.* Harvard Business Review Press.

Quiz Questions

Select the best answer for each of the following questions.

1. Leaders can handle crises if they understand that:
    a. conflict is normative and a fundamental characteristic of human behavior.
    b. an early warning system may provide false cues that should be ignored.
    c. a systematic approach seldom works due to the nature of each event.
    d. each event should be addressed immediately before the crisis actually occurs.

2. Crises in health care are stimulated primarily by:
    a. a cataclysmic event.
    b. natural disasters.
    c. simple human events.
    d. human-made war.

3. Which skills are prerequisites for 21st century leaders dealing with crises:
    a. financial management skills.
    b. adaptive and predictive skills.
    c. those surrounding immediate actions.
    d. day-to-day normative operation skills.

4. Leaders who manage within a crisis mode everyday:
   a. generate workplace energy that stimulates others to work productively.
   b. understand the connection between crisis management and crisis leadership.
   c. help people deal effectively with crisis.
   d. are not prepared for legitimate crisis.

5. Humans shape their organizations by directing interactions related to:
   a. culture and politics.
   b. finance and collaboration with other healthcare centers.
   c. technology and products.
   d. peaceful co-existence rather than conflict.

6. During crises, understanding complexity enables leaders to:
   a. understand that they cannot control direction—they must set autonomy aside.
   b. focus on using today's technology rather than innovations.
   c. distance themselves from non-crisis decision-making.
   d. control variables affecting human interaction.

7. Which of the following statements is correct?
   a. The higher the complexity of an organization, the fewer crises they may experience.
   b. The higher the complexity within organizations, the higher the intensity of potential crisis.
   c. The lower the complexity of an organization, the less likely it needs to adapt to crisis.
   d. The lower the complexity within organizations, the easier it is to manage change.

8. Effectively managing change means:
   a. leaders focus on creating internally adaptive environments and forgo focusing on external environments.
   b. leaders focus on creating externally adaptive environments and forget to focus on internal environments.
   c. leaders create an internally and externally adaptive environment.
   d. leaders adapt to crises as they arise, as it is impossible to plan for an adaptive environment.

9. Adaptation to change involves:
   a. being willing to alter routines.
   b. maintaining historical rituals.
   c. maintaining previous communication channels.
   d. being willing to alter the patient experience.

10. Broad-based social, political, and economic shifts that are immediate and create crisis often have a:
    a. longer response time.
    b. low level of risk that doesn't affect normal work.
    c. need for nonsustainable responses.
    d. shortened response time.

11. In adaptive organizations, workers understand that:
    a. ritual is normative.
    b. change is ever-present.
    c. process activities are constant.
    d. stability is expected.

12. To thrive in crises, leaders should:
    a. avoid surprises that could affect the organization.
    b. hold off on using strategic tools that may not lead to recovery.
    c. develop resources to adapt to crisis, not just react to it.
    d. anticipate new factors that might affect the organization's work.

13. The vitality and viability of a team's work is based on:
    a. awareness of external events outside the focus of the team's control.
    b. awareness of internal circumstances directly affecting the team's performance.
    c. function and action by team members.
    d. high-quality outcomes of the team's activities.

14. Which of the following statements about team performance is *false*?
    a. An effective team will handle crisis encounters better than one that lacks integration.
    b. The efficacy of team interactions is critical to smooth functioning of the team.
    c. Team members who work well with others can be effective despite lacking other qualities.
    d. Team flexibility is limited when members are ineffective in communicating competently.

15. Which of the following options reflects a "team outcome"?
    a. Effectiveness in completing practice expectations
    b. Achievement of a goal
    c. Development of a deliverable team
    d. Competency in team-driven processes

16. When confronting crisis events, good process infrastructure:
    a. does not necessarily relate to goals and objectives.
    b. can create chaotic activities initially.
    c. is not related to stability and a solid frame of reference.
    d. gives direction and meaning to individual work.

17. During crisis, competence is an important process factor because:
    a. issues of competence are minimized during critical moments.
    b. it is heightened as long as leaders provide direction.
    c. it is usually missing and, therefore, effective work is minimized.
    d. lapses in identifying and managing issues of competence may compromise work.

18. A cybernetic model for responding to crisis:
    a. is intermittently rigid and flexible based on needs.
    b. has processes that are cyclical/continuously fluid.
    c. is stagnant due to uncertain times.
    d. has intermittent processes that can be quickly revised as needed.

19. Which statement best represents a strong service core?
    a. Encouraging business opportunities that may alter the mission.
    b. Understanding that business ventures need to be disciplined with mission and purpose.
    c. Facilitating innovative options that can take the organization down a new path and purpose.
    d. Affirming that work that is not aligned with vision and values is important if it has meaning to workers.

20. Contemporary chaos and complexity theory characterizes complex human systems and organizations as:
    a. self-organizing and spontaneous.
    b. predictable and deterministic.
    c. stable and ordered.
    d. systematic and controlled.

21. Which of the following does *not* refer to leaders' roles in "triggers" of imminent change?
    a. Read signals
    b. Draw inferences from signals
    c. Revise work group dynamics
    d. Determine the potential impact on the organization

22. Strategic environmental scanning providers leaders with:
    a. tools and processes to predict essential change.
    b. reinforcements without the need to stay current with systems changes.
    c. diverse innovations that can improve circumstances.
    d. honest feedback about process work and employee challenges.

23. The degree and specificity of future change can be determined by:
    a. shifts in political power in the U.S. Senate.
    b. noticing a lack of emerging technology.
    c. shifts in economics related to healthcare reimbursement.
    d. noticing that there is stability in work conditions.

24. To ensure sufficiency in adaptation, prediction, and response, leaders must help their stakeholders assess:
    a. local trends.
    b. critical environmental changes.
    c. outdated technology.
    d. nonessential work conditions.

25. A solid crisis preparedness plan must address all *but*:
    a. strategic changes.
    b. service crises.
    c. operational changes
    d. personal unrest.

CHAPTER EIGHT

The Focused Leader: Embracing Vulnerability, Risk Taking, and the Potential to Succeed

Take comfort in the notion that we have never been in control!
—*Anonymous*

Evolved people respect differing views, understanding that life's meaning is to be found everywhere. They are open, always learning and growing. An evolved person knows that there is only one truth, but many different ways of seeing it.
—*Lance Secretan*[1]

Chapter Objectives

At the completion of this chapter, the reader will be able to:

- Understand vulnerability as a positive leadership trait.
- Identify four essential relationship skills that support vulnerable leadership.
- Discuss the process of complexity communication.
- Evaluate open communication as a means of improving leadership expertise.
- Critique vulnerable leadership as a moral imperative.

I don't have all the answers; am I a failure? Traditional organizations hold leaders to standards of rationality, clarity, and foresight—yet most leaders cannot meet these standards because they are human and face an incredible amount of unpredictability and fallible analyses of data. To be able to prosper and thrive in the current millennium, the leader must shift from the somewhat comfortable position of control to one of great uncertainty and vulnerability. In reality, uncertainty and need for vulnerability have always existed for leaders. With the current explosion of information technology and availability of information, leading using command-and-control behaviors, where power and decision-making is held by a few people at the top, is no longer adequate when team effectiveness requires their engagement in decision making. To be sure, no leader is alone on this journey.

---

[1] Reprinted by permission of Dr. Lance Secretan.

CHAPTER EIGHT The Focused Leader: Embracing Vulnerability, Risk Taking, and the Potential to Succeed

The importance of focus on the work at hand has never been greater in light of the increased activities and need to become more vulnerable and open to uncertainty as a way of leading. According to Goleman (2015), managing our distractions instead of letting them manage us can lead to increased focus using a mindfulness approach. This chapter discusses the nature, processes, and strategies to embrace vulnerability. As always, it is important to recognize the interconnectedness of the multiple aspects of emotional and cognitive leadership behaviors.

Leaders of postmillennium quantum organizations must facilitate the activities of organizations effectively in an environment in which control and direction are uncertain. They must be mindful of the idea that uncertainty is the norm and that one cannot know everything there is to know. They must be willing to take risks, recognize that their colleagues come from a wide range of backgrounds and experiences, and realize that they will never obtain a complete picture, no matter how accomplished their communication with others. Finally, they must use new strategies based on vulnerability principles if they are to succeed in facilitating a healthcare system that is effective.

In the Industrial Age, leaders were expected to be in control. Whether chief executive officers or case managers, they were viewed as being in charge and in possession of the information that consumers and employees wanted and needed. According to the classical theories of management, good leaders knew everything and could do everything better than anyone else. They held all the information necessary for operating the organization, and shared this information with employees only when appropriate.

Today things are much different. Information is currently available to the masses and in great quantities, minimizing any leader's potential for being in control of anything. Furthermore, all leaders have limitations, and as they move through the chaos of the transition into the Information Age, they typically experience feelings of defenselessness, inadequacy, and fear, leading to disengagement and a search for courage. Leaders, to act with vigor in this time of great uncertainty, can stop protecting themselves from being vulnerable and engage in their vulnerability to lead more effectively.

Leadership Fitness in the New Millennium

The leadership fitness profile is very different from the leadership role of the past, which was basically one of command and control. In the new millennium, leaders find themselves in an environment of great uncertainty, and to navigate in this environment they need to be comfortable with taking risks, being vulnerable, and stretching the boundaries of current thinking and current practices. They also need to coach employees to develop the same performance characteristics. Engaging the staff to work collectively to interpret the events of change in a way that makes sense of them is essential for success.

Vulnerability, risk taking, and stretching are required for several reasons. First, the present is very different from the past, and the skills that will be needed in the coming age, the Information Age, are very different from those needed in the Industrial Age. Past practices of bureaucratic command and control cannot be assumed to be effective in a new environment in which the distribution of knowledge has been radically altered and the skills needed to manage the

> **Point to Ponder**
>
> Becoming vulnerable is a growth process—a process without a roadmap—yet one that opens up endless opportunities.

environment are undeveloped. The quantum leader, besides exemplifying the spirit of incompleteness, must shift from managing content to guiding process and outcome over and over again until order finally emerges.

Second, the leaders of the healthcare professions need to maintain a focus on creating a new framework for each profession, a framework that allows them to understand and create the future rather than sustain the past. As part of this process, they need to scrutinize the relationships between the professions, examine the specific services provided by each profession, and assess the value of these services in the marketplace. The services that add value will be retained, and those that do not will be eliminated.

> ### Group Discussion
> Compare the behaviors of classical management and those of vulnerability leadership. Examine the practices of coaching, facilitating teams, building relationships, and empowering others in each model.

Vulnerability

In the Industrial Age, vulnerability in a leader was seen as a weakness. Indeed, the word *vulnerability* tends to conjure the idea of susceptibility to physical or emotional injury or to corrupt influence. This type of vulnerability is very different from the type required of leaders in the Information Age. The essence of *vulnerability*, as the term is used in this text, is openness to others and to new ideas (**Exhibit 8-1**). It encompasses being able to do the following:

- Examine long-held beliefs and change one's mind without feelings of inadequacy.
- Recognize personal limitations and strengths.
- Work from a clearly defined personal identity.

Vulnerable leaders know and show their limits, whether these pertain to knowledge or to abilities. Rather than work beyond their limits, they allow people with the right kind of aptitude to assume responsibility for particular tasks. According to their mindset, their role is to create the conditions that allow employees to make their maximum contribution and simultaneously enjoy their work.

Exhibit 8-1 Leadership Vulnerability

Facilitators	**Barriers**
• Openness to new ideas	• Aloofness, arrogance
• Recognition of personal limitations	• Egotistical
• Feelings of adequacy	• Fear of losing control
• Self-awareness of strengths and weaknesses	• Fear of discovery
• Absence of ego	• Believed immunity to anxiety, fatigue, illness, and overwork
• Trust in others	
• Courage	• Perfection

Leadership vulnerability is not about weakness or incompetence. Team members and colleagues do not want leaders to be weak, ailing, or whining. They look for strength and self-confidence, but the kind of self-confidence that permits someone to share his or her limitations and not maintain a stance of immunity to anxiety, fatigue, or doubt. Leadership vulnerability is also about creating conditions that encourage safe and healthy dialogue as the way to do business.

In contrast, leaders who act out of a sense of invulnerability tend to be aloof, separate themselves from those they lead, and avoid making time for the meaningful discussion of complex issues. Their purpose in behaving in this manner is to keep control over situations and to abstain from dialogue that might lead to the revision of their chosen courses of action. Charisma, too, is suspect. There is a dark side of charisma that requires attention. Chamorro-Premuzic (2012), in *Harvard Business Review*, noted that the short-term effects of this type of leadership or charm serve to engage people; however, in the long term there are four significant downsides:

- Charisma dilutes judgment.
- Charisma is addictive.
- Charisma disguises psychopaths.
- Charisma fosters collective narcissism.

The traits and behaviors associated with invulnerability play a big role in protecting leaders' sense of control. Traditionally, leaders have feared not just losing control but also being found out. They have worried that others would discover that they are not what they seem to be, that they do not have all the answers to all the questions. Quantum leadership, on the other hand, is about the absence of ego. Quantum leaders seek exposure of their limitations as a means of improving organizational performance. According to Torbert (2000), vulnerability is paradoxically powerful. When power is exercised by a leader who remains vulnerable or open to transformation, the result is voluntary transformation in others rather than mere external conformity and compliance (or resistance). In addition, there is no point in fearing discovery or losing control because in reality no one is really in control. Relationships in a quantum organization are based on three principles:

> **Key Point**
>
> Quantum leadership is about the absence of ego, not its presence.

1. Power is a pluralist, not an elitist, commodity.
2. Diversity of knowledge, individuals, social status, and so forth is essential.
3. Personal boundaries must be clearly defined.

These principles provide the framework for developing new and more effective relationships.

Power

The notion of power has both positive and negative connotations and often produces feelings of ambivalence. Further, because power is associated with the conflicting ideas of strength, influence, coercion, and dominance, it is both difficult to understand and to use. Yet as we move into the Information Age, leaders must comprehend the nature of power and use it effectively to enhance their relationships.

First, quantum leaders consider the quantity of power to be infinite, and thus conclude that sufficient power is generally available for all individuals to exert influence, mobilize resources, and meet their goals. They view power as located in each person, not centralized in an elite group, and they treat the legitimate exercise of power as a right that belongs to everyone. These beliefs are most clearly reflected in a complexity leadership model (Uhl-Bein & Marion, 2008).

In a traditional organization, power is concentrated at the top of the hierarchical pyramid, and work is compartmentalized and controlled from that central point. The organizational power structure always benefits some at the expense of others. If anything, revisions of the structure tend to enhance the power of those who have it. In other words, leaders seldom design themselves out of a position.

> **Point to Ponder**
>
> Knowledge really is power. Intellect is a gift, but learning is hard work.

Recent notions about power recognize the impact of technology and new generational thinking (Heimans & Timms, 2014). New power, according to Heimans and Timms (2014), embraces participation of engaged peers as the driving force for the shift of power in organizations. New power is held by many, and the goal is to channel it instead of hoarding it. Old power is held by few, is inaccessible to most, and the goal is to control. The shift is from old power to new power. In old power, the focus is on consuming goods or services in the marketplace without expecting consumer involvement to develop or improve the goods or services. New power is an evolving six-stage process in which (1) consuming the good or service is followed by (2) sharing with others to gain additional content, (3) shaping the content to

---

Group Discussion

The new power model emerging reflects the advantages of peer coordination and the agency of the crowd. The importance of participation in the change and innovation processes to the under-30 generation who make up half of the world's population is evident in such innovations as Lyft, LinkedIn, and Airbnb. These innovations move from merely consuming a product or service to sharing the content (transparency), shaping or reshaping the product with new ideas, crowd funding, producing the product, and co-owning the product.

Numerous areas in health care could benefit from thinking and acting in the new power model. As group, consider one of the following situations: management of educational materials, device management, or management of union contracts. Your group may also come up with its own situation.

- What would occur at each of the six stages of the new power model?
- What are the sources of support for this change?
- What are the obstacles to this change?
- What should be the next steps with this knowledge?

Source: Heimans, J., & Timms, H. (2014). Understanding "new power." *Harvard Business Review*. https://hbr.org/product/understanding-new-power/R1412B-PDF-ENG

reflect additional ideas, (4) funding similar to crowd funding, (5) producing content, and (6) finally co-owning the content. A dramatic shift from the control of old power to the fluidity of new power best matches the current realities and opportunities in health care in many ways.

In a quantum organization, the response to centralization is not decentralization but uncentralization. Uncentralization, unlike decentralization, does not attempt to preserve hierarchical workways by subdividing and parceling out the work while hanging on to central control through the use of more and more creative accounting systems. The new organizational structure is fluid and flexible, allowing easy rearrangement of work groups to meet point-of-service needs.

To be sure, there are differing power and communication realities among organizations. In some the style of leadership is more informal and collegial, whereas in others recommendations mostly go up and orders mostly come down. The intent, however, is the same: to minimize bureaucratic control and the concentration of power and to maximize involvement while still getting the work done.

The point is not to create "nobody in charge" systems. Yet regardless of how the leadership power transition occurs, some leaders experience real or perceived threats to their power, and their instinct for self-preservation may override their concern for organizational goals.

In many cases, employees who have high expectations of leaders are quickly disillusioned by the leaders' perceived failure to meet their expectations. In fact, traditional employees discourage leaders from becoming vulnerable. This means that leaders not only must change their own mindset but also must create the conditions for employees to adapt to the new culture. As the necessary changes proceed, the resulting battles for survival are likely to cause organizational confusion and even chaos.

Authenticity Is the Key

Leadership is often described as transactional, transformation, or complexity (Gill, 2011). It is interesting to note that there is no single accepted definition or theory of leadership, nor is there an agreed paradigm for the study and practice of leadership. According to Kurtsman (2010), there is no consensus on what leadership is, how leaders develop, or how to become a more efficient leader. Despite this lack of consensus, leaders must continually ensure that their efforts facilitate meeting the needs of the organization and provide value to the stakeholders. At times leaders unknowingly adopt one style of leadership in the hopes that it will serve the entire organization when in fact the chosen theory or model may address only one aspect of leadership. No one style, however, is absolute or appropriate for all situations. This plethora of leader styles can be daunting for the emerging leader. Formal monitoring programs provide guidance and recommendations to support role development. Yet conforming to the normative leadership style of the organization or the recent literature recommendation can spell disaster for the leader. According to George (2004), great world leaders all had very different leadership styles—George Washington, Winston Churchill, Margaret Thatcher, Mother Teresa, and John F. Kennedy all led in their own unique way.

In reality, the success of the leader is more closely linked to personal authenticity, self-awareness, and genuineness than to a particular leadership style. The leader's authenticity—not the leadership style—really matters. Attempting to emulate another's leadership style can be disastrous. New leaders may desire a model of shared leadership but must understand and live the basic values in their personal lives to make shared leadership a reality. A lack of congruence between personal and professional values creates a reality gap that is obvious to team members. This gap compromises leader authenticity because the leader talks the talk of shared leadership but is unable to fully live the values consistently.

The values of the authentic leader are shaped by personal beliefs and developed through study, reflection, and dialogue with others. These values create a moral compass for the leader and provide guidance in determining the right thing to do rather than blindly attempting to emulate the style of another leader.

A broad understanding of leadership styles serves merely as background information to understanding behavior options. Being one's own person is the key to developing an authentic leadership style that is consistent with one's personality and character. Ongoing development of the leader's personal leadership style continues as the leader encounters different situations and different people.

The authentic leader accepts personal faults as well as strengths and avoids attempting to win approval of others by covering up shortcomings and thus sacrificing authenticity to gain respect from others. There is no way a leader can do everything—be on top of the incoming mail, read the most recent literature, and be responsive to everything and everyone. Attempting to be such a leader is foolhardy. According to Lencioni (2012), vulnerability is essential for building trust and requires behaviors that reflect caring about others and their success. The authentic, vulnerable leader knows what he or she knows and what he or she does not know and is content with the limits of his or her capacity. Authentic leaders demonstrate how shifting from individual skill to collective skill unlocks a group's ability to perform by sharing vulnerability (Coyle, 2018).

Integrity is closely linked to authenticity for the effective leader. In addition to personal authenticity, the vulnerable leader exhibits integrity, a characteristic that is not just the absence of lying but the presence of telling the whole truth, no matter how difficult it might be. Leadership integrity is the uncompromising adherence to moral and ethical principles. From authenticity and integrity, trusting relationships emerge.

The Cycle of Vulnerability

Learning to live and thrive in vulnerability is a lifelong journey. It is often a circuitous journey, reversing on itself and then moving forward. Learning to live and thrive in vulnerability evolves through eight stages (**Exhibit 8-2**), which interact in a cyclical process (**Figure 8-1**).

Exhibit 8-2 The Eight Stages of the Cycle of Vulnerability

1. Become vulnerable and open to new ideas. Recognize and value uncertainty.
2. Choose to take risks that challenge the status quo.
3. Stretch organizational capability by stimulating the latent potential of employees.
4. Live the new capacity.
5. Evaluate the outcomes.
6. Course correct as needed.
7. Cherish the resulting new knowledge.
8. Begin the cycle again.

CHAPTER EIGHT The Focused Leader: Embracing Vulnerability, Risk Taking, and the Potential to Succeed

Figure 8-1 The Cycle of Vulnerability.

Becoming Vulnerable

The first stage in the cycle involves recognizing the value of being vulnerable. You need only enroll in a computer class with a teenager to discover the value of vulnerability—the value of being open to receiving new ideas about how to use a computer. By admitting you are uncertain and not all-knowing, by being willing to put aside long-standing mental models, you open yourself to the possibility of incredible growth and rewards.

Frustration and fear typically fuel the search for certainty, a search that wastes significant time and effort. In any organization, situations and relationships are usually too complex to be predictable, and therefore a degree of uncertainty is unavoidable. If fear of the unknown is allowed to rule, the result is organizational inertia and continued reliance on past practices. Despite believing in the need for change or in the savings to be gained from a new technology, leaders place too much emphasis on the failure of past innovations and sit back and do nothing.

Employees, as well as leaders, long for certainty. Formerly, securing a position in an organization meant getting employment for a lifetime. This is no longer true. As organizations face more challenges than ever before, employees face more uncertainty, particularly about the security of their jobs. As a consequence, they experience additional stress as well as feelings of isolation. In struggling to find a new vision, they become frustrated and often panic. What they should do instead is learn to tolerate and respect the discomfort of their uncertainty and thereby unleash their creativity in the interests of organizational change.

Quantum leaders give up the quest for certainty and discover the benefits of admitting fallibility. One benefit is that leaders can expend their efforts in designing the future rather than becoming petrified by feelings of panic and loss of control. After all, leaders never have possessed a crystal ball capable of predicting the future. Leadership judgment is called judgment because certainty is missing. Besides judgment, what leaders can use is creativity. To do this, though, they need time for thinking, for designing the future. Unfortunately, many leaders deny they have any extra time. Most believe they are working at their highest level of productivity and are unable to fit in additional work, especially if it is merely inventive headwork.

The common occurrence of unpredictable challenges places significant demands on leader creativity and imagination. Striving to understand and mediate uncertainty is the most appropriate and logical approach for leaders rather than working to eliminate variety and hope for stability. Working to achieve stability is irrational given the complex nature of healthcare work. According to Weick and Sutcliffe (2001) and Sutcliffe (2011), recognizing the complex nature of organizations, detecting incredibly weak warning signs, and taking strong decisive action when appropriate are the hallmarks of a high-reliability organization (HRO). HROs have gained credence for their ability to become highly reliable in minimizing errors and thereby increasing patient safety. In addition, HROs have achieved greater stakeholder engagement, time savings, and cost efficiency. These organizations demonstrate the ability to build effective practices and identify unexpected events early on and then respond to these unexpected events in ways that are adaptive rather than destructive. Leaders of HROs thrive in vulnerability, identify different approaches to issues, demonstrate resilience, and take risks in addressing situations in nontraditional ways.

The reality is that their organizations suffer severely unless they make the time to engage in creative thinking—deferring to collective expertise instead of individual expertise. In some cases, new employees have the extra time and energy to explore possible innovations and reforms. More often, the necessary time can be found by building in systems that focus on what is not working or has potential to fail (i.e., that fail to make a difference in patient care) and correct them. The time formerly spent on unnecessary tasks or workarounds can then be used to think creatively and work toward constructing a vision of the future.

Taking Risks

The second stage requires leaders to begin to take risks. Much like vulnerability, risk taking is not viewed as a classical leadership behavior and is rarely welcomed or encouraged. Instead, it is seen as increasing the organization's exposure to unforeseen hazards and to the loss of net income.

> ### Group Discussion
>
> Taking risks is avoided all too often. Fear of speaking one's mind, sharing a controversial position, or discussing negative patient events are often framed as "appropriate" behaviors. In light of the negative fantasies of losing one's job—it seldom occurs—identify at least three times you would have liked to share information or ideas but did not for fear of negative feedback. Discuss the issues and identify what really might have happened. Then do the unthinkable, share your ideas with the person you wanted to share them with—what happened? What can you learn from this process of checking out risk-taking fears?

Classical leadership behavior encompasses strategic planning and the purposeful review of ideas. This plan provides organizational direction in order for individuals to make decisions on the fly, which might seem risky. However, the ability of an organization to navigate a complex landscape and one that is full of uncertainty requires risk, and individuals need the knowledge that they are safe to take risks because others share the risk with them. Shared risk requires the democratization of knowledge where no one individual holds all the knowledge, all individuals and disciplines bring unique abilities to a team, and each must be willing to take risks to rapidly pool their knowledge and abilities to solve problems and advance a strategic direction. These same individuals interact enough to know each other's abilities, discuss improvements and failures, and seek alternative perspectives and ideas. When this occurs, risk really doesn't feel like risk, it is the norm. Too often leaders are reluctant to express ideas for fear of retaliation or rejection. The fear comes when the leader has feared risk because of the unknown consequence. Engagement of risk is essential to confronting challenge and advancing innovation, and replacing leader reluctance or fear with engagement in the vulnerability that comes with risk is essential in complex environments such as health care. Leaders must become willing and proficient in sharing opinions and assessments, communicating with the media and others external to the organization, and providing feedback when negative events occur. Leaders must not only develop competence in these three areas, they must become experts and resources for those with whom they work.

Efforts by quantum leaders to reverse the practices of institutionally imposed powerlessness, which expects nurses not to assert themselves individually or collectively, will continue the journey to optimal authenticity. Overcoming this silence leads to increased personal authenticity and greater public awareness of the importance of the role of nurses and all other healthcare professionals and safer patient care. As greater personal and professional authenticity emerges, feelings of low self-esteem, powerlessness, and lack of collegial support can only decrease. Reversing the spiral of silence begins with regular discussions of situations within the three key situations that identify specific events in which silence negatively affects open and honest communication.

Organizational structures that focus on improvement by individuals providing patient care sets the context to learn how to take risks because it involves making small changes to transform existing practices and business models. Expertise plus the expectation for improvement enables small groups of clinicians to make changes with big goals in mind and to evaluate the changes efficiently. In addition, the clinicians' skills are stretched with little risk to the organization. Support for constant improvement minimizes the chance that the organization will drift into inertia. Risk becomes the norm, change is internalized as essential for survival, and employees gain new experiences and develop new skills.

> **Key Point**
> Leadership judgment is called judgment because certainty is missing.

Embedded in improvement processes is the expectation that leaders routinely challenge the status quo—indeed, seriously challenge it, which means not asking questions out of idle curiosity but looking carefully at current dogma and raising issues that open the door to transformation. For quantum leaders, examining the work of their organizations is not a meaningless exercise but is intended to guarantee accountability and make certain that all work is value producing. Asking the unaskable questions about structure, principles, and customs requires an ease with vulnerability and an openness to and passion for new realities (**Exhibit 8-3**).

When leaders ask the unaskable, they are ostensibly inviting employees to mention the unmentionable, which the employees can perceive as very risky, especially when the leaders' body language says, "Do not raise difficult issues." Brusque or otherwise unwelcoming behavior must be replaced with genuine openness so that the employees feel safe and the inquiry into problems can be fruitful and lead to growth. Although decisions made under conditions of incomplete information sometimes fail to have a positive outcome, leaders must be willing

---

Exhibit 8-3 Risk Taking

- Encourages creativity
- Supports improvement
- Requires continuous evaluation
- Allows for mistakes
- Requires vulnerability
- Requires resiliency
- Is required of leaders
- Is inconsistent with classical leadership behaviors

---

to risk changing course if there are good reasons to do so. No one knows the future for certain, as shown by the many mispredictions perpetrated by supposed experts. (Perhaps none is more famous than the implicit prediction regarding the future course of movies that was contained in the question asked by Warner Brothers in 1927: Who the heck wants to hear actors talk?)

Some risky decisions have paid off well. Consider the cash register, which was introduced in the late 19th century by Patterson as a help in cash management and as a means of double-checking the honesty of sales clerks. Patterson took an incredible risk in challenging the status quo, and indeed at first everybody resented the product. Owners, for example, refused to have this "thief catcher" in their stores. Patterson had to use great leadership skills to convince others to accept his idea and to motivate his salesforce to sell the product. Today, of course, no store is without one.

The role of the leader is to inspire creativity and hard work and to challenge the past as prologue, recognizing that the past is past. The work of inspiration requires not just inspirational phrases but inspirational behavior. Risk-disposed leaders encourage others by showing what can be done, not merely by sermonizing about opportunities. They also need to exhibit candor and vulnerability, to identify value in marginally successful efforts, and to allow others to take risks and experience success and failure.

Risk-disposed leaders develop a very high level of self-discipline that allows the processes of risk taking to evolve. A strong sense of commitment can be more valuable than intelligence, education, luck, or talent. Leaders adept at taking risks neither surrender nor overreact to crises or marginally successful efforts; they regroup and return. They take stock of the situation, often pulling back temporarily (but not too long) while they plan the next steps. They realize that sometimes it is best to put aside personal feelings and let bygones be bygones. Finally, they focus on the present and the future, both of which offer perils and possibilities, rather than on the past, about which nothing can be done.

Resiliency is the key. Leaders must be resilient to manage the uncertainty and inherent risks that are features of the leadership role. They must act with confidence, purpose, and enthusiasm rather than hesitation and self-doubt. To manage risks through resiliency, they must apply determination and energy, inspiring those around them at the same time.

Rational Risks and Negative Fantasies

Negative fantasies often cause leaders to become paralyzed or reluctant to take risks. In reality there is little, if any, chance for such fantasies to be realized. Perhaps the most common negative fantasy in health care is the perception that one will be fired for taking risks and speaking

CHAPTER EIGHT The Focused Leader: Embracing Vulnerability, Risk Taking, and the Potential to Succeed

> ### Group Discussion
>
> The 3D printer provides innovative products and challenges many of our current assumptions. In a recent TED Talk, Dr. Anthony Atala describes the printing of a human kidney (http://ed.ted.com/lessons/printing-a-human-kidney-anthony-atala). Review the TED Talk. Given these advances, discuss the implications of this new technology as it relates to healthcare services. Consider the impact of 3D printing of kidneys on the following:
>
> - The need for dialysis units
> - The need for transplant facilities
> - Required skills of healthcare professionals
> - The cost of health care
> - Any other ideas that could emerge from this technology

up. Individuals often worry that speaking up will have a negative outcome on their reputation, their ability to communicate openly and honestly with others, and, ultimately, the security of their position. Leaders can minimize negative fantasies through discussion with colleagues and clarification of the issue and its importance. Further, leaders can examine the issue and determine whether indeed there is rational risk involved.

The four areas in which risk is considered rational are (1) advancing the organization, (2) developing skills, (3) mandatory reporting, and (4) whistleblowing (Porter-O'Grady & Malloch, 2018). Each risk serves a different purpose:

1. *Advancing the organization:* Every organization strives not only to survive but also to thrive in the best way possible. To ensure contemporary services, the leadership team evaluates numerous programs, systems, technology advances, and products. Leaders are routinely faced with choices about clinical programs, initiation and expansion of new services, hiring, firing, selecting equipment, and prioritizing which issues are addressed and which issues wait for attention. Choices that are rational and minimize risk are those choices that are made on the basis of core values, respect for others, the safety of individuals, strategic goals of the organization, and available resources.
2. *Developing skills:* All individuals need new skills to continue to exist in the ever-changing environment. Acquiring new knowledge and skills is considered a rational risk when those skills are needed to improve job performance or for other available opportunities. Considerations should be given to personal physical capability, resources, and family obligations to support rational risk taking. Examples include developing skills in computer programs, public speaking, sports, creative arts, and personal protection.
3. *Mandatory reporting:* Many state licensing agencies require licensees to report to the licensing board the unprofessional conduct of other licensees. Protecting the public from licensees who commit repeated errors, abuse alcohol or drug substances, and/or are incompetent to do the work often requires professionals to identify issues and take risks to speak up and address the situation. This

action is not an option in many states and requires collegial support to meet this expectation. Examples include unprofessional conduct, repeated medication errors, boundary violations, and theft from patients. Mandatory reporting is a rational risk required by statute.

4. *Whistleblowing:* Whistleblowing is about righting a wrong—a wrong that is believed to be deceitful or that results in the mistreatment of others. To be sure, the need for whistleblower protection arises when the culture of the organization does not support open communication, differing opinions, and rational risk taking. Individuals believe they have not been heard on an issue or believe the public interest is compromised and there is danger to the public or the environment. The intent of the federal whistleblower act, also known as the False Claims Act, is to combat fraud and corruption and to protect those who exposed information from wrongful dismissal, allowing for reinstatement with seniority, double back pay, interest on back pay, compensation for discriminatory treatment, and reasonable legal fees. Although the whistleblower legislation is present, this approach is considered a rational risk and involves personal and professional risk regardless of the outcome.

The influence of the workplace on ethical or principled practices is significant because it may render the leader vulnerable to conflicting peer opinion, loss of colleague approval, physician conflict, and patient dissatisfaction. More often than not, leaders risk changing their relationships and reputation in creating and sustaining an ethical climate. Many organizational cultures discourage employees from challenging or disagreeing with others and label such behaviors as negative and disruptive. A culture of trust and openness, in which employees are encouraged and expected to identify and confront ethical dilemmas as a team, often requires risk taking to make the best decisions and simultaneously value employees.

Employees who participate in decision making and have access to the information necessary to make informed decisions are empowered and contribute significantly to organizational performance. A culture that fosters and reinforces the value of risk-taking behaviors is an essential characteristic of a high-performing organization. The following questions should be considered to ensure ethical decisions are made:

- Is the action under consideration legal?
- Is the action consistent with organizational policies and guidelines? If not, should a policy be developed or modified?
- Is the action consistent with organizational values?
- Am I personally okay with the proposed action?
- Would I be satisfied if someone took this action with me?
- Would the most ethical person I know do the same thing?

Determining when to take a risk is seldom straightforward and linear. Learning to fly an airplane is steeped in risk but is also supported by extensive safety processes. In addition to one's personal comfort and competence with risk taking, the context in which the risk is taking place can be either supportive or not supportive. The same risk may be viewed and managed quite differently in different organizations, with some viewing it as positive and others viewing it as negative and disruptive. Leaders are encouraged to assess their perceptions of risk taking and risk takers and work to create a culture that is open, trusting, and supportive of new ideas.

Stretching One's Capability

In the third stage of the vulnerability cycle, the leader of an organization works to stretch one's personal capability for actions. In doing this, the leader looks for new and untapped potential. Typically, this potential lies within the organization. For example, new and long-standing employees in continuing education programs represent two main sources of serviceable potential.

Despite the chaos and uncertainty in organizational operations, quantum leaders learn to mitigate and overcome their reluctance to implement new processes in the face of economic downturns and perceived dangers, including the threat of failure. This is not to say that the dangers are not real. Yet there are also serious dangers that arise when an organization fails to adapt to the changes in its environment or undergoes unmanaged change.

Risk taking serves to stretch one's capabilities. Indeed, overcoming risks by facilitating the potential of the members of the organization should become the new golden rule. The best strategy is to put new ideas out into the open and begin to design new services and products once thought unattainable. By sharing the uncertainty, leaders can increase the level of trust in the organization and strengthen the social connections, thereby raising the levels of reciprocity, information flow, collective action, happiness, and wealth.

Kellner-Rogers (1999) stated that a complex web of relationships and creating meaning characterizes all living systems, including organizations, gangs, families, and political movements. This web is not describable using neat organizational charts or flow diagrams. Even more important, it cannot be used to predict outcomes. The relationships that make up a living system display an incredible capacity for engaging in sophisticated coordinated behaviors. These behaviors, however, are seldom the result of directive leadership, strategic plans, or engineered solutions but instead usually occur when the conditions that support risk taking and creative stretching are present. In short, they emerge to the degree that the members of the organization are open, vulnerable, and willing to take risks.

Capra (1982) described the emergence of coordinated behaviors using the analogy of chemical combination. Sugar is made up of three atoms: oxygen, hydrogen, and carbon. Where is the sweetness? The sweetness is in the relationship between the atoms. It is not a quality of any of them individually but emerges in the molecule as a whole. Likewise, when vulnerability, risk taking, and stretching enrich the communal capacity of individuals, behaviors that produce positive results emerge more frequently.

In fact, less than optimal results often lead to a new and better order, as shown by the following story. In a Midwestern village at the end of the 19th century, a common orchard was used by all of the villagers to feed their livestock. Over time the villagers, despite working diligently, went bankrupt and even faced starvation. What happened? Before the collapse, each villager had thought, "The more livestock I have, the better off I will be. The feeding is free, so I will increase my herd as fast as I can." The number of livestock grazing in the orchard increased so rapidly, however, that the grass was soon depleted and the trees died. The livestock began to starve and the village faced destruction. The main problem was that the villagers all engaged in the same behavior without awareness of their interdependence and of the impact of their behavior on the village as a whole. It was by experiencing the dire outcome of their actions that the villagers were able to recognize their interdependence and to gain the power to reverse the course of events.

Living the New Capacity

The fourth step is living the new reality. Living the new reality is about trial and error, about learning what works and what does not work. Once a new path has been identified, the leader,

Group Discussion

As described in the text, at the end of the 19th century a common orchard was used to graze livestock by everyone in a small Midwestern village. Because the feed was free, everyone felt the temptation to add animals to their herd. Eventually, after a rapid increase in the total number of livestock, the grass became depleted, the trees died, the livestock starved, and the villagers went bankrupt. Obviously, new rules were needed. Who should create the new rules for use of the orchard? What strategies would you recommend to correct the situation and make the village prosperous again? How should the strategies be evaluated? What is the relevance of this case history to the role of leadership in the transition from the Industrial Age to the Information Age? Identify at least two scenarios in your organization that bear some resemblance to the case history and critique how the main issues were managed.

along with the team members, supports the unfolding of additional capacity (new work processes or services). Ideas become reality by being applied by the organization on a trial basis. For the organizational leader, living the new reality involves the following:

- Allowing the new work processes (or services) to become integrated into the system through pilot programs of tests of change
- Determining the fit between the processes and the stakeholders (patients, employees, and the entire organization)
- Accepting that unanticipated outcomes will occur, both positive and negative
- Coaching others to sustain the new knowledge
- Supporting vulnerable behaviors
- Role-modeling desired behaviors to enhance mutual trust

During this phase of the cycle, the leader and team might easily lose sight of the original purpose. The tendency is for them to become so anxious and pressured for success that they do not always examine the new processes carefully enough to determine the full range of their effects. The goal here is not to ensure the success of the new processes but to allow them to fully emerge and become integrated into the system to evaluate their goodness-of-fit (i.e., their advantages and disadvantages for the organization, the employees, and the patients).

The leader and the team must allow the new work processes to unfold, to live and breathe, rather than expecting perfection immediately.

Evaluating the Outcomes

In the fifth stage, the results of implementing the new work processes or services are evaluated. Mechanistic principles of thought view the interaction of the parts over the linear cause-and-effect relationships of individual parts. Given the nature of healthcare organizations, such principles are inappropriate for evaluating work processes and must be replaced by nonlinear evaluation models for two reasons. First, the increasing complexity of work in the Information Age minimizes the number of simple cause-and-effect relationships. Second, living systems, especially systems that encompass human beings and their behavior, cannot be understood mechanistically.

Because of the complexity of organizations, the assessment of processes and outcomes requires the use of multiple indicators and a nonlinear evaluation model such as a performance matrix. A matrix accommodates different data levels, data measures, and traditional performance measures while taking into account the limitations of cost–benefit analysis by expanding to include additional outcomes. A matrix examines multiple categories of data that represent the multiple measures that match the processes under evaluation in order to optimize decision-making (**Exhibit 8-4**).

A performance matrix provides a framework for assessing the impact of selected indicators on organizational performance and can help minimize the tendency to make a decision on the basis of a single indicator. In some situations, for instance, it might show that a course of action, despite increasing the organization's net income in the short term, negatively affects other indicators, including consumer and employee engagement and the organization's reputation, in both the short and long terms. The matrix also can be used to compare two or more options and their overall impact on the organization.

Whether the matrix is used or not, the goals of this stage of the vulnerability cycle are the following:

- Measure multiple process and outcome indicators.
- Evaluate the quality, service, and cost of the new work processes.
- Avoid simple, linear, cause-and-effect assumptions.

When the risk results in a less-than-optimal outcome, the work becomes that of course correction and remediation. The new knowledge gained from the unsuccessful effort is critical to continuing success; this information serves to inform others of a course of action that should not be repeated. Six actions are recommended when a negative outcome is identified:

1. Acknowledge that the outcome is less than expected.
2. Correct negative outcomes quickly; ensure personal safety.
3. Apologize quickly to those affected.

Exhibit 8-4 Performance Matrix

	Quality Measure	**Service Measure**	**Cost Measure**
Patient, Family, and Consumers	Feel safe Information access	Experience of care	Unit cost of service/product
Employee	Workplace safety Healthy work environment	Engagement Teamwork	Labor cost Turnover
Provider	Absence of patient adverse events	Engagement	Efficiency of patient throughput
Organization	Industry rankings	Consumer recommendation	Cost per case or visit

4. Review the goal and the selected process and identify areas of vulnerability. Be sure the work is still the right thing to do. Determine whether the goal is still appropriate.
5. Modify the process to avoid further negative outcomes.
6. Never be reluctant to abandon the goal and the process if safe and effective processes cannot be determined.

Course Corrections

In the sixth stage of the vulnerability cycle, the leader and the team must carefully examine the processes from all perspectives, looking for unacceptable outcomes and opportunities for improvement. Timely evaluations become the norm. What the leader and the team should not do is implement the new processes as if they were permanent and fully refined, hoping that no rework is necessary and that no additional costs are incurred. Continual adjustment should be the norm. When undesired results occur, the team recognizes the results and modifies the processes as needed to achieve the desired results.

Cherishing the New Knowledge Gained

The goal of this step of the vulnerability cycle is to cherish and make use of the knowledge gained. Each time a risk is taken, an outcome occurs—an outcome that may not have been anticipated. Consider the following two scenarios. In scenario A, an organization implemented a new work assignment process based on the recommendation of the staff employees. The project was more successful than anticipated. Not only were the original goals accomplished, but the professional behaviors of the employees improved and their job satisfaction levels increased (because of their involvement). In scenario B, the management team selected a reputable work management system without input from the employees. The employees did not support the system, and the costs for additional education and monitoring were much greater than anticipated. Employee satisfaction declined. Both projects were well thought out, and positive results were anticipated in both scenarios. In scenario A, the new process was retained. In scenario B, the project was discontinued. The learnings from the failed system were analyzed and retained as knowledge for future projects.

> ### Group Discussion
>
> Suppose your organization is exploring two employee retention programs. One applies to all employees, whereas the other applies only to nurses, who have an especially low retention rate. The same amount of funding is available for each program. Select indicators for the nine dimensions of the performance measurement matrix to evaluate each program, and then identify the potential positive and negative effects of each on the organization. Which program offers the greatest benefit to the organization? Explore other scenarios in which the performance measurement matrix could be applied.

CHAPTER EIGHT   The Focused Leader: Embracing Vulnerability, Risk Taking, and the Potential to Succeed

> ### Group Discussion
> The eight stages in the cycle of vulnerability present leaders with different levels of challenge. Consider two recent projects that were implemented in your organization, one believed to be a success and the other not. Using the cycle of vulnerability, determine for each project the stage at which the implementation processes were most successful and the stage at which interventions would have been especially helpful.

Point to Ponder

"Preparing an environment that will nourish creativity is, in itself, a creative activity. Spontaneity, dynamism, fun, humor, freedom from fear of failure, incentives, sympathetic values and culture, a soul space, and celebration are just a few of the essential ingredients of a creative culture. Leaders who seek to liberate the soul through creativity must establish a sanctuary in which failure is not punished but valued as a learning experience."

—Lance Secretan

Beginning the Cycle Again

At the end of the vulnerability cycle, the challenge is to identify what was valuable and what was problematic and begin the process again with the next opportunity or challenge. Repeating positive processes is as important as avoiding negative results. Although sometimes it is easy to see the value of implementing new processes or services, at other times it is difficult to discern anything more than that the implementation was not effective at this time and place. Nonetheless, leaders should always document both the positive and the negative results and try to view the implementation as a lesson in the value of vulnerability.

Coaching and mentoring employees in the development of vulnerable risk-taking behaviors are the logical next step. To guide employees toward these behaviors, a leader must first establish a culture of trust. The leader and employees must then discuss the value of risk taking and its potential impact on organizational productivity and morale. The coaching process—in which leader and employees learn together rather than alone—becomes transformative for everyone and for the organization as a whole. Guiding each other to become more vulnerable requires attention to both the content of the situation and the new relationships that emerge once the culture supports vulnerable behaviors.

Quantum leaders must develop patience to wait for the vulnerability cycle process to evolve, learn to trust in the value of fostering a vulnerability culture, and maintain their confidence in the inevitability of progress. Mutual trust evolves when the leader and employees experience the positive realities of the vulnerability cycle and when employees are valued for their efforts as well as the results of their efforts.

In addition, leaders serve as facilitators to guide employee and team member engagement rather than as directors of the activities of the employee. Facilitating is not about judging behaviors and offering advice; rather, it is about recognizing new behaviors when they occur and inviting the employees to offer feedback on their performance and perceptions of success. It is also about maintaining composure and showing tolerance, because vulnerable behaviors and risk taking are learned slowly, and employees who have yet to acquire the necessary skills may only partially finish new behaviors. Finally, it is about communicating well and developing and sustaining the kind of relationships that support new behaviors.

> ## Group Discussion
> Imagine you are a leader coaching employees in the acquisition of vulnerability behaviors. Develop a coaching outline that (1) describes the components of the vulnerability cycle, (2) provides examples of the relationships that emerge in a vulnerability culture, and (3) presents three strategies to sustain vulnerability behaviors.

New Relationships

Although much attention has been given to the differences between the Information Age and the Industrial Age, the fact is that successful leaders in all periods of history have valued information and knowledge. Being well informed with timely information has allowed leaders to facilitate the development of effective solutions to problems. Seldom do leaders rely on secondhand or outdated information. Instead, they develop networks of reliable sources to provide them with steady streams of current information. Indeed, their relationships with information sources in the organization and in the community take on ever greater significance as the availability of information increases.

Noted leadership expert Kouzes (2000) believes that, for leaders, social capital is as important as intellectual capital, if not more important. After all, leadership is about relationships. Who people know and what they can do for each other facilitates the work of the organization. This is not to say that brains or intellectual capital are not important, especially in the Information Age, but knowing is different from doing and does not necessarily translate into action. Making something happen requires having information and good relationships. Furthermore, with the opening of the floodgates of digital communication pathways, relationships are even more complex than before. Removing the traditional hierarchies of communication brings new obligations, such as the need to value diversity and personal privacy and to respect boundary setting and self-disclosure (**Figure 8-2**).

Inclusivity: Valuing Diversity in a New Way

People differ in more than gender, race, and ethnic background. People grow up in different geographical locations, speak different languages, practice different religions, and belong to different generations. In addition, people think and act differently. Some think quickly, some slowly, some are analytic, others are creative, some are detail-oriented, some prefer the big picture, some want facts, some depend on intuition, some are outgoing, some are reserved—and the list goes on. Given these differences, it is a wonder that we can relate to each other at all. Yet the diverse reality of our universe requires that we maximize our efforts to form relationships, despite the prejudices that unfortunately form because of our differences.

Labeling individuals who differ from us and profiling their behaviors may make it easier for us to function at times, but labeling and profiling create irrational biases and often prevent people from forming meaningful relationships or fracture the relationships that do become established. Creating expectations of inclusivity rather than valuing diversity provides a positive

Figure 8-2 Relationships in the Information Age.

approach to including the multiple attributes of our humanness. Thus, the benchmark for evaluating the breadth and depth of a team now focuses on openness and inclusivity rather than searching for documentation of the diversity of races, sexual orientation, and gender present in a team.

Perhaps the greatest obstacle to valuing inclusivity and developing new relationships is the common reluctance of individuals to accept change. Even when they are given a clear explanation of nonmechanistic processes, for example, and shown how these processes have led to success, many people continue to adhere to mechanistic and linear approaches and remain convinced that these would have brought about still better results. In short, these people resist admitting that the good old days were not really all that good, not even as good as today or as good as the future could be. Furthermore, because of their reluctance to change, the challenge of guiding others on the journey into the next age is monumental, and leaders can become disheartened at the prospect of leaving behind those who, for whatever reason, have cold feet. Nonetheless, if they are to lead the journey, leaders cannot afford to spend their time trying to convince everyone that the world is in fact changing.

The beauty of inclusivity it that it is continually emerging. Seeing differences as enhancements rather than as deterrents is increasingly important in the Information Age because attempts to filter out data can discourage creativity and obstruct an organization's creative potential. Keeping an open mind is necessary for gaining a richer, more complete understanding.

By contrast, in the Industrial Age creative thought was discouraged and consensus was encouraged. "Be a team member" was the slogan. The former emphasis on harmony and accord should be abandoned; instead, we need to embrace the idea that organizational success lies in transforming our notion of organization and consistency and accepting that the chaos of competition and the order of cooperation can and do coexist.

Healthcare Leadership Inclusivity

Reaching strategic goals, improving decision making, and achieving care equity are positively impacted as the diversity of leaders more closely aligns with the population served. Strategies to increase the diversity of healthcare leadership are continually discussed and offered to support the nature of inclusivity. In particular, many organizations have created executive roles to support the work of increasing inclusivity to increase numbers of minorities (11% in 2015) of executive leaders to better represent the population served (Livingston, 2018). The American Hospital Association's (2019) Institute for Diversity in Health Management provides resources such as assessment tools and current data to assist leaders in this work.

Opportunities for Change

When things go wrong, what usually goes wrong are relationships, not physical objects or processes, and these go wrong because of poor communication. Unfortunately, as a society we have very little idea how to get along with one another. Wars rage around the globe, the divorce rate is higher than 50%, and violent crime is rampant. The legal profession has been dubbed "the undertakers of relationships."

Fortunately, healthcare leaders are realizing the importance of establishing and maintaining productive relationships. In particular, current healthcare reform expectations include effective partnerships with patients, partnerships that facilitate effective engagement that positively affects health. Furthermore, although the internet is a valuable new communication tool, there are reasons to worry about its dehumanizing effects. For example, it allows people to inhabit a virtual world and spend less time relating directly to others. Although technology is necessary for leading an organization, it is not sufficient. Who one is in relationships with others may be just as important as what one does in the way of delivering technologically sophisticated care. Quality relationships are characterized by trust, the honoring of differences, clear personal boundaries, comfort with self-disclosure, and open communication—all of which confer a degree of vulnerability.

Privacy

The explosion of social media as a means of communication has made privacy a hot political issue. Historically, privacy advocates have had difficulty building support for their position. Now, social media users are becoming especially concerned about their privacy, largely because of the numerous available sources of information from social media sites and the well-known trails of e-commerce "cookie" crumbs that make it easy for companies to gather and sell customers' personal data to other companies. Recently, practices that inform consumers of their privacy rights and offer the option to opt out of further data sharing have become commonplace, as well as cautions to social media users to filter their contributions to the widely accessed social media sites.

Furthermore, whether out of boredom or curiosity, we are spying on one another like never before. Tiny wireless cameras are used not just for espionage but to detect shoplifting in department stores, and a world of websites publish our dirty laundry and private thoughts. Although people in general need to be more open to ideas, to be more vulnerable, they also understandably want barriers around their private lives. For example, few people, if any, are willing to allow the rest of the world access to all of their personal, financial, and health information. Where the boundaries lie is unique to each person, and determining what to consider private and public in the Information Age requires careful reflection.

Unfortunately, it is not a simple process to identify what will be shared with whom and at what time. For one thing, individuals do not present appropriate component parts of themselves whenever these are desired. Instead, individuals are unified wholes. Mary Parker

Follett, noted management expert, pointed out: "It is unrealistic and wasteful to organize work on the basis that a person can be abstracted from the totality of their being and put into the exercise of one particular skill, taught to perform it to a certain standard, and expect continuous performance at that level—and nothing else. One cannot disconnect themselves, leaving most of themselves at the work-gate and take in just that bit relevant to their job" (Graham, 1995, p. 75).

The lack of clearly defined personal boundaries (personal firewalls) is a major cause of relationship problems. As privacy diminishes, the importance of personal boundaries increases. Personal boundaries are different for each individual, and creating effective boundaries requires a healthy sense of identity. Boundary violations often run rampant in organizations. Saying no is frowned on. Yet excessive overtime, for instance, violates employees' family boundaries. The best course of action is to respect assumed or articulated boundaries until permission is given to cross them.

Personal boundaries include physical, mental, and spiritual boundaries. In general, a person's physical boundaries extend beyond the person's skin to encompass a space surrounding his or her body. Hugging or standing too close is a violation for some and welcomed by others. A person's physical boundaries also pertain to his or her possessions, money, time, and energy. Touching personal belongings in someone's office may be viewed as acceptable or as a violation. Mental boundaries pertain to beliefs, emotions, and intuition. They are violated, for example, when people are told they do not have the right to feel and appropriately express their emotions. Spiritual boundaries pertain to people's self-esteem, their sense of identity, and their relationship with a higher power. Destructive criticizing, yelling, and uttering abusive words are violations of spiritual boundaries.

> **Point to Ponder**
>
> Leaders have always been set on stage, in sight and view of the whole world. The internet puts the leader under the microscope for all to see in the finest detail.

Traditionally, boundaries and boundary violations in health care have been assessed from a patient–caregiver perspective. The point is that the patient is especially vulnerable by virtue of illness or injury and is dependent on the clinician for help, whereas the clinician has access to sensitive information about the patient and may uncover medical problems that the patient normally would share only with intimate friends. Given the imbalance of power, the clinicians have very clear responsibility to delineate and maintain appropriate boundaries.

The power imbalance between managers and employees creates similar expectations. In any relationship between a manager and an employee, both are responsible for delineating their personal boundaries, a task that is an essential step in creating an effective working relationship. Lack of boundaries blurs the purpose of the relationship, creating an ambiguous situation in which harm to either person may result. In addition, uncertainty is unnecessarily increased, to the detriment of the relationship and the entire organization. For far too long, command-and-control leaders have unwittingly violated the personal boundaries of employees without their consent—not with malicious intent but to ensure that the work of the organization was completed in a timely manner. The challenge for leaders today is to avoid dwelling on the rights and wrongs of past practices and instead to move forward and create the conditions in which personal boundaries are acknowledged and respected.

> ### Group Discussion
> You have accounts on four social media sites: LinkedIn, Facebook, Twitter, and Foursquare. Create a list of the advantages and disadvantages of these sites for you personally. How will you ensure control of your information for each site? If your information is compromised on any of these sites, how will you course correct to regain the level of information control desired?

Self-Disclosure
No relationship can develop fully until the participants expose something of their deeper selves to each other. Revealing oneself to others—one's thoughts, feelings, and intentions—is about telling one's story. Self-disclosure leads to greater understanding, trust, compassion, and commonality—in short, to a better relationship.

The idea that self-disclosure is valuable is often difficult to embrace, especially in a business context, because it runs contrary to classical management theory. In traditional organizations, people who stand around talking about matters unrelated to work are seen as wasting time. The obsession with efficiency is an obstacle to appreciating the value of strengthening relationships through casual conversation.

Self-disclosure is based on trust, on having total confidence in the integrity, ability, and good character of the other person. In other words, the person making the personal disclosures must believe the other person reliably follows through on commitments, has the competence to carry out his or her responsibilities, is emotionally balanced, and consistently chooses the "right" action.

Relationship Skills
In establishing relationships with employees and helping them develop a vulnerable and open style of behaving on the job, leaders must not assume that the employees have well-honed relationship skills. In fact, many employees, like many leaders, have less-than-adequate skills. Relationship skills, unfortunately, are not necessarily learned by growing up in a family. Many adults, because of how they were raised, have developed patterns of behavior that obstruct learning and accountability (e.g., conflict avoidance and assuming a victim attitude). In addition, many have failed to acquire the skills needed to cope with change, deal with personality differences, and communicate effectively.

Rather than becoming Information Age aliens, quantum leaders learn when to spend time building relationships and when to focus on tasks. In a healthy organization, the distinction between performing tasks and building relationships becomes blurred. For one thing, the latter can be used to develop the relationship skills needed to incorporate vulnerability and open communication into the organization's work and grow its capacity. Developing these skills takes time as well as a strong commitment on the part of leaders. In addition, leaders can enhance the effectiveness of these skills by using the principles of complexity communication.

Complexity Communication

In sharp contrast to traditional hierarchical organizational structures, the new organizational structures allow for communication in multiple pathways, up, down, across, and circularly, with a minimum of midlevel layers between executive management and staff. Using information networks, organizational staff in different divisions communicate and collaborate with each other in a moment's time. Multidirectional communication is the norm rather than the exception to support interprofessional collaboration and partnerships (Sherwood & Horton-Deutsch, 2015).

In many organizations the entire focus is on sending information, which is only one-third of the communicative interaction. The assumption is that the receiver understands what the sender intended. This assumption is often wrong, and the full exchange should include the sending of information by one person, its reception by one or more people, and, finally, a confirmation of their understanding.

Complexity communication is presented as an evolving process to illustrate the specific behaviors involved (**Figure 8-3**). It requires sensitivity to the myriad interrelationships and interdependencies that are characteristic of a quantum organization. It is based on three behaviors: critical listening, critical questioning, and critical thinking. The term *critical* here should not be taken as having a negative connotation; it is intended to have roughly the same meaning as *analytical*. This process is continually iterative and dynamic.

Critical Listening

In a conversation each listener has the responsibility to get the message, but often listeners are too busy thinking about what they want to say to listen carefully enough. People often understand only half of what is said to them. Being vulnerable requires expert listening skills—skills that many people obviously cannot claim.

The greatest challenge for listeners is to "still the mind," to stop the self-talk and mental rehearsing of what they intend to say when it is their turn. Stilling the mind is also about dismissing mental models, at least temporarily. Its consequences include allowing listeners

Figure 8-3 Communication Leads to Collective Mindfulness.

enough time to formulate enduring and just solutions and minimizing the tendency to seek quick fixes.

Our deeply held internal images of how the world works have a powerful impact on how we listen and react to information. Putting aside our perceptions of power, money, gender, culture, physical appearance, and so on is simply impossible. Nevertheless, leaders who listen with an open mind and create the conditions for employees to do the same see better outcomes from their decision making.

Another challenge is to deal with information overload. Some individuals want to tell everything they know or at least provide more information than the listener needs, which puts a strain on the listener. The listener must then listen even more carefully to discriminate between what is worth retaining and what is not. Managing information is not an easy task, but it is essential for effective and efficient communication.

Critical Questioning

Lawyers are schooled never to ask a question that they do not already know the answer to. Vulnerable leadership requires the opposite. The purpose of critical questioning, or asking for significant information, is to check individual perceptions of an issue or situation and render it more manageable. Leaders in the Information Age need to ask new types of questions, including questions about progress, value, and satisfaction. Asking for clarification is also a good way to minimize misinterpretation.

The wise leader never leaves a meeting without going through a checkout procedure. This procedure involves asking the participants questions such as the following: How do you think the meeting went? Did we accomplish what you thought should be accomplished? What was accomplished?

Asking questions about the value of work done ensures that all of the work planned or completed will in fact make a difference. Examples include these: What difference will this work make? To whom will it make a difference? At what cost?

Questions about the skills and roles of employees are also important. Do the skills of the employees match the needs of the marketplace? Is there a need to eliminate or add job duties? Are the organization and the community better off because of the services or products provided?

In asking questions like the preceding, leaders attempt to learn more about those being queried and their perspective on issues related to their work and the organization. In the fast-paced world of health care, leaders run the risk of overgeneralizing from past experiences, and asking lots of questions can help prevent this mistake in reasoning. Unfortunately, listening is not always easy for leaders.

> **Point to Ponder**
>
> "Rest assured, no matter how bad it looks, I will not judge you until I have heard your side. Once a leader puts expedience above fairness, his reputation and integrity crumble away like something rotten."
>
> —Elizabeth I

One of the keys to critical questioning is to refrain from offering advice or commentary to the person being questioned. Most leaders are comfortable providing guidance to others, and they readily give advice. Critical questioning requires something more—the gift of an ear. Asking questions garners the questioner more information if the respondent is allowed to express pertinent opinions. Examples of questions leaders might ask are listed in **Exhibit 8-5**.

> ### Group Discussion
>
> Staffing is the largest expense for most healthcare organizations. One reason is that the uncertainty of patient care needs requires a healthcare organization to have sufficient staff on hand to cover upward swings in care delivery, including emergency situations. Use the principles of vulnerability and complexity communication to create an effective and efficient staffing system that incorporates staffing by ratios and/or patient acuity. Discuss the advantages and disadvantages of the system. How can you be sure that the right clinician is with the right patient at the right time? Is the highest quality care provided at the lowest cost?

Exhibit 8-5 Examples of Critical Questions

- What is your understanding of this situation?
- Why is this important to you? To others? To the organization?
- Which issue do you think this situation is related to: technical, systems, or people related?
- What do you need to know to make a decision on this issue?
- What assumptions do you think others have made about this situation?
- Who else cares about this issue as much as you do?
- This sounds very rational. What do people believe about it?
- This sounds very emotional. What do people feel about it?
- What are the choices in the situation?
- What would you find helpful in this situation?
- What might we be missing?

Receivers of information, or listeners, need a safe space to ask clarifying questions of the senders. In other words, the open exchange of information depends on the existence of a safe forum. If the sender of a message feels threatened by the receiver asking questions about the message, the resulting hostility can quickly end the questions and cause a breakdown in communication. If the receiver feels unsafe asking questions about the message, the resulting silence could easily be misinterpreted as agreement and understanding. When leaders misconstrue the absence of questions as acceptance and understanding of their messages, they commit a grave error.

For some leaders the challenge is different. Those who are steeped in the classical command-and-control leadership culture rarely ask questions to gain information. In their view, they are expected to be experts on all matters related to their role and are reluctant to ask for information for fear of exposure. Although their concern about looking less than competent is generally unfounded, they still are not able to listen very well or feel comfortable asking for advice from others. In the new age, their main challenge is to allow themselves to become more vulnerable and hence more open to input from others.

Critical Thinking

The ability to think critically has long been recognized as a necessary management skill. What is different in complexity communication is the sequence of events. The process begins with critical listening, followed by critical questioning, and then critical thinking. It does not make sense to engage in analysis before listening and asking questions to clarify content so that all vital data can be considered. Further, complexity communication begins with the individual and extends to the team so participants can assimilate information and then reach a logical conclusion as a team, not individually.

Critical thinking encompasses the following components:

- Analyzing the use of language
- Explicating assumptions
- Formulating problems
- Weighing evidence
- Evaluating conclusions
- Discriminating between arguments
- Justifying claims
- Clarifying values

Critical thinking is helpful for seeking deeper meaning, validating perceptions, and setting priorities. The proper attitude for engaging in critical thinking is a mix of reflective skepticism and tolerance for ambiguity. Openness is essential for examining evidence. Too often people proclaim they are thinking critically when in fact they have prejudged the issues, and their discussion supports preconceived notions rather than exploring the range of available options. Managing the complexity communication process requires a more critical or analytical style of thought and communication.

For many leaders and employees, engaging in dialogue runs counter to the prevailing culture within their organizations—a culture that instead fosters internal competition and sets hierarchical limitations on who can contribute to the decision-making process. These leaders and employees find it especially difficult to recognize and practice openness and self-disclosure, suspend judgment, and promote collaboration as ways of increasing collective intelligence. In complexity communication, it is normal to view disagreement as an essential aspect of dialogue and to avoid suppressing differences merely for the sake of preserving the peace. Although intensely painful at times, learning the necessary skills and engaging in complexity communication dialogue have a value that can hardly be overstated.

Developing dialogue skills and communicating with others based on the belief that every person is of value but has a limited view represent an overwhelming challenge. In this type of communication, careful listening is integrated with questioning for clarification, and then messages are analyzed using critical-thinking skills. Many leaders are quickly able to develop the three distinct skills of listening, questioning, and thinking but have difficulty with sequencing the application of the skills. Leaders commonly think or make a decision first (often before all the information is presented), request information and clarification second, and then listen as the final step—the fire–aim–ready approach. Despite the fast-paced work environment, which hinders contemplative communication practices, quantum leaders recognize the benefits of complexity communication and coach others to use the associated skills to mediate the internal competition and reinforce new and more effective behaviors.

Collective Mindfulness

Complexity communication skills are especially important in health care, where the potential for catastrophic outcomes, should employees fail to communicate, can be significant. Given the critical nature of the services they provide, healthcare organizations often develop what is known as the power of collective mindfulness, a phenomenon described by Weick and Sutcliffe (2001). Collective mindfulness is the capacity of groups and individuals to be keenly aware of significant details, notice errors in the making, and have the shared expertise and freedom to act on what they notice. These are all characteristics of highly reliable organizations.

Consider the case of a patient who is experiencing cardiac arrest. A team of nurses, respiratory therapists, and physicians quickly assembles, prompted by a prearranged code call. Within minutes the patient's heart rate is stabilized, respiratory function is restored, and the team disperses. Those unfamiliar with emergency departments might believe the actions of the health professionals had been tightly scripted and well-rehearsed. Rather, the professionals all knew their particular role, had experienced similar situations in the past, and had only to listen to what was happening, ask for additional necessary information, and think through and integrate past experiences with the current event to perform the rescue.

To be effective in potentially catastrophic situations, health professionals depend on their mastery of standardized routines and on complexity communication at its best. They listen intently and with full presence, question only for clarification, and intervene as a finely tuned unit.

Collective mindfulness is not limited to clinical situations. It is evident in many types of situations in which there are complex interpersonal relationships. Consider healthcare staffing. Healthcare leaders are continually challenged to deliver reliable services in the face of fluctuating conditions, such as shortages of qualified employees and reductions in reimbursement. Quantum leaders create a culture that allows employees to be flexible (but in orderly ways) and to focus energy and expertise where and when they are needed. They can then use the employees to assist in dealing with the difficulties that arise by creating strategies that address the appropriate issues.

Hidden within the spirit of collective mindfulness is the essence of vulnerability—being open, searching for new solutions, taking risks, trying new strategies, retaining what works, and discarding what does not work. What emerges is a delicate balance of processes that encourage continuous learning and improvement, while at the same time promoting order and reliable performance, a very powerful combination.

> ### Group Discussion
>
> Select two teams, one composed of experienced employees and the other composed of newer employees. Consider an emergency situation in which a patient is experiencing chest pain. Compare the two teams with regard to their working relationships, communication skills, and ability to prioritize and make decisions. How can you use this information about each team?

Strategies for Cultivating Leadership Vulnerability

In this section, two strategies for fostering vulnerable or open leadership are proposed: open communication and syndication. Both strategies have inherent risks and require leaders to stretch current thinking. Although many other strategies support open leadership, these two are designed to begin the process of changing mental models and moving to practices that fit with the work of the quantum organization.

Open Communication

Some leaders have confused dialogue with behind-the-scenes consensus building and decision making. Making decisions before all the information is considered leads to poor outcomes and decreases trust in the integrity of the decision-making process. Although according to the classical management model conducting business in informal settings such as the dining room and the golf course may have some merit, recent advances in information technology have brought both challenges and opportunities to the way business is conducted. In particular, by aiding in the removal of secrecy and increasing the ease of dialogue they support the open communication model.

The open communication model is based on the same principles as open meeting laws (**Exhibit 8-6**). The idea behind these laws, which have traditionally applied to meetings of public bodies, is that publicizing meetings and conducting them openly maximizes public access to governmental processes. All 50 states have enacted some type of legislation to recognize the public statutory right to openness in government. The laws require meetings of public bodies to be conducted openly and for notices and agendas for such meetings to be provided to the public. Open meetings expose the conduct of the business of government to the scrutiny of the public and prevent decision making in secret, thereby

---

Exhibit 8-6 Basic Principles of Open Meeting Laws

1. A meeting is considered to be a gathering that can occur not only in person but also through technological devices.
2. All meetings of a public body shall be open meetings, and all persons so desiring shall be permitted to attend and listen to the deliberations and proceedings.
3. An "open call to the public" is permitted but not required. The purpose of an open call is to allow members of the public to address the public body on matters not listed on the agenda.
4. Executive sessions will be used to seek legal advice and review confidential records. No votes are taken in executive session.
5. Appropriate notice of each meeting will be given (usually not later than 24 hours before the meeting), and the agenda and meeting location will be posted.
6. For each meeting, there will be written minutes or a recording that will include an accurate description of all actions proposed, discussed, or taken and the names of members who propose each motion.
7. The minutes or a recording of any meeting, except an executive session, must be open to public inspection no later than 3 working days after the meeting.

Data from Vermont Secretary of State. (2019). A Guide to Open Meetings. https://sos.vermont.gov/media/vpnbxckz/a-guide-to-open-meetings-january-2019.pdf

ensuring that appointed members of boards and commissions truly serve as representatives of the broader community and that the actions taken are in the best interests of the community.

The open communication model applies the principles of open meeting laws to organizations, based on the belief that the work of any organization belongs to all its members and that encouraging open communication enhances organizational effectiveness and capacity. The principles focus on the manner in which members communicate and make decisions, and their overall goal is to increase the fairness of decision-making processes and prevent them from being influenced by off-the-record communication between decision makers and others. The following seven principles, if followed, increase the incidence of open dialogue, improve trust among employees, and decrease bureaucratic processes:

1. The business of the organization shall be conducted during open meetings, which are defined as gatherings of people physically, telephonically, or electronically. This principle requires that issues brought before a committee are discussed in the presence of all members of the committee. It is not appropriate to discuss any topic without involving all the parties. Ex parte communication considers only one side of a situation, and as such violates the first principle of open communication. Email communication, telephone conversations, and casual dialogue at social gatherings about committee meeting topics are not allowed. The intent is to eliminate selective collaboration and prevoting on issues before the actual meeting. Decision making that is inclusive from the start results in decisions that, because everyone is highly invested in them, are more likely to succeed.
2. The date and time of each meeting, its location, and its agenda shall be posted. Publicizing this information allows unofficial but interested members to learn the issues to be covered in the meeting and to discuss them with other members ahead of time. It also helps eliminate the chance that decisions will be made in secret. In the meeting itself, only issues identified as being on the official agenda are discussed, which means that no surprise or unanticipated issues are dealt with. Although posting meeting information may be cumbersome at times, it minimizes the chances of reactive decision making.
3. Every meeting shall be open to all persons desiring to attend and listen to the deliberations and proceedings. The intent of this principle is to remove even the appearance of secrecy. It is based on the belief that the satisfaction felt by employees, along with their job performance, is highly correlated with their involvement in decision making that directly pertains to their work.
4. Every meeting shall include a "call to the attendees" to allow members of the organization or the community a defined allotment of time in which to address the official members on matters discussed. Although dialogue on the issues is restricted to official members of a committee, other attendees should be afforded an opportunity to react to what the official members say. Allotting a specified amount of time for comments keeps the meeting from running past its scheduled end. In addition, the official members are not required to respond but are requested to consider the additional information when making decisions.
5. Executive sessions shall be used for the purpose of seeking expert advice or reviewing information defined by law as confidential but not for the taking of votes.

Some types of information, such as performance evaluations and salary and wage data, are protected. In executive sessions, issues involving confidential information are discussed, but no voting or decision making occurs.

6. Each meeting is documented by written minutes or a recording that includes an accurate description of all actions proposed, discussed, or taken and the names of the members who voted for each motion. Documenting the work of a committee fully prevents decision makers from hiding behind the cloak of the summative vote count. It also forces decision makers to own their opinions and makes them accountable to the membership at large. Minutes serve as a historical record of the decision-making process.
7. The written minutes or the recording of any meeting except an executive session must be open to inspection no later than 3 working days after the meeting. Ensuring that a record of discussion in the meeting is available to all interested parties in a timely manner again helps lift the shroud of secrecy.

Interestingly, the two most common violations of open meeting laws are discussion of agenda items without the full board or committee present (ex parte) and inappropriate use of the executive session. The same violations should be expected during implementation of the open communication model because collaboration and prevoting on issues have been a traditional practice in organizations, as has the use of executive sessions for dealing with matters of organization-wide concern.

Syndication

The second strategy for cultivating leadership vulnerability is organizational syndication, which is basically a way of structuring business to tap latent potential. Based on the recognition that information is now widely available, syndication uses resources outside of an organization to benefit the organization.

Organizations, according to Dee Hock (1999), are extremely good at some things, are very good at many things, but are not good at everything. In fact, organizations are pathetic at some things. Although much organizational work is believed not to be amenable to syndication, significant work elements might be, especially those at which organizations are pathetic.

Syndication, which originated in the entertainment world, is now beginning to define the structure of e-business. It involves the sale of the same good to many customers, who then integrate it with other offerings and redistribute it, similar to the way television programs or news stories are managed.

Syndication is a radical new way of structuring business (**Table 8-1**). It requires leaders to rethink their strategies, to reshape their organizations, to change the way they interact with customers and partner with other entities, and to pioneer new models for collecting revenues and earning profits. Integrating syndication into an organization is similar to creating a "chaordic" organization, as defined by Dee Hock (1999). Hock is credited with devising a new concept of organizations based on the belief that chaos and order, competition and cooperation, can be harmoniously blended. He conceived of a global system for the electronic exchange of value, and the result was VISA International, which is owned by 22,000 member banks that compete with each other for 750 million customers and honor each other's transactions across borders and currencies.

TABLE 8-1 Business in the Syndicated World

	Traditional Business	Syndication
Structure of relationships	Linear supply and demand	Loose weblike networks
Corporate role	Fixed	Continually shifting
Value added	Dominated by physical distribution	Dominated by information manipulation
Strategic focus	Control scarce resources	Leverage abundance
Role of corporate capabilities	Sources of advantage	Products to sell
Role of outsourcing	Gain efficiency	Assemble virtual corporation

Reproduced from Werbach, K. (2000, May–June). Syndication: The emerging model for business in the Internet era. *Harvard Business Review*, 90. Reprinted by permission. The Harvard Business School Publishing Corporation. All rights reserved.

> ### Group Discussion
>
> A group of healthcare organizations has decided to apply the syndication model to its employee development program. Imagine you are on the team creating the product to be syndicated. Using the principles of syndication, your team has been assigned the work of content originators. Describe the content origination process and continue to model development with the creation of packaging and distribution plans for the education program. What are the advantages and disadvantages of syndication as a way of developing and implementing programs? Who would support or oppose the syndication model? What performance measures could be used to evaluate it? How is syndication in this situation similar to the concept of "new power"?

Chaordic organizations present an unambiguous challenge to the traditions of independent organizations by bringing into existence an interconnected international reality once believed impossible. They also offer courage to those considering syndication for selected services or products. At the moment, the chaordic model is mainly a learning aid, however, and cannot be quickly imprinted on existing organizations.

Syndication is based on the realization that needed expertise is often found not inside an organization but beyond its boundaries. In a syndication network, the roles of originator of content, syndicator or packager of content for distribution, and distributor of content to customers are quite different from the traditional roles of content developer and distributor of content to employees.

In a syndication network, the content originator has greater responsibility and accountability than in traditional organizations. In some situations, leaders have established collaborative initiatives that can be moved to the syndication level. Health centers for indigents, school health education and treatment clinics, hospice centers, and training programs developed through cooperation between communities and financiers are candidates for syndication. Because of their need for standardization of services (to ensure quality), operational cost savings, and conservation of capital, each could be syndicated to create a greater network without substantial duplication of effort. The role of the originator is to assess and consolidate the work of many products into a single product desired community-wide.

The second key role, that of syndicator, encompasses packaging the content and managing the relationships between originators and distributors. The syndicator's goals include achieving consistency of products and services, uncovering user expectations, and supporting the established relationship between product users and the syndication processes. Time-limited agreements would support state-of-the-art products and services that provide appropriate quality at the lowest cost because failure to meet the standards would cause users to turn to other syndicators.

Finally, the distributor is responsible for delivering the goods from originators to users. As the virtual world develops, many more information services and education programs are likely to be distributed through the internet. Additional examples include a 911 response alternative of sending a mental health professional (instead of law enforcement) to some 911 calls or the addition of Healthy People 2020 tools to health system websites.

It is no longer cost-effective for every organization to provide every service. Not only is it costly, but individual organizations lack the necessary concentration of expertise. The syndication model offers opportunities for current providers of services to generate revenue through a shared process as designated originators. Designated originators provide the content of their expertise to the product and become co-owners of the syndication model. If syndication became common in health care, those organizations with significant expertise could earn income as a result of contributing to the origination process, whereas those with limited expertise could have access to standardized state-of-the-art products for a reasonable cost.

Is There a Choice?

Are leaders obligated to develop a vulnerable leadership style? Do they need to replace closed leadership behavior with open leadership behavior? The obvious response is yes, there is no choice, the value of vulnerability is too conspicuous to deny. The move into the Information Age requires different skills and knowledge than those required in the Industrial Age.

However, some leaders may have difficulty making the transition. Some, for example, might support the concept of open leadership, but because of the perceived threat in admitting to a lack of answers or information, they might be resistant to living the new behaviors. They also might have great difficulty in creating a culture supportive of open leadership because their failure to walk the talk of vulnerability hurts employee morale and lowers the level of trust within the organization.

Thus, the best strategy for leaders right now is to critically assess their personal status and their ability to assimilate vulnerable behaviors and integrate them into their performance. Acquiring the skills needed to implement the open leadership model is a long-term process that requires understanding, commitment, and persistence. Ethically, developing open leadership skills is the right thing to do. In addition, as successful behaviors emerge, leaders will see some of the benefits to be gained from changing to a better model for the times.

Conclusion

Currently, it is nearly impossible for a single person to know more than 10% of what there is to know about a particular topic. This is most disconcerting to leaders who have worked and studied diligently to know as much as they can. Unfortunately for these leaders, it is even apparent to their colleagues that they do not have all the answers. In addition, they have no chance of catching up because information continues to accumulate too rapidly. The good news is that everyone is in the same situation; no one ever has all the answers.

The new challenge for leaders is to become comfortable managing the information that is available—to become competent as information access finders and relationship makers. Furthermore, as this chapter points out, the best approach to leadership today is to understand that the high speed of change, among other factors, makes total control impossible, and to therefore accept that vulnerability and open communication are required. In addition, throughout the journey of learning to become openly vulnerable, leaders necessarily will become competent in managing uncertainty, encouraging risk, valuing diversity, and communicating with others based on principles of complexity and respect for privacy and personal boundaries. Increasing vulnerability increases leadership excellence, but no leader can achieve this desirable result without significant commitment and effort.

Chapter Takeaways

1. Leadership vulnerability is a positive leadership trait, and while difficult to engage, it results in more transparent leadership practices.
2. Relationships in health care are the essential foundation of quality care.
3. The cycle of vulnerability provides a simple, yet comprehensive framework for experiencing change and innovation.
4. Understanding the concepts of old power and new power increases understanding of the impact of generational thinking and the availability of technology.
5. Complexity communication elements—stilling the mind, seeking greater understanding and interpretation—support mindfulness in a high-level manner.

Case Study 8-1

Positioning for Positions

Everest Health System is located in the Midwest and is the largest healthcare system in the region, with 3 large acute care hospitals, a mental health hospital, 2 smaller community hospitals, and a rehabilitation hospital. In addition to the inpatient facilities, the corporate structure of Everest Health System owns a physician group with 10 outpatient clinics distributed over the large metropolitan area of nearly 3.2 million people. Everest also contracts with an independent group of physicians who are recognized as "Everest physicians" and share in negotiated group insurance rates for inpatient and outpatient services. In addition, Everest has an outpatient sports medicine and rehabilitation center, an outpatient MRI diagnostic center, 2 outpatient surgical centers, a cancer center, and a standalone infusion therapy center. The 3 large acute care hospitals are all Magnet designated, and 2 are recognized with the Planetree designation as well.

All of the chief executive officers (CEOs) of the inpatient and outpatient centers report to an executive vice president for patient care, and the chief operating officers (COOs) and chief nursing officers (CNOs) report to the CEOs at their respective facilities. Being a progressive healthcare system, the executive VP for patient care desires to develop an Institute for Nursing Excellence, an idea that also appeals to the executive for philanthropy because there is a potential donor who might be willing to fund the new institute. An outside consultant has been hired to facilitate the development of the new institute. It is decided that the membership of the newly formed institute will consist of the CNOs and the directors of research and development for each of the inpatient facilities who report to each of the CNOs.

During the first few months, the consultant facilitates the meetings. The group spends considerable time and process to identify what they consider to be the characteristics of an Institute for Nursing Excellence. Using this as a foundation, they developed a mission and vision statement and created a professional practice model that would serve as a conceptual model that could be used to articulate the purpose, mission, and vision of the institute internally and externally. After these foundational documents were developed, they decided to focus on meeting the recommendations of the Institute of Medicine's *Future of Nursing* (2010) report and look for opportunities to improve measures of nursing quality across the system. After 8 months of meetings, the CNOs met privately and decided to lead the meetings themselves and terminate the services of the consultant. One of the CNOs of the larger acute care hospitals volunteered to be the leader of the group.

Over the next year, the group worked on developing a strategic plan with measures for expected deliverables for quality, research, education, and nurse-sensitive indicators. The CNO leader also developed a job description for a director for the institute that was approved by the full membership. The position description was written to indicate that a doctorate in nursing was strongly preferred and that the applicant should have previous experience in nursing leadership positions. There was considerable discussion about the title of the position, with several options considered, such as director, vice president, and executive vice president.

Another area of consideration was the reporting structure for the new position. Several concerns were raised among the members, but these were not openly discussed in the meetings. Some of the CNOs were concerned that if the new position reported to the executive VP of patient services, the position might evolve into a chief nurse executive (CNE) position for the entire healthcare system and that they might be required to report to this person in the future instead of the hospital CEO. The CNOs indicated they don't want this new person to "interfere in the operations of their hospitals" and "tell them how to run their business." The directors of research and development also were concerned that they, too, might be required to report to this new centralized position; some of the directors prefer to report at the entity level rather than the system level. There was significant discussion about the new person reporting to the CNO in current institute leadership role because this structure would elevate that person above the other CNOs.

After several months of discussing the pros and cons of reporting structures, titles, and levels of authority for the new position, the job description was written to place the position one level below the CNOs with wording that the person would report to the entire CNO group. The position was viewed by the CNOs to be at an equal level of the directors of research and development. The position was then posted for recruitment.

A few applications were received, but they were reviewed first by the CNOs in their regular CNO meetings before they were shared with the entire institute membership. Applicants who seemed appropriate were interviewed by phone by the CNOs and then vetted to the entire institute membership for a second phone interview or a face-to-face interview. It soon became apparent that most applicants with strong leadership experience were uneasy about a position that reported to a "group" instead of to one individual, and because most applicants had been CNOs or directors of nursing schools, they were not satisfied with the title "director" instead of "vice president." Months of debate ensued with no resolution to the reporting structure, title for the position, or selection of applicants willing to take such a position.

Because the new position remained unfilled for more than 18 months, the "interim director" position was rotated among the CNOs, but the directors of research and development were not considered in the rotation. With months of tenure in the interim director role, the lead CNO was in the spotlight for interviews and collateral materials developed to showcase the Institute for Nursing Excellence. This led to some of the CNOs voicing concern that the interim director CNO was "taking all the credit" personally for the institute's accomplishments without sharing the recognition and awards among all of the CNOs.

Over months of meetings, evidence of nursing excellence (publications, research, certifications, and newly earned degrees) were collected from each respective entity by one of the directors for research and development and published in a document highlighting nursing excellence at Everest Health System. The funding received from the major donor was used to provide nursing scholarships, and the group met to develop the application process, selection criteria, and the selection process. The money was distributed in scholarships for applicants bridging the associate degree to baccalaureate, the baccalaureate to master's, and the master's to doctorate. The institute membership seemed to work well together when given a specific task to accomplish.

The directors of research and development talked among themselves and voiced concerns that they felt that the institute had lost its vision and that the CNOs were controlling the work of the institute without recognizing the contributions or value that the directors brought to the institute. As issues were discussed at the institute meetings, any observer could see rolling of eyes and other nonverbal expressions of discontent among the members. Some members were meeting outside of the institute meeting to analyze what they believed was the "true agenda" of some of the CNOs. Some members expressed that they believed that decisions were made from a fear perspective: fear that hiring a real leader for the institute at the vice president or executive VP level might compromise the CNOs' power or disrupt the existing CNO reporting structure.

Communication among the group was guarded; positions on issues were calculated; and there was little transparency in expressing real feelings about important issues. When there was an application from and interview of a nationally known nursing leader for the position, the group began to speak of elevating the position to a VP level, but the reporting structure remained with the position reporting to the institute CNO leader. The applicant subsequently rescinded his application, and he stated that "he perceived that the group was not working well together and he was not willing to take a position at a director level that reports to a group as contrasted to an individual."

Questions

1. What is your perception of the forces that may be at play among the institute members?
2. What might you do as an institute member to facilitate a higher performance among the group?
3. What might be the risks, gains, and personal vulnerabilities in trying to redirect the group?

4. How might outcomes be different if there was more vulnerability and transparency among members?
5. What would be your vision of what could be done to create an exemplar Institute for Nursing Excellence?
6. If you were a CNO, using the six stages of the cycle of vulnerability, what might you do to try to facilitate change in the group dynamics?
7. How might collective mindfulness help the group to achieve the original vision for the institute?

Case Study 8-2
Taking the Next Step

Ashlee has worked at Midwest Medical Center for the last 10 years as the director of medical surgical services. She has really enjoyed this role, and has led her team of nurses to accept many new changes to improve their scores in patient satisfaction and physician satisfaction. She has prided herself on advancing the skills and competencies of her direct reports (nurse managers), and has encouraged them to become certified in their nursing specialty areas. Ashlee also meets with the general staff at least once a month and provides information to them relative to the progress toward the nursing division's overall goals and other hospital information. She makes every attempt to meet with the staff of both days and nights and make certain that she has a presence with the staff during their unit meetings at least once a month.

Ashlee is well liked by her direct reports and all of the staff in general. Her managers have an opportunity to provide input into Ashlee's annual performance appraisal, and they frequently cite examples of how Ashlee has supported them and helped them to grow in their roles. On the annual employee opinion survey, the nursing staff of Ashlee's departments comment that she is visibly present on the unit and open to discussing issues of concern with them. Ashlee is very comfortable in her role and has a good working relationship with the other nursing directors and directors of other hospital ancillary departments and specialty areas. Ashlee has no desire to change her position or leave the organization, but she is constantly looking for ways to create new energy for herself in the workplace. Occasionally, the chief nursing officer (CNO) asks Ashlee to assume responsibility for other nonnursing departments as the interim director until a replacement director can be hired, or Ashlee is asked to assume the leadership of various project task forces for the organization. Ashlee has a great relationship with her CNO and looks to her as a mentor in her own career. The other directors indicate their appreciation for the chief nursing officer as well.

Ashlee is surprised one day in the Nurse Executive Council when the CNO announces that she will be leaving Midwest Medical Center in the next 30 days because she is relocating to another state with her husband, who has assumed a very prestigious position in one of the major universities there. The CNO announces that she has been selected as the chief operating officer (COO) of the Northwest University Medical Center, which is a huge promotion for her as well. The CNO announces that the Human Resources department will be placing advertisements in local and regional newspapers, in major nursing management journals, and on the organization's website for a replacement CNO. She also suggests that the directors consider applying for the position themselves because they are familiar with the organization and the strategic vision for the nursing division.

Chapter Eight The Focused Leader: Embracing Vulnerability, Risk Taking, and the Potential to Succeed

Ashlee leaves the Nursing Executive Council with mixed feelings—sadness at losing her personal mentor and conflicted with internal confusion as to whether she should apply for the position herself. She had never thought of herself as leaving her current position, and she begins to question her capabilities and skills for a CNO position. She is certain that at least one other director will apply for the position because he has often talked about wanting to be the CNO in an organization. For the next few days, it seems that Ashlee can think of nothing else but the CNO position. She tries to visualize herself in the role and consider all of the responsibilities that the role would entail. She knows that applying for the role would be a risk because she would be leaving a very comfortable position and moving into a position that would require new skills, new relationships with other healthcare executives, and a much broader scope of responsibilities.

She also feels the risk of applying for the position and not being selected. How would this look in the eyes of her colleagues? How would this look in the eyes of her staff, who have been as supportive of her as she has been of them? At times her mind is filled with the negatives of the role and all that could go wrong. She is aware that there is a constant threat of union organization because many of the other hospitals in the city are already under union contract. Midwest Medical Center is the only hospital that has not been organized. She is also painfully aware of the financial pressures that she would have to assume in the CNO role, and she has observed the current CNO struggling with budget cuts, managing negative budget variances, and advocating for the needs of the nursing department. Ashlee wonders if she has the skill and capabilities to be successful in negotiating budget needs for nursing with the chief financial officer and other executives.

At other times Ashlee's head is filled with visions of what she could accomplish as a CNO. Although she had considered returning to school for her PhD in nursing, she delayed those plans for personal reasons. Now she really regrets that decision. Although the position description for the CNO indicated that a PhD was preferred, Ashlee wondered if the applicants with a PhD would have preferential consideration. On the other hand, she realizes that she has an excellent reputation in the organization as a visionary leader, and her department is nearly always in compliance with the organization's performance goals and other important metrics such as HCAHPS scores and nursing-sensitive indicators. Ashlee knows that although she has experienced many past successes, she would need to stretch her own capabilities to be successful in the CNO role. Being a positive person, she tries to envision herself in the role and rehearses in her mind the steps that she would need to take to lead the nursing division successfully. It is a huge risk and opportunity, and she is feeling the weight of her own advice to others in coaching them to stretch and expand themselves in assuming new roles. She has often told others to allow themselves to become vulnerable to grow personally and professionally. Now she remembers her own advice to others, and her advice is cogent to her as well.

Ashlee's colleague applies for the CNO role, and she learns that there are at least two other outside applicants who have previous experience as CNOs at other organizations. One of these outside applicants also has a PhD in Nursing Administration. Now Ashlee is all the more conflicted as she considers her own decision and evaluates her own capabilities for the role. She decides to talk over this important decision with trusted friends and colleagues inside and outside of the organization. Many encourage her to step forward and apply for the position even though she is comfortable in her current role. Realizing that she doesn't have much time to ponder this decision, Ashlee finally decides that she should throw her "hat into the ring," and she applies for the position.

After talking with the Human Resources representative, Ashlee is slated to interview with members of the executive team, physicians, nursing director representatives, and other divisional leaders. She also meets individually with the CEO and the COO, and then in a group interview with the entire executive team. Ashlee tries to prepare herself for the individual and group interviews by reviewing the vision and strategy of the hospital and updating her knowledge of some of the current financial challenges faced by the hospital in the new healthcare economic environment. Ashlee has a strong vision of nursing and its role in maximizing the patient-centered experience of patients and families who are served by the hospital. She discusses her goals of improving nurse–physician relationships in an effort to ensure positive patient outcomes and opportunities for change that would not only improve the nursing work environment but would also enhance the organization's success in meeting the hospital's goals.

In the interviews, Ashlee discloses a lot about herself, her personal goals, and her goals for nursing. She indicates that she has a very positive relationship with many of the leaders in the organization. One of the more difficult questions that she has to address is to describe an innovation she has done to achieve a desired program or goal for her department. Ashlee carefully considers before she speaks, but then describes an example of planning and implementing a program where nurses and physicians round together and include the patient in the discussion of the plan of care. She indicates that at first physicians were very reluctant to participate in the collaborative rounds, and she describes the strategy that she used to first listen to their concerns and those of the nurses. She discusses how she identified champions of the change process and used the nurse and physician champions to facilitate the acceptance of the process by those who were more reticent. She also describes how she measured the change using a collaborative behavior scale and nurse and physician satisfaction scale before and after the implementation of the collaborative rounding approach. Ashlee suggests to the interviewers that she believes strongly that measuring the results of change is critical to demonstrate the effectiveness of the change to others, building trust for future changes. The implementation of the collaborative rounding process resulted in an improvement in patient satisfaction scores and in collaborative behavior, nurse satisfaction, and physician satisfaction scores.

In one of the interviews, Ashlee is asked whether she truthfully feels that she has the capabilities to fulfill the role of the CNO because she doesn't have experience as a CNO. At first Ashlee is a bit intimidated by the question, but she thinks carefully before she answers. She explains she is highly successful in her current role and is viewed as a visionary leader in the overall hospital organization. She also indicates that she would have some learning and developmental needs, but she feels confident that she could work with her executive colleagues, the nursing leaders in the organization, and her peers to enhance her skills and competencies in the role. She thinks that it is best to be honest about her development needs in the new role but indicates that she is willing and able to advance herself and to provide value to the organization as a new CNO. After the interviews are completed, Ashlee wonders whether she should have expanded on her past successes rather than being so open and honest about her development needs for the new role. She silently hopes that she has not lost the position because of her honesty, but she feels that it is important that the selection team sees her as an individual who could carefully assess her own strengths and weaknesses for such an important position.

Questions
1. What do you think about Ashlee's decision to apply for the CNO role?
2. How would you have answered the question if you were Ashlee and were asked about your capabilities to fill the CNO role?

3. How did Ashlee show her vulnerability as a leader in considering the CNO role and in her answers to the interview groups?
4. What are the areas of vulnerability that Ashlee will face as a new CNO?
5. What do you perceive to be Ashlee's areas of strength and areas that need development?
6. What challenges and obstacles do you think that Ashlee might encounter if she were selected for the role of CNO?
7. If you were on the interview team, how would you vote when Ashlee is considered against her competitors for the role?
8. Would you have preference for an applicant who had past experience as a CNO, an applicant who had a PhD in nursing, or an inside applicant who had experience with the hospital and the current nursing division's vision for the future?

References

American Hospital Association. (2019). *Institute for Diversity in Health Management*. https://www.aha.org/websites/2015-06-01-institute-diversity-health-management

Capra, F. (1982). *The turning point: Science, society, and the rising culture*. Simon & Schuster.

Chamorro-Premuzic, T. (2012). *The dark side of charisma*. HBR Blog network. http://blogs.hbr.org/2012/11/the-dark-side-of-charisma

Coyle, D. (2018). *The culture code*. Bantam Books.

George, B. (2004). The journey to authenticity. *Leader to Leader, 31*, 29–35.

Gill, R. (2011). *Theory and practice of leadership* (2nd ed.). SAGE.

Goleman, D. (2015). *Focus: The hidden driver of excellence*. Harper Collins.

Graham, P. (Ed.). (1995). *Mary Parker Follett—Prophet of management: A celebration of writings from the 1920s*. Harvard Business School Press.

Heimans, J., & Timms, H. (2014). Understanding "new power." *Harvard Business Review*. https://hbr.org/product/understanding-new-power/R1412B-PDF-ENG

Hock, D. (1999). *Birth of the chaordic age*. Berrett-Koehler.

Kellner-Rogers, M. (1999). Changing the way we change: Lessons from complexity. *Inner Edge, 1*(6), 18–22.

Kouzes, J. M. (2000, October). Link me to your leader. *Business2.com, 10*, 292–295.

Kurtsman, J. (2010). *Common purpose: How great leaders get organizations to achieve the extraordinary*. Jossey-Bass.

Lencioni, P. (2012). *The advantage*. Jossey-Bass.

Livingston, S. (2018). Fostering diversity for the next generation of healthcare leaders. *Modern Healthcare*. https://www.modernhealthcare.com/article/20181013/NEWS/181019970/fostering-diversity-for-the-next-generation-of-healthcare-leaders

Malloch, K. (1999). The performance measurement matrix: A framework to optimize decision making. *Journal of Nursing Quality, 13*(3), 1–12.

Porter-O'Grady, T., & Malloch, K. (2018). *Quantum leadership: Creating sustainable value in health care*. Jones & Bartlett Learning.

Secretan, L. H. K. (1997). *Reclaiming higher ground: Creating organizations that inspire the soul*. Macmillan Canada.

Sherwood, G. D., & Horton-Deutsch, S. (2015). *Reflective organizations: On the front lines of QSEN and reflective practice implementation*. Sigma Theta Tau.

Sutcliffe, K. M. (2011). High reliability organizations (HROs). *Best Practice & Research Clinical Anaesthesiology*, *25*, 133–144.

Torbert, W. R. (2000). Exercising vulnerable power. *Inner Edge*, *3*(4), 19–22.

Uhl-Bein, M., & Marion, R. (2008). *Complexity leadership: Part 1: Conceptual foundations*. Information Age.

Weick, K., & Sutcliffe, K. (2001). *Managing the unexpected: Assuring high performance in an age of complexity*. Jossey-Bass.

Werbach, K. (2000, May–June). Syndication: The emerging model for business in the Internet era. *Harvard Business Review*, 90.

Suggested Readings

Axelrod, D. (2000). *Elizabeth I CEO: Strategic lessons from the leader who built an empire*. Prentice Hall.

Bell, C. R. (2005). The vulnerable leader. *Leader to Leader*, *35*, 19–23.

Bly, R. (Ed. & Trans.). (1981). *Selected poems of Rainer Maria Rilke*. Vintage.

Brown, B. (2012). *Daring greatly*. Avery.

Cleveland, H. (1972). *The future executive: A guide for tomorrow's managers*. Harper & Row.

Cranley, L. A., Doran, D. M., Tourangeau, A. E., Kushniruk, A., & Nagle, L. (2012). Recognizing and responding to uncertainty: A grounded theory of nurses' uncertainty. *Worldviews of Evidence-Based Nursing*, *9*(3), 149–158.

Crenshaw, J. T., & Yoder-Wise, P. S. (2013, February 24–27). Creating an environment for innovation: The risk-taking leadership competency. *Nurse Leader*, *11*(1), 24–27.

Cukan, A. (n.d.). *Caregiving: Fighting a culture of fear*. http://www.upi.com/Health_News /2006/02/14/Caregiving-Fighting-a-culture-of-fear/UPI-38431139947951/

Diorynck, B., Hannes, L., & Grant, T. S. (2017). The role of individual and collective mindfulness in promoting occupational safety in health care. *Medical Care Research and Review*, *74*(1), 79–96.

Krass, P. (Ed.). (1998). *The book of leadership wisdom: Classic writings by legendary business leaders*. Wiley.

Margolis, J. D., & Stoltz, P. G. (2010, January–February). How to bounce back from adversity. *Harvard Business Review*, 87–92.

Murphy, L. G. (2012). Authentic leadership: Becoming and remaining an authentic nurse leader. *Journal of Nursing Administration*, *42*(11), 507–512.

Porter-O'Grady, T., & Malloch, K. (2012). *Leadership in nursing practice: Changing the landscape of health care*. Jones & Bartlett Learning.

Quinn, R. E. (1996). *Deep change: Discovering the leader within*. Jossey-Bass.

Rooke, D., & Torbert, W. R. (2005, April). Transformation of leadership. *Harvard Business Review*, 67–76.

Rosen, R. H. (2008, Fall). Embracing uncertainty and anxiety. *Leader to Leader*, 34–38.

Shirey, M. R. (2012). How resilient are your team members? *Journal of Nursing Administration*, *42*(12), 551–553.

Shirey, M. R. (2019). Integration of authentic leadership lens for building high performing interprofessional collaborative practice teams. *Nursing Administration Quarterly*, *43*(2), 101–112.

Werbach, K. (2000, May–June). Syndication: The emerging model for business in the Internet era. *Harvard Business Review*, 85–93.

Wong, C. A., & Walsh, E. J. (2019). Reflections on a decade of authentic leadership research in healthcare. *Journal of Nursing Management*, *28*, 1–3.

Youngblood, M. D. (1997). *Life at the edge of chaos: Creating the quantum organization*. Perceval.

CHAPTER EIGHT   The Focused Leader: Embracing Vulnerability, Risk Taking, and the Potential to Succeed

Quiz Questions

Select the best answer for each of the following questions.

1. Vulnerability is an essential leadership trait for the quantum leader. Which of the following is its major effect?
   a. To expose the leader's weaknesses to others in the organization
   b. To improve the leader's ability to manage information
   c. To reduce the leader's authority and control
   d. To improve the leader's ability to uncover multiple perspectives on an issue

2. Uncertainty in organizations results in a wide range of reactions from leaders. What do most leaders in quantum organizations believe about uncertainty?
   a. Uncertainty is normal.
   b. Uncertainty is the cause of errors.
   c. Uncertainty is a deterrent to creativity.
   d. Uncertainty is surmountable.

3. Nonlinear evaluation of work is the norm for quantum healthcare organizations. What does the nonlinear evaluation of a work process look at?
   a. The cause-and-effect relationships of the process
   b. Outcomes that occur repeatedly
   c. Multiple outcomes
   d. Multiple process participants and multiple outcomes

4. The recognition that uncertainty and chaos are present in all organizations is changing the nature of strategic planning. Which of the following tactics can be used to increase the utility of the planning process?
   a. Decreasing the timeframe under consideration
   b. Adapting initiatives
   c. Adding team members with different perspectives
   d. Increasing the attention given to specific measurable goals and objectives

5. Complexity communication leads to several important results. Which one of the following is a result of complexity communication?
   a. An increased focus on the sending of information
   b. Collective mindfulness
   c. Greater participation of team members
   d. More risk taking

6. New strategies are needed for leaders to provide health care in an environment that is unpredictable and changing rapidly. What is the strategy of open communication designed to do?
   a. Prevent hasty decisions.
   b. Increase team member participation in meetings.
   c. Increase trust in the decision-making process.
   d. Eliminate confidential information.

7. A leader's understanding of his or her personal boundaries, privacy needs, and self-disclosure limits is an important new tool in the leader's toolbox. What does this tool allow the leader to do?
   a. Set limits with employees.
   b. Share feelings and expectations in a meaningful way.
   c. Develop a clear sense of his or her identity as a precursor to relationship building.
   d. Avoid conflict and support team processes.

8. A leader's relationships or social connections have increased in importance as a means to which end?
   a. To facilitate the work of the organization
   b. To increase the leader's visibility
   c. To interpret information
   d. To manage conflict

9. Privacy is a continuing concern for healthcare leaders. How is it best controlled?
   a. By government agencies
   b. By each individual
   c. By eliminating communication on the internet
   d. By developing coded communication

10. Syndication is a new way of using healthcare resources creatively and cost-effectively. What is one of its main disadvantages?
    a. Syndication is expensive.
    b. Syndication requires an increased number of employees.
    c. Syndication has not been used extensively in the healthcare field.
    d. Syndication results in the sharing of information.

11. The importance of focus as a leader includes all of the following, *except*:
    a. to develop multitasking expertise given the complexity of healthcare demands.
    b. to fully understand the specific message being delivered.
    c. to increase one's abilities to filter out distractions.
    d. to engage in meaningful dialogue that leads to the resolution of issues.

12. Which of the following best describes leadership fitness?
    a. Be fully present in mind, body, and spirit.
    b. Be prepared to embrace uncertainty as a vulnerable, rational risk taker.
    c. Be prepared to embrace uncertainty and engage in rational and irrational risk taking.
    d. Be prepared to stretch one's capacity as a leader.

13. Vulnerability is:
    a. a positive leadership attribute that leads to increased transparency.
    b. about susceptibility to negative influences.
    c. reflective of internal weakness and a poor performance history.
    d. a positive trait that encourages others to protect important data.

14. Charismatic leaders have often been sought after and embraced as critical to success. What are the drawbacks of charisma in leadership?
    a. Charismatic leaders are self-centered and avoid employee engagement.
    b. Charismatic leaders tend to create cults of followers rather that cultural depth.
    c. Charismatic leaders have been known to be narcissistic or mentally ill.
    d. All of these statements are true of charismatic leaders.
    e. None of these statements are true of charismatic leaders.

15. Authentic leadership is best described as:
    a. behaviors of truth-telling that is similar to transformational leadership.
    b. a personal style that is necessary for shared governance.
    c. personal authenticity and congruence of professional and personal values.
    d. routinely sharing strengths and personal shortcomings.

16. The cycle of vulnerability identifies stages of experience vulnerability. It does *not* include:
    a. risk taking and project evaluation.
    b. reflection on risk-taking success and selection of the next project or risk.
    c. evaluation of the impact of risk taking on patient care.
    d. taking risks designed to focus on the use of innovation tools.

17. Taking risks in healthcare can be either rational or irrational. Why are rational risks necessary in health care?
    a. To protect employees from harm
    b. To improve communication openness and effectiveness
    c. To overcome feelings of discrimination and powerlessness
    d. To develop skills or engage in whistleblowing

18. Which of the following is the best description of *new power*?
    a. It is a new style used by the millennial generation to advance technology.
    b. It embraces participation and the evolving process of using goods and services.
    c. It is an approach to change that requires skilled collaboration.
    d. It is a fad developed by researchers to recognize the impact of technology.

19. Leadership judgment evolves over time as individuals gain experience in leading. It includes all of the following behaviors, *except*:
    a. being certain about decisions.
    b. analysis of multiple perspectives before selecting an option.
    c. using the cycle of vulnerability as a framework to monitor risk taking.
    d. integration of experiences, recommendations from others, and personal values.

20. The innovation of the 3D printer could have dramatic impacts on many healthcare processes. Which response best describes the impact of the 3D printer?
    a. It is an innovation that will have a moderate impact on the supply of human organs.
    b. It is an innovation that will shift the work of clinicians to more technical practices.
    c. It is an innovation that has the power to transform complex supply-and-demand dynamics.
    d. It is an innovation that will shift in-patient services to ambulatory services.

21. Stretching one's capability is best described as:
    a. engaging in risky behaviors that involve unsafe situations and potential harm.
    b. engaging in new behaviors to expand one's level of competence or to add a new competency.
    c. engaging in new behaviors that include both rational and irrational risks.
    d. reinforcing recently learned skills.

22. In the cycle of vulnerability, one of the steps is living the new reality. The purpose of this phase is:
    a. to allow for a time of inactivity away from risk taking.
    b. to identify the potential for success of the new work.
    c. to allow others to engage in the new work.
    d. to engage in new behaviors for a length of time to experience and validate the new reality in multiple situations.

23. Which of the following is true of collective mindfulness?
    a. It allows an individual to fully focus on the issue.
    b. It is a dynamic in which listening, questioning, and thinking occur as a means to best understand information.
    c. It requires that negativity be removed from conversations.
    d. It is a dynamic in which reflection and listening occur to fully understand the information.

24. Critical questioning is an essential communication skill. Why is it often difficult to learn?
    a. It is natural to want to give advice.
    b. Questions that seek information usually result in yes/no answers.
    c. Reflection does not necessarily result in deeper meaning and understanding.
    d. Questioning is an invasive process that often intimidates others.

25. Strategies for cultivating leadership vulnerability include all of the following, *except*:
    a. allowing staff to attend medical staff meetings.
    b. employing the cycle of vulnerability to monitor new idea development.
    c. engaging in open communication workshops.
    d. avoiding syndication activities to protect the organization's reputation.

CHAPTER NINE

Transforming Error and Engaging Failure Toward a Culture of Safety

It is often the best people that make the worst mistakes—error is not the monopoly of an unfortunate few. We cannot change the human condition, but we can change the conditions under which humans work.

—*James T. Reason*[1]

> ## Chapter Objectives
>
> *At the completion of this chapter, the reader will be able to:*
>
> - Describe the elements of a culture of safety.
> - Describe the concept of failure as an opportunity to improve healthcare outcomes and advance innovations.
> - Describe the advantages and disadvantages of mandatory reporting and disclosure of failures and errors.
> - Compare the advantages and disadvantages of managing failure solely from a systems perspective with managing failure from an individual perspective.
> - Describe the advantages and disadvantages of remediation and discipline as interventions for minimizing error.
> - Show how healthcare leadership failures can be transformed into practices supportive of the quantum organization.

It is a wonder that more errors or failures do not occur in health care in light of the multiple and unending influences that have the potential to impact outcomes. Multiple team members, each with different values, skills, and motivations; complex equipment and technology that is continually being updated; clinical practice variation; physical space that varies from service to service; and the interrelationships of all these impede successful healthcare practices and

---

[1] From Reason, J. (2000). Human error: Models and management. *British Medical Journal, 320,* 768.

outcomes; oftentimes patients are kept safe only because of the heroics of clinicians. In addition, natural chaos emerges from healthcare reform requirements, workforce shortages, and reimbursement limitations. In this chapter, a new perspective is presented in which *failure* is introduced as the more appropriate term for events that do not go as planned or are unsuccessful. Failure is a situation in which there is a lack of success, whereas errors and mistakes assume negative intent and harmful behaviors (Davidson et al., 2017). Failures are about processes not occurring as expected; errors are about processes going wrong because an inappropriate approach or process was completed in a way that was not intended. This distinction, although seemingly minor, is important; to recognize the unintended consequences of trying something new and not getting the expected results is in fact a fruitful outcome and provides information to support innovation solutions. Each patient situation is unique, and clinical interventions are being done for the first time in many situations; the intervention, although well-supported with evidence, is new to this particular patient, with unknown results to compare with. From this perspective, there are most likely far more situations of failure than error in health care, and likely both system failure and individual failure. The important point to recognize is that both failures and errors do occur; however, failures need to be recognized as unsuccessful without bad intent, and errors need to be recognized as deviations from accepted practice that need to be corrected. Imagine a healthcare culture where systems and habits exist with a continuous quest for patient safety.

Healthcare leaders and professionals are generally fearful of making the wrong decision or doing the wrong thing. Yet the potential for failures, breakdowns, and errors in the care of patients is always present, which is why the concept of culture is important. Breakdowns can be caused by poor healthcare clinician performance, unavailability of essential resources, and systemic problems. In the best-case scenario, good systems design and the appropriate number of qualified staff serve to minimize failures and crises when the culture provides the context for safety. Healthcare leaders have the ultimate responsibility for making decisions that create safe clinical practice conditions and for responding to public pressure to improve medical care and reduce negative patient events—quantum leaders facilitate the context for safety.

Creating the Context for Safety

The collective values, beliefs, and norms that are held by all individuals of an organization determine the organizational culture. The behaviors that are practiced in a culture inform the members how the organization operates. A culture of safety exists when all levels of an organization are committed, trust each other, share beliefs that safety is important, and have confidence that their actions will yield safety for patients. A safety culture has full awareness of the complexity and the system and human factors that influence safety through an interplay of leadership, policies, and practices and establishes systems to evaluate the organization's level of reliability in preventing harm (Sherwood & Armstrong, 2016).

The context for safety requires that there is an awareness of the role system design plays when things go wrong rather than blaming an individual. The individual is only one part of the work system. A work system includes the tools and technology, how they are organized, the internal environment, the individual, and the tasks the individual performs (Holden et al., 2013). System design, or how things are designed within the work system, takes into account the limitations of individuals who work in the system or the human factors. In their meta-analysis of the culture of safety literature, Sammer et al. (2010) describe seven elements of a safety culture model that serve as the organizing framework for this chapter. The elements are (1) just culture, (2) learning, (3) teamwork, (4) communication, (5) evidence-based practice, (6) patient-centered care, and (7) leadership. It is the context and interplay of these elements that support a culture of safety.

Just Culture

The reality is that if human beings are involved, things will not always go as planned. Big mistakes, little mistakes, mistakes of consequence with adverse outcomes, and mistakes of little consequence occur every day. To be sure, not every unexpected result is harmful. Further, there are many sources of unexpected events—from human inexperience to incompetence to systemic problems. Near misses are also of concern. Although a near miss, by its nature, may not result in full-scale harm, the surrounding events offer a rich source of information to be studied as a means of avoiding similar situations in the future. Discussing near misses allows an organization to assess specific products or procedures and develop recommendations for improvement.

Just culture is an element of safety culture where a method is used to determine whether errors are an individual failure or a system failure. A just culture is characterized by trust and is nonpunitive; a blame-free atmosphere exists to encourage the reporting of error. A just culture is defined as "an environment where professionals believe they will receive fair treatment if they are involved in an adverse event and trust the organization to treat each event as an opportunity for improving safety" (Petschonek et al., 2013, p. 192). Through leveraging the knowledge of the staff closest to the work, quantum leaders establish the cultural context that ensures the conditions of a just culture, which include the following:

- An organizational responsibility to provide the systems and structures for employees to accomplish their work
- An understanding that all come to the workplace with different values and expectations
- A belief that employees are well-intentioned
- A commitment to the fact that when people feel safe to report error, improvement opportunities are revealed, and the organization can solve problems, prevent recurrence, and improve performance

The concept of trust is an important element of a just culture. The ability of members of the organization to act without fear is essential to patient safety. Disrespectful behavior and intimidation especially in situations of unequal power cannot exist. The organization, its employees, and their patients win when just culture replaces blame and punishment and removes the motivation for individuals to remain silent when their voice is key to prevention and improvement.

> **Point to Ponder**
>
> Consider what would have happened if you had allowed shame and embarrassment to overwhelm you when you fell as a baby while trying to learn how to walk. You would still be crawling!

System Versus Individual Errors

Identifying and understanding the source of mistakes or errors is an essential first step in identifying breakdowns and opportunities for improvement (**Exhibit 9-1**). Unfortunately, the information needed to achieve this step is commonly lacking, partially because those responsible

Exhibit 9-1   Key Concepts

- *Adverse event*: An injury caused by clinical management rather than by the patient's underlying disease or condition.
- *Accident*: An event that involves damage to a defined system that disrupts the ongoing or future output of that system (Kohn et al., 2000).
- *Breakdown*: Situations that unfold in undesirable ways as the result of team members' performance, the unavailability of essential resources, and system problems (Benner et al., 2010).
- *Clinician*: An individual qualified to deliver health care, including medicine, nursing, mental health, pharmacy, dentistry, etc. (National Academies of Sciences, Engineering, and Medicine, 2019).
- *Error*: The failure of a planned action to be completed as intended (error of execution) or the use of a wrong plan to achieve an aim (error of planning) (Kohn et al., 2000).
- *Failure*: Lack of success.
- *Mistake*: An error in action, opinion, or judgment caused by poor reasoning, carelessness, or insufficient knowledge.
- *Safety*: Freedom from accidental injury.
- *Harm*: "Physical, psychological, or emotional damage, without consideration of the mortality or propriety of the actions leading to it" (Wears & Sutcliffe, 2020, p. 9).

> **Key Point**
> When a mistake or error occurs, do not react immediately. Take a deep breath and share your feelings. Learn to ask questions to gain as much information as possible about the situation. Avoid the tendency to judge or criticize.

for the mistakes or errors aren't asked to participate in the discussion, are reluctant to volunteer what they know, or are not aware they were involved in an error. An incomplete analysis of the situation stalls the process and can lead to inappropriate recommendations. The quality of the information surrounding a mistake or error affects the quality and sustainability of the follow-up interventions. Once all the information is collected, the source of error can be localized, and the interactions between the individual and the system and their role in causing the less-than-desirable outcome can be examined.

Much rhetoric has been devoted to system-related causes of medical errors, partly as a result of the significant publicity generated by the 2001 Institute of Medicine (IOM) report on patient safety and medical errors. The media, policymakers, healthcare providers, and the public have all expressed concern and urged that something be done, and consequently healthcare leaders are expected to pay special attention to the system-related problems. Although the IOM report emphasized the importance of system-related factors for reducing the incidence of errors, such as safety systems, job design, and medication administration, the solution does not lie in an either/or approach (**Exhibit 9-2**).

Although the problem is not one of bad people working in health care but of good people working in bad systems, those bad systems are created by people—people who have the capacity to fix them. Further, the systems approach has the disadvantage that it:

- decreases attention to particular aspects of care, especially in the area of relationships;
- flattens out beneficial variations in practice;
- promotes a false and distorting vision of medicine as solely technical; and
- weakens the moral commitment of professionals (Benner et al., 2010).

Learning

Exhibit 9-2 Comparison of Individual and System Accountability

Individual
- Professional/legal mandates
- Emphasizes individual factors
- Emphasizes individual expertise, thoroughness, and accountability
- Views individual as locus of responsibility for errors
- Aims to assign blame and/or extract competency

System
- Human factors and work systems
- Emphasizes structure and organizational factors
- Emphasizes standards, automation, and redundancy
- Views the system as locus of responsibility for errors
- Aims to decrease guilt and increase honesty in reporting

In other words, including both system-related factors and individual factors in error analysis is important if leaders are to develop new approaches to error management that are effective and sustainable. Our drive to be the best, to have the most, and to be in control has led to substantial achievements, but it does not always bring about the best outcome for an organization, and in some cases results in failures or errors. In a just culture when the outcome is less than optimal, the leaders and employees are held accountable, not just for the adverse outcome but also for the learning with safety as the quest.

Learning

The constant attaching of blame to individuals creates a climate of fear and decreases the candid reporting and discussion of mistakes. Learning to appreciate failures and errors as a catalyst for change and improvement opens the door to unexpected opportunities. Failures and errors allow leaders to look at things differently and even revise their plans in light of their new perspective. Quantum leaders examine negative events carefully and work to minimize or eliminate feelings of shame and embarrassment—a once-common response.

Methods for evaluating error or failure provide a shift from blame to a process of objectifying the event through an apparent cause analysis (ACA) or a root cause analysis (RCA), where each element of a work system is evaluated related to its contribution to the failure. The ACA and RCA are structured methodology for analyzing an event that involves the team members closest to the work to learn about the issues that caused an adverse event. Leaders are key to success of ACAs and RCAs through demonstration of their willingness to learn. The steps of an ACA and RCA include determination of the correct method of analysis, gathering of information and mapping the process, assembling the team, identifying root causes, identifying actions, measuring success, and disseminating findings (Braaten, 2016). Clearly an RCA can only be effective if participants feel safe openly talking about the occurrence. As teams gain experience in talking with each other about errors and near misses, learning cultures will become proactive in identifying and improving potentially unsafe processes. The RCA serves as a cultural bridge to a better view of safety. The old concepts of seeing error as a

> **Point to Ponder**
>
> To avoid blaming an individual for a failure, what new or different strategies could you use that would reflect the complex nature of failures and focus on the team and the work systems?

problem of individual competency and blaming the individual for the error are replaced with a belief that the human is only one part of the work system (the other being the systems, technologies, and individuals involved), and both require evaluation and improvement.

> ## Group Discussion
>
> Reflect on a recent error that resulted in serious harm. How was the situation managed? Were there people who remained silent? Did the questions asked focus on identifying someone to blame, such as these: What is wrong here? Who was responsible for this? Or did the questions enable the organization and the clinician to learn more about the situation and be better positioned to avoid recurrences of the error? Better questions for investigating an error include these: Why is this error occurring again and again? Am I missing a lesson here? How can I turn this situation into an opportunity for growth and learning for myself and the team?

Point to Ponder

All failure is normative. It is central to the human experience and a requisite on life's learning journey.

Exhibit 9-3 lists appropriate questions to ask when a failure or error has occurred. One good example of the way failures can lead to positive outcomes is the story of the invention of Post-It Notes: A newly created glue that did not work as planned was turned into a great success—the creation of easily removable stick-on notes. As this example shows, failures may bring good fortune, and learning to trust the potential of failures to create new opportunities is the only way to move from the toxicity of a blameful culture to the productivity of an accountability culture where all clinicians can respectfully disagree or question in any situation. Psychological safety is an important element of safety culture and is defined as "a climate in which people are comfortable expressing and being themselves" (Edmondson, 2019, p. xvi).

Teamwork

The value of teamwork and collaboration has never been higher in this context of increasing disease complexity, with larger numbers of individuals with more than one chronic disease managed by potentially disconnected treatment and technology. In addition, the reforming

Exhibit 9-3 Asking Better Questions

Do Ask
- Why do you think this error occurred?
- Is there a way to avoid this occurring again in the future?
- What can the team learn from this situation?
- What might we be missing?

Do Not Ask
- Why did this happen?
- What did you do wrong?
- Who is responsible for this error?

healthcare system shift to payment for outcomes that require team contributions demands interpersonal effectiveness—a new skill for many clinicians trained to practice independently. It is the collaboration of team members that will manage the intersections of care either successfully or marginally.

No clinician ever intends to make an error or harm a patient. Health care is about helping others to manage their health, relieving pain and distress, restoring functionality, or assisting in a peaceful death. Clinicians feel a sense of satisfaction and accomplishment when a patient experiences relief, a patient's functionality is improved, or a terminally ill patient dies tranquilly. They feel the opposite—discontent and guilt—when their care results in unanticipated bad outcomes. In such a situation, the essence of their healing work has not been realized. Learning to respond to the emotional distress of an adverse event is one of the greatest challenges for clinicians.

Expecting Perfection

Health care, by its very nature, is uncertain and imperfect. The variability in perceptions and in the interpretations of clinical data by both patients and clinicians means that many decisions are partially accidental. Further, medicine is inherently experimental in that each patient has a unique set of characteristics (e.g., age, weight, metabolism, existing conditions, and behavior patterns), and care is essentially provided in a unique manner for each patient. There is never total assurance in health care, and when perfection is expected and the outcomes are inconsistent with the expectation, clinicians suffer emotional distress (**Exhibit 9-4**). Although the mind may understand and tolerate a failure, the human heart is most unforgiving when things do not go well.

Honoring Excellence

In many cases, leaders work diligently to preserve the status quo and avoid changing current processes for fear of making failures and errors. When a failure or error occurs, leaders usually act to rectify the situation immediately and return to the status quo ante. Unfortunately, their fear of disrupting existing routines discourages creativity and motivates employees to refrain from rocking the boat as well. In other words, their drive to sustain the perceived perfect present quashes their own spirit and the spirit of the employees, obstructing the potential for

---

Exhibit 9-4 Two Strategies for Handling Failure and Errors

Expecting Perfection
- Is unrealistic but is considered the proper attitude
- Creates unrealistic expectations
- Fails to consider the wide variability in patient situations
- Positions providers as scapegoats for lack of success

Honoring Excellence
- Takes into account the trial-and-error nature of health care
- Supports the evolution to best practices
- Supports continual improvement processes
- Respects the nature of human interactions
- Reinforces a positive culture of excellence

improvements. Indeed, the fear of failure or retribution that employees feel causes them to essentially "retire on the job" and reduces their productivity. The reality is that trial and error are necessary for improvements to be discovered and implemented.

When things do not go as planned, the best response is to look for the insight in the failure or error and use the information to begin to transform the ineffective practice (see Exhibit 9-3). Overcoming the common obstacles to an open culture fear of punishment for self-reporting, and fear of retaliation for reporting others' errors must be part of the strategy to honor excellence (HealthLeaders Media, 2013). It is through the continual remodeling and transforming of care that best practices or templates for excellence are uncovered. When leaders believe that perfection has already been achieved, they view modifications as inappropriate and a waste of time, thereby hindering the emergence of true excellence.

> **Point to Ponder**
>
> Expecting perfection eliminates the possibility of excellence.

Further, an important organizational dynamic emerges when leaders acknowledge that being right all the time is not even a possibility. If leaders are not highly invested in always being right, they find their employees appreciate their vulnerability and are more likely to approach them with new ideas.

Recognizing and Recovering from Failures and Errors

Nearly every spiritual tradition includes avenues to recognize and recover from negative events. The intent of each tradition is to learn from the event, to identify actions that decrease the chance of repeating the same event, and to improve performance as a result. For organizations to survive and thrive, they must develop traditions that support employees in recognizing failures and errors and rectifying their effects. This includes allowing employees to take responsibility for the impact of their actions and maintaining openness in the workplace, which is critical for reporting and discussing failures and errors and using them as opportunities for improvement (**Exhibit 9-5**).

Coaching employees through the recovery process ranges from simple one-time dialogue sessions to long-term counseling and frequent reassurance. A negative event that results in significant harm or in the filing of a lawsuit has the potential to destroy the career of an otherwise

---

Exhibit 9-5 Recovering from Failures and Errors

- Recognize the lack of clinician or leader preparation to manage mistakes and errors as opportunities.
- Develop strategies to cope with the sense of failure, disappointment, and remorse that often follows negative events.
- Create a coaching script for leaders to address serious failures and errors. The process of dealing with a serious failure or error includes the following:
  – Identifying critical events
  – Identifying opportunities for individual improvement
  – Identifying opportunities for system improvement and innovation
  – Following up on these steps by implementing changes
- Following a negative event, ask the individual how he or she thinks it will affect future practice.

exceptionally competent healthcare clinician. If the person has a hard time coping with the situation, he or she also will have a hard time learning how to prevent a recurrence of the failure or error. Getting stuck in the pain of personal grief or remorse or assigning blame to others does not prevent a repeat performance. In fact, by focusing on the negative emotions felt, the person is distracted from taking measures to solve the problem that led to the mistake. On the other hand, by focusing on what others could or should have done, the person may allay his or her feelings of remorse but may begin to feel powerless or even victimized. The ideal strategy is to accept as much responsibility for the negative event as is warranted, learn, and then go on to explore measures for changing the system in a way that reduces the chance of repeating the failure or mistake.

Given the need for transparency, effective coping strategies, and support for moving on, the work of the leader is clear. If failures are to be treated as opportunities for improvement, healthcare leaders must meet the challenge and create new structures and processes that support dialogue about failures and ongoing follow-up. The overall strategy includes the following:

- Acknowledging the sense of remorse or failure a person who committed an error might feel
- Seeking clarification from that person and providing social support
- Attempting to discover the sources of the problem
- Taking concrete actions to prevent future repetitions

In addition, healthcare leaders must create or strengthen support structures for those in litigation, because all too often these individuals are subtly ostracized by the healthcare team.

Many organizations have recognized the benefits of implementing programs that provide support to those who experience emotional distress following patient adverse events. One such innovation is RISE (Resilience in Stressful Events) peer-support program developed at Johns Hopkins Hospital. A group of peer responders provide support to a staff member who has identified a need for help to recover from the trauma of an unexpected adverse event (Edress et al., 2016). The culture of an organization that is reinforced by peer support is an indication of healthy teams, which establishes the importance of trust—doing purpose-driven work with a trusted team (Zak, 2017)—as the essence of teamwork.

Communication

Communication as an integral component of a safety culture is viewed in three ways: standard internal communication, external requirements for communication, and communication or disclosure to patient of safety events. Internal communication is largely cultural habit. First, human interactions that presume that only bosses or physician providers have all the answers, are able to give orders, or are the only ones that can determine if orders are well-executed is counter to a safety culture. Quantum leaders are those who set direction, invite input, create conditions for continued learning to achieve excellence, or contribute with crucial knowledge and insight to best support a safety culture (Edmondson, 2019). These leaders ask a lot of questions! Second, internal communication systems are implemented to force human interaction to establish concepts of redundancy for error prevention. Examples include read-back requirements by an individual receiving a verbal order from a provider, time-outs or briefings held prior to a procedure to make sure all parties are introduced and understand the correct procedure is being performed on the correct body site and on the correct patient and that the equipment and medication are in place, and bedside shift handoff, where the nurses involved with the clinical care of a patient confer at the bedside of the patient when transferring the care of said patient at change of shift. Clearly these type interactions, once habit, potentiate better team performance in many other situations as care is provided across departments and disciplines, and across settings of care. Accountabilities for effective communication cannot be limited to within a site of care such as inpatient care but should extend across settings of care to ensure that patient care information is not lost in a transition.

External communication is also important to achieve the transparency required for safety. Significant attention has been given to medical errors. The IOM report on errors, titled *To Err Is Human* (Kohn et al., 2000), elevated not only the healthcare community's awareness of this issue but also the public's awareness, because the reported statistics have implications for every single American. The report raised new issues, proposed solutions, and challenged health professionals and the public at large to work to reduce medical errors by at least 50% in the next 5 years. More recently, researchers at Johns Hopkins noted that 250,000 Americans die each year from medical errors, ranking just behind heart disease and cancer as causes of death (McKay & Daniel, 2016). The problem of medical errors remains a problem not only in occurrences but also in how they are statistically tracked in the United States.

Mandatory Error Reporting

Mandatory reporting may be a blessing for the public but could be seen as a curse by care providers. Although the consumers must be given information to assist them in choosing providers and services, not all mistakes and errors provide pertinent information or help in making such decisions. More specific approaches that support mistakes and errors as opportunity are needed, although negligence must of course be reported. The reporting of every minor incident to a state or national board does not necessarily enhance the protection of the public. Mandatory reporting serves to inform the public of mistakes and errors but can obstruct the use of mistakes and errors as opportunities for improvement. Because of the threat represented by reporting to a public body, care providers may be unwilling to declare their mistakes and errors, particularly minor ones. Further, minor incidents in which patients are not placed at risk of harm and care providers' competence is not put into question usually can be handled inside the organization. Most healthcare leaders believe that if mechanisms are in place to take corrective action, remediate deficits, and detect patterns of behavior, no additional benefit is gained from the mandatory reporting of minor incidents. In fact, punishing a clinician for a minor mistake adds to the bureaucratic burden and results in costs to the organization. The Joint Commission (TJC) established guidelines that provide healthcare organizations a structure for reporting expectations that is reserved for those events that meet the definition of a major or sentinel event; that is, a patient safety event that is not related to the natural course of illness that results in death, severe harm, or temporary harm (TJC, 2016). This is consistent with other external or regulatory bodies. The goal of external reporting is to provide a platform for interorganizational learning about major events.

Disclosure

Not only is mandatory reporting a complicating factor in mistakes and error management, so, too, is the expectation of disclosure. Morally, disclosure is the right thing to do. The ethics manual of the American College of Physicians states that physicians should disclose to patients information about procedural or judgment errors made during care if such information is material to patients' well-being. The ethics manual notes that errors do not necessarily constitute improper, negligent, or unethical behavior, but failure to disclose them may.

The act of patient disclosure is representative of the transparency characteristic of a safety culture. In addition, depending on the circumstances, the person or organization who commits the mistake or error may have an obligation to apologize for it or offer reparation. Although professional codes do not clearly state when an apology or reparation is expected, care providers in every discipline, not just physicians, may find themselves in a situation where some sort of acknowledgment of error is morally required. Other ethical issues arise with respect to disclosure. For example, care providers have argued that nondisclosure may be appropriate if the harm from disclosure exceeds the harm from nondisclosure or if the error is inconsequential and disclosure does not empower the patient. Both the Agency for Healthcare Research and Quality (AHRQ) and the National Quality Forum (NQF) have provided resources and positions on disclosing medical errors. AHRQ publishes the Patient Safety Network (2019) and provides guidelines for medical error disclosure. The National Quality Forum (2011) has also endorsed full disclosure of serious unanticipated outcomes.

The disclosure of a mistakes and errors raises certain practical issues, especially the timing of the disclosure, where and how to make it, to whom to make it, and what to expect as a consequence. However noble and right it is to disclose errors, the current litigious culture makes it challenging for care providers to willingly divulge their mistakes or errors, a problem not addressed in the IOM report. Their fear of malpractice suits and their resulting tendency to remain silent about mistakes and errors continues to keep clinicians from moving beyond the status quo of error management. In addition, the malpractice system is unlikely to change in the near future, and alternative methods of dispute resolution are unlikely to be instituted. On the other hand, changes in how mistakes and errors are dealt with should not wait until the legal system is corrected.

For one thing, care providers should be educated in how to disclose errors and how to maintain a relationship with a patient after an injury caused by a medical mistake or error. Not only are leaders challenged to create a culture that supports transparency and disclosure, but in many cases they need to provide educational processes for developing the skills necessary to handle disclosure appropriately. This requires incredible effort from every member of the healthcare team and patience for the expertise to emerge. The following is a set of guidelines for discussing errors with patients:

- Apologize.
- Disclose the harmful error.
- Explain why the error occurred.
- Explain how the error's effects will be minimized.
- Describe the steps the clinician and organization will take to prevent recurrences.
  (AHRQ, 2019)

Relationships are at the core of patient safety. Communication is the currency of relationships. Consider the historical world of health care when access to a paper medical record occurred through a human interaction. Today, the electronic medical record can be accessed from anywhere, anytime without any human interaction. This tells us that communication must be hard-wired, and in some cases, a hard-stop to ensure the human interface is used when needed to support patient safety, learn from other organizations that have had similar events, and most of all secure an honest relationship with patients.

Evidence-Based Practice

Evidence-based practice is an essential element of safety culture. Practices grounded in evidence that include protocols, checklists, and guidelines are characteristic of a safety culture. Clinical policies require close evaluation of best evidence, which is cited on the policy for reference by the users. Error prevention bundles are common as a checklist format for those tips that require prevention. **Exhibit 9-6** lists the top 10 patient safety tips for hospitals from the AHRQ (2018a).

The IOM competencies and multiple reports unfortunately do not clarify the locus of accountability for error. Recommendations for using a multifocal, evidence-driven approach are strongly encouraged. Both internal and external oversight mechanisms are recommended. Management of errors internally—in fact, nearest the point-of-service (or the point-of-error)—offers the best opportunity for continuing improvement, especially if there is a national repository of data on safety and supporting practices.

> ### Group Discussion
>
> A colleague in nursing reports the following incident to you: "I recently gave a patient the wrong medication. The patient was not affected, and I did not write an incident report because I did not want it noted in my personnel record or reported to the state board of nursing. This type of mistake happens often because most facilities are understaffed." How would you handle this situation? Do you agree with the nurse? What changes could be made to the system to support the reporting of this type of error and create opportunities to learn from the commission of errors? When should a medication error be reported to a board of nursing?

Exhibit 9-6   Top 10 Patient Safety Tips for Hospitals

1. Prevent central line–associated bloodstream infections.
2. Reengineer hospital discharges.
3. Prevent venous thromboembolism.
4. Educate patients about using blood thinners safely.
5. Limit shift durations for medical residents and other hospital staff, if possible.
6. Consider working with a patient safety organization.
7. Use good hospital design principles.
8. Measure your hospital's patient safety culture.
9. Build better teams and rapid response systems.
10. Insert chest tubes safely.

From Agency for Healthcare Research and Quality (AHRQ). (2018a). *10 patient safety tips for hospitals.* http://www.ahrq.gov/patients-consumers/diagnosis-treatment/hospitals-clinics/10-tips/index.html

Patient-Centered Care

The presence of a patient- and family-centered culture establishes the *why* of our work in health care. It extends the accountability of healthcare organizations beyond the walls of acute care to establish mechanisms to ensure that the patient benefits from traveling through the organization across settings of care and that patient health is positively impacted because the patient and his or her family interacted with the system. With the patient and family at the center, patient safety is established as the focus of all decision making. It becomes a core value, and clinicians should routinely ask, "What is best for the patient?" Knowing that a patient is well cared for fulfills the purpose of many clinicians who enter health care as a profession to serve by providing what is best for patients. The role of the patient and family in safety is evident because theirs are the faces in safety efforts. For example, instead of only reporting rates of infection, organizations could list the name of the individual patients who were harmed. In safety cultures, patients are often the source of safety awareness. Patients are involved in the procedural time out, in bedside shift handoff, and medication reconciliation. Many clinicians can account of times when the patient's involvement avoided a serious error.

The IOM, in its book *Crossing the Quality Chasm* (2001), defines *patient-centered care* as "providing care that is respectful of and responsive to individual patient preferences, needs, and values and ensuring that patient values guide all clinical decisions" (p. 40). Safety cultures use the tenet of patient centeredness as the purpose of their innovation.

Leadership

Leaders design, foster, and nurture the context by which safety is seen by all levels of the organization as a core value. Leaders reinforce a level of expectation that everyone can evaluate each other's work regardless of rank or position (Patrician et al., 2016). Leaders model the psychological safety behavior in a culture of safety and are a key element to leading an organization from one of punishment and fear to one of transparency and engagement.

Transforming a Punitive Culture

Efforts to decrease negative reactions to errors have been undertaken both within and outside healthcare organizations, including the Institute for Healthcare Improvement and TJC. It is this work that also needs to continually transform the quality and safety of organizations. Shifting the perception of errors to failures whenever possible is important so that we engage failures as a positive event, one that is intensely human and inherently essential to innovation. However, after 2 decades of improving quality and safety with system-level approaches, followed by a subsequent plateau of improvement, we now know that there is a continued accountability of leaders to also understand individual performance variation as an opportunity to improve quality and safety further (Yakusheva et al., 2020). Regardless of the source of the initiative to transform a punitive safety culture, leaders must embark on the purposeful and deliberate work of changing expectations and behaviors to support patient safety, the reporting of errors, and the engagement of clinicians in the process. The work of culture transformation does not occur quickly; time is required to establish new behaviors and build the necessary trust among individuals. Progress is directly related to the collective ability of the team to learn and improve. Once clinicians are engaged in improvement and understand how individuals and work systems are both involved in quality and safety, the quest for excellence, rather than perfection, is possible.

Remediation Versus Discipline

The way in which the accountability of health professionals is defined by state licensing boards tends to push leaders toward instituting disciplinary action against individuals who make mistakes or errors. However, the overall effectiveness of disciplining for improving practice or minimizing errors has not been substantiated. Further, state licensing boards have different reporting requirements. Some states, for instance, require only the reporting of significant errors that resulted in harm, whereas others require the reporting of all errors, including minor ones. The value of reporting minor errors with low risk for harm does not appear to be worth the trauma caused to the care clinicians.

Drawing the disciplinary line, according to Marx (2001), is the real challenge in determining when to remediate and learn from mistakes and when to discipline. He describes four behavioral categories helpful in making this decision: human error, negligence, intentional rule violations, and reckless conduct. Human error needs to be separated out from the categories for remediation because it is about individual behavior that inadvertently caused or could cause an undesirable outcome. These are all aspects of just culture covered earlier in the chapter.

The strategy of using remediation first and discipline when more than human error is involved deserves consideration (**Exhibit 9-7**). Remediation (counseling and guidance provided in a timely manner) serves to protect the care clinician's dignity and minimizes shame. In addition, remediation is consistent with the treatment of mistakes and errors as opportunities for learning new, more effective behaviors.

This strategy also makes both the system and the individual accountable for addressing mistakes and errors. The person who committed the mistake or error is expected to participate in the analysis of the event and identify alternative approaches that will reduce the chance of a recurrence. The other members of the team or work group also review the event and contribute to the list of recommendations. These individuals thereby gain insights that will help them avoid similar events. In other words, all the members learn not only from their mistakes but from the mistakes of others, which is invaluable for the individual members, the team, and the organization as a whole. This can be informal or part of an RCA.

Finally, the strategy puts the leader of the organization in the position to manage mistakes and errors without additional reporting to an outside agency. This is an advantage because the leader is best suited to manage minor mistakes and errors and work with the clinicians to ensure that these events are not repeated. Although not traditionally labeled remediators, most leaders are skilled in remediation techniques, especially the giving of feedback. By discussing the situation in private first, by being specific and focusing on the

---

Exhibit 9-7 Remediation Guidelines

Consider remediation when:
- The potential risk of physical, emotional, or financial harm to the client resulting from the incident is very low.
- The incident is a singular event with no pattern of poor practice.
- The employee exhibits a conscientious approach to and accountability for his or her practice.
- The employee appears to have the knowledge and skill to practice safely.

facts, and by following up to increase the chances of success, the leader can reduce minor mistakes and errors without causing the clinicians to feel unnecessary shame and guilt.

> **Point to Ponder**
>
> "Learn from the mistakes of others; you can't live long enough to make them all yourself."
>
> —Anonymous

Errors that carry a significant risk of physical, emotional, or financial harm or errors that show a pattern of recurrence require greater scrutiny and management. The leader should still refrain from using discipline until the system-related and individual issues are evaluated and a pattern of incompetence and/or negligence has been identified. The goal, in the "error as opportunity" approach, is always to learn from errors by focusing on the relationship between the individual and the system and by implementing appropriate revisions in the work processes. Discipline should be the intervention of last resort.

Healthcare Leadership: Issues and Opportunities

Everyone acknowledges that learning comes not only from the successful performance of an activity or practice but also from events that are not successful—from breakdowns or situations that did not go well. But most people are reluctant to reveal their failures, especially at work in front of others. The reluctance to talk about failures or errors means the whole team risks losing vital pieces of information that can be derived from looking at the situation carefully. Even worse, the likelihood that others will repeat the same mistakes increases dramatically.

Clinical failures and errors do not occur in isolation. As noted in the IOM reports, an organization's system—its structures and processes—has a large impact on the incidence of errors. Indeed, the system not only is the most important influence on the type and number of errors that are committed but also provides the greatest opportunity for improvement. It is through understanding the errors of the past that leaders can redesign the future to support the practices that minimize system breakdowns and individual mistakes.

Unfortunately, the recognition of failures and errors is not a simple or obvious process. Habitual routines of leaders and clinicians often are not based in current evidence and obviate the need to recognize failures and errors, and it is true that changing what has become established involves some short-term costs. Habitual routines are familiar, comfortable, and usually temporarily successful. However, long-term survival must be the focus. The desire of most leaders to experience stability in their work life makes it difficult for them to admit that the system is not working as well as it could be and that it needs to be revised. Quantum leaders realize that routine practices, standard operating procedures, and traditional protocols seldom meet organizational needs for any extended length of time. Constant adjustment of processes is always necessary to ensure continuous goodness-of-fit with the environment.

Traditional leaders tend to put a premium on "being right." They want to be seen as a competent, comprehensive resource, and thereby win the respect of the employees. In contrast, quantum leaders and their teams must learn to become comfortable with vulnerability, quickly acknowledging the existence of outdated processes, suboptimal choices, and leadership mistakes and to move on regardless of the investment. They must identify current practices that are not working or have become obstacles to providing healthcare services and then make adjustments so they function better. In most cases, these practices should not be looked on as errors but rather as outdated or, at best, mistakes. They simply no longer fit the organization's needs and currently fail to result in the desired outcomes, no matter how effective they were in the past (Ricks, 2012).

The remainder of the chapter consists of a discussion of five leadership situations, associated opportunities for change, and specific strategies for supporting the desired improvements. The purpose here is not to criticize or negate the work of leaders but rather to focus on common problems and stretch creative thinking to support our journey into the Information Age, where mistakes and errors are opportunity. The five situations are as follows:

1. Failure to shift to value-based healthcare services.
2. Failure to own healthcare products.
3. Fragmented leadership.
4. Dehumanization of healthcare clinicians.
5. Demanding the impossible.

Situation 1: Failure to Shift to Value-Based Healthcare Services

Dramatic changes in health care have occurred over the last 30 years, most notably in the area of reimbursement. Unfortunately, few, if any, healthcare structures have changed to the extent needed to ensure the delivery of high-quality healthcare services.

Financial resources have become the focus of clinical decision making. Financial officers work diligently to maximize reimbursement and reduce expenses, whereas clinicians do their best to deliver the comprehensive care expected by consumers. Many healthcare leaders continue to believe that good financial performance supports clinical quality in the same way as in the past. The role of finance has become so important, in fact, that in many organizations the chief financial officer (CFO) has a line position and controls processes and operations, whereas the medical director holds a staff position and offers input and suggestions but is impotent to control patient care services. Such changes in authority and decision making, although perhaps not reflected in the organizational chart, are otherwise explicitly recognized.

For many healthcare providers, these role changes interfere with the real work of the organization, and they view healthcare leadership these days as more like dealership. Health plan contract negotiations are based almost solely on actuarial data and the expectation that patients will use the least amount of services available. Further, although recognizing that both productivity and a healthy financial base are essential for survival, care providers find it disconcerting that these are to be achieved at the expense of patient care quality. In short, healthcare organizations have failed to adapt the healthcare system to the changing supply-and-demand factors and marketplace values, and this failure is the source of the incredible chaos being experienced by leaders, clinicians, payers, and the public.

Before the advent of the Affordable Care Act, the issue of value was relatively minor. Most expenses were covered by payers interested in increasing the access to healthcare services. Leaders worked to expand the types and numbers of services they offered to keep their organizations competitive. With this model, there is no accountability and no control. Not surprisingly, resources ran out, and the public rebelled against escalating healthcare expenditures. The imperative for leaders continues to be to reconnect the system with the marketplace and reestablish a balance between service (the providing of assistance), quality, and cost.

The separation of marketplace value and clinical outcomes was tolerable when no connection was expected in the marketplace. Consumers received the services provided, and the payers reimbursed providers as billed. Healthcare value in the retrospective payment system was determined by the provider, not by the patient. It is important to note that clinician behavior was not intended to diminish the importance of fiscal issues. There was simply no demand for real fiscal accountability. Clinicians were expected to provide the best of everything. They delivered as many healthcare services as possible. Functional, role, and clinical issues were of central concern, not financial issues. In fact, discussion of financial issues by clinicians was considered inappropriate and was discouraged.

Opportunity 1: Practice Within the Marketplace

As they begin the journey of shifting organizational work to support marketplace values, leaders need to keep in mind how health care got to its current state of chaos. The main causal factor is the current imbalance between the types and amount of services being provided and the dollars available for their purchase. In fact, the lack of dollars has created serious instability in the marketplace. In many organizations, changes are being implemented to shift the focus back to the provision of healthcare services within the marketplace parameters. Unfortunately, not all organizations have begun the work of transformation, and some have yet to identify the needed revisions.

Every healthcare leader must critically assess the services his or her organization provides to ensure that they are consistent with the organization's mission. Fixing marketplace errors requires a shift from managing for profit to managing for the organizational mission of delivering value-based health care. The process of fitting care to the available dollars cannot begin without an understanding of the value that is being bartered. Reducing or controlling services without a clear notion of the value each discipline contributes to clinical outcomes is like taking a shot in the dark. At best, it is an example of irresponsible leadership.

What Is Value?

It is not uncommon for leaders to be unsure of the real value of the services provided by healthcare clinicians in their organizations. Some clinicians are not sure of this themselves. Evidence must show that resources are being used efficiently to bring about clear improvements in patient conditions, increase the ability of the patients to manage their own health, and add to the patients' knowledge of their conditions and/or healthy behaviors. This is quite different from providing services as defined in a standards manual.

Determining the value of healthcare services is an integral part of quantum leadership. This value, which is defined by means of an equation containing the three elements of cost, quality, and service, is never simply a matter of dollars (Malloch & Porter-O'Grady, 1999). Instead, its calculation takes into account what is actually gained and what are the real costs. The exact equation is expressed thus: healthcare value = resources (funds and labor and supplies) + quality (appropriateness of interventions) + service (satisfaction and effective relationships).

Finding the value of a healthcare service requires healthcare leaders and clinicians to ask the following questions:

- What is the actual service provided?
- How do organizational processes support this service?
- What are the interactions between these processes?
- What impact does the service have on the patients and the community?

The answers to these questions guide leaders and healthcare providers toward wise choices—toward clinical decisions that are the most cost-effective and result in the highest-quality care being provided at the lowest cost (Pappas, 2013). The challenge for leaders is to reframe the healthcare quality issue as a value question. Again, value is defined as the result of an interactive process involving cost, quality, and service. The cost of health care in the marketplace is determined by both the available resources and reimbursement; the quality of the service is determined by the outcome of the service (i.e., how delivery of the service changes the patient's state of health); and service, which is the rendering of assistance, is partly a function of the time and manner of provision.

Within this framework, the marketplace phenomenon becomes apparent. The value equation is out of balance in that too much care is being provided given the level of available dollars—or too few resources are being applied to health care. The greatest opportunity or leverage point for changing the value equation begins with the element of service, not the cost or quality. If there are limited resources, questions such as this arise: Should the response to every sign or symptom be some type of intervention, particularly if it results in minimal or no improvement in the patient's clinical condition? What an incredibly difficult challenge it is for providers and leaders to deal with the issue of rationing, especially those schooled in the philosophy that increased access to health care is always in the public's interest. Indeed, rationing of healthcare services has traditionally been seen as incongruent with the American spirit. Of course, the reality is that it has occurred throughout history; it is just more obvious when the issue moves beyond the closed ranks of health professionals to the community at large.

The Metrics of Value-Based Health Care

To determine the value of health care, leaders and providers are faced with deciding what should be measured. What are the metrics of success? What constitutes value for the consumer? How are all the metrics interrelated? Current financial management is concerned with statistics such as net income margin, net present value, return on equity, return on investment, and return on assets. These metrics are unfamiliar to clinicians, and are very different from the metrics they see as vital, such as responsiveness to treatment, level of pain management, and wound healing.

Traditionally, the financial mindset has focused on return on investment for dollars spent. This measure has limited applicability in health care. In a return-on-investment analysis, the cost-to-benefit ratio shows the worth of spending dollars to make dollars. If the benefits of a healthcare program or service can be priced in dollars, then a cost-to-benefit analysis is appropriate, and the alternative that leads to the greatest dollar benefits for the cost has a good claim to be chosen. However, many healthcare decisions and services involve far more than simply generating income. In fact, healthcare dollars are often spent on a clinical problem to improve the outcomes of patient care, and ascribing a monetary value to a health outcome is a complex, if not impossible, task. Another issue is that cost-to-benefit analysis is not sensitive to healthcare objectives, including the psychological benefits of improved health, the psychological and physiological benefits of clean air and water, and so on.

Increasingly, healthcare leaders are switching to cost-effectiveness analysis (Buerhaus, 1998). Instead of measuring benefits and costs in dollars, a cost-effectiveness analysis uses units such as years of life saved to measure health outcomes and dollars to measure the cost of the treatment. Although a cost-effectiveness analysis cannot determine whether a single program's benefits outweigh its costs, it can be used to compare alternative programs. This approach is aligned to the expectations of the Affordable Care Act in which quality and outcomes are valued (Cosgrove, 2013). The time for recovery, number of readmissions infection rates, and medical errors will now be considered in payment models. In addition, perceptions of patients are now being considered in payment formulations using the Hospital Consumer Assessment of Healthcare Providers and Systems (HCAHPS) Survey. The quality of experiences with and communication with doctors, nurses, and support staff, quality of the environment (cleanliness and quiet), pain management, information about medications and treatments, and discharge information now enter into the quality and payment of healthcare services (HCAHPS, 2016).

It is nearly impossible to draw conclusions about services on the basis of a single metric. Multiple influencing factors must be considered in reaching decisions on allocating resources. Healthcare leaders are best advised to develop a matrix of metrics in which multiple essential indicators are considered in the evaluation of resource use. Cost-effectiveness should be measured in the aggregate from the multiple perspectives of quality, productivity, and cost and from the patient, care provider, and organization levels. Blending the cultures of finance and health care is challenging at best, but it can be made somewhat more manageable if everyone understands the common ground shared by finance and health professionals—they are all dependent on their checkbooks and their health, neither of which is able to exist effectively without the other.

Eliminating Nonvalue-Added Services

Most healthcare providers assume that every service provided is an essential service and that there are no opportunities for changing service patterns. They believe that if a service did not make a difference to the health of patients—did not add value in terms of increased well-being—they would not be providing it. Yet most providers have not examined each service to determine whether it really does affect the clinical conditions of patients, enhance patients' understanding of their conditions, or increase their ability to manage their own health. In many cases, services are provided to conform to standards but without improving patient outcomes.

Consider a patient who suffers from chronic uncontrolled diabetes. The patient is regularly hospitalized for stabilization and treatment. During each hospitalization, the patient receives diabetic education and attends two information sessions, in accordance with the established standard of care. Despite the instruction, the patient and family have never been able to commit to the required dietary changes, and they do not plan to make any changes. In this case, the diabetic education has failed to make a difference in terms of clinical stability, knowledge of the disease, or ability to manage the patient's health; consequently, it is a nonvalue-added service. Given the overwhelming workload of the clinicians, the service should be provided to this patient in an abbreviated form or possibly not at all. The patient medical record should reflect the reality of the situation—namely, that continuing education was considered but not implemented because of the lack of expected clinical effect.

When services that fail to add value are discovered, the leader must support the team in eliminating them, a daunting task at best. Fear of the unknown often overrides the need to change, feeding organizational inertia and reinforcing assumptions that the current way is the right and only way to do the work. Limited resources and concern about short-term costs can further impede progress. The leader's challenge is to create a culture in which all members are expected to continually seek better and more efficient ways of providing services and to eliminate practices that are no longer effective.

Once the leader identifies what actual services are delivered, what outcomes they produce, and what their costs are, the dialogue with managed care organizations changes dramatically. If the managed care organization negotiators want to decrease premiums, the leader can now translate the reduction into a decrease in services. Conversely, the leader can request premium increases to match improvements in patient outcomes. No longer is it expected that services remain the same despite a reduction in available dollars. Further, the amount of negotiating power is determined by the value produced rather than the number of individuals around the table or their negotiating tenacity. Decisions should be made from a consumer-value perspective.

> **Group Discussion**
>
> Consider the impact of an organization-wide directive focused on increasing personal and professional accountability. Each clinician is asked to recommend the elimination of two current policies that he or she believes are within the scope of their licensure and professional accountability. Would the value of health care increase or decrease as a result of this approach and expectation? Who might oppose the approach, and who might favor it?

Team-Based Health Care

For healthcare services and leadership practices to receive the kind of critical examination that is needed, the leader and the other team members must undergo a renewal of team spirit and show a willingness to challenge the status quo and expose the sacred cows of health care. No clinician should decide alone what to do for patients. Engaging in dialogue with each other is the only way clinicians can ensure that their value-based goals are achieved. In addition, dialogue between clinicians minimizes the potential for system breakdown and error. As collaboration increases, the team becomes more competent in frontline quality management and system repair. It is then able to monitor service value and to act as the agent in monitoring and managing system breakdowns. The quantum leader must create the context in which the necessary communication skills are both valued and expected. New models of team-based care are documenting time savings and improved efficiency with skill mix changes in ambulatory care. The addition of a second medical assistant (MA) to a primary care team was found to add patient capacity and net revenue, better patient satisfaction, and satisfaction for both MAs and providers (Hopkins & Sinsky, 2014).

> **Point to Ponder**
>
> Team training in health care can reduce patient mortality by 15% according to a new study. Team training can also reduce medical errors by 19% (Hughes et al., 2016).

Regardless of past practices, every decision made by a clinician should take into account the choices and decisions of others. In practice, clinicians seldom act as a team in implementing interventions and evaluating care, and each clinician delivers the kind of care that those within the clinician's discipline believe is best (as indicated by the discipline's established practice standards). To combat unilateral decision making and ensure a good fit between decisions made along the continuum of care, clinicians and patients must exhibit a strong pattern of communication and interaction.

Teamwork is essential for effective care coordination. As noted by the AHRQ, care coordination involves deliberately organizing patient care activities and communicating among those involved the patient's care, and teamwork is one of the major approaches to accomplish this complex work (AHRQ, 2018b).

Situation 2: Failure to Own Healthcare Products

The increasing involvement of external agencies in determining appropriate healthcare services sounds an alarm for even the most inexperienced healthcare leader. Regardless of perceived past failures of healthcare organizations to manage internal processes, the return of healthcare oversight and management to the point-of-service is needed to minimize bureaucracy and support the shift toward using errors as opportunities for improvement rather than punishment.

Perhaps the chaos of the transition from a retrospective payment system to a fixed payment system has blurred the expectations of all stakeholders. The expectation for healthcare systems is that processes are in place to ensure that services are both effective and provided within the marketplace parameters. The oversight of staffing, scheduling, pain management, advance directives, and so on by external agencies interferes with the performance and accountability of the internal leadership, yet the public call for organizations to meet the core responsibilities of error management, safe staffing, and pain management reinforces the notion that healthcare leaders have not previously been held sufficiently accountable.

Besides dealing with unclear expectations and uncertainty, healthcare leaders face intense financial pressures that distort the order of their stewardship obligations, which should be service first, survival second, and profit third. They also often are placed in ethical dilemmas in which the right decision is hard to determine, let alone carry out. As evidence of this, fraud and abuse stories have become all too common in the press. It seems that the prevalence of such stories is partly explained by the fact that leaders are in the position of desperately searching for financial revenues and sometimes choose questionable methods. Of course, not only is fraud, when uncovered, detrimental to the reputation of the organization, but the intense scrutiny that follows its discovery creates an atmosphere of mistrust between care providers, payers, and the government. Yet, although fraud is a criminal matter that must be addressed in the court system, many issues are better managed internally. The challenge for leaders is to determine which issues are best managed internally and which issues must be managed externally.

Opportunity 2: Moving from External Oversight to Internal Accountability

There is a pronounced need for less external regulation and more professional accountability within organizations. The locus of accountability for clinical quality lies within each profession, and the content is defined by its standards. The accountability for an organization's systems, structures, and processes rests with the leaders, and the content is defined by the organization's mission, vision, and values. The control or oversight of the organization's services and leadership rests with the governing board because its members understand the needs and expectations of the community being served much better than any external accrediting agency could. It should not be necessary for business and government agencies to force or direct care providers and organizations to address issues such as the high incidence of medical errors or perform their essential duties as providers of health care.

Living Accountability

Accountability-based health care is an essential foundation for the "error as opportunity" approach recommended in this chapter. To ensure accountability for system processes, expectations for performance must be clearly defined for and shared by all members of the organization, and performance that meets the stated expectations must be recognized and rewarded routinely. In addition, incompetence or failure to live the expected behaviors must be dealt with in a timely manner. All too often leaders ignore incompetence because they want to avoid confrontation. Hoping that the problem simply disappears is unrealistic and damaging to the morale of the organization, because it has the effect of lowering the performance standards. Quantum leaders are competent not only at managing incompetence but also at coaching other team members in managing incompetence. They know that managing incompetence is strongly associated with improved organizational performance and increased employee morale, as well as decreased errors.

Political Competence

Developing political skills is essential for all members of the quantum organization. In the past, healthcare leaders have played a role in devising and implementing health-related policies at the local, state, and national levels, but as organizations increase the extent of their team-based activities, political competence is a requirement for all employees involved in providing services.

Political competence is defined by Longest (1998) as the dual capacity to accurately assess the impact of public policies on one's area of responsibility and to influence public policy making at both the state and local levels. For each healthcare service offered by an organization, the organization's leaders must understand the service and try to determine the expected impact of public policies and the policies of accrediting organizations and health plans on the service. Further, each member of the organization must understand the internal policies that apply to the provision of services and know when to communicate concerns to the organization's leaders, when to use positional power to exert influence on policymakers, and when to remove or mitigate barriers to care to ensure that the services are provided.

> ### Group Discussion
>
> Healthcare providers are under pressure to discharge patients according to protocols and guidelines. When patients fall outside the guidelines, the providers must advocate for lengthier stays with insurance companies and, when their requests are denied, are put in the untenable position of discharging patients under unsafe conditions. As leader of the surgical unit, you believe patients are often being discharged prematurely, especially patients who are unsteady and not voiding well. In this situation, what is your obligation as leader? What information should you be communicating, and when and to whom should you be communicating it? What changes in practice are recommended? What rationale for these changes is likely to garner the most support?

Politically competent healthcare clinicians also are able to assist regulators and legislators in creating solutions and to describe the clinical and economic value of healthcare services to patients, purchasers, and policy analysts. Organizational policies and procedures are designed to incorporate professional standards, define expectations, and enhance service quality. When policies exist that are inconsistent with standards, contradict expectations, or impede service quality, politically competent providers can communicate the issues of concern and facilitate the revision of the policies.

Situation 3: Fragmented Leadership

Traditional healthcare organizations rely on clinical professionals to deliver the services defined by the mission, and they rely on management professionals to make the service processes more efficient and effective. Given that the clinical and management professions have different knowledge bases and values, clinicians and managers are sometimes at odds with each other. However, their differences have become increasingly problematic for the delivery of healthcare services as the environment has been affected by burdensome reimbursement constraints, increasing competition for a larger share of diminishing resources, and a lack of qualified healthcare workers. Indeed, the internal competition between clinicians and managers has negatively affected productivity and, more important, discouraged innovation.

Because of the ongoing financial pressure and competition experienced by healthcare organizations, patient care often loses out to financial priorities. In fact, left with few opportunities for reducing expenses, healthcare leaders often end up searching for ways of managing the demand for healthcare services rather than managing expenses.

Most healthcare leaders are experts on healthcare infrastructure and marketplace principles. Very few are experts on clinical care and marketplace principles. As a result, many organizations are struggling because their leaders do not have clinical competence and are making decisions solely from a financial perspective. No longer can healthcare organizations afford leaders incapable of integrating patient care needs and financial survival.

Opportunity 3: Holographic Leadership

The strategy of minimizing competition between financial and clinical priorities and increasing collaboration requires a new model of healthcare leadership. Leaders in quantum healthcare organizations need to be competent and knowledgeable in both healthcare and marketplace management. The position of chief executive or patient care administrator should be occupied by someone who has advanced clinical training (e.g., a physician, nurse, pharmacy, social worker, or physical therapist) and has expertise in the management of these clinical services. The chief executive's knowledge base should include an understanding of how services are provided, what their outcomes are, how to estimate costs, and how to determine the availability of reimbursement. A background in the business end of health care is not by itself sufficient for leading a 21st-century healthcare organization, and neither is experience as a clinician.

As the healthcare environment changes, so, too, does the set of critical leadership competencies. The new competencies reflect an integrated or holographic perspective on the healthcare experience that encompasses the technical, relational, and intentional aspects of patient care. The quantum healthcare leader must have a clear understanding of the procedural work of clinicians and must possess the skills to connect clinicians to the service and system infrastructure in such a way as to ensure that value-based care is delivered within the limits of the available resources. Health care provided without a specific intention or without effective relationships between clinicians is fragmented care, and fragmented care is no longer acceptable or affordable.

Necessarily, all operational or line positions in health care require knowledge, skills, and abilities that jointly reflect a holographic healthcare perspective. Operational positions are held by healthcare employees accountable for ensuring that the value equation is balanced. Staff positions are those positions that support the work of the organization but do not require clinical competence. In many ways, this model should suit those who were in traditional staff positions but were pushed into operational roles without being given adequate training. Such professionals (e.g., finance officers) are now expected to do what they do best without the additional burden of making decisions in areas in which they lack expertise. Experts in planning, human resources, and finance are ideally suited for staff or consultant positions, and together they can participate as team members in a shared leadership team model.

> **Group Discussion**
>
> Imagine a healthcare organization in which the leaders were competent in both clinical and management disciplines. Speculate on how the organization would be structured. What roles would be added or eliminated? Would the patient care outcomes likely be different? In what way? Would job satisfaction be affected? Summarize the advantages and disadvantages of this model.

Leaders in the new millennium must determine the most effective and efficient processes to achieve the three goals of high-quality patient care, organizational viability, and respectable profits. Given that healthcare economists focus on the supply and demand for services, reimbursement mechanisms, productivity, the impact of technology, workforce issues, market dynamics, and health-related public policy, it is incumbent upon clinicians to provide a clear description of the healthcare services and their outcomes, the time and skill level requirements for each service, and the cost of providing each service so that the economists can analyze the aforementioned factors and their relationships accurately.

Situation 4: Dehumanization of Healthcare Clinicians

The financial pressure experienced by healthcare organizations not only has affected the type and number of services afforded patients but also has altered the way organizational leaders are managing healthcare clinicians. In some cases, the clinicians perceive their treatment as uncaring and ruthless and see themselves as pawns. As evidence, clinicians can point to regular rounds of staff reductions, staffing by ratios, elimination of continuing education programs, and the use of hiring bonuses.

Workforce Reductions

The elimination of leadership and clinical positions with little or no warning seriously mars the morale of the healthcare workforce. Competent leaders and clinicians/staff are finding it increasingly difficult to rebound and find new employment. Regardless of how the termination is handled, they find it nearly impossible to live with the notion that "it's not personal, it's business" when their livelihood has been dramatically altered.

The hidden costs that result from the disruption of relationships in the workplace have yet to be measured. One hidden cost is the loss of departing employees' knowledge of the job and the other workers and the organization. Another is the reduction in needed competence and experience, which, if severe enough, can lead to a phenomenon known as failure to rescue (described later). Further, because length of employment usually determines who gets let go, newly hired employees with up-to-date skills and knowledge are sometimes eliminated in favor of employees who have minimal or outdated competencies.

> ### Group Discussion
>
> Some leaders focus on processes alone, others on outcomes alone, still others on both processes and outcomes. What are the consequences for the organization when the leader is process oriented? When the leader is outcome oriented? When the leader is both process and outcome oriented? Compare the differing effects of the three approaches. What are the advantages and disadvantages of each? Which approach fits best with holographic leadership?

To understand the harm that can occur from workforce reductions, consider the critical surveillance role played by nurses. Indeed, their vigilance is essential to rescuing many patients who have experienced a complication. In such a situation nurses must first recognize that a complication has occurred or is impending, and then they must intervene rapidly to ensure the patient's survival. When nurse staffing levels are reduced, the ability of the clinical nurses to recognize a potential or an actual problem is compromised, sometimes to the extent that they fail to save a patient who might otherwise have survived.

Another common effect of decreasing the number of competent registered nurses is the implementation of mandatory overtime. In fact, more than 70% of hospitals in the United States have formal mandatory overtime requirements. Making healthcare providers put in extra hours can push them beyond their physical limits and reduce their ability to perform competently. Tired and overworked care clinicians are poorly suited for the level of clinical surveillance required for quality patient care.

Finally, in addition to reductions in the absolute number of nurses employed, licensed personnel are being replaced with unlicensed care staff, thereby diluting the skill mix. As a cost-saving measure, the shift to employing fewer licensed care staff has not been particularly successful. Not only do the overall number of hours of care increase when the licensed hours are decreased, but the level of surveillance also declines dramatically. There is no substitute for having a reasonable number of highly trained nurses provide care to the patients.

Staffing by Ratios

Staffing levels are closely tied to the incidence of medical errors. The potential of inappropriate staffing to cause an increase in the number of medical errors is generally recognized but not always taken into account in an organization's decision making. There is little evidence to use in determining the necessary level of staffing to ensure that the quality of patient care is maintained, organizational goals are met, and the clinicians' working conditions are acceptable. Studies intended to assess the effects of different ratios of patients to registered nurses are numerous and conflicting. Thus, historical averages of hours of care provided for each patient are typically used as the basis of daily staffing.

The problem is that this technique wrongly assumes that the needs of all patients are essentially the same and, more important, that the skills of nurses are comparable. Instead, patient needs vary widely, as do levels of nursing competence. Indeed, if a historically based ratio is used, such as four patients to one nurse, the chance of a match between patient care needs and on-the-job personnel is low. For example, on some days the correct ratio for meeting patient needs adequately might be three to one, whereas on other days it might be five to one. Frustration increases for both patients and clinicians when there is no adjustment in staffing, up or down, to meet the identified needs. In addition, with improvements in surgical processes, many patients are discharged prior to midnight (the traditional measure for billing for a patient day thus used in productivity calculations). The metrics inadequately reflect the nurse workload for the care of the surgical patient that is compressed into a shorter timeframe.

Evidence-based staffing confronts leaders with two challenges. First, although clinicians often dislike ratio staffing, they have difficulty when assignment ratios vary among colleagues. For example, nurses expect to be given reasonable workloads, but even when patient acuity is lower than average, they still resist accepting an assignment with a higher-than-average patient-to-nurse ratio. Getting nurses to understand and accept assignments based on patient risk and need for surveillance instead of numbers is a challenge for leaders—and an opportunity.

The second challenge is to determine which healthcare interventions contribute to meeting patient care needs and how effective they are. The main problem is that the nature and types of interventions vary widely from organization to organization and from clinician to clinician. Valid and reliable information that demonstrates the value of each clinician's contribution is sorely needed because it improves the dialogue between clinicians and leaders and helps them find meaningful solutions to managing the workload.

Developmental Freeze

Equally demoralizing for clinicians is the inconsistency of leadership support for professional development aimed at giving them skills they need to function effectively in the changing marketplace. Elimination of funding for professional development programs, both internal and external, commonly occurs when resources become strained. The strategy of requiring employees to attend seminars on vacation time at personal expense and limiting out-of-state travel reimbursement sends a strong negative message as to the value of continuous learning to the organization.

In addition, these restrictions increase the probability of failure-to-rescue incidents and other crises. The unavoidable breakdowns that occur in providing patient care and in the organization's systems require quick responses to prevent the breakdowns from developing into full-blown catastrophes. Most educational programs focus on giving clinicians the knowledge and skills they require to meet current standards of practice, but few offer learning opportunities that would allow clinicians to develop the proper skills for responding to imminent breakdowns. As the environment changes, so do the skills and interventions needed to manage developing crises, and continuous learning is a requisite for gaining the competence to address the kind of breakdowns that are likely to occur in the present.

Hiring Bonuses

In desperation, leaders sometimes use economic enticements to recruit needed healthcare clinicians. The practice of offering sign-on bonuses is based on two assumptions—(1) that individuals usually act in ways they believe will make them better off and (2) that individuals generally believe better off means more money. The reality is that each person has his or her own preference map, and that dangling cash before healthcare clinicians does not always induce the desired behaviors. Besides money, clinicians and providers want respect, involvement in decision making, and good relationships with colleagues, among other things. The bonus model, by treating clinicians as shallow and materialistic, has the effect of disparaging them. Some clinicians, of course, respond to the enticement of a financial bonus in given situations, but most are motivated by a combination of social, emotional, and material needs, not just led by the dollar.

Sign-on bonuses also send the wrong message to existing staff, especially long-time employees, who likely feel resentment because they have not gotten bonuses for their loyalty. Sign-on bonuses therefore tend to reduce employee morale and create a revolving door that can seriously affect patient care. Further, there is no way the sign-on bonuses can neutralize the cost of turnover, which is between $5,000 and $50,000 per nurse. The assumption of sign-on bonuses is that healthcare clinicians are for sale to the highest bidder and are willing to go across the street for dollars. They thus cause competition among healthcare organizations as well.

Opportunity 4: Revaluing Healthcare Providers and Clinicians as Vital Capital

The healthcare marketplace can hardly support guarantees of lifetime employment for anyone. Yet there are other options besides discarding employees whenever marketplace demands change. In fact, some of these options, by respecting the dignity of the individual and encouraging creativity and innovation, are more likely to improve an organization's long-term performance than are cyclical episodes of mass layoffs. The challenge for leaders is to make hiring and firing decisions from a broad perspective that takes into account multiple performance indicators, not merely the monthly cash flow or short-term costs. In particular, these decisions should be based on a full consideration of the effects of staff reductions and restructuring on patient care outcomes and on the ability of care clinicians and providers to provide healthcare services efficiently and effectively.

Given the increasing documentation that experienced and credentialed employees have a positive impact on patient outcomes, other approaches to managing the workforce are indicated. The first step is to shift to a type of evidence-based decision making that considers not only financial indicators but also the intellectual capital profile of the employees. The second step is to look at both short- and long-term effects of resource decisions. **Exhibit 9-8** contains a list of studies that show the impact of staffing on patient outcomes, cost of care, and healthcare provider and clinician satisfaction.

Evidence-Based Staffing

Effective staffing is a matter not just of numbers but of mix. It requires developing new and creative strategies to manage the combination of predictable and unpredictable workloads and the availability and supply of experienced and competent healthcare clinicians and providers. Given that at least 80% of the healthcare workload is predictable and repeatable, one challenge is to develop a workforce suitable for this portion of the workload. Core staffing must meet the identified range of care needs on a shift-by-shift and day-to-day basis. The second challenge is to handle the remaining 20% of the workload—the unpredictable portion. Because the services needed are unpredictable, it is futile to attempt to plan for and manage this portion. People generally do not call ahead and schedule trauma, deliveries, and medical emergencies with any sensitivity to the time of day or the availability of care providers. The goal therefore is to build enough flexibility into the staffing to ensure appropriate care clinicians are on hand

Exhibit 9-8 Nurse Staffing and Patient Outcomes: Selected References

Aiken, L., Clarke, S. P., Cheuny, R. B., Sloane, D. M., & Silber, J. H. (2003). Education levels of hospital nurses and patient mortality. *Journal of the American Medical Association, 290,* 1617–1623.

Aiken, L., Clarke, S. P., Sloane, D. M., Sochalsi, J., & Silber, J. H. (2002). Hospital nurse staffing and patient mortality, nurse burnout, and job dissatisfaction. *Journal of the American Medical Association, 288,* 1987–1993.

Alasak, J., Tabar, N. A., & AbuRuz, M. E. (2015). Patient satisfaction with nursing care: Measuring outcomes in an international setting. *Journal of Nursing Administration, 45*(11), 563–568.

Allen, S. B. (2015). The nurse–patient assignment: Purposes and decision factors. *Journal of Nursing Administration, 45*(12), 628–635.

American Nurses Association. (2012). *Principles for nurse staffing.* Author.

Bae, S. (2012). Nursing overtime: Why, how much, and under what working conditions. *Nursing Economic$, 30*(2), 60–71.

Behner, K. G., Fogg, L. F., Fournier, L. C., Frankenbach, J. T., & Robertson, S. B. (1990). Nursing resource management: Analyzing the relationship between costs and quality in staffing decisions. *Health Care Management Review, 15*(4), 63–71.

Blegen, M., Goode, C., & Reed, L. (1998). Nurse staffing and patient outcomes. *Nursing Research, 47*(1), 43–50.

Blegen, M., Goode, C., Spetz, J., Vaughn, T., & Park, S. (2011). Nurse staffing effects on patient outcomes: Safety-net and non-safety-net hospital. *Medical Care, 49*(4), 406–414.

Boev, C. (2012). The relationship between nurses' perception of work environment and patient satisfaction in adult critical care. *Journal of Nursing Scholarship, 44*(4), 368–375.

Buerhaus, P. (2010). It's time to stop the regulation of hospital nurse staffing dead in its tracks. *Nursing Economic$, 28*(2), 110–113.

Buerhaus, P. (2010). What is the harm in imposing mandatory hospital nurse staffing regulations? *Nursing Economic$, 28*(2), 87–93.

Buffington, A., Zwink, J., & Fink, R. (2012). Factors affecting nurse retention at an academic Magnet hospital. *Journal of Nursing Administration, 42*(5), 273–281.

Buhlman, N. (2016). Nurse staffing and patient-experience outcomes: A close connection. *American Nurse Today, 11*(1), 49–55.

Cairns, L., Hoffmann, R., Dudjak, L., & Lorenz, H. (2013). Utilizing bedside shift report to improve the effectiveness of shift handoff. *Journal of Nursing Administration, 43*(4), 160–165.

Cathro, H. (2013). A practical guide to making patient assignments in acute care. *Journal of Nursing Administration, 43*(1), 6–9.

Chaiken, B. P. (2015, September/October). Using patient acuity to drive health flow. *Patient Safety & Quality,* 12–13.

Cho, E., Chin, D. L., Kim, S., & Hong, O. (2016). The relationships of nurse staffing level and work environment with patient adverse events. *Journal of Nursing Scholarship, 48*(1), 74–82.

Cho, S., Mark, B., Knafl, G., Chang, H., & Yoon, H. (2017, February). Relationships between nurse staffing and patients' experiences, and the mediating effects of missed nursing care. *Journal of Nursing Scholarship, 49*(3), 347–355.

Cho, E., Park, J., Choi, M., Lee, H., & Kim, E. (2018). Associations of nurse staffing and education with length of stay of surgical patients. *Journal of Nursing Scholarship, 50*(2), 210–218.

Cimiotti, J., Haas, J., Saiman, L., & Larson, E. (2006). Impact of staffing on bloodstream infections in the neonatal intensive care unit. *Archives of Pediatric & Adolescent Medicine, 160*(8), 832–836.

Coffman, J. M., Seago, J. A., & Spetz, J. (2002). Minimum nurse-to-patient ratios in acute care hospitals in California. *Health Affairs, 21*(5), 53–63.

DesRoches, C., Miralles, P., Buerhaus, P., Hess, R., & Donelan, K. (2011). Health information technology in the workplace: Findings from a 2010 national survey of registered nurses. *The Journal of Nursing Administration, 41*(9), 357–364.

Eastabrooks, C. A., Midodzi, W. K., Cummings, G. G., Ricker, K. L., & Giovannetti, P. (2005). The impact of hospital nursing characteristics on 30-day mortality. *Nursing Research, 54*(2), 74–84.

Friese, C., & Himes-Ferris, L. (2013). Nursing practice environments and job outcomes in ambulatory oncology settings. *Journal of Nursing Administration, 43*(3), 149–154.

Griffiths, P., Recio-Saucedo, A., Dall'Ora, C., Briggs, J., Maruotti, A., Meredith, P., Smith, G., & Ball, J. (2018, January). The association between nurse staffing and omissions in nursing care: A systematic review. *Journal of Advanced Nursing, 74*, 1474–1487.

Guiliano, K., Danesh, V., & Funk, M. (2016). The relationship between nurse staffing and 30-day readmission for adults with heart failure. *The Journal of Nursing Administration, 46*(1), 25–29.

Halm, M. (2019). The influence of appropriate staffing and healthy work environments on patient and nurse outcomes. *American Journal of Critical Care, 28*(2), 152–156.

Harper, E. (2012). Staffing based on evidence: Can health information technology make it possible? *Nursing Economic$, 30*(5), 262–267.

Hickey, P., Gauvreau, K., & Connor, J. (2010). The relationship of nurse staffing, skill mix, and Magnet recognition to institutional volume and mortality for congenital heart surgery. *Journal of Nursing Administration, 40*(5), 226–232.

Institute of Medicine. (2010). *The future of nursing: Leading change, advancing health*. National Academies Press.

Kalisch, B., & Lee, K. (2012). Congruence of perceptions among nursing leaders and staff regarding missed nursing care and teamwork. *Journal of Nursing Administration, 42*(10), 473–477.

Kim, C., & Kim, J. (2018, February). The association between nurse staffing levels and paediatric nursing-sensitive outcomes in tertiary hospitals. *Journal of Nursing Management, 26*, 1002–1014.

Kim, J., Kim, S., Park, J., & Lee, E. (2019, March). Multilevel factors influencing falls of patients in hospital: The impact of nurse staffing. *Journal of Nursing Management, 00*, 1–9.

Laschinger, H. K. S. (2006). The impact of nursing work environments on patient safety outcomes. *Journal of Nursing Administration, 36*(5), 259–267.

Law, A., Stevens, J., Hohmann, S., & Walkey, A. (2018). Patient outcomes after the introduction of statewide ICU nurse staffing regulations. *Critical Care Medicine, 46*(10), 1563–1569.

Lewis, H. S., & Cunningham, C. J. L. (2015). Linking nurse leadership and work characteristics to nurse burnout and engagement. *Nursing Research, 65*(1), 13–23.

(continues)

Exhibit 9-8 Nurse Staffing and Patient Outcomes: Selected References (*continued*)

Martsolf, G. R., Auerbach, D., Benevent, R., Stocks, C., Jiang, J., Pearson, M. L., Ehrlich, E. D., & Gibson, T. B. (2014). Examining the value of inpatient nurse staffing: An assessment of quality and patient care costs. *Medical Care, 52*, 982–988.

Needleman, J., Buerhaus, P., Mattke, S., Stewart, M., & Zelevinky, K. (2002). Nurse staffing in hospitals: Is there a business case for quality? *Health Affairs, 25*(1), 204–211.

Olds, D., Aiken, L., Cimiotti, J., & Lake, E. (2017, June). Association of nurse work environment and safety climate on patient mortality: A cross-sectional study. *International Journal of Nursing Studies, 74*, 155–161.

Pappas, S. H., Woodard, J., & Davidson, N. (2015). Risk-adjusted staffing to improve patient value and financial performance. *Nursing Economics, 33*(2), 73–79.

Patrician, P., Loan, L., McCarthy, M., Fridman, M., Donaldson, N., Bingham, M., & Brosch, L. (2011). The association of shift-level nurse staffing with adverse patient events. *Journal of Nursing Administration, 41*(2), 64–70.

Prestia, A., & Dyess, S. (2012). Maximizing caring relationships between nursing assistants and patients: Care partners. *Journal of Nursing Administration, 42*(30), 144–147.

Salin, S., Kaunonen, M., & Aalto, P. (2012). Explaining patient satisfaction with outpatient care using data-based nurse staffing indicators. *Journal of Nursing Administration, 42*(12), 592–597.

Serratt, T., Harrington, C., Spetz, J., & Blegen, M. (2015). Staffing changes before and after mandated nurse-to-patient ratios in California's hospitals. *Policy, Politics & Nursing Practice, 12*(3), 133–140.

Shang, J., Needleman, J., Liu, J., Larson, E., & Stone, P. (2019, May). Nurse staffing and healthcare-associated infection, unit-level analysis. *The Journal of Nursing Administration, 49*(5), 260–265.

Shin, S., Park, J.-H., & Bae, S.-H. (2018, May–June). Nurse staffing and nurse outcomes: A systematic review and meta-analysis. *Nursing Outlook, 66*(3), 273–282.

Sibler, J., Rosenbaum, P., McHugh, M., Ludwig, J., Smith, H., Niknam, B., Even-Shoshan, O., Fleisher, L., Kelz, R., & Aiken, L. (2016, January). Comparison of the value of nursing work environments in hospitals across different levels of patient risk. *JAMA Surgery, 151*(6), 527–536.

Swiger, P. A., Vance, D. E., & Parician, P. A. (2016). Nursing workload in the acute-care setting: A concept analysis of nursing workload. *Nursing Outlook, 64*, 244–254.

Trepanier, S., Early, S., Ulrich, B., & Cherry, B. (2012). New graduate nurse residency program: A cost-benefit analysis based on turnover the contract labor usage. *Nursing Economic$, 30*(4), 207–214.

Wei, H., Sewell, K., Woody, G., & Rose, M. (2018). The state and science of nurse work environments in the United States: A systematic review. *International Journal of Nursing Sciences, 5*, 287–300.

Zhu, J., Dy, S., Wenzel, J., & Wu, A. (2018, February). Association of Magnet status and nurse staffing with improvements in patient experience with hospital care, 2008–2015. *Medical Care, 56*(2), 111–120.

to respond quickly to an unscheduled event. Meeting these two challenges requires two very different philosophies regarding staff availability and compensation.

To regain the respect and support of employees, leaders must learn to lead clinicians to achieve patient outcomes consistent with the organization's strategic priorities. When there is a gap between the organization's needs and what the employees are able to offer, change is indicated. How this change is managed is crucial for the organization. Leaders and employees must enter into a dialogue to reach a clear understanding of the organization's responsibility to support continued development for clinicians while at the same time expecting clinicians to obtain knowledge and credentials that enhance their performance and engagement. Collaborative dialogue between employees and leaders on how to respond to changing needs leads to a more stable workforce and greater employee satisfaction.

Staffing for Patient Needs

Attempts to devise accepted national standards for nurse-to-patient ratios have yet to produce meaningful recommendations, and with good reason: facility case mix indices, reimbursement plans, and available support services vary widely. Further, the standards would set average numbers for meeting patient care needs, and these needs, by virtue of their unpredictability, cannot be met by using average numbers for daily staffing. In most organizations, daily patient needs vary at least 20% above and below the average, and it is possible that at no time do the actual needs exactly equal the average. In fact, using average numbers in planning the daily staffing discounts the range of nursing activities that are needed to respond to different case mixes.

Revising the nurse-to-patient ratio daily is essential for minimizing discrepancies between patient needs and clinician capacities. In some organizations, valid and reliable patient classification systems have been used to determine patient care needs on a shift-by-shift basis. The information gathered becomes the basis for daily staffing and long-term scheduling. Once a

Group Discussion

In many organizations, when staff reductions are needed, those with least seniority are eliminated rather than those with greater seniority. Seldom is consideration given to the specific skills and credentials of those who are let go. Review the following research data and create a plan to manage the next round of staff reductions in your organization:

- Compared with other healthcare clinicians, certified nurses report fewer adverse events, have higher patient satisfaction ratings, and are more effective communicators and collaborators with other clinicians.
- An extra hour of nursing care is related to fewer urinary tract infections, a decrease in pneumonia, and a decrease in the probability of postoperative blood clots.
- As the number of medical residents, registered nurses, registered pharmacists, medical technologists, and total hospital personnel per occupied bed increases, mortality rates decrease.

Should the plan take into account employee longevity? If so, how? What effects on patient outcomes should the new model be expected to have? Who will support the new model, and who will oppose it?

representative sample of patient care needs that reflect the full range of needs is determined, the average nurse-to-patient ratios can be calculated. These ratios serve as standards, although they can become problematic when used for shift-to-shift staffing because they are not sensitive to fluctuations in patient needs, technology, and procedures required and are mostly grounded in counting tasks the nurse must do. Some analysis on staffing to patient risk for adverse event has shown operational benefits when nurse ratios are adjusted based on the patient's risk (Pappas et al., 2015).

In determining daily patient care needs and the proper number and mix of clinicians, leaders can consider the dynamic interaction of the economic factors, technology, and labor availability. The greatest hope for developing valid standards lies in understanding the interrelationships of nurse-to-patient ratios and patient needs (intensity and acuity).

Shared Accountability for Learning

Healthcare clinicians have an interest in continuing to acquire more knowledge and develop new skills throughout their career life, and the organizations that employ them share this interest. In fact, investing in their employees is a way for organizations to invest in the future, and therefore it makes sense for any organization to create programs that recognize the professional development efforts of its providers and clinicians. The providers and clinicians, on the other hand, should be willing to make a commitment to continue working for the organization as a quid pro quo. It is not unreasonable for an organization to expect a promise of 5 years of employment in return for tuition support for a higher education degree. Similarly, if an organization compensates a clinician for attending a conference or pays the registration fees, the employee should be expected to share new information with the healthcare team. The terms of any agreement must be determined before the investment.

In cases where employees pay for their own continuing education and show improvement in their performance because of their educational efforts, they can rightly expect the organization to recognize their increased ability through some form of compensation, such as an increase in salary. Employees should not suppose the organization will reward educational efforts that fail to affect their performance.

Situation 5: Demanding the Impossible

Healthcare clinician assignments are increasingly complex and sometimes overwhelming. Indeed, feasible assignments are the exception rather than the norm. Clinicians, nurses in particular, frequently are demoralized by being asked to do more than they are capable of, and for many the gap between what is being requested and what is possible has grown wider.

The limitations and inflexibility of current staffing and scheduling systems, coupled with the pressure to minimize costs, have prevented leaders from adequately supporting clinicians and providers who have been given arduous assignments. At best, these clinicians and providers receive encouragement and sympathy; at worst, they are berated for their inability to manage the workload. Although not the intent of leaders, the result is that employees feel abandoned and mistreated, they seek assistance outside of the organization, and the relationship between the employees and leaders becomes increasingly adversarial.

It is disconcerting for the profession and the community at large to observe clinicians who believe themselves abandoned by the leaders of the organizations for which they work. Exhortations to do one's best are no longer able to counter the professional discouragement felt by clinicians. As a result, some clinicians and providers have become openly critical of the health professions, discouraging others from joining or even leaving themselves for another. Encouragement rests in the fact that health care, particularly nursing, is a desirable profession for the millennial generation.

Opportunity 5: Managing the Needs–Resources Gap as a Team

Even using the most reliable and valid patient classification systems, leaders rarely match actual patient care needs and staff resources, including hours of staff time. Because some gap between needs and resources is almost inevitable, the challenge for leaders is to create effective systems for managing the gap.

Providers and consumers must engage in a dialogue to identify more precisely clinical care needs, desired outcomes of services, and available resources. In addition, if they discover a gap between needs and resources, they must reevaluate these. Attempting to provide all services regardless of the available resources, as has been the practice in the past, is irresponsible.

Much of the difficulty in identifying and managing the needs–resources gap stems from the failure of society to decide whether health care is a right or a privilege. Until society reaches a verdict on this issue, confusion will reign. As clearly as can be determined, health care is a cross between a right and a privilege—a right when you fit the parameters of the government, and a privilege when there is limited access and nonemergency services are involved. Several strategies offer help in minimizing the gap between healthcare needs and staff resources:

- Ensure that the system used to estimate patient care needs is valid and reliable.
- Eliminate nonvalued-added services. After carefully examining all services to determine how they affect outcomes, eliminate those that generally fail to have a positive effect.
- Delay noncritical functions until staff resources are available. Some interventions, to be effective, depend on the delivery of services at precise times. Other interventions are not time sensitive and can be delayed without compromising the overall treatment. Most medications cannot be delayed, but daily treatments can be moved to the next shift.
- Reexamine previous efforts to call in additional clinicians, and move staff from unit to unit to uncover opportunities for putting personnel to better use.

Currently, the responsibility of managing the needs–resources gap is placed on individual clinicians, increasing their feelings of abandonment. Further, providers are often expected to administer decisions made elsewhere and on the basis of economic factors—decisions that frequently put patients and families at risk. The preceding strategies can be used by individual clinicians to the best of their ability. The most common strategy is to eliminate or delay services, and each clinician uses his or her personal criteria in deciding whether to use them because open discussion of the associated issues has been discouraged. Failure of clinicians to manage their assignments is generally viewed as a sign of incompetence rather than as a sign of system overload. The challenge faced by healthcare leaders is to shift management of the needs–resources gap from the individual to the healthcare team—and ultimately to the community, if need be. Accountability for managing the gap must be elevated to the collective level so that healthcare clinicians, healthcare leaders, and the community can work together to find solutions.

> ### Group Discussion
> Consider a situation in which a unit is short two nurses. Using the principles of variance management, develop a plan to address the gap. Answer the following questions: When should the discussion about the gap occur? Who should be present? Identify the strategies that will be used (e.g., eliminate nonemergency-related work, request nurses to work overtime, stop admissions). How will the actions taken be documented? What future discussion will occur to avoid the same situation or to prepare for managing a similar situation?

Highly Reliable Organizations and Safety Culture

The former way of thinking about our cultures when addressing error and failure was to blame individuals and only focus on safety when a serious event occurred, resulting in a culture with low trust and disengagement. The concept of high reliability is to establish a context of health care where there is leader and clinician ownership, creating a trusting, just culture with continuous focus on near misses and unsafe conditions with a quest to eliminate harm to patients. Born in the aviation and nuclear power industries because of the high risk and high complexity of the work, high-reliability concepts were adopted by health care to aid in preventing failure by implementing processes to manage complex work and technologies. The organizing principles and practices of highly reliable organizations (HROs) include the following:

- *Preoccupation with failure*—operating with a chronic wariness of the possibility of unexpected events; asking what could go wrong here
- *Reluctance to simplify*—deliberately questioning assumptions and refusing to explain away situations
- *Sensitivity to operations*—ongoing quest to understand the human and organizational factors of the work being done, the team member capabilities, and available resources
- *Commitment to resilience*—developing capabilities to cope with, contain, and bounce back from mishaps because people talk about them and learn from them
- *Deference to expertise*—decision making migrates to those individuals with the most expertise with the problem regardless of authority or rank (Sutcliffe, 2011)

Establishing the social and relationship foundations of reliable performance is an important step in health care, and quantum leaders are prepared to respond. When the HRO practices are bundled, the ability to make weak signals visible and adaptable to intervention occurs (Sutcliffe et al., 2017). HRO principles alone will not eliminate errors, but like many organizational interventions, the leaders' application of these practices will improve health care.

Conclusion

It is not errors that are the problem, but how we respond to errors when we forget that errors are natural—natural as long as there is any shred of humanness present. By keeping in mind that errors are natural, we are more likely to recognize that errors, besides causing inconvenience or hardship, offer opportunities for improvement. Unfortunately, most leaders view errors as solely harmful and believe it is their responsibility to discipline those who commit them. They therefore look for someone to blame and possibly punish, and this is the problem. The punitive approach to error management encourages secrecy and discourages analysis of the situation and development of strategies to avoid repeat errors.

Any changes to the current system have the potential to threaten the established power base of leaders. The structure of power and the organizational culture often bias the perspectives of those who benefit from the existing system. Alterations in the organization's structure and the roles of its members may increase the power of some members and reduce the power of others. Some resist reward systems or metrics that diminish their status and authority within the organization. Nevertheless, shifting from a culture of blame to an open culture in which error is perceived as an opportunity for improvement requires leaders to reconsider how power is perceived and used in the organization. Punitive power becomes passé and intolerable, whereas the power of dialogue emerges as the propulsive force driving the organization toward success. Leaders must learn and adapt to concepts of making sure the information closest to the work is available at all times, not just when error occurs.

Managing errors as opportunities and improving our services without debasing our values and subverting our commitment to public safety remain important challenges. The presentation of the five leadership errors discussed in this chapter is intended to heighten readers' awareness that many long-held practices may no longer be effective. The opportunities discussed are just a few of the many available to creative healthcare leaders—opportunities waiting only for discovery and testing. One of the opportunities that is currently prevalent, the opportunity to reframe the work of health care using a value-based model with high reliability, can only serve to enhance a system in which partnerships among patients, families, and clinicians work to empower the patients to manage their own health.

Finally, even when things are going wrong and mistakes abound, trust in your journey and look for the lesson to be learned. Find the gift in the goof!

Chapter Takeaways

1. Failure is normative; it is a part of the process of discovery and innovation.
2. Managing failures and errors requires evaluation of both individual behavior and system infrastructure adequacy.
3. Recovering from failure and error requires a conscious effort to recognize the situation, explore the dynamics, and develop strategies to modify processes to prevent recurrence.
4. Remediation is preferred to discipline when human failure occurs; discipline is indicated when there is negligence, intentional rule violations, or reckless conduct.
5. All healthcare failures present opportunities not only to correct the situation but also to embrace innovation and transform practices.

Chapter Nine   Transforming Error and Engaging Failure Toward a Culture of Safety

Case Study 9-1
So, What Is Really Broken Here?

Central Valley Hospital is a well-respected community hospital that provides a comprehensive array of medical and surgical services and maternal newborn services. The hospital has been recognized with Planetree and Magnet designations and is viewed in the community as one of the top hospitals for excellent services. Employees generally view the culture of the hospital as very positive, and management has implemented a multifocal strategy to enhance employee, physician, and patient satisfaction. The mission statement, values, and behavioral standards are posted openly where they can be seen by all, and every employee's performance expectations and performance appraisal include an evaluation of how that person lives the expected values and behavioral standards. The values include integrity, trust, honesty, professionalism, patient centeredness, and excellence.

Central Valley has an active quality department that reviews all patient and organizational outcomes and meets with department leaders to discuss ways of continually improving outcomes. There is significant emphasis on "excellence," and managers at all levels of the organization are evaluated on their ability not only to meet financial budget targets but also to meet various quality indicators and national benchmarks.

Reyna is a manager in a 32-bed general medical unit, and she has approximately 150 part-time and full-time employees who report to her. Reyna reports to the vice president of medical surgical services, who, in turn, reports to the chief nursing officer (CNO). Reyna has a Bachelor of Science degree in nursing and is currently in her second year of the graduate program in nursing with an emphasis on nursing administration. She has enjoyed her classes on leadership theories and their application in the healthcare setting, financial management, quality and program evaluation, and a practicum that focused on just culture, patient safety, and quality improvement using tools such as Lean and Six Sigma. Reyna tries to apply much of what she learns in the school setting to her daily work.

Every year Central Valley disseminates the results of the employee opinion, physician satisfaction, and patient satisfaction surveys to the management team. Feedback regarding the national benchmarking quality indicators such as NDNQI and CalNOC data is shared with the nursing management team. Reyna and her nurse manager colleagues appreciate the openness of the organization in sharing the results with them, but talking among themselves they realize how much stress is created when they receive results that do not meet expected standards. Reyna is faced with a decline in scores on the patient satisfaction, employee satisfaction, and culture of safety surveys. She attributes the decline of patient satisfaction to recent changes in the dietary department that have resulted in delays in tray delivery and a remodeling project on the unit that has created unexpected noise during the day.

She has also evaluated potential causes of the decline in employee satisfaction and identified a trend that has occurred annually with lower employee satisfaction scores during the months of July through October. During these months, the patient census and average patient acuity are higher than all other months in the year. Reyna does everything she can to ensure adequate staffing and to be visible and available to the staff more than usual during these times. She is surprised to see the decline in the culture of safety scores, and she begins to investigate potential reasons for the decline by talking with the staff to get their perspective on why they scored specific items so low. Reyna feels that she is held accountable for scores without being in control of all of the factors that cause staff and patients to score the surveys so low.

At a recent nursing leadership meeting, the directors announced that all managers who did not meet the targeted levels on the patient satisfaction, physician satisfaction, employee opinion, and the culture of safety surveys must prepare a report outlining their strategy to correct the problems and ensure that upcoming surveys demonstrate an improvement.

In her meeting with the director, the director is even more critical about Reyna's performance as a nurse manager in allowing these declines to occur. She tells Reyna that her performance is under scrutiny and that corrective actions need to be taken immediately to improve the scores; Reyna must demonstrate changes immediately on the unit to improve the situation. Needless to say, Reyna feels completely deflated at the end of the meeting and feels unfairly blamed and unsupported by her director. When she reflects back on her classes on just culture and leadership, she questions her director's approach with her. She feels that her director should do more to support her and give her encouragement and direction in improving the survey scores and in changing the potential causes of the problems that contribute to the dissatisfaction of staff and patients. When she discusses the situation with her colleagues, those who report to her same director experience the same concerns. Other managers with different directors indicate that their directors partner with them in identifying methods to continually improve scores on all quality indicators.

When Reyna reviews the items on the various surveys with her staff, she discovers that the staff do not have a clear understanding of the meaning of some of the questions. After discussing some of the items on both the employee opinion survey and the culture of safety survey, the staff inform her that they would have scored the items differently if they understood the meaning of the items. She begins to wonder whether patients felt the same way about their patient satisfaction survey or whether their overall satisfaction rate was unfairly weighted with their discontent with the noise factor and the late meal trays as contrasted to their overall level of satisfaction with their nursing care.

Reyna feels more frustrated than ever being held accountable for survey scores that contained items that are not in her control to change and improve. She also is frustrated with the attitude of her director, who seems to blame her for the scores and offers no insight or assistance in resolving the underlying problems that are reflected in the survey scores. Reyna feels powerless and victimized in the situation. As she prepares her report to submit strategies for improving the scores, she includes the discussions with her staff about their interpretation of the wording on some of the items and outlines how she and her staff would partner in improving the workplace environment to ultimately improve the survey scores. Reyna also includes the plans that she and her staff had developed together to enhance patient satisfaction. Reyna had met with the manager of the dietary department to negotiate a solution to prevent late tray delivery, which she believes is a major contributor to patient dissatisfaction. Despite her report and strategies to improve survey scores, Reyna dreads meeting with her director and feels that she could not trust her to evaluate her fairly or to manage her up to the CNO or other executives in the hospital. Reyna believes that her director is neither living the values of the hospital nor demonstrating the principles of just culture in blaming the managers rather than partnering with them to correct situations that contribute to lower survey scores.

Questions

1. How do you feel that the director's actions influenced the culture of her department and her nurse managers' work performance?
2. If blame should be placed for the low survey scores on the patient satisfaction survey, the employee opinion survey, and the culture of safety survey, who should be blamed for the decline in scores?
3. If you were Reyna, what actions would you take to improve the scores on these three surveys?
4. If you were the director of the department, what might you do differently to facilitate improvement in the survey scores?
5. Managers are frequently held accountable for outcomes over which they do not have direct control. How can leaders influence managers in these situations to remain motivated and to continually improve the outcomes?

Case Study 9-2

It Could Have Happened to Anyone

The phone rings at 2 a.m., and Judy is immediately awakened from her sleep. As she listens to the voice on the other end, she suddenly feels sickened with the news. The assistant manager of the unit informs her that a patient has been given a large dose of insulin that was intended for a different patient. The nurse failed to check the receiving patient's armband or call the patient by name prior to administering the insulin. Because it was in the middle of the night, the patient was groggy and did not question why he was receiving medication. Now the patient was in severe hypoglycemia, hypotensive, and exhibiting cardiac arrhythmias. The patient was transferred to the intensive care unit, and the family was called and informed of the error. The assistant manager reported that the nurse was one of the more senior and experienced nurses who had an impeccable work ethic and a reputation for being one of the best nurses on the unit. She shared that the nurse was absolutely devastated about the error and nearly hysterical. The patient's physician was very angry on the phone when the error was reported to him, and he was on his way to the hospital. Judy told the assistant manager that she would come to the hospital right away to meet with the patient's family, physician, and the nurse. Before she left home, Judy phoned the department director, who also indicated that he would come in to the hospital to assist in any way possible.

When Judy arrived at the hospital, she was informed that the patient had just expired and that his family were on their way to the hospital. The patient's physician was in the ICU talking with the other physicians and nurses who tried to resuscitate the patient. The ICU physician indicated that although the overdose of insulin contributed to the death, the patient's underlying condition made it impossible to correct the hypoglycemia and to save the patient.

After speaking to the physicians, Judy went to her own unit to speak with the nurse who made the medication error. She could only imagine how devastated the nurse was feeling, so she approached her gently and with compassion in her voice and mannerisms. Judy listened to the nurse as she tearfully recounted the story of going into the patient's room and administering the medication. She acknowledged that she had not checked the patient's armband because she did not want to disturb the patient, who was sleeping. This was her first night to care for the patient who received the insulin and the patient next door who was supposed to receive the insulin. Both of the patients were men in their 70s who had the same diagnosis and who actually had similar physical characteristics and facial features. Both men had been admitted during the day and were assigned to adjacent rooms. To make matters worse their last names were similar. The nurse could hardly speak for the tears, and she was shaking uncontrollably. The assistant manager completed the forms necessary to report the incident to the hospital's quality and risk management departments. After the nurse signed the documentation, Judy suggested that she ask a family member to come and drive her home. Judy was concerned for the nurse's safety because she was completely distraught. She told her that it would be necessary for her to take several administrative days off, but she should be available to speak with the hospital attorneys and risk management.

After leaving the nurse, Judy went back to the ICU to meet with the patient's family. When she arrived there, the department director was already engaged with the family, who were both angry and devastated with the news of how the patient had been given the wrong medication inadvertently and had expired. Because the department director and social services were working with the family, Judy returned to her unit to meet with her staff and the assistant manager.

Everybody on the unit was affected by the event, and many of the nurses were in tears. The assistant manager was also feeling the pressure of the situation and was trying to coordinate the care of the remaining patients on the unit. After working to stabilize the emotions on the unit, Judy met with the department director, the CNO, the physicians, and the attorney for risk management. The required phone calls and paperwork were completed notifying the health department of the medication error and the patient's death. Everyone realized that the health department would conduct a thorough investigation of the situation, review the hospital's policies and procedures related to medication administration, and inquire as to how nurse competencies were assessed and reviewed. The hospital attorney indicated that he and the risk management team would continue to meet with the family and suggested that social work or a clinical psychologist be involved in the meetings. The CEO met with the public relations department to prepare an official hospital statement about the situation because reporters from the community television stations were already calling and requesting information about the patient's death.

Questions

1. If you were Judy, what steps would you take with your nursing staff to stabilize their emotions about the situation?
2. What should Judy do to stabilize the team culture so that they can all work well together again?
3. What steps should Judy or the hospital's leaders take with the nurse who administered the wrong medication to the patient? Should this employee be terminated as a result of the error?
4. Identify both the individual errors and the system errors that contributed to the medication error.
5. What work needs to be done by the hospital's leadership to manage the internal and external (public) reaction to the error and the patient's death?
6. What should leadership do to help the hospital recover from this error?

References

Agency for Healthcare Research and Quality (AHRQ). (2018a). *10 patient safety tips for hospitals.* https://www.ahrq.gov/patients-consumers/diagnosis-treatment/hospitals-clinics/10-tips/index.html

Agency for Healthcare Research and Quality (AHRQ). (2018b). *Care coordination.* http://www.ahrq.gov/professionals/prevention-chronic-care/improve/coordination/index.html

Agency for Healthcare Research and Quality (AHRQ). (2019). *Disclosure of errors.* https://psnet.ahrq.gov/primers/primer/2/error-disclosure

Benner, P., Malloch, K., & Sheets, V. (Eds.). (2010). Overview: NCSBN practice breakdown initiative. In P. E. Benner, K. Malloch, & V. Sheets (Eds.), *Nursing pathways for patient safety: Expert panel on practice breakdown* (pp. 1–29). Elsevier.

Braaten, J. (2016). Root cause analysis: A tool for high reliability in a complex environment. In C. A. Oster & J. S. Braaten (Eds.), *High reliability organizations: A healthcare handbook for patient safety & quality* (pp. 113–136). Sigma Theta Tau.

Buerhaus, P. (1998). Milton Weinstein's insights on the development, use, and methodologic problems in cost-effectiveness analysis. *Image: Journal of Nursing Scholarship, 30,* 223–227.

Cosgrove, T. (2013). Value-based healthcare is inevitable and that's good. *Harvard Business Review.* https://hbr.org/2013/09/value-based-health-care-is-inevitable-and-thats-good/

Davidson, S., Weberg, D., Porter-O'Grady, T., & Malloch, K. (2017). *Leadership for evidence-based innovation in nursing and health professions.* Jones & Bartlett Learning.

Edmondson, A. (2019). *The fearless organization: Creating psychological safety in the workplace for learning, innovation, and growth.* John Wiley & Sons.

Edress, H., Connors, C., Paine, L., Norvell, M., Taylor, H., & Wu, A. W. (2016). Implementing the RISE second victim support programme at the Johns Hopkins Hospital: A case study. *BMJ Open, 6:*e011708, 1–12.

HealthLeaders Media. (2013, July). *Safety stumbling blocks: Advancing clinical quality from data to decisions.* http://content.hcpro.com/pdf/content/293611.pdf

Holden, R. J., Carayon, P., Gurses, A. P., Hoonakker, P., Hundt, A. S., Ozok, A. A., & Rivera-Rodriguez, A. J. (2013). SEIPS 2.0: A human factors framework for studying and improving the work of healthcare professionals and patients. *Ergonomics, 56*(11), 2–29.

Hopkins, K., & Sinsky, C. A. (2014). Team-based care: Saving time and improving efficiency. *Family Practice Management, 21*(6), 23–29.

Hospital Consumer Assessment of Healthcare Providers and Systems (HCAHPS). (2016). *CAHPS hospital survey.* http://www.hcahpsonline.org/home.aspx

Hughes, A. M., Gregory, M. E., Joseph, D. L., Marlow, S. L., Lacerenza, C. N., Benishek, L. E., King, H. B., & Salas, E. (2016, June 16). Saving lives: A meta-analysis of team training in health care. *Journal of Applied Psychology, 101*(9), 1266–1304.

Institute of Medicine (IOM). (2001). *Crossing the quality chasm: A new health system for the 21st century.* National Academies Press.

Kohn, L. T., Corrigan, J. M., & Donaldson, M. S. (Eds.). (2000). *To err is human: Building a safer health system.* National Academies Press.

Longest, B. (1998). Managerial competence at senior levels of integrated delivery systems. *Journal of Healthcare Management, 43,* 115–135.

Malloch, K., & Porter-O'Grady, T. (1999). Partnership economics: Nursing's challenge in a quantum age. *Nursing Economics, 17,* 299–307.

Marx, D. (2001). *Patient safety and the "just culture": A primer for healthcare executives.* Patient Safety Network. http://www.psnet.ahrq.gov/resource.aspx?resourceID=1582

McKay, M., & Daniel, M. (2016). Medical error—the third leading cause of death in the US. *BMJ, 353*, i2139.

National Academies of Sciences, Engineering, and Medicine. (2019). *Taking action against clinician burnout: A systems approach to professional well-being.* National Academies Press.

National Quality Forum (NQF). (2011). *Serious reportable events in healthcare.* http://www.quality forum.org/Publications/2011/12/Serious_Reportable_Events_in_Healthcare_2011.aspx

Pappas, S. H. (2013). Value, a nursing outcome. *Nursing Administration Quarterly, 37*(2), 122–128.

Pappas S., Davidson, N., Woodard, J., Davis, J., & Welton, J. M. (2015). Risk-adjusted staffing to improve patient value. *Nursing Economics, 33*(2), 73–78, 87.

Patrician, P., Godlock, G. C., Lewis, A. S., & Miltner, R. S. (2016). Just culture and the impact on high reliability. In C. A. Oster & J. S. Braaten (Eds.), *High reliability organizations: A healthcare handbook for patient safety & quality* (pp. 139–155). Sigma Theta Tau.

Petschonek, S., Burlison, J., Cross, C., Martin, K., Laver, J., Landis, R. S., & Hoffman, J. M. (2013). Development of the just culture assessment tool: Measuring the perceptions of health-care professionals in hospitals. *Journal of Patient Safety, 9*(4), 190–197.

Ricks, T. E. (2012). What ever happened to accountability? *Harvard Business Review, 90*(10), 93–98.

Sammer, C. E., Lykens, K., Singh, K. P., Mains, D. A., & Lackan, N. A. (2010). What is patient safety culture? A review of the literature. *Journal of Nursing Scholarship 42*(2), 156–165.

Sherwood, G., & Armstrong, G. E. (2016). Current patient safety drivers. In C. A. Oster & J. S. Braaten (Eds.), *High reliability organizations: A healthcare handbook for patient safety & quality* (pp. 25–47). Sigma Theta Tau.

Sutcliffe, K. M. (2011). High reliability organizations (HROs). *Best Practice & Research Clinical Anaesthesiology, 25*, 133–144.

Sutcliffe, K. M., Paine, L., & Pronovost, P. J. (2017). Re-examining high reliability: Actively organizing for safety. *BMJ Quality and Safety, 26*, 248–251.

Wears, R. L., & Sutcliffe, K. M. (2020). *Still not safe–Patient safety and the middle-managing of American medicine.* Oxford University Press.

The Joint Commission (TJC). (2016). *Sentinel events.* https://www.jointcommission.org/assets/1/6/CAMH_24_SE_all_CURRENT.pdf

Yakusheva, O., Needleman, J., Bettencourt, A. P., & Buerhaus, P. I. (2020). Is it time to peek under the hood of system-level approaches to quality and safety? *Nursing Outlook, 68*(2), 141–144.

Zak, P. J. (2017, January–February). The neuroscience of trust. *Harvard Business Review.* https://www.emcleaders.com/wp-content/uploads/2017/03/hbr-neuroscience-of-trust.pdf

Suggested Readings

Ariely, D. (2010). Good decisions, bad outcomes. *Harvard Business Review, 88*(11), 40.

Benner, P. (2000). *Error in medicine: A complex sorrow.* Paper presented at conference, University of California–Berkeley, March 11–12.

Benner, P., Kyriakidis, P. H., & Stannard, R. D. (2001). *Clinical wisdom and interventions in critical care: A thinking-in-action approach.* Saunders.

Berkow, S., Jaggi, T., & Fogelson, R. (2007). Fourteen unit attributes to guide staffing. *Journal of Nursing Administration, 37*(3), 150–155.

Buerhaus, P. I. (2009). Avoiding mandatory hospital nurse staffing ratios: An economic commentary. *Nursing Outlook, 57*(2), 107–112.

Chang, Y., & Mark, B. A. (2009). Antecedents of severe and nonsevere medication errors. *Journal of Nursing Scholarship, 41*(1), 70-78.

Chuang, Y., Ginsburg, L., & Berta, W. B. (2007). Learning from preventable adverse events in healthcare organizations: Development of a multilevel model of learning and propositions. *Health Care Management Review, 32*(4), 330-340.

Clancy, C. (2009, September–October). Patient safety: One decade after *To Err Is Human*. *Patient Safety and Quality Healthcare*, 8-10.

Ebright, P. R., Urden, L., Patterson, E., & Chalko, B. (2004). Themes surrounding novice nurse near-miss and adverse-event situations. *Journal of Nursing Administration, 34*(11), 531-538.

Fagin, C. M. (2001). *When care becomes a burden: Diminishing access to adequate nursing.* Milbank Memorial Fund.

Hofmann, P. B. (2005, January/February). Responsibility for unsuccessful promotions. *Healthcare Executive*, 32-36.

Hyun, S., Bakken, S., Douglas, K., & Stone, P. W. (2008). Evidence-based staffing: Potential roles for informatics. *Nursing Economic$, 26*(3), 151-158, 173.

Institute of Medicine (IOM). (2004). *Keeping patients safe: Transforming the work environment of nurses.* National Academies Press.

Kalish, B. J., Landstrom, G., & Williams, R. A. (2009). Missed nursing care: Errors of omission. *Nursing Outlook, 57*, 3-9.

Lachman, V. D. (Ed.). (2006). *Applied ethics in nursing.* Springer.

Reason, J. (2000). Human error: Models and management. *British Medical Journal, 320*, 768-770.

Rosner, F., Berger, J. T., Kark, P., Potash, J., & Bennett, A. J. (2000). Disclosure and prevention of medical errors. *Archives in Internal Medicine, 160*, 2089-2092.

Silber, J. H., Williams, S. V., Krakauer, H., & Schwartz, J. S. (1992). Hospital and patient characteristics associated with death after surgery: A study of adverse occurrence and failure to rescue. *Medical Care, 30*, 615-629.

Watson, J. (2006, January–March). Caring theory as an ethical guide to administrative and clinical practices. *Nursing Administration Quarterly, 30*(1), 48-55.

Williams, L. L. (2006, January–March). The fair factor in matters of trust. *Nursing Administration Quarterly, 30*(1), 30-37.

Quiz Questions

Select the best answer for each of the following questions.

1. Marketplace value incorporates the essential factors affecting health care. Which of the following factors is *not* included in the marketplace value equation?
   a. Available reimbursement
   b. Time and type of provider
   c. Return on investment
   d. Appropriateness of clinical service

Quiz Questions

2. Errors in health care are inevitable. Given the nature of the interactions between clinicians, patients, technology, and the environment, errors should be:
    a. expected and tolerated.
    b. managed by the team.
    c. viewed as opportunities for learning and improvement.
    d. eliminated at all costs.

3. Disclosure and mandatory reporting of errors are both recommended as strategies for managing errors in health care. Why are these two behaviors incompatible?
    a. Mandatory reporting removes the safety from disclosure and makes clinicians unwilling to admit to their errors.
    b. Disclosure of errors implies failure.
    c. Malpractice cases do not allow disclosure of errors.
    d. The goal of mandatory reporting of errors is to establish blame, whereas the goal of disclosing errors is to generate an open dialogue.

4. To shift from external regulation to internal accountability, which of the following does an organization require?
    a. An increase in the number of committees
    b. Elimination of licensing requirements
    c. The commitment of the leadership to monitor and manage the meeting of healthcare standards
    d. Support from The Joint Commission

5. Cost-effectiveness analysis has been proposed as more appropriate than cost-to-benefit analysis for evaluating healthcare services. Which of the following is one of the advantages of cost-effectiveness analysis?
    a. It takes into account health outcomes and the cost of treatment.
    b. It takes into account the cost of treatment and the cost of health outcomes.
    c. It takes into account the cost of the service and the savings achieved.
    d. It uses units such as years of life saved instead of dollars to measure health outcomes.

6. Why have clinicians not been able to effectively manage the gap (variance) between patient needs and healthcare resources?
    a. It is difficult to determine the actual variance.
    b. The interventions selected by individual clinicians to manage the variance are not known to the others on the healthcare team.
    c. The individual clinician feels abandoned by the system.
    d. Ownership of the problem and the solution rests with the healthcare team.

7. What does staffing by ratio (the ratio of patients to clinicians) require?
    a. Sufficient funding
    b. A valid and reliable baseline of patient care needs
    c. Historical trend data to support the ratio
    d. Approval of the legislature

8. How do holographic leadership and fragmented leadership differ?
    a. In their basic philosophy
    b. In the skills required of leaders
    c. In the leaders' scope of responsibilities
    d. In the degree of financial expertise required of leaders

9. The process of recovering from the negative consequences of committing a medical error has not been discussed openly in the past, most likely for which of the following reasons?
    a. The emphasis of healthcare education and practice is on doing things right.
    b. The threat of lawsuits forces clinicians to keep silent about the errors they commit.
    c. Most clinicians do not need guidance in learning to live with errors.
    d. Most clinicians receive help confidentially.

10. The Agency for Healthcare Research and Quality and National Quality Forum's top 10 safety tips:
    a. are recommendations primarily focused on clinical interventions.
    b. provide both infrastructure and clinical intervention recommendations.
    c. primarily provide guidelines for medical students and residents.
    d. do not hold the force of law.

11. Which of the following is true of failure?
    a. It includes intentional medical errors and adverse events.
    b. It is a situation in which there is a lack of successful planning and execution of established protocols.
    c. It is best considered an integral element of the innovation dynamic.
    d. It always reflects poorly on the individual involved.

12. Which of the following is true with regard to expecting perfection?
    a. Perfection is desired by patients and clinicians.
    b. Perfection is not realistic when the staffing ratios are higher than budgeted.
    c. Perfection should be the gold standard for all patient care services.
    d. Perfection considers the wide variability of patient situations and clinician skills.

13. Public reaction to error/disclosure resulted in all of the following, *except*:
    a. additional complexity in the healthcare system.
    b. increased awareness of patients and families about errors.
    c. decreased errors and patient injuries.
    d. new national task forces to address safety.

14. Disclosure strategies include all of the following, *except*:
    a. allowing time for the issue to settle before discussing it.
    b. apologizing for the mistake or failure.
    c. listening to all family members.
    d. identifying course-correction plans.

15. Punitive cultures in health care:
    a. are intended to decrease errors by using punishment as a strategy to gain attention.
    b. result in cover-up of errors and blaming of others.
    c. should be considered unethical and shifted to a more positive and supportive culture.
    d. perceive punishment as an opportunity for innovative change.

16. Individual versus system accountability has received much attention in health care. Which of the following would be the most appropriate approach in evaluating errors?
   a. Disciplining individuals when a failure is identified
   b. Remediating the individuals involved as corrective action
   c. Exploring the individual's past error record and all related policies around the error
   d. Exploring the individuals and policies involved in the area of concern to determine corrective action

17. Which of the following is true of remediation?
   a. It is the preferred action when an individual is involved in a serious error for the first time.
   b. It is not supported by most state boards of nursing.
   c. It requires more time with the employee than does the time for discipline.
   d. It is not appropriate when there is a single instance of reckless conduct.

18. Which of the following best describes marketplace practice?
   a. Healthcare services available based on approved evidence-based practices
   b. Healthcare services that specifically meet the needs of the patient and are reimbursed by the insurer
   c. Providing services that are reimbursable
   d. Providing the services required for patient recovery regardless of available reimbursement

19. Team-based care is essential because clinician collaboration:
   a. results in challenging the status quo when appropriate.
   b. decreases the potential for system breakdown and error.
   c. increases the emphasis on patient goals.
   d. results in a focus on value-driven care.

20. Which of the following is true of fragmented leadership?
   a. It is the result of specialized disciplines and their need to focus on their specialty.
   b. It is necessary to allow clinicians to do their work and managers to do their work.
   c. It could result in decreased costs with team-based leadership in which clinicians and healthcare managers collaborate to create healthcare policies and infrastructure.
   d. It is more cost-effective than holographic leadership.

21. Dehumanization of healthcare works occur when individuals are treated as expendable machine parts. Which of the following scenarios is *not* dehumanizing?
   a. Annual layoffs to adjust to budget performance
   b. Allocation of educational funding based on patient satisfaction scores
   c. Small bonuses for perfect attendance
   d. Acuity-based staffing models when the census is above the 50th percentile

22. Hiring bonuses are not appropriate for the long-term retention and satisfaction of employees. Which reason best explains why bonuses are not the best recruitment strategy?
   a. They do not consider the social and emotional needs of new hires.
   b. Current employees are disenfranchised because they have not received bonuses.
   c. New hires are an unknown entity and performance has yet to be proven.
   d. It recognizes the high value of the person being hired.

23. The real problem in error management is the human emotional element and how to simultaneously address the error, coach the individual, and modify the system infrastructure to avoid recurrence. Quantum leaders should engage in all of the following behaviors to achieve positive outcomes in addressing errors, *except*:
    a. avoiding knee-jerk responses to create an impact and perception of doing something.
    b. establishing an infrastructure with resources prepared to respond to errors in a comprehensive, timely manner.
    c. engaging risk management staff to assess the negative impact on the organization.
    d. placing all involved persons on administrative leave until the error is investigated.

24. Honoring excellence in patient care services, rather than perfection:
    a. avoids mechanistic thinking and approaches to error.
    b. values the nature of complexity underpinnings of emergence and interconnectedness.
    c. is consistent with Magnet accreditation guidelines.
    d. is supported by an organization's mission, vision, and values.

25. Reporting of negative events is influenced by several factors. Which of the following should *not* be considered in reporting negative events?
    a. Licensing boards, state health departments, Centers for Medicare and Medicaid, and The Joint Commission
    b. Organizational quality councils for guidance and direction prior to reporting to any agency
    c. Consultation with the ethics committee
    d. National Quality Forum

CHAPTER TEN

The Fully Engaged Leader: Demonstrating Capacity to Sustain Relationships

> The illiterate of the 21st century will not be those who cannot read and write, but those who cannot learn, unlearn, and relearn.
> —*Alvin Toffler*

Chapter Objectives

At the completion of this chapter, the reader will be able to:

- Understand the attributes of the fully engaged leader and the relationship of engagement to organizational outcomes.
- Review the theoretical underpinnings of the emotional aspects of leadership and the challenges of integrating these concepts into leadership development.
- Explain the role of self-awareness, compassion, passionate optimism, and impulse control in the development of emotional competence.
- Describe the stages of acquiring emotional competence for the individual and for the team.
- Discuss the challenges of measuring and documenting the organizational impact of emotional competence.

The notion of engagement in health care is increasingly important in our work to optimize patients' involvement in the management of their own health care. The Patient Protection and Affordable Care Act reinforces the Institute of Medicine's call from more than 10 years ago for patient centeredness, and now mandates the use of measures to validate patient centeredness, patient satisfaction, patient experience of care, patient engagement, and shared decision making in its provisions (Millenson & Macri, 2012). Intuitively, healthcare leaders have believed that engagement is important. but have not always actualized the engagement in consistent, measurable ways. Thus, the quantum leader must provide clear expectations of not only what engagement embodies but also strategies to achieve engagement. This process begins with

CHAPTER TEN   The Fully Engaged Leader: Demonstrating Capacity to Sustain Relationships

leaders becoming more knowledgeable about engagement and then working with the healthcare team to learn to fully engage not only the patient but also the entire team.

Fully engaged leaders understand the complexities within relationships and how important they are in transformational work. In order to move from disengagement to engagement, engaged leaders act and reflect on the events and processes of leading that emphasize the short term and integrate the long-term needs of the community.

Leader success depends on a wide range of variables that relate to the work to be done, the skills and abilities of the leader and the team, the needs of the team members, the resources available, and the motivation of all those involved. This list is not all-inclusive, and it continually evolves. The right stuff of leadership may indeed have common characteristics and behaviors, but the reality is that each leader has a unique combination of characteristics, values, behaviors, and ability to get the work done. Most leaders develop their personal essence on the basis of education, experience, mental intelligence, emotional intelligence, and the ability to form meaningful relationships. The ultimate goal of the self-exploration in achieving high levels of emotional competence is to reach a state of equanimity; a state in which the spirit is balanced between suppression and identification (Young, 2016). Suppression is an unhealthy effort to cope with feelings that we are unsure about, whereas identification, the opposite, is the state in which we are fixated inappropriately on an idea or feeling and unable to move forward. Practicing equanimity allows the leader to gain understanding of experiences that free thoughts for future ideas and work (Young, 2018). This chapter presents the emerging profile of the fully engaged leader to demonstrate a greater appreciation of the complexity of leadership and the significance of engagement as a leader characteristic and to stimulate discussion of the potential impact of engaged behaviors on organizational performance and patient outcomes. A brief review of the emotional intelligence literature and processes to develop engagement and a discussion of team emotional competence are also presented.

To support the work of the organization, leaders must have not only technical management skills but also skills in managing emotions—theirs as well as those of other individuals in the organization. Emotionally competent leaders exhibit a high regard for colleagues and subordinates; an understanding of basic motivations, as well as basic justice; a willingness to take responsibility; a willingness to correct faulty situations; and a willingness to take positive, quick, and aggressive action when indicated.

Quantum leaders recognize that they have no more control over organizational outcomes than do police officers over the movement of a large crowd. The officers may be able to herd the crowd in a certain direction for a period of time, but their control over the crowd is only temporary and cursory. Leaders can no longer rely on command-and-control leadership methods. They are being challenged to shift to behaviors

> **Point to Ponder**
>
> **Engagement**
> "Employees who forge a strong emotional bond with the organization they are a part of, taking pride in what they do and speaking favorably about their employer to friends and family" (Wright, 2020, p. xxi).
>
> **Disengagement**
> Withdrawing from involvement; detachment; release from something that holds fast (The Free Dictionary. [n.d.]. Disengagement. In *TheFreeDictionary.com*. http://www.thefreedictionary.com/disengagement).

that facilitate individual performance, team effectiveness, and shared decision making. Leaders must replace traditional controlling leadership methods with coaching, mentoring, and facilitating. To do this, they must gain an understanding of the emotions and attitudes of all members of the organization and communicate this understanding to everyone else. Only when all members have an appreciation for each other's emotions and share an understanding of the goals of the organization can the real work be accomplished. In short, integrating emotional competence into the leadership model has a substantial impact on the quality of the work processes and their outcomes. The only way to move from a culture of demoralization, where clinicians go to work every day knowing they will feel like a failure by the end of the shift because of pressure to complete tasks and inadequate time (Dempsey & Assi, 2020), is to lead with emotional competence to a culture of engagement.

Managing the feeling side of the organization requires emotional competence. For leaders, emotional competence encompasses the abilities to identify, understand, use, and regulate the emotions that arise during the course of their work. Emotions in organizations are similar to emotions experienced in all walks of life and are seldom unique to the workplace or to an individual. Although it is difficult to separate emotions by setting, this chapter attempts to focus on the typical emotional experience in the workplace and the behaviors that organizational leaders tend to use to increase emotional competence.

Underpinnings of Emotional Competence

The worldview of the quantum leader differs significantly from the traditional Newtonian worldview. Leadership theory in quantum organizations takes into account the realities of dissipative (transforming or chaotic) systems. In these systems, structures that exchange energy and matter with their environment form spontaneously. Given that healthcare organizations experience continuous and complex interactions during the formation of the new structures, competence in managing the feeling side of work becomes essential. Following is a description of five quantum organization characteristics that reflect the emotional realities of human systems.

Holism

Quantum organizations are holistic rather than fragmented, which means they recognize the connectedness between work processes and individuals. Holism, as an organizational value, supports the organization's integration with the world and is inconsistent with organizational structures made up of distinct departments and processes.

Intrinsic Motivation

A quantum organization operates on the principle that human beings, by their very nature, are internally motivated. In other words, the leaders of a quantum organization use a theory Y style of management, or a style that assumes that employees are ambitious and self-motivated, and fully recognize the creativity, capability, and motivation of all members of the organization. Further, the leaders do not structure the organization hierarchically, with chains of command encompassing many levels of superiors and subordinates, and they do not believe that the members are inherently lazy and uncreative and always in need of specific directions to be productive. They believe, instead, that for members to show initiative, ownership, and high productivity, the only requisites are positive support and a context for performance. Quantum leaders also believe

CHAPTER TEN   The Fully Engaged Leader: Demonstrating Capacity to Sustain Relationships

that collective wisdom is most likely to emerge when all members are treated as if they are internally motivated to act in the organization's best interests. The belief is that individuals who are valued and encouraged to thrive create a synergistic cooperative that itself thrives.

Emergent Leadership

According to quantum leadership theory, organizational leadership emerges from the combined active engagement of all members of the organization. Thus, as the engagement of individuals in the work of the organization increases, the leadership also increases. In this view, leadership is not attached to individuals but rather occurs in the space between individuals. It is not something done by one person (the leader) to many others (the followers), and it is not a role reserved for the people at the top of the organization.

The model of leadership as emergent differs importantly from the dyadic model of leadership, which is based on hierarchical (superior–subordinate) relationships (Allen, 2000). In this latter model, leadership is treated as a solution to particular organizational problems, specifically problems of performance. An organization that uses the dyadic model tends to be equilibrium seeking and structure preserving; certainty and stability are important goals, but leadership does not expect control to be complete because they know that some degree of change is unpredictable or uncontrollable and that change in structure results in energy loss. High levels of performance occur only when a leader of superior capability defines and directs the work to be done.

> **Key Point**
>
> Leadership occurs in the space between individuals working together. It is an emergent property of their relationships, and not the management or direction of work by individuals placed in superior positions.

Treating leadership as emergent fits well with the belief that individuals are intrinsically motivated, creative, and capable. It also fits well with dissipative models of leadership, which are discussed next.

Dissipative Leadership

Whereas the traditional dyadic model of leadership considers complexity and disruption as anomalies that should be eliminated, the dissipative model views change and the disruption it brings as necessary for survival in a complex world. Organizations require leadership that knows how to manage for efficiency and results while also leading for adaptability (Uhl-Bien & Arena, 2017). Because of the complex nature of today's society, simplistic problem-solving models based on linear command and control are no longer adequate tools for managing change and enhancing adaptability. Administrative or leadership theory must be revised, therefore, to reflect the current nature of organizations as complex, dynamic, dissipative systems. Change is not merely a problem to be solved; change is.

The dissipative model of leadership rightly treats change as normal. It also favors transferring leadership responsibilities to a group process in which no specific person is in charge but every person is assumed to occupy a leadership role to some degree. It views leadership as a dynamic community-building process rather than a means for achieving organizational goals—as a process of change where the ethics (rules of conduct) of individuals are integrated into the mores (customs accepted without question) of a community. Further, in this model leadership becomes a form of participative democracy in which the actions of individuals are motivated by their own wants and needs and directed toward a perceived collective good. The focus is on the intrinsic and foundational values of individuals and the group rather than on causes and effects; leadership, in this view, is the emergent property of relationships, not the management of work by individuals placed in superior positions.

Integrated Leadership

The quantum leadership model recognizes emotional competence as an important skill, especially for leaders of healthcare organizations. Quantum leaders must possess not only intellect, analytical ability, technical skills, and appropriate experience, they must also possess the ability to understand and manage relationships, including their emotional dimension. To be fully effective, they must first master the required technical work skills; second, understand and intentionally choose those work processes most likely to achieve the desired outcomes; and third, be able to form and sustain relationships—and they must do all this in an organization in which the interdependence of individuals and work processes is recognized (**Figure 10-1**).

Traditional leadership job descriptions generally do well defining the necessary product- or service-specific knowledge, skills, and abilities. As for the second requirement, choosing the appropriate work processes, leaders often find it difficult to determine which interventions or processes achieve the organization's goals efficiently. The object is to define and commit to value-based interventions. Too often organizations use long-established processes that are outdated and do not contribute to reaching the desired outcomes in any way.

Consider the myriad times healthcare clinicians monitor and record vital signs and no intervention follows. Why perform these activities with such frequency? Perhaps it is just because "we've always done it this way." The reality is that taking vital signs, although it requires skilled clinicians, seldom contributes to the outcome. Indeed, the need to show that taking vital signs frequently has real benefits for patients deserves consideration. Clinicians are reluctant to give up long-held practices for fear of losing critical data and the legal ramifications, but given the serious shortage of healthcare workers, any and all practices that do not obviously contribute to better patient outcomes should be evaluated for elimination. Leaders, especially in this new age, must ensure that resources are appropriately allocated and that the work of each individual is aligned with the goals of the customers and the organization. In

What
Technical intelligence:
Knowledge of the
service content

How
Relational intelligence:
Connecting the technical
with the personal

Where
Intentional intelligence:
Value-based goals

Figure 10-1 The Components of Leadership Effectiveness.

> **Key Point**
>
> Principles of emotional competence:
> - The individual members of an organization are interconnected and interrelated.
> - The individual members perceive their work as natural and a source of fulfillment and growth.
> - Creativity is inherent in the individual and in the collective wisdom of each team.
> - The individual members are motivated to contribute to meaningful goals and focus on self-esteem and self-actualization.
> - Leadership emerges from the combined active engagement of all members of the organization, not from the activities of a single individual.

fact, all members of the organization must become skilled in selecting interventions that further the organization's mission.

Purposeful (intentional) use of time, labor, and equipment is closely related to the third requisite, developing and sustaining relationships to support work processes. Proficiency at building rapport among members of the organization is increasingly seen as an essential leadership skill; effective relationships, it is now recognized, can substantially improve performance. It is also recognized that effective relationships require the participants to have some understanding of naturally occurring human emotions. The nature of emotional competence required by leaders (and others) is discussed in the following section.

Nature of Emotional Competence

Traditional leaders tend to look on the meaning or feeling side of leadership as its soft side, the work that is often subjective and difficult to teach or measure. Emotional competence is more than a list of attributes. It is a collection of perceptions, behaviors, knowledge, and values that, for instance, enable a leader to manage meaning between individuals and groups within an organization. For healthcare leaders, emotional competence involves the interpretation and translation of personal feelings into the processes of the workplace. The key concepts of cognition, competence, emotion, intelligence, and volition are defined in **Exhibit 10-1** to assist in understanding the essence of emotional competence. The characteristics and behaviors that exemplify emotional competence include the following:

- Self-awareness
- Openness to new ideas
- Knowledge appreciation
- Compassion
- Presence
- Mindfulness
- Nonverbal emotional competence
- Passionate optimism
- Resilience
- Passion through balance
- Impulse control

At times leaders become over focused on the style and behaviors of leadership to the extent that a member's style (Myers-Briggs type or DiSC) is provided on the employee badge. Both leaders and employees become focused on the style of decision making at the expense of the

> **Exhibit 10-1** Key Concepts
>
> - *Cognition*: Pertains to mental processes of perception, memory, judgment, and reasoning.
> - *Competence*: The state of having suitable or sufficient skill, knowledge, and experience for some purpose.
> - *Emotion*: The affective side of consciousness in which joy, sorrow, fear, and so on are experienced. Emotions are distinguished from cognitive and volitional states of consciousness.
> - *Intelligence*: The capacity for learning, reasoning, and understanding; aptitude in grasping truths, relationships, facts, or meanings; mental alertness and quickness of understanding.
> - *Volition*: The act of willing, choosing, or resolving; the exercise of the will.

desired outcomes. Although it is certainly relevant to know, for example, that some individuals are ENTJs (extraversion, intuition, thinking, judging types) and make decisions more quickly than others, this information is one piece of data and relates more to how an individual works within a team and less to their ability to respond quickly to ensure patient safety. The leadership style impacts the performance of the team in order to achieve needed outcomes by understanding each team member behaviorally and creating the team context that yields the best collective performance. The fully engaged leader ensures that focus is on the desired, value-based outcomes that support quality patient care service and that information specific to style is supportive but not the driver of processes.

Many scholars continue to offer guidelines for leadership, but there is no widely accepted, standard template of behaviors for effective leadership. Outcomes of good leadership, such as the achievement of clinical outcomes, employee satisfaction, and fiscal stability, which integrate and reflect the unique values, beliefs, and skills of the organization, have been identified more consistently than behaviors have. Regardless of the approach or theoretical underpinning selected by the leader to guide the development of interpersonal or relationship skills, the process of development must always be directed to the outcomes; processes must never overtake the significance of the desired outcomes. As previously noted, working to identify one's decision-making style and focusing on the need for expression of that style in deference to achieving organizational goals are inappropriate. The goal is to understand one's style, integrate it into the group decision-making process, and achieve the desired goal (Gill, 2011).

Although it is difficult to describe or measure the relational work in the world of organizations, its absence is usually very obvious. When negative outcomes result from the lack of the relational aspect of leadership, for instance, these can be described very clearly by nearly every leader. In a systematic review of leadership styles and outcomes, Cummings and colleagues (2018) concluded that there was strong support for relational leadership styles (transformational, resonant, authentic), instead of task-focused leadership, in order to promote an engaged nursing workforce that yielded desired organizational outcomes. They include the negative consequences of disregarding others as unique individuals, discounting the feelings and values of others, and being abrasive to or ignoring others, all of which tend to cause alienation and loss of support. A leader may accomplish the technical side of a task quickly and in an exemplary manner, but a failure to consider the feelings and interrelationships of those involved usually prevents the outcome from being sustainable and diminishes the commitment and motivation of the team in the future.

Self-Awareness

When leaders know what works for themselves it enhances their ability to understand what works for others in similar situations. In fact, self-knowledge is an important pillar of emotional competence. To achieve self-knowledge, leaders need to understand the quality of consciousness they bring to the workplace and recognize that, although they cannot always control events, they can control their thoughts. The ability to self-regulate allows for meaningful expression of ideas at the appropriate time. In many ways, this competency also reinforces personal humility to be open to the ideas of others.

They also need to realize that individuals each have unique patterns and perceptual filters that affect their interactions with others. This is not to suggest that every individual requires a psychoanalytical evaluation. The point is that leaders need to appreciate that they each have a preferred style of interacting, have their own sources of motivation and energy, and have unique ways of perceiving information and determining which types of information to consider. Leaders (and others) also have different communication styles (e.g., open, confrontational, assertive, and withholding) and different decision-making styles (e.g., autocratic, collaborative, participative, and consensus building). Numerous assessment tools are available to help leaders determine their degree of assertiveness, their type of creativity, and their styles of collaborating and communicating. (**Table 10-1** presents examples of behavioral assessment categories.)

Self-awareness is also about developing an understanding of and appreciation for ambiguity and paradox. Although uncertainty or ambiguity can have a positive value, not everyone is comfortable with the lack of clear and certain pathways. Learning to live with paradox or seemingly contradictory ideas where multiple paths are essential becomes a significant challenge for the leader trained and experienced in the command-and-control leadership model because they believe in a single path. Yet leaders today must recognize that paradoxical situations are a normal part of the organizational landscape and do not necessarily have to be resolved through compromise. For example, contradictions and uncertainty create opportunities for leaders to explore perspectives that differ from theirs and to be confronted with new ideas and feelings. In short, far from being calamitous, paradox, much like conflict, offers formerly hidden benefits to the organization that is open to profit from it.

The leadership role as it relates to relationships has a paradoxical aspect. Although people generally have a need to belong to a group for support and for reference, research indicates that effective leaders, despite spending most of the work time in contact with others, tend to have minimal need to belong to a specific group. Leaders instead tend to be self-reliant and

TABLE 10-1 Behavioral Assessment Categories

	Emotional Competence			
Source	Categories			
Astrology	Water	Fire	Air	Earth
Hippocrates	Melancholy	Sanguine	Phlegmatic	Choleric
Jung	Feeler	Intuitor	Thinker	Sensor
Merrill, Wilson, and Allessandra	Amiable	Expressive	Analytical	Driver

are comfortable acting as a dissenting voice or challenging the status quo. This is not to say that leaders do not create and sustain meaningful relationships. Rather, recognizing that integrating subjective meanings into the leadership dataset is essential for achieving optimal outcomes, emotionally competent leaders use both personal relationship data and organizational data to inform their decisions. Note, however, that this is very different from aligning with specific partisan perspectives or choosing sides in decision making.

Collins (2001) found that powerful leaders often possess a paradoxical mixture of personal humility and professional will. The combination of humble unpretentiousness and fierce, even stoic, resolve is at odds with the traditional image of leaders as larger than life. This union of modesty and willfulness has some obvious merits as a leadership style, especially for leaders in the coming age. Among other things, leaders who are both modest and willful tend to act with a clearly expressed openness to others, place people and their feelings first, recognize the positive and negative aspects of the current reality, sustain their faith in the organization's potential for success, channel their energy into the organization, and are disposed to develop successors rather than leave the issue of succession unresolved. They appreciate the traps inherent in short-term success and false optimism, and they are inclined to foster organizational learning because of their healthy skepticism of their own accomplishments. Besides documenting this unusual combination of leadership values and priorities, recent research has shown that overwhelming improvements in organizational performance can result.

Openness to New Ideas

Leaders who understand their own decision-making and communication styles find it easier to appreciate other perspectives. They thus can take better advantage of the fact that every healthcare organization, because of its range of individuals, teams, and disciplines, is a repository of multiple viewpoints on everything needed to create cost-effective services, from the content of the services to the processes for designing and delivering them.

In addition, such leaders, by considering other viewpoints, can achieve a higher level of emotional competence, which includes the ability to listen to what others have to say and integrate what is important into the organization's collective wisdom. Sometimes, because of the fast-paced, results-oriented environment in which they function, leaders are forced to learn how to maintain suffering silence, which is a form of listening in which the emotions that obstruct listening and the objective evaluation of ideas are suppressed.

Knowledge Appreciation

For leaders of quantum organizations, self-knowledge and openness to the opinions of others are closely related to the perception that new information is essential for growth. Necessarily, besides developing a thirst for new knowledge, leaders also must acquire the ability to filter out insignificant information. In the current data-rich age, far too much information is available on the internet, and more passes through every leader's hands. Filtering and managing new information nonetheless reinforces the undeniable passion of leaders to make a difference.

> **Point to Ponder**
>
> Without feelings of deep sympathy and respect for others struck by misfortune and a genuine desire to alleviate suffering, patient care service would be no more than a robotic endeavor for caregivers.

CHAPTER TEN   The Fully Engaged Leader: Demonstrating Capacity to Sustain Relationships

The greater a leader's self-knowledge and openness to new ideas, the greater the leader's confidence in making decisions. Emotionally competent leaders make decisions readily and enthusiastically, not because they believe they are always correct, but because they understand that there is always a risk of error and that progress cannot be made without taking action. In fact, they strongly believe that unsuccessful outcomes or errors are opportunities for improvement and not something to be avoided or eliminated.

Compassion

Compassion is another main pillar of emotional competence. In health care the emotional intensity surrounding trauma, birth, suffering, and dying makes compassionate service the intended norm. Clinicians and patients have indeed come to recognize the importance of understanding and sharing one another's feelings, including joy, sorrow, and all the emotions in between. Further, compassion fosters the kind of personal involvement that is necessary for clinicians and patients to develop strong and effective relationships and for clinicians to apply their objective (technical) knowledge and skills.

Interestingly, the powerful urge of clinicians to alleviate patient distress cannot prevent them from objectifying patients when they discuss patient issues. The patient becomes a medical condition instead of a person. In contrast, clinicians who are emotionally competent learn to integrate the objectivity of the gallbladder disease with the subjectivity of the patient and to perceive the patient's unique needs and feelings about the disease and its impact on the patient's functionality. The patient remains a person and is not referred to as a room number or a diagnosis.

In many ways, compassionate patient care is similar to compassionate leadership. For instance, the leader attempts to integrate the subjective, which here encompasses the relationships between the members of the organization, and the objective, which encompasses the work to be accomplished. In addition, although leaders should sympathize with employees who have suffered a misfortune, they should refrain from attempting to resolve the employees' issues. Offering guidance and reassurance is appropriate and consistent with the principle of personal accountability, but attempting to manage another's situation is paternalistic and disempowering. The emotionally competent leader develops the ability to express sincere sympathy when an employee experiences adversity but does not cross the line into paternalism. The challenge is to integrate the subjective and the objective—to remain personal in the relationship with the employee while also considering the organization's needs and the employee's accountability for doing his or her job. In meeting this challenge, the leader avoids objectifying the employee (e.g., treating the employee as an attendance problem).

Consider this common situation. An employee with repeated absences is disciplined by a leader on the basis of an established attendance policy. The leader's goal may be compassionate leadership, yet the objective policy is allowed to get in the way. To act with compassion, the leader needs to inject subjectivity into the equation, which can be done by exploring the surrounding events (the context of the absences) and the employee's feelings. Compassionate leadership emerges when the leader looks at both the personal information and the objective needs of the organization to find an equitable solution. This is not to say that it is okay not to hold the employee accountable for meeting the expectations of the organization. In fact, compassionate leadership is a broad enough concept to include dismissing the employee if the employee fails to make a sincere effort to do his or her job.

As shown by this example, compassionate leadership is sometimes hard to achieve. It is especially hard to achieve in a traditional organization, where workforce numbers and productivity targets are determined by the chief executive officer (CEO) and handed down to managers for implementation. In difficult times the CEO usually mandates a reduction in the workforce using one of two approaches. In the first approach, the CEO keeps distant from the process, causing the employees to view him or her as callous. In reality the CEO may be very compassionate, but by not becoming directly involved in the process he or she inadvertently appears indifferent. In the second approach, the CEO, having identified the workforce reductions to be implemented, remains involved and available during the communication and early implementation stages. As a result, the employees perceive the CEO as compassionate and caring.

Presence

For any leader, being present—especially being available following any decision that has positive or negative implications for others—shows that the leader is connected with the employees and is willing to participate with them in a common journey. Leaders with a low degree of emotional competence tend to be visible in the workplace after announcements of pay raises or new benefits packages and noticeably out of town when decisions that negatively affect members of the organization are first publicized. Involvement in managing the impact of all decisions shows that the leader is committed to the employees, is willing to claim ownership of the decisions, and is sensitive to the varied meanings of the decisions for the employees. Absence, by contrast, conveys that the leader is uninterested in the impact of difficult decisions on others and is afraid of claiming the decisions. Leaders must realize that it is not only their technical skills or verbal communication that makes a difference, but that it is also their ability to show that there is someone at the top who cares about what is happening.

> ### Group Discussion
>
> Imagine that in the midst of a recent blizzard, a healthcare organization experiences a serious staffing shortage. Because the storm is forecast to continue, the employees who are at work wonder whether they should inform the leadership team of the shortage. At what point, if at all, should they contact the senior leaders? When should the senior leaders be required to be present at the organization? How would the leaders' actions likely affect the willingness of others to attempt to come to work? What impact would the leaders' presence have on the employees' morale? How long will the employees remember the presence or absence of the leaders?

Employees who are facing layoffs will search for the linkage between the (objective) financial goals of the organization and the (subjective) impact of the workforce reduction on their lives. In such a situation, the employees interpret the leader's physical presence and availability for dialogue as compassionate leadership. Note that this does not negate the importance of the role of other leaders at the work unit level; yet employees facing adversity seek to connect their subjective reality (e.g., the reality of being out of work) with the personal (subjective) responses of the chief decision maker.

CHAPTER TEN   The Fully Engaged Leader: Demonstrating Capacity to Sustain Relationships

Mindfulness

The emotionally competent leader is mindful of recurring situations, the past reactions of members of the organization, and the implications of these reactions. As a result, the leader is able to identify certain patterns of behavior and develop skill in understanding and interpreting these situations as guidelines for future behavior. Significant research and publications on mindfulness provide clarity and value of this concept (Good et al., 2016). Mindfulness in management literature is described as cognitive flexibility and clear-minded attention to novelty; attention coupled with meta-awareness or an apprehension of the current state of mind that monitors focused attentiveness (Dreyfus, 2011). In essence, leaders interpret the emotional reactions of individuals in recurring situations and ensure that that they are present or attentive when another such situation arises. For example, a disaster of any kind requires the physical presence of the leader to support the employees emotionally. Seldom is the presence of the leader needed—or even desired—for the technical work of a disaster, rather the presence is needed for experiential processing. The leader should have no question as to the significance of his or her presence when employees are emotionally affected.

Mindfulness is also essential in the development of leadership wisdom. Reflective questioning to gain self-awareness and understanding of situations where the leader is involved is a practice of mindfulness. Questions such as "What about the group meeting bothered me?" or "Did I handle that conflict with curiosity and respect?" help leaders gain wisdom with regards to their leadership approach and effectiveness (Pesut & Thompson, 2018).

Nonverbal Emotional Competence

A leader's physical stance and actions transmit nonverbal messages and can arouse positive or negative emotions. Imagine a group of people standing together in such a way as to invite new participants. Now imagine a group standing close to each other in a closed circle and speaking in hushed tones. The message sent by this arrangement is that newcomers are not welcome. Again, an extended arm, a handshake, and the offering of physical space are friendly behaviors, whereas turning one's back to an approaching person, folding one's arms, and speaking in hushed tones are inhospitable behaviors. The former convey feelings of acceptance, whereas the latter are rejecting and exclusionary. Or consider the unexpected entry of a competitor into a group of highly antagonistic opponents. The conversation may stop altogether or verbal confrontation may ensue, depending on the emotional state of all the parties. Emotional reactions are pervasive in any situation in which people are present, and dealing with these reactions requires great compassion and self-awareness.

Passionate Optimism

Amid the complexities and unending demands, healthcare leaders often find it difficult to remain enthusiastic about the work to be done, and they may find it easier to see the cup as half empty rather than as half full. They may therefore need the refreshment afforded by reminiscing about the beginning of their careers, when their deep concern for patient care was the driving force of all their actions. During this earlier period, besides acting out of altruism, they undoubtedly believed they could truly make a difference. In fact, as new professionals, they were focused on understanding the seriousness of each patient's condition and identifying the treatment most likely to result in a favorable outcome. In spite of the challenges, hopefulness was their modus operandi. Emotionally competent leaders retain the passion of their early healthcare experiences and work diligently to guide others in developing and cherishing the same spirit of passionate optimism. This is not to say that they are immune to discouragement or unrealistic about the future. All leaders experience disappointment and disillusionment, but emotionally competent leaders recognize that successes and failures are both normal and that times of disappointment eventually give way to times of breakthrough and achievement.

Maintaining a positive mindset means holding positive images rather than negative images and viewing all situations as blessings and/or opportunities. When the results are not desired or anticipated, leaders should look for lessons to be learned and value the information gained. A positive mindset stands in sharp contrast to a pessimistic worldview, which fosters passivity and a general unwillingness to take appropriate action in the face of adversity. Pessimism depletes the life force of all involved. Even in the worst of circumstances leaders are challenged to find positive meaning for themselves and the members of the organization. And when positive meaning cannot be found, the most logical source of encouragement becomes each individual's support system, including family and friends.

Resilience

Many leaders have acquired the skill set needed to manage personal disappointments and to coach others in the management of their disappointments. Traditionally, individuals who receive bad news are expected to deal with it outside of the workplace. Yet when a team jointly addresses the disappointments of individual team members, productivity is likely to be enhanced and work disruption minimized. Further, allowing time for the team to process disappointments and create effective coping strategies strengthens the emotional competence of the team.

Passion Through Balance

Creating or restoring passion for work typically has a subtle impact at the outset, but eventually the results become obvious. Passion often emerges from situations that seem overwhelming. Given the current rate of change and innovation, few can keep pace to their satisfaction. There is far too much knowledge available and not enough time or skill to winnow out the unneeded information. Reestablishing a proper balance requires a new filter for consciousness, a filter that allows leaders to sift through information and select only what is pertinent to the issue at hand. Also, leaders can find new comfort in accepting their limitations and the impossibility of reviewing all there is to know. They can also find comfort in realizing that if out-of-the-ordinary information is needed, it probably is available through the internet. Establishing a balance between information input and available time is one component of the total equation, and

> **Point to Ponder**
>
> Thoughts on resilience:
>
> - Resilience is the capacity to cope with unanticipated dangers after they have become manifest and to learn to bounce back.
> - To be resilient means being able to come away from the event with an even greater capacity to prevent and contain future errors.
> - Resilience is the capacity for improvisation, which allows the organization to expand exponentially not only with the range of actions in its repertoire but also the range of potential threats it can foresee.
>
> —Karl Weick and Kathleen Sutcliffe
>
> Reproduced from Weick, K., & Sutcliffe, K. (2000, Summer). High reliability: The power of mindfulness. *Leader to Leader, 21*, 33-38. © 2000 John Wiley & Sons. Reproduced with permission of John Wiley & Sons, Inc.
>
> "Resilience is the ability to grow from adverse events and find meaning in them" (Southwick & Charney, 2018, p. 8).

it helps in creating the space needed for passionate optimism. Establishing a balance between work and personal life is another prerequisite for passionate optimism.

Passion is more easily sustained when working from a place of purpose where there is alignment with the leader's work and what the leader values. Passion is enabled when the conflict between personal life and work life is minimal. Emotionally competent leaders act to ensure that employees do not feel they have to hang their personal values at the door when they come to work. Although the purpose of their activities is to assist the organization in meeting its goals, only when these goals are congruent with the employees' personal values will their enthusiasm survive. If there is a conflict between goals and values, the best strategy is to bring the conflict and the employees' feelings into view and work to minimize the conflict. Failure to address such conflicts quickly depletes the energy of the organization.

Noted leadership expert and philosopher Peter Russell postulated that in the past it was difficult for people to develop passion and happiness because they had scant material possessions and few career options (Russell, 1993). For example, in preindustrial times 97% of Americans worked on the land. Life was hard and food was scarce. There was no central heating, and the water was not always healthy to drink.

Today, in contrast, grocery stores offer a bounty of food, department stores are filled with clothing and other goods, and hot or cool air is available with the push of a button. If we are unhappy or lack passion, therefore, the probable reason, rather than the absence of something external, is that we are experiencing an inner lack of meaning or sense of personal purpose. Society tells us that to overcome our unhappiness we must do something to meet an external need—buy new clothes or a new car or eat a well-prepared meal—but the void remains. As a consequence, people increasingly recognize that what they are missing is meaning in their life. Meanwhile, the drive for more technology and more material goods continues to accelerate. The challenge is not to negate the value of material well-being, but to make a place for passion—to use emotional competence to create a balance between the material and the emotional sides of life.

Impulse Control

Full emotional competence includes impulse control, or self-regulation—the ability to temper negative emotions. Emotionally competent leaders know how to share feelings appropriately and maintain dignity. Managing emotions is not the same as lacking emotions. Even the most emotionally competent leaders experience feelings of anger and frustration, but they are able to mediate and reframe them to minimize the misuse of energy. The common expectation is that the fundamentals of impulse control were developed in childhood and that anger and frustration are thus managed in a healthy way. Unfortunately, not every individual grew up in a family in which healthy impulse control strategies were handed down. Many instead learned patterns of behavior that were obstacles to personal growth and accountability, such as conflict avoidance and assumption of a victim attitude. These individuals need new skills and behaviors to function in high-stress environments.

As the need for emotional competence becomes more apparent, organizations are developing personal growth and development programs not only for leaders but for all employees and even members of the community. Not surprisingly, attendees of such programs identify non-workplace roles, such as that of parent, spouse, friend, and community member, to which the skills they learn can be profitably applied.

Leaders are expected to achieve personal impulse control and also to acquire the skills to coach others to develop and maintain impulse control. By generally remaining composed and positive in attitude, leaders are better able to support group processes and contribute to the accomplishment of the organizational work. They can still express strong and passionate feelings, but they keep themselves from losing control. Maintaining their cool also allows them to better manage other individuals who become emotionally upset or agitated. If someone does begin to get overly excited, an emotionally competent leader can respond in such a way as to deescalate the loss of control and minimize the chance of emotional fireworks that destroy relationships.

Interestingly, self-control manifests largely in the absence of obvious outbursts. Being unfazed under stress and handling a hostile person without lashing out in return are indications of self-regulation and the ability to manage negative emotions. Controlled emotional behavior avoids misinterpretation of events through the lens of anger and minimizes the chance that a benign comment will lead to skewed perceptions through hostility. Mindfulness practices of self-reflection aid the leader to mature this ability further.

Related Concepts

Several concepts related to emotional competence—emotional intelligence, character, and integrity—are helpful in understanding its underpinnings and significance. Although none is equivalent to or subsumed under the concept of emotional intelligence, each applies to the same set of phenomena. For example, although the concept of character is much broader than the concept of emotional competence, a person's character—the traits that form that person's nature—directly affects the person's ability to become emotionally competent. In general, an emotionally competent leader possesses a high level of emotional intelligence, a strong character, uncompromising integrity, a strong moral conscience, and an optimistic outlook on life.

Emotional Intelligence

Goleman (1998) has done groundbreaking research on the nature of emotional intelligence and its importance as a factor in achieving personal excellence. Emotional intelligence, according to Goleman, determines our potential for learning the practical skills of emotional competence. The five elements that make up emotional intelligence are as follows:

1. Self-awareness is the ability to recognize and understand one's moods, emotions, and drives, as well as their effect on others.
2. Self-regulation is the ability to handle emotions so they facilitate rather than interfere with the work to be done. People with this ability are conscientious, able to delay gratification to pursue goals, able to control or redirect disruptive impulses and moods, and prone to suspend judgment and to think before acting.
3. Motivation is a passion to engage in work for reasons that go beyond money or status. It leads to a propensity to pursue goals with energy and to persevere in the face of setbacks and frustrations.
4. Empathy is the ability to understand the emotional makeup of other people. It allows a person to develop rapport with a broad diversity of people and to treat them according to their own emotional reactions.
5. Social skill is a proficiency in managing relationships and building networks. People with this skill can read social situations accurately and find common ground and build rapport.

Recent variations in the descriptions of emotional intelligence (EI) have raised concerns for some scholars. Some believe that the significance of EI has been overstated because of the lack of evidence supporting the relationship between emotional intelligence and workplace success (Vitello-Cicciu, 2002), whereas others documented the benefit of EI when hiring nurse managers because of the positive influence emotionally intelligent leaders have on the quality of nursing practice and patient outcomes (Spano-Szekely et al., 2016). Despite the criticisms of the lack of conceptual clarity and overriding behaviors, the basic notion of EI continues to enlighten many leaders about the complexities of emotions and their impact on the workplace. By its nature, emotional intelligence is a complex phenomenon subsuming theories of emotion, motivation, behavior, intelligence, organizational behavior, and neuroscience. The intersections and overlapping of one's feelings, sense of purpose, knowledge, and attitude vary widely and often unpredictably. New perspectives and new approaches to further engagement and expertise in relationship building can still be learned from the study of the emotional intelligence literature.

Emotional competence, like other kinds of competence, is the possession of certain skills, learned or unlearned. As indicated previously, emotional intelligence, like other kinds of intelligence, is the potential to learn new skills. Emotional agility is when the leader is flexible with thoughts and feelings so the leader can respond optimally to daily situations in complex environments (David, 2016). Thus, a person who has emotional intelligence has the potential to learn how to be emotionally competent, whereas a person who has emotional competence already possesses a fair number of the appropriate skills.

Character
The term *character* is ambiguous. First, it can refer to the aggregate of features and traits that form the individual nature of a given person. The term has that meaning in such sentences as "What is her character?" and "He has a bad character." The term can also be used as a synonym for moral fortitude, as when we tell someone, "Show some character." To say that a person has character in this latter sense is to say that the person has the moral fortitude and discipline to exemplify the highest virtues of his or her time.

Integrity
Integrity is the quality of being morally upright and always acting openly and honestly. Individuals who have integrity consistently act on their own values in all situations and do not hide critical information, break promises, or fail to fulfill commitments. Commitment to the journey that requires leaders to be emotionally competent and fully engaged is not always valued. Significant pressures emphasize the technical work of strategic planning, budgeting, and controlling. Time and energy to develop relationships or the soft side of leadership are viewed as luxuries, given that they are not believed to be necessarily related to the net income margin. Developing the people skills of leadership—regardless of which label or attribute is attached to them—provides the most effective vehicle for sustained learning to occur through the recognized power of the collective emotions of the team. It is through people's full engagement with their work that the measurable, sustainable results of satisfaction, quality outcomes, and strong net income margins are achieved. Organizations continue to struggle not only to recognize the quantifiable value of emotional competence but also to inexorably link these attributes to technical leadership processes. Continual reinforcement and demonstration of these relationships is a never-ending process for engaged and enlightened leaders.

Emotional Risks of Leadership

All leadership decisions are inherently uncertain and have the potential for error. But even if a leader fully understands that mistakes are unavoidable and accepts that he or she will make some wrong decisions, the emotional impact of making an error can be devastating. Historically, leadership education programs have offered participants little preparation for managing miscalculations and missteps. The emphasis has been on success, not failure.

The emotional effects of failure that leaders face on a daily basis cannot be eliminated. They can only be managed. In essence, the reputation of the leader is continually at stake. To manage emotional risk, leaders need a high level of emotional competence, including self-awareness, compassion, passionate optimism, and resilience. They typically must use their emotional competence to deal with issues such as lack of feedback, inconsistency in the reactions of stakeholders, and employment insecurity, all of which have the power to cause confusion and emotional turmoil.

Lack of Feedback

Honest feedback given to a leader and recognition for work accomplished fuel the leader's passion for doing his or her job. Both are highly valued and sought after by most leaders (and also by most employees). On the reverse side, a lack of performance feedback causes stress and undermines the leader's confidence. So does a lack of acknowledgment from a supervisor, whether positive or negative. Not knowing where he or she stands with the supervisor is emotionally draining.

In addition, the more uncertain the leader becomes about his or her performance (because of the lack of feedback), the more likely the leader is to lose confidence in his or her decision-making ability, and the more likely the supervisor is to continue to withhold feedback, leading to a cycle of uncertainty and negative emotions. Failure to create the ideal team, to achieve clinical goals, or to meet financial targets results in damage to a leader's ego. In such cases, timely feedback is critical to reversing negative outcomes, learning from the undesired outcomes, and relieving the leader's emotional stress.

Inconsistent Feedback

Imagine that the department practice council develops a plan for patient restraint management with the intent of ensuring patient safety and meeting regulatory requirements. When the plan is presented to the hospital practice council, the council quickly reviews and approves the plan, but the critical care clinicians recommend numerous revisions and withhold their endorsement. The leader of the department practice council, faced with such different stakeholder responses, is likely to feel confused as well as less confident in his or her abilities. Yet the leader should keep in mind that, all too often, actions that are successful in one situation are ineffective in others, with no apparent explanation. In other words, the wide-ranging responses that different individuals or groups can have to the same action might appear as an impenetrable mystery that challenges a leader's ability to lead, but in such situations it is healthy to avoid being overly self-critical and to minimize the emotional insult. The best strategy is to focus on the context of the actions and reactions and to recognize that the values and goals of the stakeholders can vary widely, resulting in widely differing responses. In the case at hand, the leader's task includes not just creating an appropriate plan but understanding and managing the context in which the plan is proposed.

Employment Insecurity

In the typical organization, leaders serve at the will of the organization and can be removed without much notice or explanation. An employment contract helps in managing the processes of separation, but it cannot prevent the emotional damage that results from the removal. Regardless of the health of the individual's ego, the experience is devastating. Expecting a leader to view the discharge as a business decision and not as a personal judgment is insulting and dishonest. Whenever someone's professional relationships are severed, membership in an organizational team is canceled, or income is eliminated, it is, in fact, very personal.

Being discharged from a job or position often results in serious emotional trauma. In fact, heightened sensitivity to the experience can be seen as the downside of emotional competence. If the leader avoided all feelings and emotions, he or she actually could view the discharge simply as a business issue. The reality is that situations that negatively affect any part of an individual's life are personal and often painful. Compounding the problem for healthcare leaders is that people in health care are expected to provide care rather than receive care. Thus, it is very difficult for them to handle being in need of support, sympathy, and compassion.

Although the emotional effects of uncertainty and employment insecurity are not unique to health care, the values of clinicians, especially the importance they place on caregiving, cause them to have heightened emotional sensitivity and often heightened vulnerability to emotional upset. Among the consequences are that clinicians, especially those who are emotionally incompetent, are predisposed to experience great stress, suffer a loss of confidence and passion, and feel incredible turmoil and disappointment. The solution to being exposed to emotional risk is to develop significant emotional competence. In addition, a leader undergoing an employment crisis can mitigate the resulting depression and sense of devastation by keeping in mind his or her skills and abilities and past performance and achievements.

Benefits of Emotional Competence in Health Care

Relational work—does make a difference in health care. That is not a controversial claim. But leaders are often unsure how the value of relationships can be substantiated and translated into organizational effectiveness and a better bottom line. Traditionally, leaders have examined care delivery from a purely technical perspective. However, the processes involved in providing care encompass both technical (quantitative) and human-related (qualitative) attributes. Thus, a holistic perspective, one that includes quantitative and qualitative measures, is needed for evaluating care delivery.

Leaders know that technical skills are necessary for producing products and services and are essential for success. Leaders also know that defined goal-directed (intentional) behaviors are essential. More recently, they have begun to realize that the relationships among members of the organization have an impact on effectiveness. Yet all too often they fail to see the interconnections between the technical aspect of work, the intentional aspect of work, and the relationships among the workers. Only when leaders integrate the workers' essential technical skills, their goal-directed activities, and their ability to form meaningful relationships does optimal organizational effectiveness result (see Figure 10-1). In addition, treating the work to be accomplished as a nonreducible unit of service shifts the evaluation focus from the parts to the whole, where it properly belongs.

> ## Group Discussion
> The three components of integrated leadership—the technical, relational, and intentional—offer a framework for optimizing the use of resources. In a recent committee meeting, a new benefit for child care was introduced and added to the benefits package at the request of an influential board member. The benefit offers a fixed per diem reimbursement amount to pay for child care provided to the children of employees. It is uncertain whether employees are interested in or will use this benefit. It is also uncertain how the value of this benefit will be assessed. Analyze the addition of this benefit from the perspective of the three components of integrated leadership. That is, identify the technical, relational, and intentional considerations that pertain to it. Based on the discussion of these considerations, recommend whether to add the benefit or reject its inclusion into the benefits package.

The value of emotional competence is evident in nearly every interaction in an organization. For instance, effective leaders possess a high degree of self-awareness, compassion for others, self-control, resilience, and passionate optimism, and this powerful combination enables them to achieve the most challenging goals and enlist others in completing the organization's work. Yet it is difficult not only for the leaders themselves to measure the value of passion and emotional competence, but also for board members, who tend to neglect these in the selection of CEOs, especially where the financial stakes are substantial.

Focused Hiring
Increasing evidence exists that choosing a leader should involve more than finding the candidate with the best history of financial performance, stock pricing, expense management, merger experience, and workforce reductions. Many boards, however, still believe that if a candidate's achievements are notable, especially in the financial area, they cannot go wrong in hiring that candidate. The problem with this strategy is that many executives who have succeeded because of their financial acumen lack the requisite emotional competence and fail to listen to others, develop meaningful relationships, share honest feelings, and empathize with others—their leadership can harm organizational performance rather than improve it. In particular, their way of handling subordinates might easily cause an increase in turnover and a decrease in market share and net income. Cases in which this has occurred confirm a relationship between the emotional competence of an organization's leader (soft skills) and the organization's financial measures (hard skills).

The cost of turnover continues to be a challenge. In many job categories the cost of turnover and replacement for one position exceeds $50,000. With healthcare annual turnover rates averaging 15% to 20%, the annualized costs are significant. In addition, although many organizations assume the greatest turnover is at the staff level, in fact the greatest turnover is at the middle management level.

Staged encounters of the formal interview process seldom reveal the real nature of any job applicant. Finding an applicant with the right fit requires spending extensive time evaluating

Exhibit 10-2 Interviewing for Emotional Competence

These questions are asked of both the candidate and the representatives in the current work environment. Interviewing team members compare responses for consistency and fit with the organization.

Directions: Select the most appropriate response.

	Strongly Disagree	Disagree	Agree	Strongly Agree
1. Does the candidate have the ability to manage disappointment?	❏	❏	❏	❏
2. Does the candidate listen to others' ideas?	❏	❏	❏	❏
3. Does the candidate value the contributions of team members?	❏	❏	❏	❏
4. Does the candidate hold others accountable for their performance and promises?	❏	❏	❏	❏
5. Is the candidate comfortable delegating important tasks to others?	❏	❏	❏	❏
6. Does the candidate energize others?	❏	❏	❏	❏
7. Does the candidate spend time communicating the organization's vision and purpose?	❏	❏	❏	❏
8. Do members of the organization trust the promises of the candidate?	❏	❏	❏	❏
9. Is the candidate interested in the concerns of employees?	❏	❏	❏	❏
10. Does the candidate share information willingly and in a timely manner?	❏	❏	❏	❏

the most promising candidates before hiring by reviewing credentials, prescreening the candidate, and then asking the right interview questions. Then, once the candidate with the greatest potential for success is selected, extensive time is required to integrate him or her into the organization. The more time spent with the candidates before hiring, the more likely the candidate with the best fit is hired, the less likely that person is to leave the organization, and, as the new hire becomes more acculturated over the first year, the greater the job satisfaction he or she experiences. New interviewing processes and different types of questions are needed to identify the chemistry between an applicant and the members of the organization (**Exhibit 10-2**).

Succession Planning

Another opportunity for leaders to use emotional competence is in succession planning. Organizations are wise to ensure that the integrated skill sets of all leadership hires, not just the top leaders, are consistent with their needs both present and future. The skill sets and characteristics desired for leadership positions should be clearly defined and shared within the organization for aspiring and existing leaders. Succession planning should not be left solely to chance or placed in the hands of a single department or organization leader. An intentional process should be used to identify and develop successors based on assessment data of incumbent high-potential leaders plus retirement predictions and existing pipelines of the existing workforce. In order to effectively identify high-potential leaders, it is important to separate concepts of manager and leader as different roles and skill sets. In addition, the prevailing attitude in some organizations of "derservability," or individuals who deserve to be leaders due to employment longevity or because of an individual's clinical expertise, should be separated from the requirement of the ability to lead as the most important prerequisite (Jones, 2018). Hiring from within has a positive organizational impact on retention and engagement when high-performing employees see a path to their own development and success. The greatest success comes when organizations make a strategic commitment as a job expectation of current leaders to develop future leaders. Along with this expectation comes the formalization of mentoring programs and enriched leadership development programs that develop the leaders for future leader requirements (Fray & Sherman, 2017).

There is also threat when a leader undermines the effectiveness of succession planning. This calls on the emotional competence and wisdom of other incumbent leaders to address this leader's behavior. Undermining could manifest as a leader who doesn't really want to leave or a belief that no one is as good as them so they choose a less talented successor (Dattner & Chamorro-Premuzic, 2016). These leaders don't mentor others and prevent their successors from developing their own abilities or finding their leader presence because the incumbent leader wants them to carry on an old leadership style, which may not be a fit for where the organization needs to go. Succession planning is needed, and when supported by resources that aid in attracting and developing new and experienced leaders, experienced leaders commit to serve as mentors in order to contribute to their leadership legacy.

Higher Productivity

Significant opportunities for increased productivity exist when emotional competence becomes an attribute not just of individual members but of the entire team. Given that the real work of an organization occurs within a team framework, the greater the ability of team members to truly work together, the greater the positive impact on organizational performance. Note that working together involves more than cooperation, participation, and commitment to goals. The team members must exhibit self-awareness, compassion, passionate optimism, and impulse regulation if they are to achieve their desired outcomes. According to Druskat and Wolff (2001), team success lies in the fundamental conditions that allow effective task processes to emerge and cause members to engage in these processes wholeheartedly. Three conditions—trust among members, a sense of group identity, and a sense of group efficacy—are essential to effectiveness. Without these, teams simply go through the motions of cooperating and participating, and members hold back rather than fully engage, reducing the level of effectiveness.

Healthcare teams that recognize the interconnectedness of members and acknowledge the unique contributions of each to the delivery of services make substantial contributions to the achievement of organizational goals. Specifically, they help improve patient care outcomes, implement strategies in a shorter time, apply new knowledge as it becomes available, use organizational resources more productively, problem solve more creatively, and manage work processes more effectively. According to Orsburn et al. (1990), most organizations experience a 20% to 40% increase in productivity when employees are deeply involved in their work. Self-directed teams serve as organizational change strategies to empower staff, gain job satisfaction, and improve feelings of autonomy over patient care (Maurits et al., 2017; Vito, 2019).

Selecting and mentoring individuals for team membership using the principles of emotional competence reinforce the benefits of effective teams. The goal is to select members who are not just team players but who also bring to the team varied interests and skills. To do this, it is helpful to look at the results of self-assessment exercises used to assist members in learning about themselves and other team members. These exercises can provide information about behavior patterns and the filters people use in their interactions with others. Understanding the unique characteristics of different team members facilitates the team's work and makes it timelier. Information on the following usually can be easily obtained:

- *Decision-making style*: Some individuals consider information and ideas objectively and logically, whereas others tend to be more subjective and value oriented.
- *Motivation*: Some individuals are energized by dealing with the outside world and thrive on personal interactions, whereas others are more comfortable thinking and reflecting and are disinclined to share an idea until comfortable with it.
- *Processing*: Some individuals require facts and step-by-step processes and focus on the present, whereas others are more comfortable with insights and intuitions and focus on the future.
- *Orientation to outside information*: Many individuals need information so they can predict and plan, whereas others tend to be comfortable with little information and letting things happen.

If all the team members are aware of each other's behavior patterns, interests, and background, the team will work together more effectively and plan for future membership. For instance, if a behavior pattern is missing from the team (e.g., the reflective pattern mentioned under "motivation" in the previous list), the team can try to identify candidates who possess it. The team can also target candidates likely to offer a range of ideas or who have the skills to facilitate the team's work.

In addition to providing guidance in the selection of members, emotional competence increases the probability that team members will hear each other's concerns and understand each other's feelings. By taking time to consider matters from each member's perspective before making a decision, the team, besides being able to incorporate the different perspectives into the final decision, recognizes each member's importance, thereby improving the members' morale and willingness to cooperate. This process is very different from calling for a majority vote in the interest of expedience. Teams with high levels of emotional competence understand that consideration of the views of each member is a requisite of sustainable decisions. They try to obtain a consensus rather than majority agreement to ensure that all team members are behind the decision. The intent is never to remove the emotion from the process but rather to hear every member to create trust and ultimately foster greater participation among members.

Coaching Upward

Coaching is a valued method of developing skills, but it traditionally has been used almost exclusively by superiors to assist those subordinate to them. The most challenging type of coaching—and the one ordinarily overlooked—involves providing feedback to those individuals with greater authority. As the members of an organization become more emotionally competent, coaching upward becomes less challenging and is embraced more readily. Once the halo of infallibility is removed from the most powerful positions in the organization, those

Group Discussion

Sharing feedback upward (to superiors) provides information about an individual's impact on another individual similar to downward (subordinates) or sideways (to peers) feedback. The CEO of your organization has scheduled a leadership retreat at a time when the staffing is seriously low. The topic of staffing does not appear to be of interest to the senior leaders or at least is of less concern to them than other topics. Together with your team, create a plan to discuss this situation with the CEO. The goal is to give feedback to the CEO, a person with more power, authority, and/or experience than you. In the best-case scenario, the feedback will enhance the effectiveness of the retreat and ultimately improve the organization's performance. The risk is that the feedback may be rejected by the CEO and may negatively affect your relationship with the CEO. You can use the following list of steps to guide your preparation for the "coaching upward" meeting:

1. Describe the situation (topic).
2. Agree on the specific objective of the session.
3. Share your assessment of the situation. Why is a change needed? How will the CEO benefit from the change? How will the organization benefit from the change?
4. Validate your assumptions with the CEO. Ask for comments.
5. Invite suggestions from the CEO.
6. Suggest possible solutions. Cover the full range of options.
7. Select a course of action.
8. Agree on the course of action. Identify the timeframe for the expected change.
9. Identify specific steps to achieve the change.
10. Commit to action. Thank the CEO for his or her willingness to examine the issues and work to make the organization more effective.

in other positions can use the skills of coaching upward to give appropriate feedback, often averting serious negative outcomes as a result.

People generally appreciate constructive, timely, and sensitively delivered feedback that can be put to practical use. Despite this, people who give feedback frequently are tentative and unsure that what they are doing is appropriate. Giving feedback completes the circle of communication and further advances the work of the organization in a positive manner.

Developing Emotional Competence

Effective and accomplished leaders can possess natural or inherent ability and likely also acquired leadership skills, including emotional competence. These latter skills are acquired through development programs complemented with focused coaching, time, and experience, as seen in many succession planning programs.

Exhibit 10-3 presents a five-stage model of development based on the Dreyfus and Dreyfus (1996) skill acquisition model as a framework for understanding how leaders obtain emotional competence incrementally. Each of the five skill levels is described to assist readers in assessing

Exhibit 10-3 Individual Emotional Competence Skill Levels and Behaviors

- Novice (detached observer)
  - Formally educated in the principles of emotional competence
  - Aware of personal interaction styles and behavior patterns
  - Has not held a formal leadership position
- Advanced beginner (active participant)
  - Has increasing self-awareness but limited openness to the ideas of others
  - Tends to be judgmental
  - Has increasing confidence in ability to participate and make decisions
  - Begins to think and feel simultaneously; not always certain of the meaning of events or if there is a connection between an event and another's emotional reaction
  - Is easily discouraged and not always optimistic about the future
- Competent (integrated with the process)
  - Has emerging compassion for others
  - Exhibits authentic presence in teamwork; listens actively and critically to others
  - Is able to think and feel simultaneously and acknowledge the feelings of others
  - Gives both positive and negative feedback (a requirement of effective communication)
  - Is increasingly open to others' ideas
  - Gains comfort in challenging the status quo
  - Begins to develop the ability to control impulses
- Proficient (therapeutic engagement)
  - Has emerging sense of optimism and ability to manage negative emotions
  - Is able to read or experience chemistry between people (e.g., recognizes allies, identifies who to trust, and recognizes nonsupport or hostility)
  - Understands the meaning of relationships
  - Has a positive but realistic attitude; believes in the team's ability to accomplish the work to be done
  - Believes integrity is an essential characteristic
  - Has emerging passion for the process and the relationships among team members
  - Inspires others with passionate spirit and commitment
  - Begins to develop resilience to negative events
  - Exhibits increasing impulse control
- Expert (dialogic engagement)
  - Demonstrates self-awareness and utilizes self-assessment information to improve personal performance and to support and understand team members
  - Possesses strong resilience to the negative realities of the workplace and coaches others in developing similar skills; able to manage difficult information
  - Is able to think and feel simultaneously
  - Is open to others' ideas and viewpoints
  - Actively seeks opinions from team members on their task processes, progress, and performance
  - Actively coaches and mentors new members as well as current members
  - Exhibits well-developed impulse control

their own level of emotional competence and in continuing to mature toward the highest skill level. The following subsections describe the levels of emotional competence in more detail, and behaviors that demonstrate emotional incompetence that individuals sometimes exhibit and should seek to eliminate are discussed in an upcoming section.

Novice Stage

In the first stage, the individual, despite having formal education in leadership, has no experience in the application of leadership knowledge and skills. The novice is a detached observer of the processes of leadership and, in regard to emotional competence, has at most a personal awareness of interaction styles and behavior patterns.

Advanced Beginner Stage

The advanced beginner is finally engaged in a leadership role, testing the knowledge and skills gained during formal education. The focus is on developing competence in coaching and mentoring and in relationship management. Although the advanced beginner's level of self-awareness is increasing, his or her main goal is to demonstrate personal competence and ensure satisfactory work. The advanced beginner is starting to think about group processes and how to integrate the emotions of others but is not always certain of the connections between an event and another's emotional reaction.

The advanced beginner spends little time or attention on understanding the reactions of others in the setting. Also, he or she is not always open to the ideas of others and tends to be defensive or judgmental. The advanced beginner is starting to become more confident as a decision maker but is discouraged easily and is not always optimistic about the future.

Competent Stage

In the third stage, the individual is more experienced as a leader and is beginning to develop compassion for others. The individual can think about issues and simultaneously have feelings and acknowledge the feelings of others. He or she also now develops the ability to be present physically and mentally, attend to conversations with authenticity, and listen to and ask questions of team members with sensitivity to their emotions.

The individual is increasingly compassionate and open to the ideas of others and is less judgmental than previously. He or she also exhibits a greater ability to control impulses and begins to feel comfortable challenging the status quo.

Proficient Stage

Team leaders often hit an invisible wall at the competent stage and do not make it to the proficient stage. If this happens, the teamwork becomes rote and frequently is ineffective. Long-standing teams that meet without adding value to healthcare outcomes fit this category.

A team leader who reaches the proficient stage is noticeably more comfortable in the role and has a better grasp of the influence of relationships on team activities. The proficient leader can think and feel simultaneously and read the chemistry among people, recognize allies, identify who to trust, and sense where nonsupport or hostility is present. This leader is beginning to develop the ability to manage incivility and conflict and is generally optimistic, including about the team's ability to accomplish its work. Only rarely is the individual discouraged or negative about the future. Passionate optimism—the integration of a positive outlook and wholehearted commitment—becomes the norm. Finally, the proficient leader has increasing control over impulses and is developing resilience in the face of difficulties or crises.

Expert Stage

The leader at the expert stage uses self-assessment information to improve personal performance and to support the other members of the team. Thinking and feeling simultaneously is the only way the expert leader knows how to act. As an accomplished team member, the expert leader not only is open to new ideas but also seeks input from others. The expert leader actively coaches and mentors new members as well as current members in developing expert emotional competence skills. As a passionate optimist, the expert leader is highly resilient and at the same time possesses sophisticated impulse control.

Emotionally Incompetent Behaviors

In journeying toward full emotional competence, people exhibit behaviors indicative of emotional incompetence. Given that incompetence is often easier to describe than competence, the following examples of emotional incompetence are presented as a means of indicating what emotional competence is.

Acting as Devil's Advocate

All too often, people consider an issue or situation from the self-appointed position of devil's advocate. In most such cases, people assume this perspective for lack of self-awareness and understanding of their own point of view. They hide behind the role for any number of reasons—usually known only to them. Common reasons include lack of information, inability to support an idea while unsure how to express nonsupport, and desire to block the decision-making process.

Displaying a Bad Attitude

People who have a difficult time participating in work processes often display negative behaviors ranging from grumbling to shirking. They usually do not understand that such behaviors impede progress and decrease the overall morale of the group, or, if they do, they might refuse to acknowledge the effects of their actions on others or dismiss their behavior by claiming, "That's just the way I am."

Displaying a Superior Attitude

An individual with a superior attitude responds to comments with indignation and criticism. The individual also usually does not recognize the adversarial nature of his or her responses and their impact on others but views them as a necessary means for getting the entire group to understand its inadequacies.

Tolerating Errors

Tolerating errors or undesirable behaviors implies these are accepted. In many cases, the tolerance results from the inability of those in charge to react and correct the errors or behaviors and/or the organizational culture's lack of support for managing problematic behaviors. When an individual fails to meet the relevant behavioral standards, managers and others in the organization must use the situation as an opportunity to reinforce the organizational culture and build better relationships.

Failing to Balance Work and Relaxation

Often leaders find themselves spending more time at work and less time at home, believing that the operation of the organization is more important than other priorities. Further, they commonly believe their presence is required for productivity to occur. They thus wind up spending excessive hours at work and neglect the other parts of their lives, including recreating with family and friends. The focus on work tasks is characteristic of the advanced beginner level of emotional competence, whereas achieving a balance between work and family and community is characteristic of the expert level.

Team Emotional Competence

In creating team-level emotional competence, a team builds on the skills of the individual members and focuses on itself as a collective. The assumption is that the members have at least a basic understanding of team processes such as setting common goals for the team, communication, and developing trust. It is through these processes that the team members begin to feel confidence in each other and in the team as a whole, reinforcing successful team behaviors. Team emotional competence, like the individual variety, usually is developed incrementally in a five-stage process (**Exhibit 10-4**).

Exhibit 10-4 Team Emotional Competence Skill Levels and Behaviors

- Novice (detached observer)
  - Team is newly formed and consists of independent participants.
  - Members have no prior relationships with or knowledge of behavior patterns and emotions of other members.
- Advanced beginner (active participant)
  - Group guidelines are developed and understood by members (this transition stage reflects the shift from the use of individual power to integrated goals and unified or shared support for goals).
  - Group cohesion is beginning to develop.
  - Team is mainly focused on meeting processes.
  - Team behavior patterns are beginning to emerge.
  - At times, the team is overwhelmed and easily discouraged.
- Competent (integrated with the process)
  - Members are increasingly self-aware and sensitive to communication dynamics between members.
  - Team establishes realistic ground rules.
  - Members understand each other's skills and emotions.
  - Team routinely requests feedback from every member at the beginning and the end of the meetings.
  - Outcomes of the team's work are evident.
- Proficient (therapeutic engagement)
  - Team members understand the goals of the team and the relationship of their work to that of other teams in the organization.
  - Team members seek feedback from others in the organization following team meetings and bring feedback to the next meeting.
  - Team is passionate about its work and optimistic that it can make a difference.
  - Team shows tolerance for character failings.

(continues)

Exhibit 10-4   Team Emotional Competence Skill Levels and Behaviors (*continued*)

- Expert (dialogic engagement)
  - Team members understand the team's goals and how they relate to the organization and community at large.
  - Team consists of experienced and mature members.
  - Team is able to integrate local and national regulations into its work.
  - Team often makes recommendations and moves beyond its specific assigned tasks to create better options for the organization.
  - Team terminates itself when it is unable to add further value to the organization.

Novice Stage

A novice team consists of individuals coming together for the first time for a newly defined purpose. The members know very little, if anything, about each other and typically do not share common feelings or values—or if they do, they are not aware of their commonalities at this point. A novice team's focus is on understanding the purpose of the team and setting the ground rules.

Advanced Beginner Stage

In this stage, the team becomes more cohesive through establishing how to carry out meeting tasks such as setting agendas, recording the minutes, and ensuring that the ground rules are defined and followed. Jockeying for power often occurs at this level, but it tends to end once the team develops feedback skills and gets into the habit of recognizing the contributions of each member. The team makes a conscious and deliberate effort to (1) shift from valuing power as traditionally used to foster empowerment and (2) develop an awareness of the behavior patterns of each member. However, the members evidence little openness toward substantive ideas and dialogue. Their focus is on task completion and agenda management. They also are discouraged easily and are uncertain as to their ability to create meaningful change.

Competent Stage

A competent team is a compassionate team, and its compassion is reflected in its willingness to discuss every member's issues of concern. The team members have moved from trying to acquire individual power to acting as an authentic collective. They not only show themselves capable of thinking and feeling simultaneously but also acknowledge each other's feelings and integrate them into the team's overall work. In addition, they set and follow ground rules that are realistic and support the team's work. The coaching and mentoring they do with each other are intended to foster behaviors that aid the team, rather than to develop skills that are useful only outside of the team. Finally, the team's level of trust in itself grows, and the members begin to challenge the status quo and consider alternatives to the way things are currently done.

As with individual emotional competence, there is often an invisible wall between the competent and proficient stages. Teams at the competent stage can meet the requirements for standard success but find it impossible to become passionately optimistic while recreating the future or to maintain resilience in the face of negative events. They accomplish the assigned work but seldom move beyond the assigned boundaries.

Proficient Stage

As the emotional skills of the team mature, the team develops a sense of passionate optimism about the future. A proficient team differs from a competent team in considering the needs and priorities of the whole organization as integral to its work. All the members are aware of and understand each other's behavior patterns and use these patterns in developing a consensus on issues, encouraging each other to discuss difficult issues, and addressing the emotions that these issues tend raise. At this stage, the team members recognize each other's character failings as inevitable and work to restore the integrity of relationships.

Expert Stage

For a team to arrive at the expert level of emotional competence is a highly desirable but rare event. An expert team is purposefully coached and mentored and requires ongoing support and validation if it is to be sustained. At this level of performance, the team not only embodies all the characteristics of the proficient team but also considers the needs and priorities of the organization and the healthcare community and ensures that proposed team actions are congruent with the organization's culture and politics.

The members are aware of individual, team, and organizational emotions as an interactive whole. As a team, they have established norms that strengthen their ability to respond effectively to the kind of emotional challenges a group confronts on a regular basis. These norms are directed toward three goals: creating resources for working with emotions, fostering an affirmative environment, and encouraging proactive problem solving. In addition, the expert team embodies resilience to the realities of the environment. Finally, the team members, besides being individually aware of their inward- and outward-directed emotions and able to regulate them, jointly develop a level of group mindfulness.

Causes of Team Dysfunction

Teams that have existed for a long time commonly acquire behavior patterns that can render them inefficient or nonproductive. For instance, they often leave assignments incomplete, allow malcontents to continue griping, pay scant notice to habitual tardiness and absenteeism, and go off on tangents that have little to do with their intended work. Each team has a natural life span, and when its work is completed it should be disbanded or assigned another project.

It is also important to realize that a team may move along the developmental trajectory at an irregular rate and may even regress, such as when its membership and goals change. Further, it is common for a team's development to inexplicably halt before the proficiency stage, in which case the team never gets to the point of integrating its work with that of the organization, much less with the environment or the community at large.

The reforming healthcare system and the associated changes in revenue streams can serve as a threat to the relationship between teams and senior leaders. Even competent, proficient teams are impacted when the balance of providing high-quality care and stable reimbursement is disrupted as in the current healthcare markets.

Before the reimbursement levels were reduced, healthcare teams, although not yet at the proficiency level, were aware of the needs and feelings of all individuals, and their emotional performance could be rated as competent. Their work had two focuses: providing high-quality patient care and maximizing reimbursement. When reimbursement decreased, the teams fell even further short of taking into account the goals of all members (or the goals of the organization as a whole) and thus never reached the proficiency level.

In many ways the course of events described resembles Levy's (2001) Nut Island effect. The Nut Island story is about a team of competent, highly committed employees who performed a vital behind-the-scenes task. The team was adept at organizing and managing itself. Its self-sufficiency was taken for granted by senior management, and when it asked for help or tried to warn of impending trouble, it was ignored or put off because senior management, looking at its history of success, would assume it could handle the current situation. Consequently, an adversarial relationship began to develop between senior management and the team. Unfortunately, the team reacted in a way that worsened the problem. The team made it a priority to stay out of management's line of sight, which led it to deny or minimize problems and avoid asking for help. Eventually, the team began to make up its own rules to enable it to fulfill its own mission—apart from the mission of the organization as a whole.

At this point, both senior management and the team had distorted views that were very difficult to correct. The team members believed they were the only ones who really understood their work and were unwilling to listen to outsiders attempting to help solve their problems. Management remained disconnected, believing that no news was good news. Only a significant external event could change the course of events. Neither the senior managers nor the team members considered the meaning of their work within the context of the entire organization or the marketplace. As a result, the team's level of emotional competence decreased dramatically.

Connecting with Generations of Workers

Workforce composition has always included different generations of workers and varying beliefs, values, and expectations. The emotionally competent leader recognizes the impact of each generation and works to understand the defining characteristics of each and ensure that all are respected. Too often, the generation of the leader is proffered as the only acceptable behavior for all generations. Each generation is characterized by historical, political, and social events that share core values, work ethics, and economic movements of its members. The collective personality of each generation serves as a reference point from which to comprehend how life experiences affect core values and influence one's work. Generalizations of worker profiles should be avoided, given that the traits are often overlapping between generations and anecdotal. However, understanding the basic distinctions of each generation is helpful in creating engagement strategies and supporting policies. Current workforces include five

Group Discussion

The Nut Island story encompasses a number of issues, including lack of teamwork, insensitivity to a team's context, and disharmony between the feelings of individuals in the local setting (the team members) and individuals at the system level (the senior managers). Use this story to elucidate adversarial relationships that exist between leaders and departments in your organization. Identify at least three strategies to mitigate the friction or hostility between the parties using emotional competence as the framework. What outcomes would you select as measures of the effectiveness of these strategies?

generations: matures or traditionalists born between 1928 and 1945; baby boomers born between 1946 and 1964; generation Xers born between 1965 and 1980; and generation Yers (Millennials) born between 1981 and 1997 (Fry, 2016) and now Generation Z, born in 1997 to the current time (Dimock, 2019).

Measuring Emotional Competence

Most healthcare organizations know how to measure and document clinical outcomes, financial results, and market share. Most, however, are very uncomfortable assessing factors such as behavior patterns, compassion, passionate optimism, and impulse control. The reality is that individuals tend to measure what they are comfortable with and ignore those areas they are not comfortable measuring. Given that at least four characteristics have been identified that reflect emotional competence, individuals and groups have the opportunity to measure their level of competence in handling their own and others' feelings.

> **Point to Ponder**
>
> The way to gain a good reputation is to endeavor to be what you desire to appear.
>
> —Socrates

First, individual leaders should consider developing a reputation assessment and management survey (**Exhibit 10-5**) to help them formally manage their reputations. Many forward-thinking leaders have done reputation management informally on the assumption that how others perceive them influences their ability to affect organizational operations. By creating a personal sensitivity process for gathering accurate feedback, a leader can learn about his or her effect on others and gain useful information for developing a reputation management plan. Both self-perceptions and the perceptions of others provide a helpful perspective on one's effectiveness.

Self-knowledge allows leaders to begin the journey toward the highest level of emotional competence. In many organizations, leaders use a 360-degree evaluation to gain additional information about their leadership abilities. Although feedback from superiors, peers, and subordinates is important, the source of the feedback must be identified to reinforce the importance of trust and honest communication. Further, such assessments need to contain items for measuring behaviors and characteristics that reflect emotional competence, including self-awareness, compassion, passionate optimism, self-regulation, and resilience.

To help measure the emotional competence of teams, specific items related to self-awareness, compassion, passionate optimism, self-regulation, and resilience should be

---

Exhibit 10-5 Reputation Assessment and Management Survey

1. Am I trustworthy?
2. To what extent do I trust others?
3. Do I practice what I preach?
4. Do I tell people who need to know what I am thinking and why I am acting in a particular way?
5. Am I dependable?
6. Do I listen nondefensively?
7. Am I able to find the grain of truth embedded in a criticism?
8. Am I visible and available when things are not going well?
9. Am I perceived as a hard worker?
10. Do I value the contributions of team members?

included in employee satisfaction and patient satisfaction surveys. The integration of individual and team information provides an overview of the emotional competence of the organization.

Conclusion

We live in complex times. To be successful, we need to think and feel simultaneously and to acknowledge our feelings and those of others. The goal of the quantum leader is to learn as much as possible from the past and gracefully and soundly move to more appropriate methods of leading the work of organizations. These methods include acting in ways that build relationships and are sensitive to people's behavior and emotions to increase their active engagement with their work.

The ability to manage feelings is a skill no leader can be without. The first step toward gaining this skill is to understand what is important not only to oneself but also to others in the organization. Ignoring the feelings and behaviors of others is a sure way to impede progress. Although progress is usually incremental at best, quantum leaders always have an eye on the future while holding onto their passionate optimism as a sacred gift.

Chapter Takeaways

1. Efforts to increase employee engagement with the work and people of health care are essential leadership activities.
2. The increasing science of relationships supports the work of effective relationships.
3. Emotional competence includes not only emotional intelligence but also the ability to practice and become effective emotionally.
4. Moving from a competent to an expert in emotional competence requires intense self-awareness, resilience, openness, and willingness to coach future healthcare workers.
5. Emotional incompetence is easy to recognize but difficult to change in spite of the incredible benefits of doing so.

Case Study 10-1

Managing a Team When the Stakes Are High

Mary is the director of case management and has six managers who report to her. In Mary's hospital and healthcare system, case management has a direct interface with the financial department, and Mary reports directly to the chief financial officer (CFO). She also interfaces with the payer side of the business, which includes contract negotiations with various state and federal payers, HMOs, insurers, self-insured employer groups, and the hospital's own self-insured/managed care group. In interfacing with these various groups over the years, Mary has improved her competencies in interprofessional collaboration and negotiation. It hasn't always been easy balancing the needs of the patients with the financial demands of the payer groups, but Mary has astute business skills that position her well in hard-nosed discussions related to cost, profits, quality, and more demand than the system can supply.

Case Study 10-1

The skills of the managers who report to Mary are quite varied. Two of the six have earned their master's degree in nursing and are relatively new to their roles and case management. One of the other direct reports has an MBA and came from the payer side of the business. The other three have been in their roles for a number of years, and although they perform well, they rarely show the initiative to "think outside the box" or advocate for patients when the patient need is not strictly within the prescribed guidelines. These three individuals work well together, but they do not seem to interface well with the other members of their team. When Mary meets with them individually, she hears stories of how they do not trust the other three, who have more education than they do but less experience in case management. In the meetings Mary observes these three and notices that they rarely speak up or contribute unless they are directly asked a question. Their body language and eye contact clearly indicate that they are disengaged from the rest of the group.

On the other hand, the three members of the team with more advanced education and less experience have many questions and need reassurance about their decisions with patients who need special considerations. Although they are eager to make patient-centered decisions, they are uncertain how far they can push the limits in negotiating with payers for additional coverage or equipment for patients. The manager with the MBA is very confident in his skills and is highly regarded by Mary's boss, the CFO. The manager speaks the "financial language" with ease, which impresses the CFO. The two of them often joke and laugh with one another, and clearly a strong relationship has formed. Mary not only observes her manager's very confident demeanor, she also recognizes that he demonstrates a very superior attitude when working with the others on her team. Because of his financial background, he often acts as the devil's advocate when innovative ideas are brought forward for discussion within the group. He has absolutely no tolerance for the three more senior individuals, whom he regards as being unprepared for their roles because of their lack of a master's degree and specifically their lack of financial knowledge. For the most part it seems as if he disregards much of what they say when they occasionally speak up in the team meetings. He often laughs when others are speaking or becomes engaged in other activities such as reading his emails or texts on his mobile phone.

One of the less experienced managers is very sensitive emotionally, and when pushed, it almost seems as if she is ready to cry in the team meetings. Of course, it doesn't take long for the MBA manager to take advantage of her vulnerability and relate to her in ways that increase her level of discomfort. He nitpicks every presentation she makes to the point that it drives her to tears, which appears to be very entertaining to him. Mary has assessed that the sensitive manager has the competencies and knowledge necessary to be successful in the role, but her inability to keep her emotions in control seems to detract from how others perceive her competencies. The CFO has frequently made comments to Mary about how this sensitive manager is the weakest member of the team, which requires Mary to advocate for her on several occasions. The CFO has put subtle pressure on Mary to terminate this individual because he perceives her to be very weak and incompetent. Mary has coached the manager frequently in their individual meetings about her need to develop a stronger "business face" and has tried to determine the underlying cause of the manager's lack of self-confidence because she has significant knowledge and understanding of case management. She has asked the manager to engage in some self-assessment and self-reflection related to her emotional intelligence and to work with the hospital's Employee Resource Center to develop ways to improve her self-confidence and to adapt her behavior in ways that would make her less vulnerable in group situations.

With new requirements and stricter guidelines in place with the hospital's designation as an accountable care organization, Mary's department is pressured to achieve better financial outcomes while also improving patient satisfaction levels. Her department is also held responsible for preventing 30-day readmissions that will penalize the hospital's reimbursement from Medicare. Mary realizes that her only hope for success is to improve the individual functioning of each of her direct reports and to improve the team's ability to work as a high-performing team. It is clear that every member of the team is at a different level of knowledge and experience in case management and at very different levels of emotional intelligence. When Mary assesses her team, she recognizes that she has one bully in the group who is overconfident about his own skills, completely unaware of how he comes across to others, but highly skilled in his financial understanding and case management. At the other end of the continuum, she has an individual who has the knowledge and skills of case management but who lacks self-confidence and is highly sensitive to any criticism or questioning of her knowledge base. The three less educated case managers have formed a subgroup that refuses to engage with the other members of the team because they do not trust the others. It appears that Mary only has one strong manager, who is less experienced in case management, but who demonstrates a high level of emotional intelligence, desire to learn the role, and willingness to engage with all members of the team including the bully. It's clear to Mary that the team is completely dysfunctional and that she needs to develop a strategy to help this group either develop as a highly functioning team or replace some of its members with new individuals who are more willing to work as a team to meet the organization's goals.

Questions

1. How do you feel about Mary's assessment of her direct reports' job competencies and emotional competencies and their ability to work together as a team?
2. If you were Mary, what steps would you take to improve the team's level of functioning?
3. How should Mary manage the bully on her team given that he has the most expert knowledge of the financial side of case management and is highly regarded by Mary's boss, the chief financial officer?
4. What should Mary do to help the manager who is emotionally sensitive and easily brought to tears in the team meetings?
5. If you were Mary, how would you manage the three more experienced individuals who have opted out of the team's membership and who are boycotting any participation in the team meetings?
6. Mary highly values the one manager who has job knowledge but less experience and who displays the highest level of emotional intelligence. How could Mary ensure her continuing success in her individual role and use her to facilitate growth for the team?
7. Using Goleman's (1998) conceptual model of the four elements of emotional intelligence, describe Mary's level of emotional intelligence.

Case Study 10-2

I See You and You See Me, But Do I See Me?

It is absolutely clear to Bob that his colleague Karen has no clue as to how she comes across to others. The two of them are directors in a large metropolitan hospital, and competition among all the directors for resources, recognition from the chief nursing officer (CNO), and the potential for promotion is fierce. Bob really likes Karen and would love to help her gain more insight into her interactions with others and how she perceives herself in these interactions. He has watched her time and again in the Directors Council interrupting others, using sarcastic language, and demonstrating counterproductive body language and facial expressions when others present their perspectives on controversial issues. In Bob's opinion, Karen is a very effective leader for her managers, but he wonders whether she exhibits some of the same behaviors in her meetings with her managers. It seems like Karen's managers are satisfied in their roles and have a good relationship with Karen, but Bob can't be sure. He really is uncertain whether he should speak to Karen about how she is being perceived in the Directors Council, or whether he should just let it go because it isn't really his issue. On the other hand, because of their friendship, Bob feels compelled to try to help Karen gain more self-awareness and read the faces of other individuals around the table for feedback on how they are reacting to her comments and how they perceive her.

The entire director team recently participated in a 360-degree analysis of their individual skills, competencies, and behaviors in their respective roles. Input from their peers, subordinates, and supervisors was received, analyzed, and developed into an overall analysis of their strengths and areas that need to be developed for them to be successful in their roles. Bob is not certain how Karen fared with the 360-degree analysis, but he suspects that some of their peers may have been critical of her behaviors. He wonders whether he should ask Karen to join him for coffee to discuss their respective assessments, but he is not sure if she would value his openness about the situation. Bob is clear that he is not willing to discuss the matter with their boss, the CNO, because he does not perceive her to be a good leader. Although it would be her role to coach Karen and encourage her to use the hospital's resources to improve her self-awareness, Bob fears that the CNO would use the information against Karen.

Bob has spent considerable time reviewing his own results from the 360-degree assessment and has reflected on the positive and negative feedback regarding his own skills and competencies. He was pleased that his subordinates perceived him as being a very authentic leader who is committed to the employees, engages them in decisions, and is physically present in both crisis and positive situations. His subordinates perceive him to be very open and easy to engage in conversation and indicated that he values them in their roles as nurses. Although he could not determine where the input came from among the executive team, he was highly rated for his resilience and nimbleness in managing crises and other difficult situations. He seemed to be highly regarded for his character and integrity among his colleagues as well as his subordinates and supervisors. An area that was noted for further development included the need to improve his ability to find a balance between his work and personal life because he was perceived to be a "workaholic," which had affected his personal life adversely. Those who knew Bob well realized that he had recently gone through a separation with his significant other. Other areas that Bob needed to improve were his ability to listen nondefensively when others were critical of his proposals and his ability to identify and develop some of his subordinates for a viable succession plan. Bob recognizes that he has a tendency to do everything himself instead of encouraging others to participate in activities to gain knowledge and experience to prepare them for future leadership roles. Although Bob was busy taking notes about how he could improve his own performance, he was constantly reminded of his dear friend Karen and his uncertainty about how he could most effectively help her to gain more self-awareness and improved emotional intelligence.

Questions

1. How do you think Bob can most effectively help Karen, or do you think that it is none of his business?
2. What level of emotional competence do you think that Bob demonstrates in his work with his subordinates, supervisors, and colleagues?
3. What level of emotional competence do you think that Karen demonstrates with her colleagues on the Directors Council and with her direct reports?
4. Based on the information provided in this case, how would you assess the CNO's level of emotional competence? Based on your assessment, should Bob realistically use her as a resource to coach Karen?
5. Develop a script that Bob might use to talk with Karen and give her feedback about her interactions with her colleagues on the Directors Council.

References

Allen, K. E. (2000). Leadership as an emergent property of individual and group interaction. *Inner Edge*, *3*(6), 20–21.

Collins, J. (2001). Level 5 leadership: The triumph of humility and fierce resolve. *Harvard Business Review*, *79*(1), 67–76.

Cummings, G. G., Take, K., Lee, S., Wong, C. A., Paananen, T., Micarini, S. P. M., & Chatterjee, G. E. (2018). Leadership styles and outcome patterns for the nursing workforce and work environment: A systematic review. *International Journal of Nursing Studies, 85,* 19–60.

Dattner, B., & Chamorro-Premuzic, T. (2016, September 15). A CEO's personality can undermine succession planning. *Harvard Business Review.* https://hbr.org/2016/09/a-ceos-personality-can-undermine-succession-planning

David, S. (2016). *Emotional agility.* Avery Publishing Group.

Dempsey, C., & Assi, M. J. (2020). Nursing engagement. In J. Cabral, T. H. Lee, & M. Wright (Eds.), *The engaged caregiver: How to build a performance-driven workforce to reduce burnout & transform care* (pp. 113–129). McGraw Hill.

Dimock, M. (2019). *Defining generations: Where millennials end and generation Z begins.* Pew Research Center. https://www.pewresearch.org/fact-tank/2019/01/17/where-millennials-end-and-generation-z-begins/

Dreyfus, G. (2011). Is mindfulness present-centred and non-judgmental? A discussion of the cognitive dimensions of mindfulness. *Contemporary Buddhism, 12,* 41–45.

Dreyfus, H. L., & Dreyfus, S. E. (1996). The relationship of theory and practice in the acquisition of skill. In P. Benner, C. Tanner, & C. A. Chesla (Eds.), *Expertise in nursing practice: Caring, clinical judgment, and ethics* (pp. 29–47). Springer.

Druskat, V. U., & Wolff, S. B. (2001). Building the emotional intelligence of groups. *Harvard Business Review*, *79*(3), 81–90.

Fray, B., & Sherman, R. O. (2017). Best practices for nurse leaders: Succession planning. *Professional Journal of Case Management, 22*(2), 88–94.

Fry, R. (2016). *Millennials projected to overtake baby boomers as America's largest generation.* Pew Research Center. http://www.pewresearch.org/fact-tank/2016/04/25/millennials-overtake-baby-boomers/

Gill, R. (2011). *Theory and practice of leadership* (2nd ed.). SAGE.

Goleman, D. (1998). *Working with emotional intelligence.* Bantam.

Good, D. J., Lyddy, C. J., Glomb, T. M., Bono, J. E., Brown, K.W., Duffy, M. K, Baer, R. A., Brewer, J. A., & Lazar, S. W. (2016). Contemplating mindfulness at work: An integrative review. *Journal of Management, 42*(1), 114–142.

Hardin, B. (2014, August 14). The four different personality types. *Constantly Learning.* https://blog.bretthard.in/the-four-different-personality-types-9366bfefde16

Jones, B. (2018). Creating a culture of promoting from within. *Dimensions of Critical Care Nursing, 38*(1), 50–53.

Levy, P. F. (2001). The Nut Island effect: When good teams go wrong. *Harvard Business Review, 79*(3), 51–59.

Maurits, E. E. M., de Veer, A. J. E., Groenewegen, P. P., & Fancke, A. L (2017). Home-care nursing staff in self-directed teams are more satisfied with their job and feel they have more autonomy over patient care: A nationwide survey. *Journal of Advanced Nursing, 73*(10), 2430–2440.

Millenson, M. L., & Macri, J. (2012). *Will the Affordable Care Act move patient-centeredness to center stage?* Robert Wood Johnson Foundation. https://www.rwjf.org/en/library/research/2012/03/will-the-affordable-care-act-move-patient-centeredness-to-center.html

Orsburn, J. D., Moran, J., Musselwhite, E., & Zenter, J. H. (1990). *Self-directed work teams.* Business One Irwin.

Pesut, D., & Thompson, S. (2018). Nursing leadership in academic nursing: The wisdom of development and the development of wisdom. *Journal of Professional Nursing, 34*(2), 122–127.

Russel, P. (1993). *The white hole in time: Our future evolution and the meaning of now.* Harper Collins.

Southwick, S. M., & Charney, D. S. (2018). *Resilience: The science of mastering life's greatest challenges.* Cambridge University Press.

Spano-Szekely, L., Quinn Griffin, M. T., Clavelle, J., & Fitzpatrick, J. J. (2016). Emotional intelligence and transformational leadership in nurse managers. *Journal of Nursing Administration, 46*(2), 101–108.

Uhl-Bien, M., & Arena, M. (2017). Complexity leadership: Enabling people and organizations for adaptability. *Organizational Dynamics, 46*(1), 9–20.

Vitello-Cicciu, J. M. (2002). Exploring emotional intelligence: Implications for nursing leaders. *Journal of Nursing Administration, 32*(4), 203–210.

Vito, R. (2019). Self-directed teams as an organizational change strategy to empower staff: A teaching/learning case study. *Human Service Organizations: Management, Leadership & Governance, 43*(2), 146–151.

Weick, K., & Sutcliffe, K. (2000, Summer). High reliability: The power of mindfulness. *Leader to Leader, 21*, 33–38.

Wright, M. (2020). Introduction. In J. Cabral, T. H. Lee, & M. Wright (Eds.), *The engaged caregiver: How to build a performance-driven workforce to reduce burnout & transform care* (pp. xvii–xxxi). McGraw Hill.

Young, S. (2016). *What is equanimity?* https://www.shinzen.org/store/what-is-equanimity

Young, S. (2018). *The science of enlightenment: How meditation works.* https://www.shinzen.org/resources

Suggested Readings

Barsh, J., Cranston, S., & Craske, R. A. (2008). Centered leadership: How talented women thrive. *McKinsey Quarterly.* http://www.mckinsey.com/insights/leading_in_the_21st_century/centered_leadership_how_talented_women_thrive

Bennis, W., & O'Toole, J. (2000). Don't hire the wrong CEO. *Harvard Business Review, 78*(5), 171–176.

Brousseau, K. R., Driver, M. J., Hourihan, G., & Larsson, R. (2006). The seasoned executive's decision-making style. *Harvard Business Review, 84*(2), 111–121.

Buchanan, L. (2004). The young and the restful. *Harvard Business Review, 82*(4), 25.

Contu, D. (2009). Why teams don't work. *Harvard Business Review, 87*(5), 99–105.

Davis, P. D., Hensley, S. L., Muzik, L., Comeau, O., Bell, L., Carroll, A. R., Sathre, R., Brumfield, V., Ledoux, L., Bhojani, M., & Douglas, M. K. (2012). Enhancing RN professional engagement and contribution: An innovative competency and clinical advancement program. *Nurse Leader, 10*(3), 34–39.

Duchscher, J. E. B. (2004). Multigenerational nurses in the workplace. *Journal of Nursing Administration, 34*(11), 493–501.

Dyer, W. (1976). *Your erroneous zones.* HarperCollins.

Forsyth, S., & Parish, M. (1999). The practical side of emotional intelligence. *Inner Edge, 1*(5), 9–11.

Grayson, M. A. (2005). Generation X, Y, Zzzz. *Journal of Nursing Administration, 35*(7/8), 326–327.

Hansen, M. T. (2009). When internal collaboration is bad for your company. *Harvard Business Review, 87*(4), 83–88.

Hansen, M. T., & von Oetinger, B. (2001). Introducing T-shaped managers: Knowledge management's next generation. *Harvard Business Review, 79*(3), 107–116.

Jones, C., & Gates, M. (2007). The costs and benefits of nurse turnover: A business case for nurse retention. *Online Journal of Issues in Nursing, 12*(3), 2.

Lancaster, L. C., & Stilman, D. (2002). *When generations collide: Who they are, why they clash, how to solve the generational puzzle at work.* HarperCollins.

Mecklenburg, G. A. (2001). Career performance: How are we doing? *Journal of Healthcare Management, 46*(1), 8–13.

Menkes, J. (2005). Hiring for smarts. *Harvard Business Review, 83*(11), 100–108.

Porter-O'Grady, T., & Wilson, C. K. (1998). *The health care team book.* Mosby.

Safian, R. (2012, November). Secrets of the flux leader. *Fast Company*, 96–107.

Sandberg, J. (2001). Understanding competence at work. *Harvard Business Review, 79*(3), 24–28.

Smola, K. W., & Sutton, C. D. (2002). Generational differences: Revisiting generational work values for the new millennium. *Journal of Organizational Behavior, 23*, 363–382.

Vestal, K. (2005). The ugly truth: Some managers are just inept. *Nurse Leader, 3*(4), 11, 16.

Vestal, K. (2012). Which matters: Employee satisfaction or employee engagement? *Nurse Leader, 10*(4), 10–11.

Wheeler, P. A. (2005, January/February). The importance of interpersonal skills. *Healthcare Executive*, 44–45.

Quiz Questions

Select the best answer for each of the following questions.

1. Emotional competence is based on specific principles. Which one of the following is *not* consistent with these principles?
    a. Holism
    b. Newtonian principles
    c. Theory Y behaviors
    d. Emergent leadership

2. Leaders have resisted the notion that emotional competence is an essential leadership characteristic. What is the most likely reason for this resistance?
    a. The difficulty of measuring and evaluating the impact of emotional competence
    b. The lack of theoretical support for the concept of emotional competence
    c. The cost of integrating emotionally competent behaviors into an organization
    d. The lack of employee support for the idea that emotional competence is important

3. What are the four attributes specific to emotional competence?
   a. Self-awareness, integrity, passionate optimism, and compassion
   b. Self-awareness, passionate optimism, character, and impulse control
   c. Self-awareness, compassion, passionate optimism, and emotional intelligence
   d. Self-awareness, compassion, passionate optimism, and character

4. Integrated leadership is a synergistic combination of technical, relational, and intentional skills. What does this combination lead to?
   a. Emotionally competent individuals and leaders
   b. Optimal resource use and positive patient outcomes
   c. Additional costs to the organization
   d. Improved employee satisfaction

5. Self-awareness—the understanding of one's behavior patterns and preferences—is a fundamental characteristic of emotional competence. Among other benefits, which of the following does it lead to?
   a. Passionate optimism and compassion
   b. Impulse control
   c. Openness to others and an appreciation of paradox
   d. Character and integrity

6. The emotional risks of leadership are ever present and cannot be ignored. Which of the following is a source of emotional risk faced by leaders?
   a. Lack of timely feedback
   b. Lack of an employment contract
   c. Unacceptable levels of employee dissatisfaction
   d. Sharing decision making with team members

7. Emergent leadership is one of the underpinnings of emotional competence. How does emergent leadership differ from the dyadic model of leadership?
   a. The organizational chart for emergent leadership is a matrix.
   b. Emergent leadership eliminates the need for a CEO.
   c. Emergent leadership is based on the principle that high levels of organizational performance depend on the presence of a strong leader who defines the work of the organization.
   d. Emergent leadership is based on the principle that high levels of organizational performance depend on the engagement of the members in the work of the organization.

8. Impulse control is one of the hallmarks of the emotionally competent individual. How does an individual develop this skill?
   a. The person reframes negative feelings when necessary to maximize the use of his or her energy.
   b. The person learns how to apologize sincerely.
   c. The person recognizes conflict as normative.
   d. The person works to eliminate emotions in the workplace.

9. Focused hiring is a way of selecting new employees that:
   a. eliminates the need for external search firms.
   b. decreases leadership turnover.
   c. focuses on the fit between the candidates and the organization.
   d. identifies the candidate with the greatest potential for integrating into the organization successfully.

10. Individual emotional competence develops gradually through the novice, advanced beginner, competence, and proficiency stages to finally arrive at the level of expertise. What can individuals who have reached the competence stage do?
    a. Think and feel simultaneously while considering the opinions of others.
    b. Project passionate optimism for the work of their profession.
    c. Control their impulses effectively.
    d. Coach others in the development of emotional competence.

11. Team emotional competence develops through the same five stages as individual emotional competence. What can a team that has reached emotional proficiency do?
    a. Understand the skills and emotions of all team members.
    b. Orient its work toward meeting the needs of the community.
    c. Orient its work toward meeting the goals and needs of the organization.
    d. Integrate local and national regulations into its work.

12. Patient–clinician engagement can positively impact patient outcomes because of the following. Which one is the *least* supportive?
    a. Evidence-based practice support.
    b. Establishment of trust.
    c. National legislation mandates.
    d. Clear expectations and processes are identified to determine the desired patient goals.

13. The state of equanimity provides opportunities to:
    a. suppress uncomfortable issues in the short term and deal with them at a more appropriate time.
    b. minimize stress and increase spiritual balance.
    c. conserve energy and increase capacity to consider new ideas.
    d. develop effective relationship skills.

14. Emotionally competent leaders view motivation as:
    a. an expectation belonging to each individual.
    b. something that a leader is accountable to do with each team member.
    c. a process that is developed by each individual when they are engaged in goals that are mutually important.
    d. dependent upon an individual developing effective engagements ambitions and interests.

15. Dissipative models of leadership are exemplified in all of the following, *except*:
    a. caregivers are required to develop and implement solutions to clinical challenges.
    b. clinical managers are required to address disruptions within 24 hours and provide solutions for caregivers.
    c. day-shift employees identify appropriate policies for night-shift employees.
    d. change can be identified and guided by any employee in the organization.

16. Effective relationship skills require time for development and multiple experiences to validate an effective or ineffective relationship. Which response reflects effective relationship skills?
    a. Emerging emotional competence
    b. Disregard for others as unique individuals
    c. Abrasive behavior to others; always apologizes
    d. Impulsively shares great ideas with the team

17. A leader's impact on others is important for the leader to understand for all of the following, *except:*
    a. role modeling may in fact be advancing negative behaviors.
    b. expectations for positive behaviors may be contradicted by leader behaviors.
    c. nonverbal emotional competence behaviors do not influence others.
    d. passionate optimism is often interpreted as aggressiveness.

18. Behaviors that reflect a lack of openness to new ideas include all of the following, *except*:
    a. ignoring certain individuals in group discussions.
    b. requesting any further comments from others at the end of a discussion.
    c. avoiding on-the-spot spontaneous discussions.
    d. scheduling time for regular discussions.

19. Which of the following is *not* a rational/evidence-driven reason for learning new information as a behavior of emotional competence?
    a. Effective decision making requires state-of-the-science information.
    b. Maintaining knowledge content similar to provider knowledge is necessary for equitable partnerships.
    c. Attending education sessions for certification provides focused content for learning.
    d. Review of recent literature often negates current practices.

20. Examples of compassionate leadership behaviors include all of the following, *except* that:
    a. sharing experiences of joy and sorrow strengthens team member engagement.
    b. feelings of deep sympathy are required to health care.
    c. sensitivity to other's feelings results in overfriendly relationships.
    d. subjectivity is often necessary to fully understand the dynamics of another's behavior.

21. Interviewing to determine an individual's level of emotional competence:
    a. includes assessment of resilience, impulse control, and self-awareness.
    b. includes assessment of openness, mindfulness, and passionate optimism.
    c. helps in determining the applicant's fit with the organization's culture.
    d. All of these are correct.
    e. None of these are correct.

22. Mindfulness research indicates the presence of:
    a. cognitive flexibility, clear-minded attention to new ideas, and sensitivity to the environment.
    b. attentiveness to new information and the nonverbal displays of being present.
    c. cognitive flexibility, presence, and focus during large meetings.
    d. openness to the feelings and interactions of all members of the healthcare team.

23. Inappropriate nonverbal behaviors are most accurately described as:
    a. being more powerful than verbal behaviors in making an impact.
    b. inferring inaccurate realities or intentions of the one sending the nonverbal signal.
    c. reinforcing positive activities so others know what behaviors are acceptable.
    d. being most powerful when the individual has high levels of self-awareness and compassion.

24. Resilience is best described as:
    a. the capacity to cope with unanticipated dangers and bounce back to a state of equanimity.
    b. the ability to fend off negative influences and react assertively to prevent further challenges.
    c. the ability to manage personal disappointments at work.
    d. an attribute of emotional competence that does not include improvisation.

25. Feedback from leaders is essential and contributes to:
    a. recognition of an individual's accomplishments and areas for improvement.
    b. decreased confidence in decision making when mistakes are made.
    c. the leader's reputation for fairness within the organization and community.
    d. employment security with benefits for team members.

CHAPTER ELEVEN

Toxic Organizations and People: The Leader as Transformer

> In a controversy the instant we feel anger we have already ceased striving for the truth, and have begun striving for ourselves.
> —*Buddha*[1]

Chapter Objectives

At the completion of this chapter, the reader will be able to:

- Identify the common sources of toxicity and dysfunction in healthcare organizations.
- Analyze long-standing leadership behaviors that negatively affect organizations.
- Describe the negative impact of toxic organizational practices on employee performance.
- Explore the nature of career entrenchment and career adaptability as polar opposites and their potential to coach employees in organization engagement.
- Critique the 10 principles for minimizing organizational toxicity.

Health care is a complex industry with so many interacting parts that it is difficult to predict how the system will behave and respond to change. The complexity of the industry is also reflected in the organizations that comprise the industry. Many organizations thrive in the complexity because they have achieved focus, whereas others struggle because they have not addressed internal complexity of values alignment, decision making, and effectiveness and health of teams—all functions of a quantum leader. Because survival is dependent on an organization's ability to change, leaders find themselves increasingly challenged by dysfunctional and toxic people and situations who perhaps have done well in the old system but have not adopted the skills and abilities to function in the emerging environment. This can result in dysfunctional behaviors of various degrees that can affect organizational effectiveness in a range of ways.

---

[1] Lundin, W., & Lundin, K. (1993). *The healing manager: How to build quality relationships and productive cultures at work.* Berrett-Koehler.

Chapter Eleven Toxic Organizations and People: The Leader as Transformer

This chapter discusses dysfunctional behaviors that typically impair healthcare organizations, including antisocial behaviors, toxic mentoring, and neurotic and self-defeating behaviors. It also discusses organizational practices that are prone to dysfunction and organizational characteristics that reinforce dysfunction. To mitigate the negative impact of dysfunctional behaviors, the chapter presents 10 principles designed to minimize organizational toxicity. These principles focus on reversing the dysfunctional behaviors of leaders and guiding them toward more appropriate practices that can transform dysfunction into health. Future leaders will move away from directive mechanisms to lead through influence, refine ways to remain close to their teams, and establish social processes that provide direction, alignment, and commitment (Center for Creative Leadership, 2018). These mechanisms will expose dysfunction of individuals, and the quantum leader must be ready to address any element of the organizational culture that does not support effectiveness.

Increasingly, health professionals ask themselves the following questions: If healing is my profession and contribution to society, am I as healthy as I would like to be? Why are so many of my colleagues feeling the impact of moral distress and burnout? Shortages of available workers, patient and system complexity, and the uncertainty of a financing system that demands productivity all continue to fuel the disfranchisement of health professionals. Employees are reluctant to trust one another and must be coaxed to interact. Clinicians frequently are conflicted over whether to give care or withhold it. Many believe the care that is given is substandard, incomplete, and sometimes even harmful. The environment these problems create tends to suppress the humanitarian purpose most entered the caring professions to fulfill and inadvertently kills cooperation, creativity, and professional joy. Much is at stake, with as many as 43% of clinicians showing signs of emotional exhaustion, depression, and burnout (Brigham et al., 2018). An important national journey to learn about and address clinician well-being and resilience is underway, and local activities using this emerging evidence are essential to improving the current state of the health of our healers. The National Academies, in particular, have taken action to address clinician well-being and resilience (https://nam.edu/initiatives/clinician-resilience-and-well-being/).

The complaints of colleagues, along with the newspaper headlines, might suggest that healthcare organizations are more toxic and in greater distress than are many of the patients receiving healthcare services. Far too many health professionals, particularly leaders and point-of-service workers, are missing the energy and collaborative spirit that mirror health. Their psyches have been assaulted too severely and for too long by neurotic leadership styles, dysfunctional group processes, inappropriate superior–subordinate bonding, and abandonment. These unfortunate toxicogenic practices need to be swiftly reversed because they are destroying the vitality of healthcare organizations and professions.

Some may be tempted to attribute the distress of healthcare workers solely to changes in reimbursement policy and to look for the solution in a more palatable financing structure. The reality, however, is that the toxicity of healthcare organizations is not just a matter of reimbursement. Indeed, the silver lining of the prospective payment and managed care models may be that they can help expose the subtle yet pervasive toxins currently harming the healthcare system.

Healthcare organizations, for example, have been plagued by a delivery model in which clinicians spend much of their time performing disempowering activities to meet regulatory requirements, and while they are not resistant to change, they are challenged to know the appropriate change to make. These factors, along with the increasing challenge of financing care and a philosophy of things first and people second, cause organizational toxicity and nullify the essential values of healing and restoration of health. The job of organizational leaders is to identify the toxic behaviors and develop strategies to minimize their effects. Rather than attempting to determine who the guilty parties are—individuals or organizations (or both)—the challenge is to move forward and create the kind of culture that will lead to organizational health.

Some of the main differences between toxic and healthy organizations relate to issues of control, conflict, and adaptability. For example, an organization in which the level of toxicity is high can be characterized in this way:

- The leaders' approach to leadership is directive, and the employees are widely subject to forces outside their control because they have lost their critical problem-solving skills and ability to think.
- Because of their lack of control, the employees are more susceptible to illness and isolation.
- The leaders and employees try to decrease or suppress conflict rather than accept it as normal and useful when channeled toward innovation or team cohesiveness.
- The employees tend to become stuck and lose their ability to change.

> ### Group Discussion
>
> At the next team meeting, ask employees to identify at least two toxic behaviors in the organization they believe should be changed. Consider the following questions: Can you clearly and objectively define the problem? If you were in charge, how would you change behaviors to make them less toxic? What indicators would you use to measure the change in behaviors?

In contrast, a healthy organization has the following characteristics:

- Leaders foster the interdependency of teams.
- The organization depends on group process and decision making where decisions are made at the appropriate level in the organization to accomplish its work.
- The employees are engaged rather than stressed.
- The leaders and employees recognize conflict as normal and treat instances of conflict as opportunities for gaining information and planning and implementing improvements.
- Individuals and groups become facile at adapting to changing circumstances.

Cultures Depend on Healthy Individuals to Help Patients Heal

Healing and hope are the responsibilities of the clinicians who practice in healthcare organizations, and organizations are responsible for living their values, which often include respect, justice, ethical practice, compassion, and inclusivity. Paradoxically, the cultures of healthcare organizations have not always created or sustained the well-being of these clinicians—opposite to their primary mission. Healthcare executives must move away from the leadership styles that made them successful in the hierarchical healthcare systems of the past to a new approach that creates a context for positive, nontoxic cultures to exist in today's complex organizations. This evolution of leadership style recognizes the substantial impact of informal networks, external pressures, and human behavior on an organization (Uhl-Bien et al., 2008).

Any culture in which the culture itself has a negative impact on individuals' health is a toxic culture. Toxicity can come from the people, the work itself, the behavioral norms that have developed, or any combination of these environmental factors. Signs of a toxic system include evidence of overwork leading to a breakdown of team communication; hyper competitiveness; and pressure to cover, hide, or downplay aspects of an individual's identity to fit into a work culture (McKee, 2019). In these situations, teams stop collaborating. When individuals stop speaking up, blame each other, and lose trust in each other and their leader, the impact on patient safety and the well-being of the team can be severe. Marginalized safety occurs when teams have a low level of professional ownership over their work.

How Does Toxicity Develop?

Health care's complexity surfaces in today's cultures and work environments. It would seem basic to view the work of healthcare teams as simply completing the tasks of patient care; however, the realities of shorter patient throughput, staff turnover, and pressure to achieve financial targets for unit operations and patient volume all require dynamic interactions within teams and can fuel dysfunction. The introduction of the electronic medical record (EMR) shifted patient care from a team orientation to more of an individual practitioner activity. As a result, opportunities for social interaction among team members declined. Consider when paper records were the norm—clinicians would share the record and enter their information about a patient on a single document. It was common, in that era, to hear team members negotiating with each other to use the chart! Individuals had a lot of practice managing internal team dynamics. With the EMR, this human interaction has disappeared because each clinician works independently. When human interaction doesn't occur in the course of daily work, leaders must create structures for interaction that strengthen the team. When today's leaders fail to see the signs of community, their teams become vulnerable to toxicity. Complexity factors potentially cause toxicity when formal and informal leaders are not aware or capable of intervening to eliminate or, at the least, minimize the impact of environmental stress and create opportunities to re-emphasize that patient safety depends on relationships. When relationships fail, individuals don't speak up, lose trust in each other, and favor individual agendas over team effectiveness.

Complexity science offers a way to understand how leaders of complex systems can identify and work to prevent team toxicity (Weberg & Fuller, 2019). The way individuals communicate, interact, and behave in organizations can differentiate a highly performing team from one that is toxic. Leaders of complex systems recognize the impact of the interaction and behaviors within their teams aggravated by a healthcare system full of risk and uncertainty on an organization. These same leaders intentionally interact to identify patterns that signal toxicity, and intervene with purpose.

How Leaders Shape Culture

Given the right conditions, most clinicians will do excellent work, which is why cultural health is so important. Some of the conditions that indicate cultural health include regular communication, daily interactions, recognition of excellence, encouragement of personal growth, and information availability. Leaders in these cultures are comfortable with vulnerability and often engage their teams in solving problems. Being involved in crafting solutions to common problems serves as positive attractors for the team. When these conditions are absent or intentionally withheld, there is a void that creates distraction leaving the team vulnerable to toxicity.

Every team resembles a magnetic ball rolling toward a destination. In a positive culture, the team rolls past distractors on the right or left, resisting the urge to be pulled off course. Sometimes, less significant factors can force the team from its trajectory slightly but the team's momentum pulls them back to its initial path. However, larger distractions can disrupt the team, causing the ball to veer off course completely—either temporarily or permanently (Weberg & Fuller, 2019). Understanding the culture, the presence and power of positive and negative attractors, and the impact of communication on a team can help leaders be intentional about their daily team interactions (**Table 11-1**).

TABLE 11-1 Influencing Attractors as a Nurse Leader

Attractor (Stressor)	Factors That Strengthen Toxic Attractor (Team Begins to Deviate)	Factors That Weaken Toxic Attractor (Team Stays on Trajectory)
Reorganization or turnover	Silence or avoidance Generic or vague announcements No input from team on how to adapt to change	Transparent information Frequent "micro" updates Illustrate the impact of new work Engage team in change planning and decision-making process
Significant workload increase	"Doing more with less" Wishing for more time Ambiguity in length or scope of increase Leader not present in the work	Reallocation of resources Team-based solutions Describing time bounds of temporary increases Leader helps team in completing the work
Urgent high-stakes issues (legal, business, safety, human resources)	Secrecy and opacity of information Not addressing cause Exaggerating urgency or impact Blaming employees for a leadership failure Crisis is the norm; the team never moves past immediate needs to long-term goals	Focused resources Review of system impacts Debriefing ways to avoid in future Transparency in impact Clear responsibilities and roles to address issue

Reproduced with permission from Weberg, D., & Fuller, R. (2019). Toxic leadership: Three lessons from complexity science to identify and stop toxic teams. *Nurse Leader, 17*(1), 22–26. Copyright Elsevier.

Leadership Polarity Dominates

Individuals watch their leaders to see how the leader responds to change and how the leader communicates information to the team to engage them in decisions. Relationships within the team, as well as those between the leader and the individual team members, are essential to helping the leader identify the negative attractors at play in the team's daily lives. When the leader knows the members on an individual basis and has familiarity with their strengths, purpose, and goals, the leader can unite the team behind shared purpose and goals.

In addition to providing intentional leadership tailored to team members' individual motivation, executives themselves can serve as attractors—either positively or negatively. A positive leader attractor brings and keeps the team on course by serving as a consistently accurate and reliable source of information. Leaders who are negative attractors oversee teams whose confusion about priorities leads it off course. In addition, negative attractor leaders often create unhealthy rivalries, which can yield unproductive conflicts within the team (Carucci, 2018).

Millennial Nurses Crave Connection

Emerging evidence validates the importance of leaders' understanding millennial nurses' needs, because this demographic group makes up the largest portion of the nursing population. Millennial nurses themselves have told us they need to belong to a team and make connections with their patients to thrive professionally (Mahoney, 2016; Thew, 2019). Without those two conditions of employment, millennial nurses' job performance suffers. A leader who provides opportunity for team-based belonging and a strong connection to patients strengthens the engagement and fulfillment of this dominant demographic group of nurses.

Millennial nurses often view their professional contribution to patient care as the completion of a series of tasks—even though they yearn to connect with patients (Thew, 2019). Seeing the profession solely from a task perspective makes them feel emotionally empty. In this situation, millennial nurses not only fail to realize their valuable contribution to patient care, but they note that they fail to feel like a nurse. Leaders who recognize the linkage between practice and emotion can incorporate mechanisms for engagement in discussions about patients and improvement in care processes to encourage the patient connections millennial nurses value.

The primary mission of health care is to facilitate healing—of patients and of the healthcare professionals caring for them. In highly functioning organizations, the healing of patients can also heal clinicians. Stories that reflect this concept are ones where a clinician facilitated a patient's wishes for a peaceful death, or interpreted lab results that told a patient that he would recover from a catastrophic accident, or when a clinician at a bedside, thinking all was lost, felt a frail hand touching her arm. Reclaiming healing as a core aim requires recognizing the key vehicles to healing that inhibit toxic conditions: proximity, mutuality, resilience, and kindness (Awdish & Berry, 2019). Recognizing the threats to healing and prioritizing these four intersecting principles can transform an organization.

- *Proximity*: Incorporate the team into decision making to ensure that patient empathy is present.
- *Mutuality*: Share power, because no one has all the answers or owns all the facts.
- *Resilience*: Allow space for clinician resilience to support patient resilience.
- *Kindness*: Foster a culture of trust.

Individuals in organizations where there is a culture of trust are more productive, have more energy, collaborate better with their colleagues, and stay with the organization longer (Zak, 2017). These desirable results stem from individuals' substantial engagement with the organization and its mission. Engagement can be seen in strong connection with work and colleagues, the feeling of value that comes from being recognized as a real catalyst to the organization's advancement, and the self-worth associated with acquiring new knowledge. Doing purposeful work with a trusted team creates an ongoing sense of joy (Zak, 2017). Joy and trust both serve as important counterbalances to toxicity. The urgent need to eliminate toxicity correlates to the growing complexity of health care. Leaders must set out to lead in such a way as to be the organizational source of success and cultural well-being.

Toxicity in an organization can affect employees both physically and emotionally. Indeed, the field of psychoneuroimmunology has documented links between feeling states and physiological responses. The emotions associated with caring—namely, hope, love, and joy—have been identified as ingredients in the remission of disease, whereas loss of hope or love and the failure to adequately cope with stress have been identified as factors in both the onset and exacerbation of the symptoms of major illness (Moraes et al., 2018). In other words, the lack of caring or nurturing may be a primary causative factor in disease. Surely, there is a relationship between the lack of organizational caring and nurturing and the level of organizational toxicity. There are never adequate resources on a dysfunctional team.

> ## Group Discussion
>
> In organizations, there is a healthy middle ground between an overabundance and a deficiency of the appropriate type of support—resources or relationships. From this perspective, consider whether there is a shortage of healthcare workers in your organization. Ask team members the following questions: Is there an excess of employees who are less-than-average performers? Is there a shortage of employees with appropriate skills (clinical and relational) to meet the contemporary needs of the organization? What are the missing skills? Develop a plan that focuses on improving the skills and increasing the sense of community among employees. What indicators of organizational performance will be used to measure progress?

Organizational toxicity is often unnoticed at the onset but slowly emerges as cynicism, declining morale, loss of creativity and engagement, and lower productivity. If its emotional component is not addressed, it can leave a toxic residue, preventing a complete return of function. The broken spirit is difficult to heal; that is, the unresolved or buried anger and resentment remain and thwart organizational efforts.

Often, the organizational response to toxicity mirrors the primitive response of granuloma formation. In the case of granuloma formation, the body does not deal with the underlying injury but instead walls it off with a fibrous deposit of cells. The injury merely appears to be mended, and no additional healing occurs. So, too, can an organization seal off a dysfunctional component while believing that it is taking proper corrective action. Unfortunately, this

> **Key Point**
>
> If you are not the master of your spirit and permit yourself to be demeaned, you are going to get sick unless something changes.
>
> Lundin, W., & Lundin, K. (1993). *The healing manager: How to build quality relationships and productive cultures at work.* Berrett-Koehler.
>
> As clinicians, advocacy for practice models that celebrate and respect our contributions and nurture our physical, emotional, and spiritual well-being are essential to reduce caregiver suffering.
>
> Rushton, C. H. (2018). *Moral resilience: Transforming moral suffering in healthcare.* Oxford University Press.

response prevents the organization from developing strategies for avoiding similar types of dysfunction in the future and also impedes work processes that should involve the dysfunctional component. The unresolved organizational conflict, like a granuloma, persists and affects every related decision in the future.

Toxic Behaviors

When an organization provides services in ways that subtly work against its values and stated goals, it violates its fundamental covenant with its employees and the community. At the same time, the organization's leaders and other members reinforce negative beliefs about the organization and further entrench the dysfunctional behaviors. The resulting toxic interactions become destructive to effective relationships.

Toxic or hostile work environments are recognizable not just by the presence of screaming, flaring tempers, and abusive language but also by the less noticeable but often more damaging quiet demoralization that occurs. Unilateral decision making, the ignoring of requests, and the avoidance of unpleasant issues cause substantial toxicity, specifically, employee discontent. Furthermore, although chronically angry individuals and controlling supervisors regularly reinforce the toxicity, careless insensitivity to the impact of one's actions on others is one of the main causes. The organizational culture, which of course has an enormous impact on decision making, leadership style, strategy formation, and organizational change, can be influenced in subtle and complex ways by invisible long-standing psychological forces hidden from the individuals who experience them. These covert forces all too often produce organizational outcomes that appear to be extremely irrational and dysfunctional.

It is the complex, long-standing interdependencies between stakeholders that create both healthy behaviors and toxic behaviors that are difficult to untangle and remedy. Toxic behaviors within an organization seldom are the result of one individual process gone awry, but rather are the culmination of many dysfunctions that form a syndrome of organizational pathology. Similar patterns of strategic and structural defects can be as dramatic and bold as they are toxic. If one top executive uses a neurotic leadership style, others adopt similar behaviors. The result is a poorly functioning self-defeating organization.

This is not to deny that some mildly dysfunctional traits and behaviors can occur in moderation without causing significant difficulties. Most individuals exhibit low levels of shyness and depression and have a few irrational fears and suspicions. Major problems occur when these dysfunctional traits and behaviors dominate relationships between individuals.

The following discussion presents 10 sources of organizational toxicity to help readers gain an understanding of its dynamics and formulate strategies to decrease it (**Exhibit 11-1**). Note that the distinction between the toxic behaviors of individuals and organizational toxicity is artificial because the work of individuals acting as a team is in fact the work of the organization.

Toxic Behaviors

Exhibit 11-1 Ten Sources of Organizational Toxicity

1. Vertical authority structure
2. Inequitable reward and recognition practices
3. Abuse of power
4. Lack of respect for the workforce
5. Failure to manage unmotivated employees
6. Tolerance of antisocial behavior and incivility
7. Toxic mentoring
8. Inconsistency and dishonesty
9. Imbalance between work and personal life
10. Advocacy gone awry

Vertical Authority Structure

The structure of an organization reflects the levels of authority and decision making and can often be a source of organization toxicity. Structures that are flat provide employees easier access to leaders and allow for more autonomy in decision making. Organizations with a vertical authority structure frequently operate with few decision makers and multiple layers of authority, reducing the autonomy and involvement of individuals closest to the work of the organizations. Such a vertical structure restricts communication because directives must be handed down from the chief executive level to the staff through multiple layers of middle managers, inhibiting two-way dialogue about the decisions. In the complex healthcare environment, it is impossible for decision making to rest with only a few individuals; rather, a decision-making structure is needed that facilitates accountability, deference to expertise, healthy dialogue, ownership, and creativity.

Vertical organizations establish clear localization of decision making at fewer and higher levels. Leaders often become obsessively vigilant because of their belief that subordinates and competitors cannot be trusted to act without the leader's intervention. Their paranoia also leads to the centralization of power and to excessive control over individuals and decision making, which at times can contribute to workplace bullying. These organizations suffer from too much leadership control, too many rigid procedures, too much documentation, and too much attention paid to monitoring employee activities, including productivity. Leaders in a

Group Discussion

The authority and decision-making structures in an organization can be paralyzing to progress and timely integration of evidence into practice. Describe the approval processes and number of individuals involved and the timeline for approval for the last four policies that affected your work. Once this information is identified, develop a strategy to eliminate non-value-added steps and propose a new process for the organization. What are the obstacles to eliminating all clinical policies and holding each licensed clinician accountable for state-of-the-art practice within the organization?

vertical organization typically fear change and steadfastly defend ritualistic behaviors out of a desire for security. In addition, employees in an organization where decision making rests with only a few individuals results in the reluctance of employees to think on their own because they are accustomed to a leader doing that for them.

The corporate culture in a traditional vertical organization typically suppresses individual creativity. Managed like a monarchy, this type of organization infantilizes its employees by expecting near-blind obedience. The rare exceptions tend to be organizations that have adopted a shared leadership model as a needed replacement for the traditional command-and-control model.

Vertical organizations recognize that creative people are expressive people but do not allow employees to be expressive at work. Creativity threatens the status quo, and it is in maintaining the status quo that vertical leaders feel most secure. Furthermore, as a result of the suppression of creativity and independent thought at work, employees develop a desire to be managed, nourished, and protected by a leader, and their misplaced awe for the leader can prevent the organization from achieving the psychological safety needed to benefit from the opinions and thinking of the workforce. Psychological safety is broadly defined as a climate in which people are comfortable expressing and being themselves and is a key element of safety culture (Edmondson, 2019).

The separation of individuals into departments and divisions rather than functional units further reinforces power differentials. In this model, the core processes are specific to each department and are focused more on meeting departmental needs than on recognizing that customers cross multiple departments and see their care as horizontal instead of vertical. Vertical leadership in the delivery of horizontal care rarely meets customer needs. In identifying key steps toward higher-value empathic health care, Lee (2016) identifies that teams are the real units of healthcare delivery and must use the social network to enhance their effectiveness.

When considering what it takes to thrive in a complex, uncertain world, stability of the work environment is critical. Constantly shifting configurations of departments and individuals instead of formal, clearly bounded teams shakes the foundation of the vertical organization. The frequent changes in team size and membership hinder the development of expert team behaviors. Also, the threat of losing organizational positions because of anticipated mergers and acquisitions has in some cases caused senior leaders to move in opposite directions, harbor personal agendas, and be minimally compatible with each other. As for the employees of a vertical organization, when greater productivity is expected at the same time that resources are decreased, they unsurprisingly become angry and disillusioned. The survivors of layoffs are frequently less productive and develop poor job attitudes. Yet the essential vertical structure is often retained. Power is retained at the top and distributed through departmental leaders, breeding toxicity. The psychological safety that is essential to establish a culture where individuals are comfortable expressing and being themselves is a distant dream.

Inequitable Reward and Recognition Practices

Another toxin found in most organizations is inequitable pay. It is important to note that few people are ever satisfied with their level of compensation. Nonetheless, most individuals recognize that resources are limited and are only seeking equitable compensation. Compensation practices become toxic when rewards and recognition are inequitable or inconsistent.

The process of evaluating an employee and rewarding them for performance can be challenged by organizational limitations on annual compensation packages that must also respond to market adjustments for categories of employees, including nursing. These annual adjustments result in equal but sometimes minimal increases for all employees. Employees who do the requisite work, attend only mandatory continuing education programs, and miss work occasionally (although staying within the normal range) are awarded the same increase as are employees who receive numerous thank-you letters from patients, attend external continuing education programs, have perfect attendance, and participate on committees.

The challenge of using limited available dollars to pay employees appropriately for their different levels of effort is rarely taken up by leaders. Rather than awarding 0% to mediocre employees and 10% to exemplary employees, leaders use the across-the-board approach so that everyone gets something. Seldom are other nonfinancial rewards, such as preferred scheduling, used as alternatives for rewarding excellent performers. Nonfinancial recognition is an important consideration, and it must be equitable as well. Subjectivity in selection of individuals to receive public recognition or attend national conferences could also be a source of jealousy and erode team cohesion and should be replaced with objective, transparent processes for selection.

Compensation continues to be highly subjective, particularly at the senior level. Compensation for leaders is based more on market standards and on their performance as team members. Consequently, compensation practices can cause mistrust, particularly when the senior executive's compensation is disproportionately greater than that of the entry-level employee.

Group Discussion

Compressed pay ranges and limited dollars for reward and recognition continue to challenge leaders in their efforts to recognize staff. In collaboration with members of your team, revise the current reward and recognition system or create an entirely new one. Make sure the system you design does the following:

- Separates the compensation process from the performance evaluation process
- Awards nothing to employees who have a mediocre performance rating
- Includes nonmonetary rewards, such as preferred scheduling, weekend or holiday preferences, and inclusion in decision making
- Uses objective measures of performance to determine the effect of nonmonetary programs on employee satisfaction and turnover and on patient outcomes

Abuse of Power

The third toxin is abuse of power. Because the highest turnover occurs at the middle-management level, leaders are often in search of qualified candidates to fill positions at this level, often selecting expert nurses with little or no leadership experience. In such cases, intentional leader development must occur because, left unmonitored, the leader's performance could negatively impact the team and kill the spirit of this aspiring new leader. An authoritative leadership style is sometimes the default style of a new leader and can be a source of workplace bullying. In short, the wrong or inexperienced person has been promoted to a leadership position, and then, with title and power in hand, manages people instead of leading them. Nearly every organization faces the challenges of quickly finding candidates with adequate experience to fill leadership positions and then guiding them to become effective.

Indeed, the toxicity mainly results not from the appointment of inexperienced managers, but from the failure to intervene early in the process of assisting appointees to develop the skills needed for their positions.

When a new manager belittles staff members in front of patients or other staff members, communicates by memo rather than face to face, changes policies without input from others, and is rude and thoughtless, the staff members soon take on similar behaviors with each other. Some individual staff members may attempt to communicate the issues to the manager and the manager's supervisor, but any dialogue among the staff, the new manager, and the supervisor typically results in assigning blame—of the new manager by the staff and of the staff by the new manager—because effective communication is not a core competency in vertical organizations. Eventually, the staff members resign or transfer to other areas without making clear that their reason for changing employment was the lack of collegiality and of a respectful and caring work environment. The senior managers generally assume the staff members were seeking better salaries, better schedules, shorter commutes to work, or desire to return to school, and fail to recognize the true reason, allowing the toxicity to continue and intensify.

Mandatory Overtime

Another example of abuse of power is mandatory overtime. Although health care by its very nature involves the delivery of vital services that cannot be turned off and on in line with the availability of staff, mandatory overtime in a predominantly female profession raises significant issues, such as the difficulty of meeting both professional and family responsibilities. Nurses often feel exhausted and discouraged when they leave work, powerless to effect changes to ensure safe patient care, and overburdened by the overtime they are expected to put in. Like the shoemaker's children who had no shoes, healthcare workers have no health—or are being slowly stripped of the healthy balance between work and personal life they once had.

Intolerance Toward Diversity and Inclusion

Because communication technology and supersonic travel have made the world smaller, the diverse peoples of the world are able to share ideas and learn new approaches to a multiplicity of tasks. Yet healthcare organizations have commonly failed to integrate the multiple cultures of their staff members and patients (e.g., by not giving due consideration to their dietary habits and religious beliefs) and include them in decision making and dialogue so that all contributions are valued. Many have also been reluctant to actively seek diverse perspectives by including representatives from all gender and age groups in essential work teams. Instead, stereotypical executives continue to develop strategic, human resource, and budgetary plans. Thus, despite educational programs designed to minimize discriminatory practices, more proactive efforts to increase the diversity and inclusion of the entire workforce are needed. This is especially important given that some communities served by the predominantly white healthcare workforce are on average more than 30% nonwhite.

Lack of Respect for the Workforce

Leaders of vertically operated healthcare organizations have been known to view staff members as expendable—as the cost of doing business. They have been known to objectify their employees and give them minimal consideration. There are even examples of how the business of health care depends on exploiting doctors and nurses who, because of their professional beliefs and purpose, will most always do the right thing for their patients even at a high personal cost (Ofri, 2019). The good news is that many employee-focused organizations address this head on; however, in toxic organizations, the exploitation continues. In toxic organizations, employees often feel powerless and completely dependent. Employees who do not like the organization will become disengaged and seek an exit strategy.

Lack of respect takes many forms, from obvious rudeness to subtle discourtesy. It can include not responding to employee requests, dismissing new ideas with a smile, refusing to discuss issues that are important to employees, and exhibiting a general lack of manners, such as failing to say "thank you." It can also take the form of incivility, which is also referred to as bullying, lateral or horizontal violence, and harassment. Incivility not only harms the nurse but also will likely harm patients (Makic, 2018).

To be sure, the price of incivility is high. According to Porath and Pearson (2013), incivility hurts both morale and the bottom line. Data specific to decreased work effort, decreased time spent at work, decreased quality of work, lost time avoiding the offender, and taking frustration out on others have been quantified and examined from numerous perspectives.

Failure to Manage Unmotivated Employees

The fifth toxin is one that haunts even the best leaders. Finding the time and energy to work with unmotivated career employees can be overwhelming. The difficulty is not in recognizing suboptimal performance but in continuing to work with these employees despite minimal success at guiding them to do better. The lifetime career syndrome—lackluster performance by career employees unexcited or burnt out by their jobs—is one of the impediments to efficiency that leaders are required to deal with regularly.

New expectations regarding employment have emerged during the last 20 years. Organizations are not prepared to enter into lifelong partnerships with individuals. No longer can an individual expect a durable commitment as a condition of employment. The trend is for the terms of employment to be congruent with the needs and financial resources of the hiring organization. When these needs or resources change, the employee's roles and responsibilities are likely to change as well. Rather than firing these employees, managers often continue to invest in them in the hope that the support given to them will reverse their attitudes.

Some organizations will recognize the opportunities, whereas toxic organizations will resort to old ways to manage the workforce. Many organizations are in fact burdened with workers who want to leave but, for a variety of reasons, stay nonetheless. Department managers and directors often whisper among themselves, cursing the organization's flaws, but stay on because they are afraid to leave or because the pay, if little else, is excellent. Furthermore, if they left, they would have to sacrifice imminent salary increases, paid holidays and vacations, and retirement benefits. Yet they do not identify with or feel emotionally attached to their current position, and they do nothing about changing the situation.

Research by Carson and Carson (1997) confirmed that career entrenchment and career entrapment are actual phenomena of organizational life. Career entrenchment is the tendency to stay in a vocation because of the investment already made, psychological preservation, and a perception of few career opportunities. Entrenched or entrapped employees have an established way of life, usually have good salaries, and know the challenges of the workplace. Leaving their jobs would create uncertainty as well as loss of identity and loss of income. Career entrenchment perpetuates itself because when an employee becomes reconciled to staying in a career despite unhappiness with it, the employee is likely to invest further in the career, becoming more entrenched.

Exhibit 11-2 Career Entrapment Behaviors

Exit: An active strategy in which an individual leaves a career to change fields, retire, or withdraw from the labor force.

Voice: An active strategy in which an individual constructively tries to improve conditions through verbalization of concerns.

Loyalty: A passive strategy in which an individual passively but optimistically waits for conditions to improve.

Neglect: A passive strategy in which an individual allows conditions to deteriorate through reduced interest and effort, tardiness or absenteeism, increased errors, and ineffective use of working time.

Reproduced from Carson, K. D., & Carson, P. P. (1997). Career entrenchment: A quiet march toward occupational death. *Academy of Management Executives, 11*(2), 62–76.

Individuals who are dissatisfied with their career usually engage in one of four coping strategies to manage the associated stress: leave the career, openly discuss entrenchment with their employer, remain loyal to the organization while hoping for improvement in the future, or retire on the job (**Exhibit 11-2**).

People choose to enter a career based on their interests, preferences, and evaluation of opportunities. Once a person has selected a career, he or she then invests money and effort to achieve success. Typically, the person will periodically look at whether the career chosen truly offers adequate opportunities for meeting the person's needs and achieving his or her goals. If it appears to do that, the person will continue to invest in the career. On the other hand, if it does not, the person may change careers, especially if the level of investment to date has been low (a high level of investment might incline the person to remain in the career to justify the investment).

In the steady-state career prototype, an individual selects a career in late adolescence or early adulthood using a minimal amount of information, is trained in the career, and maintains the necessary performance skills for remaining in the career. Interestingly, some careers in which a high proportion of the professionals fit the steady-state model, including nursing, teaching, social work, and law enforcement, often result in burnout. Daily confrontation with human suffering and death in conjunction with lack of autonomy, heavy caseloads, increased regulation, inadequate salaries, and frequent interpersonal conflicts understandably cause many individuals in these careers to want to escape.

Career entrapment occurs when a person is deeply entrenched in a career because of prior investment in career development, psychological attachments, and a sense of obligation. Among other things, the emotional bonds forged in coworker relationships and the intimacy of a mentor–protégé relationship may be difficult to give up. As the career tenure lengthens, the person spends greater energy rationalizing the decision to stay and convincing himself or herself that success is within reach. The person also may experience social pressure to continue in the current field or have a low propensity for risk taking (a career change obviously carries risks, including the risk that the new career may be no more fulfilling than the last).

Paradoxically, whereas dismal labor and market conditions and high unemployment negatively affect turnover, they can positively affect the process of changing careers. The pressures of depressed economic conditions often provide the impetus for entrapped or entrenched employees to seek other employment opportunities. Further, an economic crisis can cause an organization to retrain employees, thus providing them a chance to escape unfulfilling positions.

Individuals who experience career dissatisfaction and distress are susceptible to anxiety, anger, and depression. The anguish of boredom and tedium associated with work tasks often lead to rumination, resentment, melancholy, and an accompanying sense of hopelessness, with negative consequences for the organization.

Those organizations that will thrive will recognize important trends in the industry. First, millennials are almost twice as likely to become nurses as the baby boomers were (Auerbach et al., 2017). The embrace of the nursing profession by millennials is because they regard nursing as a career where they have the opportunity to change roles and jobs and organizations in order to meet their needs for achievement and work–life balance. Organizations that view this positively and make nursing skills transferrable, offer many options for nurses, and shorten the learning curve for nurses to get to the next level will succeed. Some organizations have viewed concepts such as tours of duty (Hoffman et al., 2014) as a way to achieve the trust and individual abilities that millennials seek. A tour of duty represents a commitment by the employer and the employee to a specific mission or mutual investment to preserve the flexibility that both employers and employees need to adapt to a rapidly changing world.

> ## Group Discussion
>
> What is behind the resurgence of interest in nursing, the focus on healthy work environment, the emerging millennial workforce, or the demand for nurses in the reforming healthcare system? Together, the cyclical nursing shortage, the willingness of nurses to recruit others into nursing, and the emerging roles for nurses have provided promise to the challenge of maintaining a viable healthcare workforce. Create a flow chart of the nursing supply that reflects these conditions and any others that you believe impact the nursing workforce. Where are the leverage points for increasing the supply? Where would you begin? What resources are needed? What outcomes are to be expected from the interventions you recommend?

Leaders often have to manage individuals they do not particularly like. Not every member of the team is friendly, thoughtful, and courteous. In fact, according to Gallo (2013) in a *Harvard Business Review* blog, many team members are irritating; they perform their work adequately but are not easy to work with. Such interpersonal issues should not always be looked at as negative but rather as an opportunity to seek out the positive in the individual(s), reflect on the annoying behavior (it can be something that reminds you of another negative situation), or be sure your evaluation standards of performance are not biased against the unlikable individuals.

Tolerance of Antisocial Behavior and Incivility

Much has been written about deviant or antisocial behaviors in the workplace. Bullying, incivility, harassment, lateral or horizontal violence, withholding effort, and stealing are of obvious concern because they reduce group effectiveness by threatening safe and interprofessional teamwork. These disruptive behaviors serve to intimidate, undermine, and demean individuals, and the failure of leaders to recognize antisocial behaviors as inappropriate and eliminate these behaviors has a negative impact on the social climate and the general moral conduct of employees and ultimately will impact optimal, safe patient care (Makic, 2018).

According to Robinson and O'Leary-Kelly (1998), the social context largely determines how employees think and feel about aspects of their work environment and how they behave. In particular, a positive relationship exists between a given individual's level of antisocial behavior and the level of antisocial behavior of his or her coworkers. This should come as no surprise because individual group members working in a shared social environment receive similar social cues (cues perhaps indicating that certain types and levels of antisocial behavior are acceptable). In addition, when a new employee enters an established group, the extent of the group's antisocial behavior affects how likely the newcomer is to develop similar behaviors. Typically, the newcomer adjusts his or her personal behavior to fit the work environment or eventually leaves the organization. Indeed, the longer an employee remains in a group, the greater the chance he or she will behave in accordance with the group's standards of behavior. Dealing effectively with antisocial behavior can differentiate a toxic from a healthy organization because nothing is more destructive than a leader's failure to manage the obvious negative and destructive behaviors of an individual or team. Employees hear value-based proclamations for performance and integrity; what is observed is contradictory to those values and beliefs, thus eroding organizational trust. Another factor that affects the antisocial behavior level of a group is the degree of task interdependence (i.e., the extent to which the group members must coordinate their individual efforts). Enhanced interaction allows the members to more easily acquire the social information that determines their subsequent behavior. In other words, the higher the level of interaction, the greater the likelihood that group members will take each other as role models.

A quantum leader must have a behavioral understanding of the context of the work environment and how the team communicates and manages conflict—that is, whether the conflict is constructive or destructive (Kim et al., 2015). The ability to manage conflict through communication can determine the ability of teams to internally manage antisocial behavior and develop prosocial strategies that draw individuals together (Dzurec et al., 2017). When power differences exist, or when an individual that is different from the team norm perceives they have an inferior status, and the power gradient is not managed through good communication and removal of perceptions, team function declines. When teams can resolve conflict through communication, antisocial behavior is less likely to influence the team. Further, the use of concepts such as cognitive rehearsal as a shield for lateral violence can also serve to address antisocial behavior. Cognitive rehearsal is a behavioral technique consisting of three parts: (1) providing didactic instruction about incivility and lateral violence, (2) rehearsing specific phrases to address incivility and lateral violence, and (3) practicing the phrases to become adept at using them (Griffin & Clark, 2014). An example is as follows:

Uncivil behavior: Use of nonverbal behaviors such as eye-rolling, making faces, etc.
Verbal response: "I see from your facial expression that there may be something you wish to say to me. It is OK to speak to me directly" (Griffin & Clark, 2014, p. 540).

Continued focus on the work environment is essential to ensure organizational, including employee, health.

Toxic Mentoring

Mentoring has long been extolled as a means of guiding the development of inexperienced employees, but not all mentoring results in the growth of the mentee. Some leaders in fact believe that mentoring is an ill-conceived method of continuing past practices—ill-conceived because it obstructs necessary adaptations to changes in the work environment, the marketplace, and society at large. Complex organizations depend less on the development of a leader and more on the development of leadership that emerges from the interaction of individuals and groups. A form of toxic mentoring then would be where a wise elder mentored an individual with antiquated wisdom gained from the mentor's past without regard of how organizations need to change. An effective mentor would need visibility of how the leader interacts within a team to develop organizational cultures and systems and not how organizational life is ruled by leaders.

Toxic mentoring can also result when an aspiring leader seeks to please an experienced leader that he or she has idealized. If the mentor (the experienced leader) does not assist the mentee in developing his or her own identity and leadership style, the mentee could be misled into following the established path of the mentor. The main danger here is that once the mentor is no longer on hand as a guide, the mentee might become empty and powerless and unable to progress.

Another hazard of mentoring occurs when an experienced leader idealizes an aspiring leader and places unrealistic hopes on him or her. The mentor then gives the mentee overly ambitious assignments that frequently remain uncompleted. Finally, some mentors attempt to transfer their defense mechanisms to their mentees or at least convince them of the need to approach situations from a defensive and hostile posture rather than a posture of openness and inquiry. In such cases, the mentoring process is more a cloning process than a means of growth and development.

The point that aspiring leaders must keep in mind is the need to take the initiative rather than travel the same old route, to be decisive rather than defer to a higher authority, to expose themselves to failure rather than make peace with mediocrity, and to seize opportunities rather than retreat from them.

From a somewhat different perspective, toxic mentoring exemplifies the negative side of transferring one's experiences. It is impossible to approach new people or situations with a blank sheet, so we use our past experiences, positive or negative, and the stereotypes we have inherited to fill the pages (**Exhibit 11-3**). A good mentor tries to keep the slate as clean as

---

Exhibit 11-3 Toxic Stereotypes

- Female leaders cannot understand financial situations and cannot sustain company solvency.
- Older leaders cannot be effective because they do not have technical competence.
- Younger leaders cannot hold senior leadership positions because they do not have enough experience.
- Members of our church will make better leaders because we know we can count on them.
- Avoid members of certain ethnic groups when selecting new leaders because some are too expressive.
- Overweight leaders will never concentrate on the business of the day.
- Avoid selecting leaders for your committee who require too much time to make decisions because they think too slowly.

possible. The mentee needs to make personal assessments and form personal opinions using his or her own emerging leadership lens to avoid unconscious bias.

Toxic mentors typically base perceptions not only on current practices but also on early childhood experiences. They make judgments about individuals and situations before examining the circumstances and the available data. They often put forth negative profiles of individuals that include derogatory references to the individuals' gender, age, culture, mental capacity, physical stature, or religion.

Effective mentoring is truly circular in nature. Sharing experiences from the past with aspiring leaders is as important as sharing experiences with colleagues and superiors. Mentoring upward, sideways, and downward reinforces the importance of lifelong learning and makes the point that wisdom and insight are not limited to those with tenure. The healthy mentor encourages self-assessment, open and nonjudgmental examination of issues, and reevaluation of decisions as new information becomes available.

Rather than selecting and promoting others of their own image, experienced leaders need to ensure that aspiring leaders gain an appreciation of the substantial personality differences that leaders can exhibit and the importance of diversity in personality and methodology for creating optimal solutions.

Inconsistency and Dishonesty

Leaders frequently add to the toxicity in an organization by being inconsistent in word and action and by not practicing the transparency they ask of their teams. In general, employees respect and are willing to follow leaders who act in accordance with their values, principles, and beliefs. When a company identifies balancing work and leisure as a goal, it usually focuses on the employees' time at work and develops initiatives giving employees flexibility in their work hours. But if the company at the same time is not filling vacancies and is asking employees to do more with less, the added flexibility is counteracted by the extra 5 or 10 hours of work that each employee must put in weekly. The company's message becomes ambiguous, and the employees feel that the executives just do not get it because opportunities for dialogue are not available. Ambiguous or contradictory messages are quite common and usually sow confusion and distrust. The recipients of these messages begin to feel angry, insecure, and entrapped. For instance, if one employee has a clearly superior performance review but is given the same compensation as mediocre performers, the contradictory message—performance both counts (because it is measured) and does not count (because superior performance is not compensated)—likely demoralizes the employee with the outstanding record.

Although people are ordinarily uncomfortable with conflict, their discomfort reduces their opportunities to learn more about the differing positions and viewpoints of colleagues. This in and of itself is enough to support the notion that conflict should be considered normal, but there is another very important reason. People's lack of comfort with conflict and confronting the truth has resulted in the "white lies of leadership" syndrome. White lies, in fact, have become all too common in performance reviews, the selection of candidates for positions, and explanations for downsizing given to employees (Malloch, 2001).

The performance review process continues to be a struggle for most leaders, especially identifying strengths and areas for improvement in an honest and meaningful way. Reviewers find it difficult to discuss inadequate performance openly and kindly, particularly if the deficiencies have been persistent and have never been addressed. Leaders generally wish for performance problems to disappear from lack of attention so that they do not have to deal with the issue or engage in uncomfortable dialogue. To avoid confrontation, leaders sometimes rate mediocre behavior as above standard or, to equalize the distribution of a limited compensation package, they routinely rate the performance of all employees as above standard. Regardless of their intent, these types of misevaluations are forms of dishonesty.

Truth telling is also difficult when a job candidate is not picked for the position. Unselected candidates are often told the chosen candidate had better credentials, more experience, or more education. Although this may be true, there is usually more to the decision. Factors such as personal appearance, aggressiveness in the interview, or nonsupport from a colleague often play a role in the selection process, but information about such issues is rarely shared, preventing the candidate from learning how to better prepare for the next interview. Holding back critical comments, even if done out of kindness, takes control away from employees and can be seen as a form of autocratic leadership behavior.

Finally, leaders often tell white lies when explaining decisions to downsize or eliminate positions. Most often they claim the decisions are not personal or about the employees' competence but rather based on financial considerations. The truth is that downsizing is often used to weed out mediocre or dissident employees. It is also used as a way to cover the effects of poor management, such as when leaders fail to adapt to incremental changes in the marketplace or neglect to retrain employees to meet emerging needs. Nothing is more destructive to the morale of an organization than the chronic recycling of human beings, especially in an industry that espouses health as its service.

Imbalance Between Work and Personal Life

For many people, the boundary between work life and personal life has all but collapsed with the advent of the internet. Technology has opened new doors to new experiences, and the condition of being without something to do is almost inconceivable. Individuals today spend much of their time learning new ideas or deciding what to do next. Being in demand is a sign of importance and value, and new communication technologies allow people to seek out and contact each other at any time.

Perhaps high-speed living is toxic to human beings. So much time can be put into arrivals and departures that not enough is left over for the experiences themselves. Raising children, developing relationships, and creating art are not tasks that lend themselves to being done speedily and efficiently. The high-speed world of technology has separated individuals from contemplation and slow-knowing—the process of reflecting creatively rather than relying on the mere analytical horsepower of technology. The amazing data-analyzing capabilities of computers have turned contemplation into a seemingly old-fashioned pastime. The focus is on problem solving. Dwelling on issues to see whether they might lead to deeper issues is seen as inefficient and self-indulgent. The simple act of mindfulness, the process of bringing one's attention to what is occurring in the present moment and being aware of our personal thoughts, in contrast to rehashing the past or anticipating the next moment would seem to reestablish some balance in activities more representative of our humanity instead of a sole dependency on technology.

What we know is that neither technology nor efficiency can acquire more time for anyone. Time is not something one had or lost; it is what one lives in. For most of us, there is never enough time. The real challenge is to develop a balance between work and personal life and to work to maintain the desired balance.

The challenge of finding enough time to function effectively in work and at home can be greater for female leaders. Because organizations desire the senior management profile to reflect the composition of the marketplace, more women are in executive and leadership roles. The problem experienced by female leaders is that some women remain the primary family managers and spend nearly twice as many hours on household and childcare responsibilities as men do. The conflicts of interest created by playing a leadership role and acting as a mother make it challenging for women to remain as executives while meeting their full responsibilities in one or both areas and suffering a noticeable lack of balance between work and personal life. More flexibility in the workplace and stronger domestic partnership is essential to bring about a true balance of work and life.

Recently, clinicians advocated expansion of the three aims for improving healthcare systems, originally created in 2008. The aims (improving the experience of care, improving the health of populations, reducing per capita costs of care) were expanded to also include improving the work life of healthcare clinicians and staff as foundational to achieving the first three aims (Berwick et al., 2008; Bodenheimer & Sinsky, 2014). Extensive nursing research provides leaders insights into how to create the appropriate context of work to promote the health of workers (Adams et al., 2018), and it is believed that nursing efforts to improve the work environment translate to all disciplines. The elements of the work environment that are important include effective leadership, support for practice autonomy, good communication, and strong interdisciplinary relationships (Adams et al., 2018). These elements can provide a blueprint to achieve an appropriate work–life balance and help prevent the toxicity that many organizations suffer from.

> **Point to Ponder**
>
> Stanford University developed the professional fulfillment model for healthcare professionals. According to this model, the interaction and balance of a culture of wellness, efficiency of practice, and personal resilience are essential to achieving professional fulfillment.
>
> Shanafelt, T., Swensen, S. J., Woody, J., Levin, J., & Lillie, J. (2018). Physician and nurse well-being: Seven things hospital boards should know. *Journal of Healthcare Management, 63*(6), 363-369.

> **Point to Ponder**
>
> Extremes of up and down are interrelated. Excessiveness ushers in disorder and disaster, which lead to burnout and fatigue as we walk the way of personal destruction. In leading others there is nothing better than moderation. Leisure is good, yet too much can lead to restlessness and boredom. Work is important and beneficial, yet in abundance it can cause havoc in other aspects of life. Avoid the temptations of overdoing and overextending, no matter how enticing and attractive the pulls and lures might be.
>
> Brief quote from p. 155 from Huang, C. A., & Lynch, J. (1995). *Mentoring: The Tao of giving and receiving wisdom.* Harper Collins. Copyright © 1995 by Chungliang Al Huang and Jerry Lynch. Reprinted by permission of Harper Collins Publishers.

Reactive Advocacy Gone Awry

Health professionals find solace in serving patients and acting as advocates for them, but advocacy, when it is reactive, can sometimes be a source of toxicity. Consider the following scenario. The family of a patient in a critical care unit recognized that all interventions were futile and informed the nurses and attending physician they wished to cease treatment. Keeping the patient comfortable was their only goal at this time. On the next shift, the consulting physician examined the patient and determined that he needed respiratory support. The physician then proceeded to intubate the patient. Given the power and reputation of the physician, no staff member challenged his actions, even though they were contrary to the family's wishes.

On the next shift, the returning nurse realized that the wishes of the family had been violated and called the attending physician, who, in turn, removed the respiratory support. The nurse expressed a feeling of accomplishment, although she was concerned about creating conflict with the consulting physician because she had gone over his head.

Advocacy leadership in health care is a proactive process. Its purpose is to create the conditions for patients to receive the care they desire. It involves much more than removing the barriers as they are identified; in fact, the goal of advocacy leadership is to avoid having barriers in the first place. Unfortunately, reactive advocacy is the kind of advocacy that has become commonplace in our world of ambiguous values. When traditional leaders take action to alleviate unhealthy situations, they feel accomplished and complete, despite often failing to identify or address the basic problems.

Widely touted theories of transformational leadership are based on the belief that leaders have the power needed to transform a low-performing organization into a high-performing organization. This belief is itself based on the classical model of system control, which is inconsistent with the concept of organizational transformation. If one knocks down an anthill and rebuilds it, that is restructuring, not transformation. If the ants sprout wings and move to the trees, that is transformation. Thus, a quantum leader who is truly a transformer needs to approach the organization from a very different perspective—in other words, to avoid change strategies that amount to merely rearranging current structures, policies, procedures, and reward systems. Rather, a transforming leader creates a new and improved system that allows individuals to contribute to their fullest potential to deliver the most effective health care possible. And there can be no idea of asserting control in the traditional sense but facilitation of individuals to create and improve the system.

Caring leadership behaviors are an important part of transformation. They have the potential to improve team dynamics, engagement, and the capacity for caring for others. These behaviors are often seen as affirmative words, tangible gifts, gestures that show colleagues they are cared for, and time to talk about challenges and concerns (Baggett et al., 2016). Kindness at the foundation of advocacy can interrupt trends of toxicity and serve to improve organizational outcomes (Padilla, 2017). The final challenge for quantum leaders is to avoid the obvious trap of believing that organizations are inherently toxic and that their job is to eradicate toxic behaviors wherever they are found. A shift to appreciative leadership allows leaders to focus on instances where things are going right, where quality is increasing, where patients are satisfied, and where teams perform effectively (Bushe, 2014). The quantum leader's main focus should be on appreciative leadership, recognizing new beliefs and behaviors, understanding their implications, and integrating those that appear to be beneficial into current practice.

The solution to the problems that plague health care today lies in building bridges between the disciplines and recognizing the imperative to practice in such a way that environment–health connections receive primary consideration. Physical healing takes place through a multifaceted process in which the fabric of the body repairs and regenerates itself. So, too, can organizations heal.

Ten Principles for Minimizing Toxic Behavior in Organizations

The first step in minimizing the negative effects of dysfunctional behaviors is to recognize that these behaviors exist and that their elimination requires a commitment to discarding the toxic past and redefining what should be. One of the reasons that effective organizational change is often so difficult is that it involves taking authority, status, prestige, and security away from those in power, threatening their self-image and provoking resistance. But there is no other choice because many of the toxins originate in misplaced authority and power.

For the work of transformation to begin, the organizational culture must support, as its main value, the common good rather than self-interest. Organizations steeped in bureaucracy and paternalism experience a difficult transformation requiring persistent effort. For others, the journey may be somewhat less complex and traumatic. The model of seven evolving levels of organizational culture described by Barrett (1995) can serve as a guideline for organizations in monitoring their progress on the journey toward supporting the common good (**Exhibit 11-4**). Although these levels are progressive, an organization might regress at different times in the journey.

> **Key Point**
>
> *Healing manager*: A person who helps others grow emotionally and intellectually—the emotional pathway from chaotic relationships to total quality relationships.
>
> Reprinted with permission of the publisher. From Lundin, W., & Lundin, K. (1993). *The healing manager: How to build quality relationships and productive cultures at work.* Berrett-Koehler.

Exhibit 11-4   Seven Levels of Corporate Culture

1. *Survival consciousness*: The organization is focused on profits and typically uses an autocratic, uncaring, manipulative, and fear-driven culture.
2. *Relationship consciousness*: This is a benevolent, paternalistic culture with a focus on internal communications, loyalty, and friendship. Fears at this level can lead to internal competition, blame, and manipulative culture.
3. *Self-esteem consciousness*: The focus is on a desire to be a high-performing organization. The organization has a hierarchical power structure with goals of efficiency through systems and processes, best practices, productivity, and quality. Strong results orientation.
4. *Transformation consciousness*: The focus is on self-discovery, continuous renewal and learning, and teamwork. The organization begins to focus on equality and diversity. Strong goals orientation.
5. *Internal cohesion consciousness*: The focus is on shared vision and values, integrity, trust, creativity, transparency, empowerment, and integrity. Efforts abound to create conditions for cohesion, community spirit, and mutual accountability.
6. *Making a difference consciousness*: The focus is on strategic partners and alliances. The organization engages in voluntary environmental and social audits to promote social awareness and to provide support for the local community and businesses, employee fulfillment, coaching, and mentoring. The search is for long-term sustainability.
7. *Service consciousness*: The organization contributes to service to humanity. The focus is on social responsibility, future generations, the long-term perspective, ethics, compassion, and humility.

From Barrett, R. (2011). *Liberating the corporate soul* (pp. 61–67). Routledge/Taylor & Francis Books.

Exhibit 11-5 Ten Principles for Minimizing Dysfunctional Behaviors

1. Know thyself.
2. Walk the talk.
3. Be willing to listen.
4. Value the truth of the whole.
5. Empower employees.
6. Build relationships on respect.
7. Act as an agent of transformation.
8. Screen job candidates for dysfunction.
9. Expect accountability and ownership.
10. Reward value-adding behaviors.

Exhibit 11-5 contains a list of 10 principles useful for combating toxicity in an organization. By following these rules, discussed subsequently, leaders can reduce the potency of the sources of toxicity described earlier or eliminate them entirely.

Principle 1: Know Thyself

For the leader of an organization, the most important rule for minimizing dysfunction is to know what he or she stands for and what behaviors he or she finds unacceptable. Barrett (1995) makes the point that whatever a person identifies with, that person cares for. When people identify with family members, they give them support. When they identify with their environment, they protect and nurture it. When they identify with their organization or their work unit, they give it their very best. Further, when they enlarge their sense of self by identifying with their organization, they develop a greater sense of responsibility toward it and link its welfare with theirs.

Knowing yourself is more than identifying your patterns of decision making. It includes identifying your values, your outlook on life, and the importance you place on integrity and work ethic. The leader who believes that employees are basically honest, hardworking, and optimistic about the future is quite different from the leader who believes that employees do only what they absolutely must, tend to be less than truthful, and are typically negative about the future. The leaders who create the future fall into four types—the learner, who is determined to keep learning as fast as the world is changing; the disruptor, who knows when it is time to disrupt themselves by separating from the pride of the most recent accomplishment; the optimist, who is always excited about what the future holds; and the experimenter, who dares greatly, understanding there is no success without setbacks (Taylor, 2017). These are quantum leaders.

Leaders need to listen to what others have to say about them and to look carefully at their style of communication and the way they treat point-of-service workers. The words others say about them are not always

> **Point to Ponder**
>
> Passion is manifested in a commitment of energy and a personal investment in an effort so strongly felt that adversity cannot diminish the effort. Passion sees the leader through those inevitable times of toughness, darkness, and slow change.
>
> —Tim Porter-O'Grady (2000)

easy to swallow but cannot be ignored. As leaders, they are honor-bound to respond and make the changes necessary to improve their reputation. By gaining the ability to practice authentically, the quantum leader's reputation builds through honest relationships with his or her followers because the leader values their input and positively and truthfully promotes openness and support for the employees, thus improving team performance through mutual passion.

Leaders must look at themselves, confront their emotions, and acknowledge the perceptions of their employees. When an intimidating senior manager says to an employee, "I want to know how you see me," the employee might be reluctant to answer honestly out of fear of retaliation. If a leader discovers that others are afraid of being open, he or she must make the effort to eliminate the toxic behaviors that cause their fear. A self-assessment can enable leaders to gain an appreciation of unexplained discrepancies between how they are viewed by colleagues versus how they are viewed by family and friends. At work, even though people look the same, what they become in the eyes of others is seldom the same as how they are perceived in their personal life. It is possible, for example, for an individual to be considered competent outside of the workplace but incompetent at work, and vice versa. Although self-assessment and dialogue with others can clarify paradoxical perceptions, they cannot eliminate the disparities.

As leaders journey through the self-assessment process, they may find that meditation is useful for relaxing and regaining a healthy balance. Relaxation is not just the relief of tension but the foundation of self-healing abilities. By learning to relax and reflect, people build confidence in their ability to control their body, feelings, and thoughts. They become aware of having more choices in how to react and how to feel. They also become more aware of what kinds of things, people, and thoughts tend to produce tension—an important first step in learning to deal with these sources of tension constructively. In addition, relaxation interrupts habitual negative thought patterns and allows the leader to be present with others.

Principle 2: Walk the Talk

The second rule for reducing toxicity is to walk the talk—to act in accordance with expressed values. If leaders did in fact walk their talk and consequently did listen to employees, would it be necessary to have suggestion boxes? If they really had an open-door policy, would they have to sell it so emphatically? Building trust between two individuals requires the words and actions of each to be congruent. The trust that leaders acquire by walking their talk encourages innovative behaviors by employees, minimizes the potential for discrepancies between expectations and reality, reinforces their perceived integrity, strengthens the confidence that employees have in the appropriateness of future interactions, and reinforces the bond between the leaders and employees.

In times of chaos, the importance of constancy of values increases. Although the healthcare environment and marketplace present regular challenges for health professionals, the mission and values of health care remain unchanged. The values of respect, compassion, confidentiality, patient advocacy, accountability, competence, continuing knowledge development, supportive work environments, and collaboration remain constant beacons of light for those who work in the field.

Creating a team (or committee) to act as the conscience of the organization could assist all employees in evaluating their success at walking the talk. The committee, an extension of the traditional ethics committee, would provide an ongoing critique of leadership decision making to ensure that the decisions chosen are consistent with the values and norms of the organization. In addition, it could give careful consideration to potential conflicts between formally stated organizational values and unavoidable financial or business pressures, as well as issues related to all types of harassment, coercion, and discrimination.

As an example, recent downsizing efforts, despite organizations' professed respect for the dignity of all individuals, resulted in a significant loss of dignity by the employees who were laid off. If instead these organizations had used their power appropriately, acted to protect human rights and dignity, and taken organizational and societal issues into consideration at the outset of their decision making, they could have responded to the financial pressures in a way that minimized the negative impact on employees and thus minimized the resulting organizational toxicity.

Given that the traditional contract between employers and employees—in which long-term job security is traded for loyalty—is becoming extinct, a new contract needs to be fashioned to ensure that employees are not victimized or wind up working in a trustless environment. In other words, the employer–employee relationship needs to be reconceived. Although it is true that promises of long-term employment and associated benefits are inappropriate in the current marketplace, employers and employees should openly and honestly discuss the nature of the work, expected changes that affect the work, and ways in which employees can remain useful to the organization. If an employee leaves the organization, the termination of employment should be the result of a mutual decision rather than a unilateral act by either the employer or the employee.

Principle 3: Be Willing to Listen

Active listening is not just a matter of hearing; listening is an authentic connection. Good listeners take time to get to know their employees, are empathetic, and are very good at connecting with people and building trust. The leader who is an expert at listening believes that every employee is a source of unique information critical to the organization's success. It is about a relationship between the leader and the employee.

Group Discussion

If you could whisper one thing in the ear of your organization's leader, what would it be? Would it concern specific toxic behaviors? Look at what other people in your group would want to whisper. Would their questions and comments be similar to these?

- Why don't you react to that behavior?
- Give us a sign that you understand and truly care about employees in our organization.
- Why have you not fired that person?
- How do I know whether you are satisfied with my performance?

Consider the differences and similarities in the questions and comments and identify at least two strategies to correct the problems you have identified.

Shared leadership is one leadership model that is especially conducive to active listening—and to healthy dialogue. Also conducive to active listening is the horizontal organizational model, in which teams of individuals are involved in organization-wide, cross-functional core processes.

Listening is an essential part of effective problem solving and decision making. Leaders in quantum organizations use active and critical listening skills to gain a full understanding of problem situations. To acquire the depth of understanding they need, they must explore multiple issues and gather myriad data, both of which begin with critical listening.

Principle 4: Value the Truth of the Whole

The power to be gained from understanding both sides of an issue often goes unappreciated. Instead, an individual will strive to have others believe and support a particular point of view—his or her own. In the quantum organization, understanding multiple perspectives and balancing differing opinions are particularly helpful for arriving at optimal decisions. The challenge for the quantum leader is to cherish the fruitful opposition between order and creativity and to escape the grip of either/or thinking. Multiple perspectives are essential for understanding the whole. Often, the whole truth is a paradoxical joining of apparent opposites, and if the whole truth is desired, the opposites need to be embraced as a unit.

Finally, the leadership team should have room for a whole constellation of personality styles to ensure the effectiveness of its decision-making practices. Healthy organizations typically seek to include a broad variety of leadership personality styles so that multiple perspectives can be considered and no single one can dominate in the creation of strategies and structures, thereby minimizing the potential for groupthink.

Respect for individuals is paramount. Microaggressions are the everyday verbal, nonverbal, and environmental slights, snubs, or insults, whether intentional or unintentional, that communicate hostile, derogatory, or negative messages to target persons based solely on their marginalized group membership. These must be eliminated and respect must prevail if we truly value the truth of the whole (Druck et al., 2019).

Principle 5: Empower Employees

Leaders of quantum organizations work to empower employees and ensure that they have the freedom to make suggestions, grow and mature, and become sensitized to themselves and others. The corporate social democracy they practice is much different from the corporate elitism associated with centralized power. Instead of the chief executive and managers thinking for everyone, all individuals in the organization think. Instead of a mission statement being handed down, all employees should participate in the creation of the organization's vision, mission, and values because they do the work and deserve the right to define these critical elements.

Leadership expertise is easily identified in action but difficult to describe in its richness. The wisdom of leaders is similar to the clinical wisdom of clinicians described by Benner et al. (1999). It includes the essential skills of grasp (comprehension), inquiry, and forethought. Leaders who want to serve as transformers need to acquire this wisdom.

Obtaining these skills requires significant leadership experience. Leaders who have this level of experience become expert at problem identification and solving and can act in situations that are ambiguous, underdetermined, unexpected, and/or markedly different from their preconceptions. Grasping involves making qualitative distinctions, doing detective work, recognizing changes, and developing relevant knowledge bases. Inquiry involves knowing what questions to ask. Expert leaders learn to use their knowledge, experience, and intuition to anticipate crises, risks, and vulnerabilities that may affect the organization or its employees.

Forethought is another component of leadership wisdom that emerges after significant experience dealing with common situations and unanticipated events. It is basically the ability to anticipate likely eventualities and to take the appropriate actions—an ability seldom articulated despite the fact that it is pervasive in the everyday actions of expert leaders. These leaders subconsciously project possible situations that may result from particular conditions. Then, by being extra attentive and by using their ability to recognize patterns and sense the relevance of events, they are able to prepare the organization for the most probable of these situations.

Empowering employees is a career-long journey of mentoring. The goal is to transfer leadership wisdom not only to aspiring leaders but to all employees. Along this journey, expert leaders provide tools for employees to do their jobs well and to help them feel successful. They try to create a culture of respect based on the belief that employees who feel successful and appreciated in the workplace truly leave their work, both physically and mentally, at the end of the day and are thus better able to manage their time and achieve and maintain a healthy balance between work and personal life.

Zacher et al. (2015) identified the importance of career adaptability as a means to address career entrenchment. Becoming unwilling to look at the future or stuck in a job or role can be mediated with purposeful strategies that assist employees in more successfully managing their careers. Four areas to focus on include recognizing concern for the future, reinforcing individual perceptions of control over one's own development, curiosity about other career opportunities, and instilling confidence in employees to believe they can realize career goals and solve problems in managing their careers. Recognizing these strategies to enhance career adaptability in an open manner prior to a crisis situation reinforces transparency, respect, and valuing of employees.

Principle 6: Build Relationships on Respect

Each and every interaction among employees and between employees and patients should be directed toward achieving therapeutic outcomes. Relationships characterized by disrespectful behavior, insulting language, or emotional harm cannot be tolerated. Respect for employees is an expectation that is never open to discussion. No individual ever has the permission to be rude or abusive to any other individual. The fundamental right of every person to be treated in a manner that reflects the inherent value of human beings is the guiding principle of all human relationships.

Following are rules that leaders should keep in mind to help ensure that their relationships with employees and the relationships among employees are essentially therapeutic:

- Behave so as to preserve every person's dignity.
- Encourage employees to talk with each other to learn more about each other's opinions before reaching a conclusion.
- Encourage self-improvement.
- Give employees feedback on their performance.
- Be open to new ideas.

- Encourage employees to do their best.
- Compensate employees fairly for the work they do.

These next rules apply to the relationships between care providers and patients. Because their purpose is likewise to help ensure that these relationships are fundamentally therapeutic, they need to be followed by the care providers:

- Probe to uncover the rationale for any decision that a patient makes.
- Recognize that family members and friends can have a significant impact on a patient's ability to manage his or her own health.
- Consider a patient's cultural beliefs before providing care.
- Consider a patient's spiritual beliefs before providing care.
- Empower patients to avoid unnecessary dependency or overtreatment.
- Recognize that clinical and behavioral outcomes affect each other.
- Support a patient's choice to use culturally based healing practices.
- Be fully present and listen to each patient.
- Assist each patient to develop or sustain his or her ability to cope with life situations.
- Identify each patient's feelings about his or her illness and expectations for recovery.
- Encourage patients to participate in self-care programs.
- Recognize that a patient's choices should guide the plan of care.

Principle 7: Act as an Agent of Transformation

Quantum leaders encourage employees to be self-reliant and to take charge of their careers, not only their current jobs. They assist employees in overcoming the negative effects of career entrenchment or entrapment, such as dissatisfaction and ineffectiveness. Quantum leaders also do the following:

- Encourage employees to voice concerns and work collaboratively to identify and address dissatisfaction.
- Do not threaten retaliation when employees express negative emotions or opinions.
- Recognize discrepancy between ideal career progression and reality.
- Seek to transform career pathways into a progressive career management program.
- Recognize that employee loyalty has advantages and disadvantages (e.g., loyalty can be merely passive and result in skill atrophy, boredom, and depression).

In addition, quantum leaders encourage employees to engage in extra-role activities that are not directly compensated but that can decrease employee stress while simultaneously benefiting the organization. Acting as a mentor outside the organization is an example of extra-role citizenship work that can decrease the frustration of entrenched employees while reducing stress and meeting affiliation needs.

Quantum leaders understand that entrenched employees who attempt to cope with their career issues through loyalty or by acting as a constructive voice do contribute to workforce stability and reduce turnover costs. These employees often can be jarred from their entrenchment by giving them the opportunity to be involved in special projects, by permitting job rotation, by facilitating downward or lateral moves, by training them in cross-functional roles, and by allowing temporary reassignments (**Exhibit 11-6**).

Exhibit 11-6 Organizational Strategies to Minimize Career Entrenchment

- Offer generous severance pay packages to fund employees' explorations into new careers.
- Offer tuition reimbursements and time off for employees to attend classes while still employed.
- Give employees time to rotate to other positions in the organization so that they might explore another career option within the relatively safe confines of the organization.
- Discourage linear career paths and emphasize psychological success.
- Ensure that employees do not feel as though they are violating the organization's trust as they investigate new career options.
- Allow employees who leave in good standing to return if their new career plans fail.

Exhibit 11-7 Interviewing to Minimize Toxicity

1. What are your preferences for assignments, delegating, and managing authority?
2. How frequently do you believe feedback and updating of work are needed?
3. What is your major frustration in your current job? What are the major frustrations in the jobs performed by those you have supervised?
4. What would make you comfortable in overriding my authority and decisions?
5. What type of people and financial support do you require to ensure that your job is done well?
6. Has there been a time when you contributed to a positive organizational culture? If so, explain.

Career development programs can assist employees in using the "constructive voice" approach to dealing with career entrenchment. Retraining and redeployment programs further assist employees in managing their careers and thereby help the organization sustain its viability. Employees in organizations that avoid career management are less likely to discuss career issues affecting their performance.

Finally, when all else fails, it may be necessary to remove an employee who has retired on the job. Employees who have lost the motivation to develop and grow become increasingly less productive and focus on noncareer activities at the expense of the organization. They therefore need to be counseled to seek employment opportunities outside of the organization.

Principle 8: Screen Job Candidates for Dysfunction

New employees represent a significant investment for the organization, and job candidates require more scrutiny than they currently receive. To help in screening job candidates, leaders should identify specific dysfunctional behaviors that have a negative impact on organizational performance and, with the assistance of human resource experts, should develop new approaches to interviewing and selecting employees. The 10 principles for minimizing toxic behaviors under discussion in this section are likely to be useful in these endeavors, as are the 6 questions presented in **Exhibit 11-7**. In addition, these questions are appropriate for ongoing use to prevent or decrease dysfunction among current employees. Getting regular feedback from employees about their assignment preferences and current frustrations assists leaders in developing a good working relationship with them.

Principle 9: Expect Accountability and Ownership

Accountability is more than the background against which everyday decisions are made. In fact, the way in which accountability is created, negotiated, communicated, and evaluated lies at the heart of an organization's operations. Unfortunately, years of entitlement philosophies have created workers who park their brains at the door and are comfortable with being rewarded for simply showing up. Accountability is doing what you are expected to do because someone expects it of you. Organizations that expect only accountability will end up with a workplace where people do only the tasks that are listed in their job description and never take initiative to go above and beyond (Tye & Dent, 2017).

Accountability systems, to function properly, require the clear delineation of individual behaviors and supporting management practices. Both individual accountability and system accountability are necessary to support the values of integrity and transformation and to foster therapeutic relationships. Individuals in a quantum organization are not threatened by the expectation for accountability but rather need accountability and ownership to perform at a high level. Quantum leaders seek ownership in their people—doing what needs to be done because the person expects it of him- or herself and the results of their actions and the relationships they have are more important than completing only the tasks of their work (Tye & Dent, 2017).

Principle 10: Reward Value-Adding Behaviors

The opportunity now exists for leaders to shift the focus from return on investment to cost-effectiveness and to create new rules that lay the groundwork for value-based reward and recognition programs. First and foremost, healthcare leaders are called on by the economic community to use resources in a way that ensures healthcare value. Care providers can no longer give the best of everything without any financial accounting.

Healthcare leaders and providers are now required to examine services within the value equation. If resources are limited, does every patient symptom require intervention, particularly if little or no improvement in the patient's clinical condition is likely to result? Just to ask this question is a challenge for providers and leaders schooled in an environment characterized by increasing growth of and access to the healthcare system. Provision of as many services as possible was the sign of the successful leader. Unfortunately, there was no accountability and no control in the fee-for-service payment system. The result is well known: the exhaustion of resources.

Healthcare services need to be appropriate to the conditions being treated, focused on outcomes, and consistent with the wishes of the patients and families being served. The buyers and users of health care want to know they are getting value for the resources expended. They want to know that something good or better will happen because of the purchase of healthcare services—that the users' health will be improved. They also are demanding that the choices made by care providers are rational and based on evidence.

Given the expectations of buyers and users, healthcare leaders need to create an organizational context that supports the desired services and directs the rewards and recognition of the organization toward efforts that can meet these expectations. In addition, the success of care providers in improving the health of patients or community members and in managing their own health needs to be recognized and rewarded.

In a quantum healthcare organization, the care providers work to ensure the following:

- Patients experience an improvement in their clinical condition, possibly including increased physical functioning, greater tolerance of activity, improved ambulation, and/or reduced pain.

- Patients improve their ability to care for themselves, including performing wound care, taking medications on schedule, maintaining a nutritious diet, and eliminating properly.
- Patients learn more about their condition and its treatment, including their own treatment regime, appropriate procedures, potential complications, and emergency interventions.
- Patients are aware of the elements of a healthy lifestyle, including proper nutrition, weight management, activity, stress management, sleep, safety, infection control, and disease screening.

The main tasks of the leaders of a quantum healthcare organization include:

- Hiring and developing a workforce capable of achieving the patient outcomes listed previously.
- Retaining and continuing to develop the clinicians needed to meet the organization's future needs.
- Creating a system in which clinicians and leaders can influence the context of care provision based on their understanding of what is needed and what they are capable of doing (e.g., clinicians and leaders both need to actively intervene to improve communication, understand potential situations likely to unfold, and alter the context as necessary).
- Fostering therapeutic relationships among leaders, clinicians, and patients that focus on the values and beliefs of the patients, develop the inner capacities of the patients and providers, involve patients in decision making, and make room for self-responsibility.

Organizations might find it helpful to use the topic of organizational health and ways of minimizing behavioral dysfunction as the theme of a leadership retreat. In such a retreat, the participants could be challenged to define organizational health and identify toxins in their department or the organization as a whole, and then consider strategies to reduce the toxicity using the preceding principles.

Conclusion

To counteract the toxicity that currently exists in healthcare organizations, it is the leader's role to ensure that humanity is present in the workplace. There is nothing easy, however, about creating the proper context for providing healthcare services. An organization is an open system consisting of inputs, throughputs, and outputs, all of which can be healthy or toxic. The work of delivering care is complex and emotional. Clinicians deal with human beings at their most vulnerable times, which requires of the clinicians a high level of personal involvement and commitment.

What is terrifying about dysfunctional organizations is that employee emotional pain is accepted as a natural phenomenon. Employees are expected to live with discomfort as a condition of employment. The real mystery is the continual denial by leaders of a connection between employee pain and service quality. It seems to escape many leaders that employee dissatisfaction leads inevitably to patient dissatisfaction and that, conversely, there is a correlation between engaged employees and gratified patients. Even when they accept this correlation, leaders find it difficult to create the conditions and practices that increase both employee and patient satisfaction.

The aim of leadership is not to create a workers' paradise but rather to engender an organizational culture that allows for organizational transformation and for the employees' performance to live and grow. It is the obligation of the leader of a healthcare organization to push toward organizational health so that the will of the patient is respected. To do this, the leader needs to demonstrate a willingness and ability to cultivate self-transformation, as well as transformation in others, on a continuing basis.

The obligations of leaders and employees are interconnected. Neither group can be successful without both of them meeting their responsibilities. Leadership is never an either/or situation. Further, leadership is a rational service performed by rational people directed toward achieving sensible organizational objectives. However, these rational people carry with them past experiences laden with neurotic styles, negative transference, superior–subordinate entanglements, and untenable strategies. Not surprisingly, unless the leaders recognize this and foster appropriate behaviors, the result is persistent dysfunction.

Finally, leaders need to forget about ever finding enough time. There is never enough time for all the things individuals want to do. Rather, the challenge is to find a healthy balance between the things of importance: work, family, and other personal interests, including personal and professional growth.

Chapter Takeaways

1. Identifying and minimizing organizational toxicity reinforces a healthy, healing environment.
2. Leaders often unwittingly engage in toxic behaviors and, once identified, can course correct.
3. Organizational toxicity impacts not only employees but also patients and the community.
4. Facilitating career adaptability for unmotivated or entrenched employees positively impacts organizational morale and perceptions of accountability.
5. Principles for minimizing toxicity can be used to address challenging situations by moving from subjective notions to objective approaches to change.

Case Study 11-1

Toxic Incivility at the Unit Level

Jeannie Walker just accepted a job as nurse manager for the ortho-neuro unit of a large community hospital. She recently graduated with her master's degree in nursing with an emphasis on nursing leadership in healthcare settings. Excited about the new role and opportunities to influence positive changes on a nursing unit, Jeannie was not at all concerned when the human resources officer mentioned that the last three managers on the ortho-neuro unit left the position after 12 to 18 months. Jeannie had lots of clinical experience, and now armed with all that she had learned in graduate school, she was confident that she would be able to handle the management of the 32-bed unit with a staff consisting of 120 full- and part-time employees. The human resources officer had told her that half of the staff were long-term employees, but the other half were fairly new to the unit. There seemed to be a lot of turnover among newer employees, but the long-term employees had worked on the unit an average of 20 years.

Jeannie had aspirations of leading her unit in collaborative governance and hopefully influencing other directors and managers to begin the Magnet® journey.

During her first few weeks in the role, Jeannie discovered a lot of facts about the staff and the care delivery model. With a nurse-to-patient ratio of one nurse to four patients and one nursing assistant for every eight patients, the unit seemed to be reasonably staffed for the expected workload required for patient care. She also discovered that only 35% of the nurses were prepared at the baccalaureate level, 55% had attained an associate's degree, and 10% had a diploma in nursing. There was a strong ethnic mix as well, with nearly 30% of the nurses educated in foreign countries such as the Philippines (20%) and India (10%) and others who were second-generation immigrants from the Philippines (30%), the Middle East (10%), Canada (7%), and Germany (3%) educated in the United States. The remaining 20% were American born and educated. Jeannie also discovered that the unit was experiencing a higher than hospital and national average rate for hospital-acquired infections (HAIs), patient falls, and medication errors. Nurse satisfaction levels were the lowest of all of the nursing units at the hospital, and if this was not enough, the patient and physician satisfaction levels were also lower than the hospital average. Jeannie was surprised by these quality indicators, but she attributed the poor performance to the need for a consistent, strong, and visionary leader who would inspire the staff to work together and improve these quality indicators. She felt up to the challenge to transform this staff and voiced this commitment to excellence to nurses at her first staff meeting. After an energetic and inspiring "state of the union" address accompanied by her vision for the future, Jeannie was a bit surprised that the staff remained absolutely stoic and had no response to her plans to create a collaborative governance structure with unit councils providing staff input into decisions affecting nursing and patient care. Perhaps it was because she was new?

Over the course of a few months, Jeannie tried to establish a Unit Practice Council (UPC) and a Research and Evidence-Based Practice (REBP) Council, but few of the staff volunteered to participate on either of the councils. Jeannie sought a handful of nurses who she believed would be strong leaders and talked with them about her vision for empowering the nurses through council involvement. She was shocked to hear a resounding "no" from the nurses, who shared that they were afraid to participate. The repetitive answer from many of the nurses was "I only want to do my job and go home." As Jeannie inquired more and more, she discovered that the staff were extremely fractionated into cultural groups who did not like to integrate or communicate any more than absolutely necessary with other cultural groups. Not only were the nurses in firm social cliques, but the more senior nurses on both shifts had first preference for scheduling, patient assignments, and lunch breaks. They refused to take assignments to orient new personnel or to be preceptors for nursing students. Because they were such a powerful group, they seemed to make the decisions for all of the staff. If any of the nurses from other cultural groups voiced a complaint, they were the ones who were canceled first for scheduled or overtime shifts or received the most difficult patients for an assignment.

Jeannie learned that there was often open conflict among the nurses with name calling, accusations, threats, and retaliations. Evening shift nurses accused day shift nurses of being "lazy," not completing patient care assignments, or leaving the bulk of work to the evening/night shift nurses. Day shift nurses complained that night nurses were "sleeping on the job" and not properly assessing patients or documenting appropriately. To make matters worse, several of the physicians joined in with their own complaints and accusations that "these nurses are the worst of any unit in the entire hospital," "they don't know anything about ortho-neuro patients," and "they call all hours of the night for trivial things." After a few weeks of hearing all the complaints from multiple sources, seeing the negative unit quality indicators, and refereeing a number of conflicts among nurses and physicians, Jeannie felt completely overwhelmed. She mentioned to a comanager, "I feel like the man in the circus who spins plates on a bunch of poles all at once. He has to keep dancing around just to keep a plate from falling down and breaking."

Jeannie tried many of the ideas she had learned in class about managing interpersonal conflict, using change theories as a framework for change and leading intergenerational and intercultural workgroups. She met with nurses individually and in groups. She tried to create a shared vision of what the future could be. She reread the chapter "Toxic Organizations and People" in *Quantum Leadership* and tried to remember class discussions of others who had witnessed similar situations in their clinical experiences. She remained confident that collaborative governance would be the best option for correcting many of the problems on the unit.

The entire unit of nurses seemed reluctant to change and seemed to have absolutely no interest in a collaborative governance structure. Because the hospital was under a union collective bargaining contract for nursing, the union shop steward, Angelina, asked for a meeting with Jeannie.

Angelina explained that the nurses as a collective whole did not support moving to a collaborative governance structure, nor did they want input into unit decisions. "This is the job of management and not of staff nurses," Angelina explained, and she advised Jeannie to cease from trying to change the unit.

Jeannie faces huge and complex challenges with her new role as nurse manager. It is clear to her that change is critically needed to ensure optimal patient outcomes and to create a work environment that is safe and healthy for the nursing staff.

Questions

1. Using the principles discussed in this chapter, describe the stakeholders in this case; then, take on the perspective of each stakeholder group and analyze the case from that perspective. How would you transform this unit from a toxic work environment to a healthy, supportive work environment?
2. Identify the players who are the power holders and how they use that power to influence the whole unit.
3. Describe the various issues that complicate the case. How are these issues interrelated?
4. Take on the role of Jeannie, and describe how you might manage this situation and transform the unit.

Case Study 11-2

The Ambivalent Leader: Reporting to the Lion or the Lamb?

Julie has been the executive director of the Maternal–Newborn Service for 5 years and reports to a chief nursing officer (CNO). The four other executive directors of service-lines include Tim, who is the executive director of Medical-Surgical Services; Janice, who is the executive director of Critical and Emergency Services; Fred, who is the executive director of Surgical Services; and Gabriella, who is the executive director of Rehabilitation and Outpatient

Services. All of the executive directors with the exception of one are about the same age (mid- to late 30s or early 40s), educated at the master's in nursing (MSN) level (except for Julie, who has a PhD in nursing leadership), and have significant clinical experience in their service-line areas. Janice is in her late 20s, has a master's in business administration (MBA), and is also quite experienced in critical care services.

The five executive directors work well together as a team, but do not respect the opinion, direction, and leadership of the CNO, who has been in her position for 30 years. The team perceives her to be out of date, although the physicians at the hospital are quite supportive of her. They often meet to determine ways they can work around her to accomplish their individual and collective goals. The CNO reports to the CEO, along with the chief financial officer (CFO) and the chief operations officer (COO). The CNO, CEO, CFO, and COO have all worked together for approximately 7 years. The rest of the executive team has little interaction with the executive directors, with the exception of the budget season when the executive directors work closely with the CFO and COO to develop and negotiate the budgets and approved number of full-time equivalents (FTEs) for each clinical area.

One summer, Julie goes on vacation, and while away she receives a call from Gabriella, who informs her that huge changes have taken place. The president of the healthcare system has terminated the CEO and the CNO and has hired a new CEO. The new CEO was a CFO and COO in his previous employment, but has no experience as a CEO. He has a master's degree in hospital administration.

The reporting structure has also been changed. All of the executive directors, the CFO, and the COO will all now report directly to the new CEO. There will not be a designated CNO because all of the executive directors will fill that role. The new changes will take place immediately. The communication to the organization and the public indicates, "Changes were needed to position the organization for growth in current and future service-lines and expansion into new markets. The CEO and CNO have decided to pursue other career opportunities."

At first Julie is very impressed with the new CEO, who is young, enthusiastic, and very financially savvy. He meets with the executive team every Monday morning to review the previous week's performance in each service-line and to share plans for the upcoming week. He meets with each of his direct reports once per month and reviews the budget, productivity, patient outcome indicators, and satisfaction levels of staff and physicians. Julie seems to appreciate the direct communication style of the new CEO.

After a few months, Julie detects a change. As budget constraints become more apparent, the executive team is requested to tighten the belt. The proposed budget for the next year must be cut 10% across the board, and the capital budget requests become very competitive. Although Julie's area has the greatest percentage of admissions and discharges as compared to the other service areas, the reimbursement rates for her patients are significantly less than that of patients in her colleagues' service areas. Due to the way contracts have been negotiated for Medicaid and Medicare patients, Julie's area actually loses money—the cost to provide the services for 48% of the patients is more than the reimbursement rate. When this issue is discussed week after week at the Monday report, Julie begins to see a change in the group dynamics among her colleagues. Janice is emerging as the most powerful of the executive directors, and her areas contribute the most to the hospital's revenue picture. Janice often "hangs out" with the CEO and the two of them meet daily at the end of the day. The other executive directors notice the change as well, but no one feels it as much as Julie.

Julie never knows what to expect from the CEO. At one meeting he can be very kind and supportive, but at the next meeting he can be accusatory, belittling, and angry that her area is losing money—not because of productivity, but because of the revenue levels. He demands that she decrease staffing levels to cut expenses, and Julie tries to explain that doing so would put the areas out of compliance with required nurse-to-patient ratios. This rationale is not received well, and more pressure is placed on Julie to reduce staffing expenses. The CEO wants her to change the staff mix, using fewer RNs and adding more nursing assistants to cut expenses. Some of the meetings are brutal, and Julie often leaves feeling "beaten" and humiliated.

Julie is upset with the CEO, but after a few hours of reflective thinking after meetings with the CEO, she blames herself, thinking she should be more prepared, better able to articulate the area's needs, and better able to manage the CEO's aggressive nature. She dreads meeting with him, but then when the next meeting comes, he is either absolutely supportive and understanding or absolutely unsupportive and aggressive. She never knows what to expect. When she spoke with her colleagues about their relationship with the CEO, they all expressed that he was fine with them. She also met with the CFO to discuss her area's revenue, expenses, and productivity levels. The CFO was helpful and explained that the biggest problem is the way the contracts have been negotiated and that the revenue level is not in Julie's control. He indicated that the hospital decided to negotiate a low rate for maternity and newborn services in order to get a higher rate for critical care patients.

The situation begins to escalate for Julie beyond the one-on-one meetings with the CEO. He begins to attack and belittle her in the Monday meetings in front of her peers, laugh at comments she makes on any subject, and makes a point of reminding her peers that Julie's area is a revenue loser. At one meeting, the CEO distributed an article that he liked from the *Harvard Business Review* but he did not give one to Julie. When she asked if he had another copy for her, he answered, "What, little Miss PhD, I assumed you'd already know all about this." Her peers said nothing, but Julie noticed that they simply hung their heads, except for Janice who was chuckling with her hand over her mouth.

Julie, at wit's end, finally confided to Gabriella that she was considering leaving the organization. She felt absolutely defeated and could never predict what to expect from the CEO. Gabriella listened carefully and then said, "Julie, don't you see what is going on here? You are the classic abused woman. The CEO beats you up and you go away blaming yourself and promising to be better. He then feels guilty and treats you better the next time, but the cycle continues over and over. Now he is becoming more aggressive and humiliating to you in public. You have a choice. You can leave, but you will never see this issue to closure and it might affect your work in the future . . . or you can choose to break the cycle."

Questions

1. Who are the stakeholders in this case? Analyze the case by taking on the role and perspective of each stakeholder.
2. Gabriella indicates that Julie is functioning in a way similar to "abused woman syndrome." Considering the 10 principles discussed in this chapter, what do you think are the dynamics among the executive directors and CEO in this case?
3. When working in such a dysfunctional relationship and organization, what do you think are Julie's best options to heal herself and manage her professional career?

References

Adams, J. M., Zimmermann, D., Cipriano, P. F., Pappas, S., & Batcheller, J. (2018). Improving the work life of health care workers: Building on nursing's experience. *Medical Care, 56*(1), 1–3.

Auerbach, D. I., Buerhaus, P. I., & Staiger, D. O. (2017). Millennials almost twice as likely to be registered nurses as baby boomers were. *Health Affairs, 36*(10), 1804–1807.

Awdish, R. L. A., & Berry, L. L. (2019, May 9). Putting healing back at the center of health care. *Harvard Business Review*. https://hbr.org/2019/05/putting-healing-back-at-the-center-of-health-care

Baggett, M., Giambattista, L., Lobbestael, L., Pfeiffer, J., Madani, C., Modir, R., Zamora-Flyr, M. M., & Davidson, J. E. (2016). Exploring the human emotion of feeling cared for in the workplace. *Journal of Nursing Management, 24*(6), 816–824.

Barrett, R. (1995). *A guide to liberating your soul*. Unfoldment.

Benner, P., Hooper-Kyriakidis, P., & Stannard, D. (1999). *Clinical wisdom and interventions in critical care: A thinking-in-action approach*. Saunders.

Berwick, D. M., Nolan, T. W., & Whittington, J. (2008). The triple aim: Care, health, and cost. *Health Affairs (Millwood), 27*(3), 759–769.

Bodenheimer, T., & Sinsky, C. (2014). From triple to quadruple aim: Care of the patient requires care of the provider. *Annals of Family Medicine, 12*(6), 573–576.

Brigham, T., Barden, C., Legreid Dopp, A., Hengerer, A., Kaplan, J., Malone, B., Martin, C., McHugh, M., & Nora, L. M. (2018). A journey to construct an all-encompassing conceptual model of factors affecting clinician well-being and resilience. *NAM Perspectives.* Discussion Paper, National Academy of Medicine, Washington, DC. https://nam.edu/journey-construct-encompassing-conceptual-model-factors-affecting--clinician-well-resilience

Bushe, G. R. (2014). Appreciative leadership. *Journal of the Academy of Nutrition and Dietetics, 114*(Suppl. 5), S26–S27.

Carson, K. D., & Carson, P. P. (1997). Career entrenchment: A quiet march toward occupational death. *Academy of Management Executives, 11*(2), 62–76.

Carucci, R. (2018, May). 3 ways senior leaders create a toxic culture. *Harvard Business Review*. https://hbr.org/2018/05/3-ways-senior-leaders-create-a-toxic-culture

Center for Creative Leadership. (2018, June 21). What future-ready leaders do differently. https://www.humanresourcesonline.net/what-future-ready-leaders-do-differently/

Druck, J., Perry, M., Heron, S., & Martin, M. L. (2019). Microaggressions. In M. L. Martin, S. Heron, L. Moreno-Walton, & M. Strickland (Eds.), *Diversity and inclusion in quality patient care: Your Story/Our Story—A case-based compendium* (2nd ed.; pp. 15–22). Springer.

Dzurec, L. C., Kennison, M., & Gillen, P. (2017). The incongruity of workplace bullying victimization and inclusive excellence. *Nursing Outlook, 65*, 588–596.

Edmondson, A. (2019). *The fearless organization: Creating psychological safety in the workplace for learning, innovation, and growth*. Wiley & Sons.

Gallo, A. (2013, August 29). How to manage someone you don't like. *Harvard Business Review*. http://blogs.hbr.org/2013/08/how-to-manage-someone-you-dont

Griffin, M., & Clark, C. M. (2014). Revisiting cognitive rehearsal as an intervention against incivility and lateral violence in nursing: 10 years later. *The Journal of Continuing Education in Nursing, 45*(12), 535–544.

Hoffman, R., Casnocha, B., & Yeh, C. (2014). *The alliance: Managing talent in the networked age*. Harvard Business Review Press.

Huang, C. A., & Lynch, J. (1995). *Mentoring: The Tao of giving and receiving wisdom.* Harper Collins.

Kim, W., Nicotera, A. M., & McNulty, J. (2015). Nurses' perceptions of conflict as constructive or destructive. *Journal of Advanced Nursing, 71*(9), 2073–2083.

Lee, T. H. (2016). *An epidemic of empathy in healthcare: How to deliver compassionate, connected patient care that creates a competitive advantage.* McGraw-Hill.

Lundin, W., & Lundin, K. (1993). *The healing manager: How to build quality relationships and productive cultures at work.* Berrett-Koehler.

Mahoney, D. (2016, April 21). Building and sustaining an engaged culture: The experts weigh in. *Press Ganey.* https://www.pressganey.com/blog/building-and-sustaining-an-engaged-culture-the-experts-weigh-in

Makic, M. B. F. (2018). A culture of civility; positively impacting practice and patient safety. *Journal of PeriAnesthesia Nursing, 33*(2), 220–222.

Malloch, K. (2001). The white lies of leadership. *Nursing Administration Quarterly, 25*(3), 61–68.

McKee, A. (2019, April). Keep your company's toxic culture from infecting your team. *Harvard Business Review.* https://hbr.org/2019/04/keep-your-companys-toxic-culture-from-infecting-your-team

Moraes, L. J., Miranda, M. B., Loures, L. F., Mainieri, A. G., & Mamora, C. H. C. (2018). A systematic review of psychoneuroimmunology-based interventions. *Psychology, Health & Medicine, 23*(6), 635–652.

Ofri, D. (2019, June 8). The business of health care depends on exploiting doctors and nurses. *The New York Times.* https://www.nytimes.com/2019/06/08/opinion/sunday/hospitals-doctors-nurses-burnout.html

Padilla, T. (2017). Kindness: At the center of patient experience strategies. *Journal of Healthcare Management, 62*(4), 229–233.

Porath, C., & Pearson, C. (2013). The price of incivility: Lack of respect hurts morale—and the bottom line. *Harvard Business Review, 91*(1), 115–121.

Porter-O'Grady, T. (2000). A call for leaders. *SSM, 6*(10), 10–12.

Robinson, S. L., & O'Leary-Kelly, A. M. (1998). Monkey see, monkey do: The influence of work groups on the antisocial behavior of employees. *Academy of Management Journal, 41,* 658–672.

Rushton, C. H. (2018). *Moral resilience: Transforming moral suffering in healthcare.* Oxford University Press.

Shanafelt, T., Swensen, S. J., Woody, J., Levin, J., & Lillie, J. (2018). Physician and nurse well-being: Seven things hospital boards should know. *Journal of Healthcare Management, 63*(6), 363–369.

Taylor, B. (2017, December). The 4 kinds of leaders who create the future. *Harvard Business Review.* https://hbr.org/2017/12/the-4-kinds-of-leaders-who-create-the-future

Thew, J. (2019, July 19). Millennial nurses need patient connection to thrive professionally, researcher says. HealthLeaders. https://www.healthleadersmedia.com/nursing/millennial-nurses-need-patient-connection-thrive-professionally-researcher-says

Tye, J., & Dent, B. (2017). *Building a culture of ownership in healthcare.* Sigma Theta Tau International.

Uhl-Bien, M., Marion, R., & McKelvey, B. (2008). Complexity leadership theory. In R. Marion & M. Uhl-Bien (Eds.), *Complexity leadership part 1: Conceptual foundations* (pp. 185–224). Information Age Publishing.

Weberg, D., & Fuller, R. (2019). Toxic leadership: Three lessons from complexity science to identify and stop toxic teams. *Nurse Leader, 17*(1), 22–26.

Zacher, H., Ambiel, R. A. M., & Noronha, A. P. P. (2015). Career adaptability and career entrenchment. *Journal of Vocational Behavior, 88,* 164–173.

Zak, P. (2017, March). The neuroscience of trust: Management behaviors that foster engagement. *Harvard Business Review.* https://www.emcleaders.com/wp-content/uploads/2017/03/hbr-neuroscience-of-trust.pdf

Suggested Readings

Carlson, R., & Shield, B. (Eds.). (1989). *Healers on healing.* Jeremy P. Tarcher.

Hardy, R. E., & Schwartz, R. (1996). *The self-defeating organization: How smart companies can stop outsmarting themselves.* Addison-Wesley.

Kets de Vries, M. F. R., & Miller, D. (1984). *The neurotic organization.* Jossey-Bass.

Palmer, P. J. (1998). *The courage to teach: Exploring the inner landscape of a teacher's life.* Jossey-Bass.

Rosenstein, A. H., & O'Daniel, M. (2005). Disruptive behavior and clinical outcomes: Perceptions of nurses and physicians. *Nursing Management, 36*(1), 18–28.

Thurston, B. (2013, July/August). #Unplug. *Fast Company,* 73–75.

Ulrich, B., Barden, C., Cassidy, L., & Varn-Davis, N. (2019). Critical care nurse work environments 2018: Findings and implications. *Critical Care Nurse, 39*(2), 67–84.

Quiz Questions

Select the best answer for each of the following questions.

1. Which of the following best describes toxic behaviors in healthcare organizations?
   a. They are behaviors and practices that work against the delivery of healthcare services.
   b. They are engaged in specifically by individuals fearful of accountability.
   c. They can usually be remedied easily once the toxins are identified.
   d. They result from established rituals rather than faulty communication.

2. Much like physical toxins that cause illness in individuals, toxic behaviors cause illness in organizations. Which of the following is true of both human illness and organizational illness?
   a. Illness results from an imbalance in the amount and type of nutrients and cleansing activities.
   b. Additional nutrients lead to the restoration of health.
   c. Routine cleansing of waste is an effective means of restoring health.
   d. Health is the absence of dysfunction.

3. What are toxic behaviors in healthcare organizations caused by?
   a. Decreased financial support resulting from the advent of managed care
   b. The personal characteristics of the leaders and employees coupled with the realities of the marketplace
   c. A lack of leadership development
   d. Poor parenting during the leaders' developmental years

4. Why are vertical organizations often considered toxic?
   a. The departments do not communicate with each other.
   b. The customer (or patient) is not the first concern.
   c. The vigilance of the senior leaders is not appreciated by the employees and other leaders.
   d. Authority and decision making are localized at the top.

5. How can the use of mandatory overtime as a management practice in healthcare organizations be characterized?
    a. It is an appropriate means of responding to staffing needs where life and death situations frequently occur.
    b. It shows an unjustifiable lack of consideration for the need of employees to balance work and personal life.
    c. It is a matter best handled through legislation at the state level.
    d. It should be up to each organization to use as it sees fit.

6. An employee who feels entrenched or entrapped may well experience hope when:
    a. the organization brings in a new leadership team.
    b. the employee is released from the expectation that he or she will perform community service.
    c. the employee is rotated to a different position to explore another career option within the confines of the organization.
    d. a new employee benefits package is implemented.

7. Tolerance of antisocial behaviors has a negative impact on the social climate and general moral conduct of employees. When can antisocial behaviors be minimized?
    a. When group interaction is encouraged and work tasks are shared
    b. When individual members of the group confront the offending employees
    c. When these behaviors are discouraged by the organization's leader
    d. When employees with a history of antisocial behavior are not allowed to join groups in which antisocial behavior is absent

8. How can individual accountability best be described?
    a. It is the ability to give the reasons for one's actions upon request.
    b. It is something that happens to or is inflicted upon an individual.
    c. It is ownership of one's behaviors.
    d. It is the process of seeing it, owning it, solving it, and doing it.

9. If leaders are inconsistent in word and action, employees:
    a. wonder whether their decisions will be respected.
    b. view regular communication as unimportant.
    c. feel a lack of support from the leaders.
    d. feel entrapped, angry, and insecure.

10. The importance of therapeutic relationships between employees and leaders is not always recognized. What is the expected outcome of such relationships?
    a. Improved communication and more productive interaction
    b. More accurate medical documentation
    c. Preservation of confidentiality
    d. Improved job satisfaction

11. Advocacy is often misunderstood by leaders, especially when efforts are expended to repair a broken system. Which of the following is the best way to view patient advocacy?
    a. As the process of creating the necessary conditions for patients to receive the care they desire
    b. As the proper responsibility of an ombudsman within the healthcare facility
    c. As a means of quickly addressing the situations in which patient requests were not honored
    d. As a desirable but often unattained phenomenon

12. Self-assessment is an essential task for a leader who wants to transform his or her organization. For this type of leader, what is the goal of self-assessment?
    a. To create a sense of identity with the organization and motivate the leader to do his or her very best
    b. To discover both positive and negative behaviors that affect performance
    c. To share personal flaws with other employees
    d. To identify continuing education needs

13. Effective mentoring for aspiring leaders is best described as:
    a. a partnership with another aspiring leader to learn about many leadership roles.
    b. a collaboration with an experienced leader of one's organization to experience multiple organization processes.
    c. an interactive process with a national leadership expert.
    d. an evolving process in which multiple experiences, guidance from many leaders in different organizations, and opportunities for leadership occur.

14. Patient care decision making that is dominated by one group of clinicians is considered toxic for the following reasons:
    a. the decision is autocratic.
    b. the contributions of team members are minimized and devalued.
    c. efficiency is the most important factor.
    d. variation is reduced.

15. The business of healing requires all of the following, *except*:
    a. positive relationships between physicians and nurses.
    b. organizational environment collaboration.
    c. adequate funding as needed by the organization.
    d. decision making at the point-of-care.

16. Abuse of power is present in all the following situations, *except*:
    a. adjustment of staffing ratios in order to meet budget targets.
    b. a nurse yelling at another nurse curing a crisis.
    c. creating documentation entries based on the time medication was due rather than the actual time given to the patient.
    d. implementing mandatory overtime during an external disaster.

17. Discriminatory practices can be addressed by all of the following, *except*:
    a. employee meal choices offered based on ethnicity of staff and patients.
    b. selecting membership for organizational committees from all departments in the organization.
    c. ensuring an all-male staff in the maintenance department to provide heavy lifting of equipment.
    d. ensuring an all-female staff in the obstetrics area when requested by the patient.

18. Career adaptability is important to organizational success for many reasons. Which is the best combination of strategies to support career adaptability?
    a. Professional development related to recognizing career successes, anticipating new career opportunities within the organization, and an orientation to future opportunities
    b. Understanding that some jobs will be eliminated and employees will lose jobs in the normal course of business
    c. Professional development specific to managing job eliminations
    d. Encouraging leaders to engage in career planning with all employees

19. Middle-of-the-road performance reviews that fail to highlight accomplishments are the result of:
    a. strong connections between the performance process and compensation levels.
    b. the lack of competence in documentation of performance.
    c. limited resources for recognition.
    d. previous average performance reviews.

20. Toxic mentoring is often not easy to recognize. Which of the following behaviors is *not* toxic?
    a. One mentor controlling the mentoring process
    b. Exploring past successes of multiple role models
    c. Focused mentoring in one organization
    d. Exploring mentor behaviors in nonrelated industries

21. "Walking one's talk" is a simple phrase often touted as the behavior to role model trust. White lies violate this trust for all of the following behaviors, *except*:
    a. providing ambiguous and contradictory messages.
    b. providing contradictory messages to allow time to fully examine issues.
    c. avoiding conflict in public.
    d. There is no good reason for a white lie.

22. Minimizing toxicity in the organization includes valuing the truth of the whole. This strategy involves:
    a. providing full disclosure to the involved individuals.
    b. understanding the pros and cons of a situation.
    c. providing the strongest supporting evidence for a situation.
    d. understanding the multiple perspectives of a situation.

23. Which of the following behaviors will *not* reduce organizational toxicity?
    a. Avoiding hurtful and open sharing of negative information
    b. Eliminating insulting and profane language
    c. Sharing negative feedback 3 months after the incident occurred
    d. Providing performance feedback on a regular basis

24. Respectful relationships with patients include all of the following, *except*:
    a. including family when the patient consents to their involvement.
    b. always including families in discussion with the patient.
    c. encouraging a malingering patient to become more active.
    d. not calling elderly patients by their first name or grandpa/grandma.

25. Accountability for one's actions on a consistent basis can be challenging. Which of the following responses in *not* toxic?
    a. Entitled practices
    b. Lack of meaningful measurement tools
    c. Unclear expectations or rationale for behaviors
    d. Daily performance documentation

CHAPTER TWELVE

Coaching for Unending Change: Transforming the Membership Community

We can succeed only by concert. It is not "can any of us imagine better?" but, "can we all do better?" The dogmas of the quiet past are inadequate to the stormy present. The occasion is piled high with difficulty, and we must rise with the occasion. As our case is new, so we must think anew, and act anew.

—Abraham Lincoln, 1862

Chapter Objectives

At the completion of this chapter, the reader will be able to:

- Recognize the key elements of coaching within a fast-paced organization in highly charged and changing times.
- Translate the characteristics of transformational coaching into the planning and implementation of new skill formation.
- Describe the needs of teams in a system and explain the importance of team leadership.
- Identify the fundamentals of the learning organization and the dynamics of learning leadership.
- Name the steps of revolutionary and innovation coaching and how it applies to the role of the leader.

Leadership, in the contemporary healthcare system, requires both an accommodation to the realities of complexity and a deep understanding of the action of complexity. In this accelerating age of complexity, no role has been more greatly challenged. The role of leader requires a whole new frame for expression. Much of the work of leaders now is directed toward helping others confront the vagaries of major changes occurring in the work and structure of the workplace. Leaders must exhibit a new set of skills to create the conditions for a new care environment that ties effective service quality directly to positive health outcomes. The mental models and performance expectations of staff require heavy retooling to ensure that they can

> **Key Point**
> Leadership requires a level of self-knowledge and vulnerability that makes the growth experience visible to others.

thrive in the new work environment. This chapter presents some of the elements of leading in this new environment and the steps necessary to get staff engaged and motivated to change and grow in a context that demands a different way of delivering health care.

Leadership is not so much who you are as what you do with who you are. Leadership is not a state of being. It is instead a set of internal tools possessed by a person with the energy and skill to use them well. Much of the work of leadership in this new century consists of transferring new skills to the people who live and work in organizations.

Because this is a time of great change, increasing complexity, and fast-moving advances in technology, with higher expectations for health in an accountable care environment, people find it increasingly difficult to meet the growing number of new demands. Social and technological forces conspire to create the conditions that affect how people work, relate, and plan for their own future. In this process, the role of leaders is to live the positive experience of change and master the ability to engage the questions and challenges that accompany change. Staff members are watching closely to see how leaders embrace and engage the challenges of change. By observing how leaders do this, staff members create a vision for their own adjustment to change. The leaders' role modeling of adjustment to change encourages staff to adapt to change and demonstrates the necessary techniques.

From Responsibility to Accountability

In in the growing demand for value-based accountable care, responsibility is no longer the key element of work performance. Historically, a worker's performance was judged to be acceptable if the worker simply did well what he or she was supposed to do. For the performance to be evaluated as excellent, the worker had to do this work and do it exceptionally well. In the 20th-century workplace, the focus on responsibility was prevalent in every aspect of the definition of work and the measurement of performance.

This focus was structured in the workplace in several ways. First, job descriptions were often laundry lists of functions and activities. In other words, they zeroed in on the activities of work rather than their product. Second, performance evaluations reviewed the work someone did—the functions of work and the ability of the person to do the work. The person's behavior and ability to get along with others were included in the list of "competencies." How well the person did the work, not whether the work was worthwhile, determined whether the person was to be specially rewarded. Third, the evaluation of work tended to concentrate on the quality of the work processes—how the work was done and how many errors were committed. It also looked at efficiency, or the amount of time the worker spent in delivering a service or product as compared with the average.

Slavish attachment to process was an earmark of the 20th-century workplace. Process improvement, process evaluation, process measurement, process effectiveness—these all concern what workers do rather than what they achieve. One reason for this may be that, in health care, the relationship between outcome and process has never been well understood.

In this 21st-century accountable care environment, work is now viewed from the perspective of its outcomes. Research has shown that focusing on outcomes alters work processes and the elements of the work. Indeed, it is now clear that all processes gain their meaning from their results or products. In other words, a process is considered valuable to the extent it relates "tightly" to the desired outcome. Much effort is now being expended on investigating the goodness-of-fit between work processes and their intended outcomes and improving the fit where possible.

In short, it is the Age of Accountability. The major role of leaders is to move people and organizations from responsibility to accountability—from a narrow focus on processes to a perspective that encompasses processes and results (**Exhibit 12-1**). In the Age of Accountability, leaders are expected to ensure that all components of the fit between processes and results come together into a complete vision of the work and its products. Among other tasks, they need to define expected outcomes for all actions and activities and to establish aggregate performance measures for evaluating the work performed by teams.

This movement toward the appreciation of outcomes requires a tremendous reorientation of the work and the workers. For the whole of the 20th century, the emphasis was on functions and work processes, whereas now it is on creating sustainability in a time of rapid technological change. Focusing on work processes is no longer a viable strategy because they have such short life spans. The appropriate goal is to define the critical integration between means and ends, products and processes. This must be done with an understanding that sustainability is not resident in the work or even the incremental product of a given process or time. Sustainability instead results from a continuum of efforts that, when connected together, indicate the journey to be taken to improve the conditions or quality of life. In fact, this is the definitive foundation of the movement from volume-based health services to value-driven health outcomes.

Accountability is internally generated. It arises first and foremost within. Specifically, accountability is the result of a person's commitment to advancing, improving, growing, adapting, and enhancing his or her life experience. Accountability is generated out of

> **Point to Ponder**
>
> Accountability requires that people have ownership of their work. The shift is from the organization holding people accountable to self-accountability. Consequently, the organization must recognize that it does not control the work that people do but simply provides the context and scaffolding within which they do it.

Exhibit 12-1 Responsibility Versus Accountability

Responsibility (20th Century)	Accountability (21st Century)
• Process	• Product
• Action	• Result
• Work	• Outcome
• Do	• Accomplish
• Task	• Difference
• Function	• Fit
• Job	• Role
• Incremental	• Sustainable
• Externally generated	• Internally generated

the energy that a person brings to the exercise of living, whether at work or in other realms of life. In addition, accountability depends on individuals' having complete ownership of what they are and what they do and their commitment to apply their talents, energies, and skills in ways that make the circumstances of life better for themselves and others.

In an organization, in particular, accountability depends on members joining in a concerted, collective effort to achieve the organization's ends. If each person brings his or her energy, gifts, skills, and knowledge to bear fully on the work to be done, the outcomes of that work are assured. Everyone in the workplace has a right to expect a commitment from all to apply themselves and use their skills and talents to the fullest. Furthermore, everyone has a right to expect that each team member (or employee in a group work context) will have a positive relationship with the other members and exhibit energy and commitment to the work and its products.

Leaders are obligated to make certain that the processes and structures needed to support ownership of the work are fully present. The structure provides the framework that enables the requisite knowledge, education, practices, performance, regulation, competency, and impact for the practice of the professional discipline. These professional behaviors directly demonstrate the successful expression of what the structure enables (Porter-O'Grady, 2020). Each of the three main components—structure, relationship, and process—should be directed toward facilitating ownership so that the organization's work can be sustained and advanced. If the energy and desire of the worker cannot be maintained, it is impossible to sustain and advance the work of the organization.

Leaders must understand and apply the principles of human action and interaction. Human beings are dynamic and complex beings. When colleagues' commitment and motivation are at high levels, conflicts and other challenges arise. The work processes in place must be designed with the understanding that such challenges are normal and to be expected. They should also be designed to anticipate these challenges and address them in a way that increases the probability of good outcomes and sustains the work and the relationships among the employees.

In accountability-based organizations, leaders must recognize that the vagaries of human behavior and relationship are normal. Leaders must be aware of the whole spectrum of human dynamics and be capable of managing these dynamics. They must have tools and techniques to maintain the energy and focus of the workplace and its members in a way that advances the work and the achievement of desirable outcomes.

One of these techniques is to establish the expectation that principles are consistently applied and that accountability is maintained. If this is made clear to all members of the organization, along with a commitment not to permit behavior inconsistent with this expectation, the members will try to live up to the expectation and act appropriately. In accountability-based work processes, members articulate and enumerate the range of acceptable practices and behaviors, and processes for creating consistency are available to help members address those issues outside the agreed framework. Membership in a work group, like membership in any other collaborative enterprise, requires that the

> **Key Point**
>
> In an organization, the leader is responsible for creating a sustainable structure for work and ensuring a good fit between the organization's goals and processes. Congruence here guarantees that the system functions as it should.

expressed expectations for the members are fulfilled; otherwise, the goals of the group are threatened or only partially achieved.

In regard to accountability, certain patterns of behavior reflect negative characteristics that ultimately impede personal expression and team interaction in the workplace (Brewer & Sanford, 2011; Hickey & Kritek, 2012; Lencioni, 2008). Which ones fall below the line and which above depends on the particular culture and context of the workplace. Members must clearly outline the two sets of behaviors to form a framework for the principles that determine the rules of engagement in the work relationship. The structure and process of leading and managing must be designed to ensure that the above-the-line behaviors are sustained. When the below-the-line behaviors emerge, the processes and methodologies in place must "click in" so that these behaviors can be addressed quickly and effectively. Quick response to behavioral variances is essential to prevent subsequent and sometimes irresolvable problems.

It must be remembered that accountability really means something. So often in the past decade accountability lost its central meaning and its impact on organizations and people. The financial scandals of the 1990s and the 2000s highlighted just how little understanding of accountability really exists. Accountability assumes that the leader accepts the full responsibility of that which occurs under the auspices of his or her leadership. It does not matter whether someone else "did the deed"; it only matters that the leader claims accountability for the actions of those for whom he or she holds leadership responsibility.

Accountability has three major elements: the right to decide and act—autonomy; the power to decide and act—authority; and the capacity to decide and act—competence. Productive accountability requires all three to be present in the role of the leader. Failure to exercise any of the three elements always results in a failure of accountability. Personal and organizational conflict result when any one of these elements is missing from the expression of accountability. Persons and organizations suffer when there is a failure to integrate or appropriately express these components of accountability in the best interest of persons and organizations.

The dynamics of relationship and work are highly complex and variable. Although it might seem beneficial for the framework for human behavior in the workplace to be permanent and unchanging, a permanent framework, besides being impractical, is inappropriate. It is within the course of relationships and interpersonal demands that the vagaries of life always have an impact. Personal patterns of behavior and changing patterns of interaction challenge the best work environment.

Good leaders "read" work situations. They assess the demands and the dynamics of intersecting and interacting variables and judge how they affect the work being done and the relationships among the workers. They know that these variables create challenges for work relationships and functions—challenges that they are required to address. Research in the area of accountable behavior and organizational considerations is ongoing. Thus, leaders need to review this research periodically to gain up-to-date information on how to ensure that work processes result in desired outcomes.

> **Point to Ponder**
>
> Typically, approximately 90% of the leadership role is devoted to managing relationships. If a leader determines that managing relationships takes up a much smaller percentage of work time than that, the leader may need to reassess her or his priorities.

> **Group Discussion**
>
> The words *responsibility* and *accountability* often are used interchangeably, but they have different meanings. Based on the analysis of accountability in this chapter, compare how to change behavior in an accountability-based organization and how to change it in a responsibility-based organization.

Transforming Work and the Transforming Worker

During the current era, the major leadership task is to change the mental model of and framework for work. In all segments of society, work and the workplace are changing too fast for most people to keep up. Leaders, therefore, must guide the transformation of work and help people adjust, as required.

For transformation to occur, a fundamental change in thinking must take place. Workers, for example, must completely reconceptualize their roles. Most people are satisfied with establishing a pattern of work and a set of rituals. Eventually, they become so accustomed to the pattern and rituals that they see them as essential to the work. Indeed, they begin to see the work from within these patterns and rituals and ultimately become suspicious of anything that threatens what has become normal for them. Despite the fact that their adherence to patterns and rituals may impede necessary changes, leaders, who are agents of change, should not criticize them.

Leaders who try to bring about certain changes often become so unhappy with people's attachment to rituals that the rituals become the visible representation of people's unwillingness to change. After all, people's attachment to the routines of work ensures that the work gets done and meets certain standards of performance. Their attachment may obstruct improvements in quality, but it does virtually guarantee performance of the work activities.

In times of transformation, leaders look to establish new patterns of work, even if the patterns soon need to be revised because of further rapidly changing circumstances. In addition, leaders often want workers to establish the same kind of attachment to a new pattern even though they complained when the workers were attached to the old patterns.

There are also organizational dangers to transformative thinking. This type of thinking is characterized by a willingness to seriously question all current processes and can threaten organizational stability. During transformation, leaders engage the staff and other stakeholders in a dialogue and hear what would normally not be expressed. In fact, to make the transformation succeed, the leaders must be open to new ideas and be willing to listen to all kinds of responses from all stakeholders. Even the thinking that underpins the changes must be subject to questioning and exploration if the implementation of new ideas is to be appropriately rigorous and thorough. The environment necessary to support transformative thinking creates a level of challenge and instability that even leaders may not be comfortable with (**Figure 12-1** and **Exhibit 12-2**).

> **Key Point**
>
> A whole body of research demonstrates that an open, inclusive, and accountable structure for work creates extra opportunities for creativity and innovation.

20th-Century work

Chaos

21st-Century work

Ordered
Vertical
Stable
Controlled

Destabilizing
Noisy
Uncertain
Fast paced

Team based
Horizontal
Relational
Integrated

Figure 12-1 Transition from 20th-Century Work. The transition involves moving through the stages of change from predominantly vertical organizations to more horizontal systems.

Exhibit 12-2   Causes of Transformation

- Destabilized environment
- Noise
- Culture of change
- Loss
- Emerging reality

- New financial realities
- Demand for new behaviors
- Work process changes
- Shifting technology
- Rapid change in work requirements (i.e., pandemic)

The process of transformation requires an environment in which creativity and change are embraced. In other words, discourse, deliberation, dialogue, consensus building, and experimentation must be viewed as safe and appropriate strategies. Leaders must first accept a comfort in the vulnerability of the leader role to enable risk taking to occur as the norm and then create an environment for creativity and change before they can expect to see innovation and engagement with change become routine in their units or services. If the staff members do not feel safe in the presence of change, they certainly will not feel comfortable making change.

Living in an environment of horizontal relationships and accountability-based controls rather than management-driven decision making and vertical controls is a different experience for all parties. The former type of environment, however, is essential for transformative thinking and acting. Very little research suggests that rigid vertical control structures lead naturally to change and innovation. On the other hand, a whole body of research indicates that an open, inclusive, and accountable work structure creates numerous opportunities for creativity and innovation.

Biology has lessons for organizational survival. Biological research shows that growth and adaptation are required for life to continue. If the environment changes noticeably because of some cataclysmic event or the accumulation of small alterations, plants and animals either adapt or cease to exist. Indeed, past changes form the foundation for future changes, and adaptation to earlier changes determines the level of adjustment to future changes.

The same is true of organizations and other forms of social life. Even minor changes can upset the delicate balance that allows certain kinds of organizations to thrive and can turn the environment instead into a threatening place. For organizations to survive in this world, many of the processes and behaviors, rituals and routines that have their foundation in Industrial Age models of leadership thinking must be replaced by new processes and behaviors grounded in understanding of complex organizational dynamics. The transition requires true leadership and a transformational format for radically altering everything that workers know and do.

> ### Group Discussion
>
> In the emerging world of health care, the major leadership task is to transform people's attitudes and insights regarding the changes that are required of them. On a flip chart, list changes that affect what healthcare clinicians must now do in a reformed system and list attitudes toward the demand for change. Order the attitudes based on their potential influence, and discuss how a healthcare leader could alter the two most important attitudes to smooth the transition to new ways of working.

Evolution and Revolution

The major difference between evolution and revolution is the rate of change—the amount of time it takes for changes to occur. Certainly, the social digital transformation, because of its high rate of innovation, is undergoing a revolution, but the resulting changes in society are occurring at more of an evolutionary pace. It takes much longer to incorporate social and behavioral changes than to implement technological advances. Yet both types of change must be accommodated, and people need to adjust at a fast rate and a more studied rate. The challenge is to know which is occurring and to attach the right rate of accommodation to the process.

Leaders in an organization need to recognize the demand for change in enough time to respond correctly—at the right time and in the right format. Of course, leaders cannot know all changes far enough in advance to allow appropriate and timely responses. Nonetheless, the chance of responding correctly is increased if leaders assess the probability of reasonably likely changes and consider the expected effects. By anticipating the kind of changes that will occur, developing an understanding of their conditions and circumstances, and passing this understanding on to the staff, leaders ensure that the staff can react appropriately. In short, leaders must be signpost readers and articulate trends clearly enough to create a picture of their impact. Contemporary trends in the funding of health care and the growth of consumerism require significant and specific changes in the context and content of clinical practice, representing the shifting requisites of an accountable care environment (Naylor & Kurtzman, 2010; Porter-O'Grady, 2013; Shomaker, 2011).

Leaders must also be transformational agents. In coaching staff members to embrace necessary changes, leaders must show the same tone, enthusiasm, and skill in adaptation they expect from others. Seeing the signposts is simply the first step in transferring the information to the staff in a way that puts accountability for response into their hands. Leaders must be able to see systemness and complexity as normal conditions of change and adaptation. Through expressing their accountability for witnessing and previewing the potential for change, leaders prepare the staff to deal with the right change at the right time and in the right circumstances.

Transformational coaching requires leaders to engage in an array of activities that move employees through the process of responding to essential changes in a way that embraces the changes and achieves desired outcomes. In fact, leaders are responsible for creating a system of response to essential changes and then creating a structure and process for these changes to occur as lived or operational experience. Transformational coaching is more of a system than a process, and in applying the components of this system leaders can ensure a dynamic, ongoing framework for adaptation and engagement.

The Learning Organization

An organization's ability to adapt to change depends on how open and responsive the social and organizational context is to change and to the dynamic processes of learning. If the organization values change and learning, the vagaries of change will be less traumatic and incidentally dynamic. Research has uncovered the rules of engagement for creating a true learning context.

Chris Argyris (2006), in a review of the research, indicated some basic criteria for success at any level of organizational learning and change. The focus must first be on behaviors and attitudes. Identifying the fundamentals of behavior and the factors that influence specific behaviors is critical for creating a context and process for change. Once these behaviors and attitudes are identified, the focus switches to the vagaries that affect particular behaviors or recurrent patterns of behavior and through them affect the way work is done or the way it is adapted to new realities (Argote, 2013; Westerwick et al., 2016).

Leadership wisdom potentiates an organization's ability to learn. Managers and supervisors draw from the skills of data analytics, conflict resolution, and other performance-based practices. In contrast, the cultivation of wise leaders yields a leader who acquires more complex and adaptive ways of thinking. Often a coach is necessary to guide a leader into this advanced space, however many move independently past a focus on personal and organizational needs fulfillment to a higher order of leadership associated with belonging and relationships serving the common good. When the leader is solely focused on survival as in the managerial function, fear and cautionary leadership behaviors prevail. Leaders who grow past this self-interest level to an emphasis on the common good develop courage and the ability to influence and evolve as visionary leaders. At this level, they learn agility and are most likely to transform because of their comfort with vulnerability and self-awareness. Leaders are then considered wise—leaders who have exceptional insight into human development, look for deeper meaning, tolerate ambiguity, have compassion, are purpose focused, and for whom purpose serves as the rudder of their actions (Pesut & Thompson, 2018). With the growth of complexity and need for continuous learning, the development of leadership wisdom is necessary. Leading teams past their own managerial behaviors is an important reason to develop leaders with wisdom. The system developed for addressing behaviors must include a mechanism for reducing the number of continuing counterproductive activities and self-fulfilling patterns of behavior that keep participants from fully engaging with the changes they must make. Behaviors that are inconsistent with both norms and expectations find room to exist if not addressed quickly and efficiently. They even stand a chance of becoming the norm, and in any case can compromise the environment and participants in a way that obstructs adaptation to the necessary changes. The noise that results creates a further impediment to the participants' ability to engage with the changes and thrive.

Focusing on the behavior of participants gives leaders an image of the mental and emotional "maps" in operation. Leaders can then use these maps as a beginning point for the process of making meaningful and sustainable change. They need to look critically at the participants' mental maps to determine the pattern of response they have helped to create. In fact, this pattern of response—the participants' theory-in-use—has a more dramatic impact on the participants' engagement with essential change than do the behaviors themselves.

When leaders approach participants to discuss their mental maps, they do need to be cautious. These maps form the contextual framework out of which behavior flows. The theory-in-use is simply the conceptual constant that the person draws on to explain, justify, and retain sufficient commitment or energy to a particular course of action. In this highly individual context, the person seeks to provide a solid values or belief foundation that can give meaning to a position or a specific action. Often, the theory-in-use is identified as the rationale or justification the person uses for his or her actions (Hu et al., 2016). This theory-in-use has only an inferential relationship to the truth. It relates more to the individual's sense of truth or interpretation or application of truth than to anything that may actually be true. Regardless, it is vitally important to the person. It is the theory-in-use out of which that person acts, and it gives a reason for the action. In this issue, leaders find that much of a theory-in-use cannot be discussed, for it concerns who the participants perceive themselves to be, even to the point of being perceived as a part of their identity. A person's role and sense of self in the role and the person's relationships with others and the organization create a foundation for the person's pattern of behaviors. However, because every person's theory-in-use is expressed in his or her pattern of behaviors, the patterns of all participants must be directly addressed if the behaviors necessary to learning, adaptation, and meaningful change are ever to be evidenced in the organization. This awareness of a person's theory-in-use helps the leader understand and address particular behaviors and gives a clearer context to an individual's personal struggle with change. This is where wise leaders are critical.

Almost every organization fails to maintain adaptability over time. The main reason is that organizations, although they might change what people do, usually fall short of changing how they think. Because the conditions of change are now so prevalent, not to change the thinking of people has ceased to be an option. Nurses, for example, must learn to practice in a world where institutional models of practice, hospital stays, and long-term patient relationships no longer define nursing practice. Nurses who complain of a lack of time for patient care have failed to realize that their grievances reflect an outmoded mental model of nursing. Hospital-based stays will continue to shorten, the aged will be cared for in ways that do not require their institutionalization, new pharmaceuticals and gene-based treatments will radically alter how patients are treated, and so on. In this instance, the role of leaders is to assail the old mental model and create a fluid enough foundation for nurses' expectations that they give up their old expectations and acquire new ones.

Physicians also need to be aware that the circumstances that have traditionally been part of medical practice no longer exist. The unilateral, responsible, but nonaccountable practice modalities that once defined medicine are disappearing, to be replaced by accountability-based, outcome-oriented, health-focused, rational, complex, and multifocal modalities. Discussions of the healthcare system are rife with the dissatisfaction expressed by physicians who say they can no longer practice the medicine they know (Wilensky, 2016). The complexity and pace of patient care require the best of multiple disciplines, not just medicine. It is impossible to provide quality care as a lone clinician. What they have failed to recognize is that the 20th-century manual and mechanical model of medicine has died. The one that is emerging, driven by all the improvements and enhancements in therapy and treatment, and growing emphasis on ensuring healthy populations, has altered forever what medicine is and how it will be practiced.

For physicians and others to enthusiastically and energetically engage with the changes affecting medical practices, leaders must confront their mental models directly and in a manner that allows the stakeholders to identify the discrepancies between what they believe and the current reality (Stanford & Wilkins, 2016).

> **Point to Ponder**
>
> Failure to thrive is not uncommon in times of great change. The main reason is that organizations, although they might change what people do, usually fall short of changing how they think.

Effective adaptability also includes leaders developing the ability to predict changes before they actually occur. This predictive skill is now as much a part of the skill set of the leader as any other recognized leadership skill. Predictive capacity calls the leader to synthesize data and information about the convergence of forces and to define the resulting conditions or circumstances. Such skill becomes less optional for leaders as the pace of change quickens and the significance of each change increases the impact on people and groups. The scope of global changes and the broad landscape of change events now call leaders to visualize the groundswell of particular events and to link it to other elements to help prepare organization members for the onset and impact of changes far in advance of experiencing them.

Over the past 35 years, shared governance has enumerated the structural components and context necessary to create the scaffolding for sustainable change and full participation (Porter-O'Grady, 2007, 2009). Now we are joining a host of contemporary leaders in declaring the importance of engagement, shared decision making, self-direction, and professional governance and urge the replacement of traditional organizational and management constructs with currently relevant models of workplace organization (Clavelle et al., 2016).

To gain a fuller understanding of how to adapt to the changes that are occurring, leaders must create an environment that fosters learning. In doing this, they should keep the following in mind:

- Learning must be oriented to the actual experience of the learners in their own environment.
- The purpose of learning is to ensure growth, improvement, and adaptability.
- People need to be empowered to take charge of the design of their own learning and to alter their roles and behaviors in response to what they discover.

- The organization must be willing to allow experimentation and risk taking so that innovation becomes a constant.
- Learning requires time, and the organization must therefore allow staff the time it needs to pursue new knowledge.
- Learning should not be accidental or incremental; an infrastructure for learning should be developed to ensure that innovation and new learning are considered an ongoing part of the way of doing business in any environment.
- People need to feel they are growing and improving. Therefore, learning should always be directed toward giving people new skills that are relevant to their job activities.

Learning can be single loop or double loop. In single-loop learning, the learning process is implemented as designed, and the outcome is achieved as anticipated. Single-loop learning deals with the apparent, the visible, and the symptomatic. In double-loop learning, the governing variables, the driving forces, the root causes, or the foundations for action are understood and applied to the process (Guzman et al., 2015). In addition, the participants are familiar with the process of learning and incorporate it into their own learning activities as an ongoing part of delivering health services. Double-loop learning is essential to sustainable solutions and enduring results.

For learning to occur, especially double-loop learning, participants must understand their own theory-in-use (or automatic reasoning processes). Most people bring their own reasoning processes and preexisting notions to any learning situation and even look for information that validates their preexisting notions. The mother of one of the authors is a smoker of many years. When confronted with the fact that long-term smoking leads inevitably to illness and death, she invariably identifies those rare creatures who are long-lived, lifelong smokers. When reminded that she can name these people because so few are still alive, the logic escapes her. Her theory-in-use forces her to identify the circumstances in which her premises and beliefs can be confirmed and reinforced, giving her, in her own mind, no reason to change her pattern of behavior.

> **Point to Ponder**
>
> Adults learn most easily when they can apply what they have learned. The best approach is to teach them on the job so that they can apply their new knowledge then and there. Likewise, they accept changes most easily when they can act on the changes immediately.

Everyone has preexisting notions and a propensity to try to validate them. Leaders (or anyone else acting as a coach) must recognize the importance of identifying and describing these notions clearly enough to address them and use them as vehicles for personal learning and change. The goal of coaching is to help people acquire new ideas that validate the experience of change and more accurately reflect the prevailing reality, ensuring they have a place in it.

Newer concepts of triple-loop learning encourage a system that supports the questioning of premises, the clarification of beliefs, and the foundation of new learning (Rowland & Hall, 2014). The infrastructure of the organization and the configuration of leadership expectations must now be aligned to ensure that past or current notions or concepts of the work do not become impediments to questioning the prevailing beliefs, practices, rituals, and routines. This becomes necessary to ensure that the organization does not become irrelevant or so inculcated in its own story and practices that it fails to see a different world and role ahead.

Group Discussion

How many of us really know why we believe what we do or act as we do? The members of the group should each identify a statement about their professional work that they believe and two reasons for believing it. What is the theory-in-use in the application of this belief? Do others understand the statement in the same way? Is it really rational to believe the statement? Helping others change means knowing your own rituals and routines and the rational basis for acting on them.

The final step in the learning process is to generalize what has been learned and reinforce it through applied action. Using new knowledge is the best way to incorporate it into the foundation on which the processes of work are built. Furthermore, integrating new knowledge into the foundation leads to additional new learning and to additional revision of the foundation, allowing workers to achieve higher levels of performance and personal satisfaction.

> **Key Point**
>
> Being open to the dynamic processes of learning and change is a requisite of adaptability. The leader is always testing the system to see how much the staff engage with the demands of change and how quickly their roles adjust to new performance expectations and the chaos and vagaries of changing the way work is done.

Leaders need to understand that for double- and triple-loop learning to occur, they must create a culture that promotes the necessary processes and risk taking. This means that every role at every level of the organization—from the very highest levels of authority to the point-of-service—must be involved to some degree in the learning process and make use of available learning tools (**Exhibit 12-3**). In other words, the organization must live the learning process in everything it does. When an organization fails to embrace learning, often the reason is that a genuine culture of learning and adaptation was not designed and structured into the life of the organization. Dynamic adaptation and learning are simply unsustainable in any organization that does not have a vibrant learning culture.

All learning is essentially individual. It begins at the personal level before it can become organization-wide. Therefore, each member of an organization must be expected to engage in learning activities, and the structure of the organization should even make it impossible for members to survive without pursuing new knowledge. The need for all members to become

---

Exhibit 12-3 Action Learning Tools

- Case studies
- Clinical exemplars
- Comparative modeling
- Computerized scenarios
- Group practice sessions
- PowerPoint presentations
- Satellite interactive sessions
- Simulation practice models
- Storyboards
- Video presentations
- Virtual classrooms

more knowledgeable is especially great now because of the reconfiguration of systems and enterprises that is occurring. Leaders, through coaching, can help staff change the language in use and find the right questions to ask—those that reflect the current reality; it is in this reality that the answers lie.

People are so strongly socialized by their past relationships and experiences that it is difficult to alter behaviors resulting from their socialization. When people come to work, their socialized behaviors come with them and are acted out. Leaders must recognize that socialization is a critical factor with regard to change and make sure it is incorporated into the structure and dynamic of learning. By engaging employees in a discussion of the effects of socialization on their behaviors and incorporating that discussion into the learning equation, leaders are more likely to foster the personal changes necessary to generate the shifts in work processes and outcomes.

Organizing for Transformation

Leaders know that behaviors do not change accidentally or on request. The context or culture of the organization or unit plays a major role in determining what behaviors occur and how they become modified. The leader of a unit, for instance, must have in place a uniformly applied set of expectations to ensure that the patterns of behavior are consistent. Further, the expectations and associated patterns of behavior must be congruent with the environmental demands that drive the work of the unit to ensure that responses to the demands are quick and appropriate. Finally, the interplay between behavior and structure must be such that the prevailing operational processes reflect it and can use this intersection as a way of advancing organizational effectiveness.

Another essential leadership task is to establish, together with the unit's members, some basic foundations for the unit's functions. To do this, the leader must continuously assess the patterns of relationship, interaction, and personal and professional behavior within the context of the expectations defined for them. In the culture of adaptation, clearly understood and consistently applied processes assure each participant that the agreed parameters are up front and continuously applied.

The leader should be aware that the purpose of these processes and structures is not to keep people happy. In many organizations, the goal of keeping people happy actually has become an impediment to making them happy. In fact, the knowledge that the leader expects employees to be happy can create conditions that ensure they are not.

Happiness is not something that can be achieved through organizational means; it is instead a personal matter. What is within the leader's purview is keeping employees motivated, invested, involved, engaged, and satisfied with what they are doing. The leader's best chance of creating an environment in which employees are all of these things is to set expectations that are high but not so high as to prevent the employees from consistently meeting and even surpassing them. These expectations and the structures and processes developed to ensure they can be met form the framework for advancing the organization's goals and those of the people who make it up.

The leader is also responsible for ensuring that certain basic requirements for learning and adaptation are in place:

- The members of the unit must be informed of the prevailing rules for personal behavior, personal interaction, and problem identification.

- Innovation must be an expectation of the workplace and of organizational learning to ensure that workers understand that contributing to their own change and that of the system is an expectation of work.
- There must be a mechanism for calling the parties to the table when a problem occurs or an issue arises. This mechanism must become the unit's normal means for first responding to problems and issues.
- There must be a routine mechanism for discussing and critically reviewing each issue that affects the staff. The purpose of this mechanism is to give the relevant parties an opportunity to play an active part in the deliberations and decision making intended to resolve the issue.
- Shared decision-making models should be used for empowering staff members and giving them a role in dealing with issues for which they are accountable.
- There must be a forum and a method of resolution for conflicts between members, concepts, plans, or processes. These conflicts should be addressed as quickly as possible. In the case of conflicts between individuals, the goal is to return the parties to a productive and active relationship with each other. If a good working relationship cannot be established, there must be a mechanism for separating the parties.
- Staff should be involved in the strategic and tactical activities of leadership. In particular, they should participate in decisions that define their future, thereby gaining ownership of their work.

> **Key Point**
> When gathering people together, the first step is to clarify the rules of engagement. Although this can be tiresome, people must be reminded of the expectations regarding interaction and communication. Deliberations break down most often because the parameters for dialogue were not determined, reinforced, and followed.

Besides building appropriate processes and structures, the leader is responsible for stimulating the members of the unit to achieve high levels of performance. This can be done through building a shared vision and helping the members see that their work is a significant part of a great enterprise. The leader must realize that everyone wants to be a part of something important and make a meaningful and sustainable difference. The leader keeps the members as focused on the purpose of their work as on its processes. The members should not become so fixed on the work itself that they lose sight of why they are doing it.

Structure is a critical element in the creation of a meaningful and motivating work environment because it provides the context for behavior and sets the parameters for how the processes of work unfold. A good structure enhances personal interaction, problem solving, learning, and adaptation and keeps alive the human dynamics that energize and give meaning to the work. In the absence of such a structure, none of this can be ensured (**Figure 12-2**).

The Critical Value of Appreciative Leadership

Appreciative leadership is generated from the foundation elements associated with appreciative inquiry. The concept of appreciative inquiry is based on the belief that the positive focus on the best, most vital, and essential values of all living persons and systems can generate shared principles and determine how to move forward together. Generally, appreciative inquiry is reflected in five basic core processes (Watkins et al., 2016):

1. *Definition*: Choosing the positive as a focus of inquiry.
2. *Discovery*: Inquiring into exceptional positive moments.

Figure 12-2 Leader's Focus in Times of Complexity. When moving through the change process, leaders must focus on core elements.

3. *Dream*: Sharing the stories and identifying generative life forces.
4. *Design*: Creating a shared vision of a mutually preferred future.
5. *Delivery*: Engaging in creativity and innovation that constructs and uses a sustainable approach to creating the future.

In an effort to engage the hearts and minds of clinicians while establishing a foundation for innovation, leaders used the concepts of appreciative leadership to create a space for dialogue and collaboration across a continuum of care to improve innovation and accountability. The outcomes from the effort include innovation directly linked to the feedback received in the forums, staff support of emerging system initiatives, appreciative leadership competencies and knowledge, and continued support for the culture of innovation and transformation at the point of care (D'Alfonso et al., 2016).

As an expressive form for appreciative inquiry, appreciative leadership creates the context, skill sets, and application of positive leadership processes and dynamics in a way that facilitates the appreciative in all elements of work and relationships (McCarthy, 2016). Appreciative leadership builds on existing positive concepts that identify the role of the leader in creating a generative context for embracing and engaging the creative and innovative dynamics related to the construction of the future (Butani & Plant, 2016). Practices associated with the positive interactions identified in significant conversations and confrontations, therapeutic interactions, and positive psychology all represent the best in the expressive characteristics of appreciative leadership (Bleich & Hessler, 2016). The tools found in those practices and processes are part of the compendium of resources that, when consistently applied, provide the opportunity to operationalize appreciative leadership.

Five appreciative leadership principles guide the translation and operation of the appreciative in the expression of the leadership role.

Appreciative Principle 1: The Relational Capacity to Mobilize Accountability

Accountability is a centerpiece of professional behavior. The leader looks for behavioral patterns that represent adult-to-adult interchanges and interactions that suggest an understanding of equity, value, and collateral relationships. Equitable communication suggests an understanding of the value of everyone within the professional practice setting and an understanding that this value drives their contribution to the organization and to all roles. Furthermore it leads to a contextual expectation for continuous dynamic engagement; a recognition that all members of the participating team have something specific and significant to offer in contributing to the value of the work of all and that each must know what that contribution is, be able to articulate it to others, and understand the level of appreciation that both self and other reflects in that expectation. It is only when self-expectation and mutual validation of it are clear that expressions of crucial accountability, the ownership of the contribution, become transparent, clear, and visible to all.

Appreciative Principle 2: Leader Self-Awareness and Self-Confidence

A sense of self and self-knowledge in the leader is not an option if respect and honor of the leader's role is to be evident in others across the workplace. Leaders must evidence their having grappled with the personal issues of confidence, potential, and growth in a way that demonstrates to others that this commitment to self-development is a challenge to others to do so in their own lives and practice. Furthermore, it requires that the leader be clear with regard to competence expectations and the integrity and consistency in understanding and accountability. The leader uses language that enables, engages, and advances exploration and understanding in a way that ultimately results in a positive outcome. All of this is represented in the person of the leader, how he or she is witnessed and experienced, as evidenced by the positive feelings and sense one has within and following an interaction with the appreciative leader.

Appreciative Principle 3: Language Expectations and Obligations

The appreciative leader understands the power of language. It is through language that we come to understand meaning, value, belief, and the character of one another. The leader fully understands the power of language and is strategic in its use, crafting questions and interactions with forethought and intention. The leader is careful to use inclusive language, avoiding all "you" statements, setting aside judgments, and placing inquiry and exploration at the center of the interaction. The appreciative leader stays forever in the "I," never in the "you." The appreciative leader uses language as an exploration, a clarification, a vehicle for understanding. Using language appropriately respects ownership for others' language, behaviors, actions, and impact. The leader never assumes ownership for others' accountability and obligations. At the same time, the leader makes clear the consequences and impact of others' expressions, always holding them accountable for what they own.

Appreciative Principle 4: Performance and the Demonstration of Impact

The fundamental aim of leadership to the organization is the achievement of strategically driven outcomes and impact. Without such drivers, the organization would have no medium or means for ensuring its sustenance and sustainability. Therefore, an important role of the appreciative leader around this requirement is the obligation for specificity and clarity of expectation reflecting decisions that were made, goals that were set, and actions that were taken. This obligation for impact and outcome requires clear performance roles, processes, and metrics that focus on and emphasize the relationship of performance to deliverables. Here again, the appreciative leader focuses on work as a value, one that is reflected in the impact it produces in the outcomes it achieves. Recognizing this relationship between work value and impact, the appreciative leader is always aware of the need to evaluate the continuum of effort and to recalibrate effort for inevitable adaptation, adjustment, and response to change.

Appreciative Principle 5: Integrity/Inclusion: The Way of Leading
The appreciative leader is always appreciative. Because this leader is available to the continuing growth in developing insight, he or she respects individual voices, never failing to sustain opportunities for their expression and contribution to work and relationships. Because the leader is appreciative, the leader re-languages error messages, changes misconceptions into positive perceptions, alters miscommunication into opportunities for understanding, and challenges inaccurate notions as a vehicle for deepening and enriching dialogue and discernment. Through these processes the appreciative leader builds collective wisdom/collaboration and positive patterns of behavior and interaction between all members of the learning/performing team; furthermore, the leader ensures the accuracy/appropriateness of information and data, sources of understanding, and resource access and use. Through the use of appreciative acknowledgment of the broad range of talents and skills across the diversity of team members, the leader uses shared leadership skills and processes to develop others and acknowledge their individual and collective roles in their mutual ownership, joint accountability, and shared contribution to valuable outcomes and work successes.

Appreciative leadership is a discipline, a skill set. It requires focused and intentional self-awareness, self-development, and mindfulness with regard to one's own leadership expression and to the relationship and impact that expression has on those he or she leads. It is a lifelong journey demonstrating the continuous and dynamic commitment to personal growth in developing leadership wisdom and, through the insights gained, refining leadership practices, advancing its applications and utility, and deepening the richness of relationships and expression in ways that make a difference to persons and organizations.

Dealing with the Lack of Time

"Not enough time" is perhaps the most widely heard mantra in the workplace today. In the past few years, it seems as if work has expanded and time has been compressed. Although time has not literally shrunk, dramatic changes during this period have affected people's perception of both time and work.

First, in general, work has become more complex. Although the purpose of a job may remain the same, what it takes to do it has changed radically. There is simply more to the job than there used to be. In health care, for example, managing the continuum of care so that the proper services are provided in a timely fashion requires communication and interaction with a whole host of professionals and use of numerous resources that are new on the scene. The need to do work speedily and effectively has also increased the intensity of the work and made time even more of a concern.

Leaders and staff need to look at the issue of time differently. For many years, work was viewed as a process that had no beginning or end. As a result, it became an end in itself, and the usual goal was simply to be efficient and do what had to be done on time. The issues are now more profound and require a different mental model for their resolution. Rather than looking for more resources or time, leaders are confronted with the questions about who should be used and how they should be used—questions about being different in a world that is changing before our very eyes. The fact is that resources, human and other, are not available in the same numbers and format they once were. The questions are no longer about more of anything. Looking for more resources, people, or time is not likely to help get more of any. The issue is no longer about doing more with less; instead, questions are about doing and being different in a changing world.

> **Point to Ponder**
>
> Leaders can have a big impact on problem solving merely by eliminating the word *more* from the dialogue. As long as people believe that more resources—more money, time, people, capital, equipment, and so on—will solve their problems, they will not put enough imagination and creativity into the mix to discover sustainable solutions. An abundance of resources can often be the enemy of imagination and creativity.

In other words, leaders are the individuals to challenge the prevailing framework. For instance, in addition to realizing that resources are finite and not as readily available as before, leaders must repeatedly point out to the staff that the value of work is embedded in outcomes, not processes. They must also recognize that nurses and physicians are challenged with having to validate their treatment decisions by providing evidence that their choices were less costly or less resource intensive than comparably effective treatments or had better results than other possible treatments could have had. For most of their years in practice, health professionals never had to prove a functional relationship between what they did and what resulted. Today, there is no future for healthcare decisions and actions for which such a relationship cannot be demonstrated.

Work in this new era requires more flexibility and fluidity than previously. The old notion that work should have fixed time and function parameters is no longer realistic. With wireless technology, a healthcare clinician can be anywhere and still be reached for advice or follow-up. When does a clinician's job really begin, and when does it really end? It is now the responsibility of the individual to determine his or her workload and availability and the extent of the work period. In the past people went to a workplace, did their jobs, and went home. Today, jobs go with the jobholders wherever they go, and no parameters define the jobs more narrowly.

Leaders must now begin to apply tools to staffing that allow the planning and utilization of staff to be more flexible. They must also consider job candidates with an eye to their skill sets and personality characteristics to ensure they increase the organization's adaptability. The notion of goodness-of-fit applies to people just as it does to roles. Scheduling around workload is now a critical method of staffing. So is contracting for workload—bringing staff members on board based on an agreed workload and paying them for the workload rather than for time and function. These methods give staff members more control over their work life and over their life outside work.

The revolution in communications gives staff members more documentation and information-gathering options, not to mention unprecedented access to each other. The hands-free earpiece or headset allows clinicians to connect with others at a wide variety of times rather than just during a few set periods (e.g., rounds). Finding someone, reading the chart, and documenting information have become easier with the new telephone and personal digital assistant devices now common in the workplace.

Because of the increase in specialization, health professionals have become more interdependent. No one can be an expert in everything, and the members of a healthcare team must identify and make use of each other's expertise, fashioning a strong clinical network in the process. The leader of the team helps the other members become more self-reliant, where appropriate, and more interdependent. Rather than being a manager in the traditional sense, the leader is instead a colleague who creates the possibilities and conditions for real advancement and learning.

Time and resource problems do not always have easy solutions, and what might work in one part of an organization might fail outright in another. The organization's leader should realize that all problem solving is ultimately local and that those individuals who own a problem must be the ones to discover and implement its solution. Therefore, the leader needs to push staff members to find their own solutions and to identify processes that work for them and can be sustained in their environment. The key here is ownership. Those in administrative areas of the organization do not know how to resolve all the difficulties that arise at the point-of-work. Rather, the staff members know how to handle problems there, and the leader's job is to engage them to cocreate the context of their work so they can own the problems that arise, apply the appropriate methods and tools to solve them, and then use the necessary means to evaluate the outcomes and sustain whatever benefits they have achieved. The leader, of course, keeps his or her eye on the results, knowing that outcomes drive all processes and that all processes are disciplined by sustainable outcomes.

> **Key Point**
>
> Staff members must be allowed to find solutions to their own problems. The role of the leader is not to solve problems for others, but to make certain that staff members have the insights and skills necessary to problem solve. A leader's one absolute unforgivable act is to take ownership for other people's problems.

Leaders are often required to play the role of coach, and they bring to this role not only insight and skill but passion as well. In fact, by exhibiting energy and drive, they encourage others to stay invested in their own activities and commitments. They act as living examples of the excitement that results from engagement with the challenges of the times.

Coaches, including leaders acting as guides or counselors to staff members, find their greatest reward in helping others develop and move in the direction they need to go. They become invested in the achievements of those they are helping to learn and experience the learners' gains as gains of their own. Issues that arise in coaching and that leaders acting as coaches in a team situation need to keep in mind are as follows:

- *Having a genuine interest in people means supporting their growth.* Every team leader therefore needs to make sure other members know and feel the obligation to advance themselves and become full participants in the process of learning and adapting. The individual team members are accountable for thriving, and the leader must always keep this truth in front of the team members' eyes.

- *Learning how to use questions to activate and assess their thought processes.* Essential for coaches is the ability to build relationships with other members. Humble inquiry (Schein, 2013) is the basis for building trusting relationships and requires the leader to refrain from telling, to learn to do more asking, and to engage in successful work-related listening. Telling implies that the other person does not already know what is being told to them and that they ought to know it. Asking temporarily empowers the other person, and it does make the leader vulnerable, but it draws the other person into the driver's seat and opens the door to strengthening the relationship. It is key that the leader listen intently and build on the information from the response. In a work environment where tasks accomplishment is more important than relationship building, this approach of humble inquiry can begin to shift the importance from tasks to strong relationships.
- *Coaching team members is not the same as raising children.* The team members are always fully accountable for their own development. The leader provides assistance in the form of tools and support but does not take on the burden of accountability for the other members' growth and advancement. The leader's role is to remind the team members of relevant expectations and parameters for action and to support them in meeting those expectations.
- *When coaching other members of a team, the leader does not take possession of their work.* Also, the leader does not own the staff's relationships and interactions or the outcomes of their efforts. The leader is alert to staff attempts to transfer ownership and must ensure that ownership remains where it belongs. The leader is like a circuit rider, moving continuously around the periphery of the team, observing, interacting, assessing, and identifying. When issues, deficits, or concerns arise, the leader is ready to transfer skills, insights, and tools to the team members in a clear way to ensure they have what they need to deal with their problems and advance their own work.
- *The team leader is not in control of the lives of the other team members or the circumstances in which they do their work.* The leader is their colleague rather than their manager, and the coaching role is one of partnership. The team leader's job is to keep the other members connected, invested, and aware and to help them develop to the point where they can operate with little outside intervention. In a transformational time, the leader is always pushing at the edges, helping the other members recognize the changes that are occurring, the issues that are arising, and the best methods for resolving them. The leader is in back, pushing the team into its reality, not in front, pulling it into his or her reality.
- *The leader is the chief learner on the team.* By modeling her or his commitment to the "way of learning" as a way of living, the leader helps create a learning culture and shows others how to embark on their own journey. The leader is always curious, searching, reading signposts, transferring information, raising issues, and pushing the parameters. The leader sees learning as a dynamic, as an essential constituent of living and relating, and becomes for the team a visual representation of learning in action.

In these times, because the work of transforming organizations is so critical, leaders in their role as coaches must exhibit the attitudes and behaviors of change and adaptation. In living the process of change, they perhaps do more to further the ability of others to handle change than they do through explicit instruction. People need to see leaders dealing with change so that they have someone rather than something to identify with. They look to leaders to humanize the experience of change by growing and adapting themselves. By seeing others who are successfully adjusting to change, they become more comfortable carrying out their own personal journey of transformation.

The Leader as Revolutionary

The healthcare system is at a critical juncture. New thinking, different models and processes of accountable care and service, and whole new technologies are pushing the system toward a huge transformation. Yet there is so much in the way—a long history of now outmoded patterns, rituals, routines, and infrastructure. To help carry out the transformation, each leader must become a revolutionary in residence.

The skills of revolution are different from those of evolution, because, in a revolutionary context, time is compressed, it is already too late, the options to thrive are significantly threatened, and leaders and personnel are almost paralyzed by their circumstances. In this case the leader of an organization has the job of initiating a number of processes so that the organization as a whole can engage with the radical changes occurring and implement adaptations in a timely fashion. Of course, the leader cannot do it alone. A coalition of like-minded revolutionaries is necessary for substantive change to occur. Indeed, the leader, acting as a transformational revolutionary, seeks to widen the circle of "conspirators" until the whole organization is conspiring to transform itself and its processes to meet current demands. This section describes several steps a revolutionary leader goes through to ensure that adaptation becomes the modus operandi of the system.

> **Point to Ponder**
>
> The only real difference between evolution and revolution is the pace of change.

Create an Argument for Revolution

The organizational leader must create a vision of the transformation, because what the transformation is and does are critical to mobilizing people. The leader thus gathers like-minded leaders within the organization to make a statement about the efforts required by the transformation—essentially a vision statement. This translational skill set is now essential for leaders to be able to refine changes in the social, political, and economic environments in a language and manner that can be understood at the point-of-service. The forces at play, the impact of events, the changing circumstances, the altered financial configurations—all these

> **Group Discussion**
>
> As a group, identify one major change currently under way in health transformation that directly affects the delivery of patient care. Make sure that the change is significant and radical. Using a flip chart, create a plan for revolution around the identified change. Identify the various constituencies and conspiracies that are necessary for building momentum. Evaluate whether the plan is revolutionary and how and where to implement it.

jointly determine how the current mental model should be revised and what needs to be done. The organizational leader then collects data to validate and refine the vision statement. The statement must show a clear connection between the conditions and the response and indicate why the conditions are so compelling as to make nonresponding a nonchoice. The vision statement must not only describe the conditions but also explain the response, citing the critical factors that influence the organization's position in the future.

Develop a Charter for the Future

After clarifying the conditions demanding transformation, the leader and his or her coconspirators must develop an agenda for the future. This can be likened to a map of the territory through which the system must now travel (the trajectory of change). The goal at this stage is not to devise a detailed program for change but to articulate the themes and signposts indicating the organization's proper direction. The charter should consist of a simple and clear point-by-point enumeration of the factors and themes of "becoming." It should contain engaging terminology so that key words and phrases such as "creating a sustainable partnership" or "building the health journey" can be pulled out and used to generate energy and enterprise throughout the organization. It should also indicate obstacles in the way of achieving the goals for which the conspirators need all of their commitment to overcome.

Build the Conspiracy

The transformation process has no meaning and will die an ignoble death if the conspiracy does not continuously expand. The charter starts to gain life when the organization embraces it as its work. The role of the leader is to make sure that commitment to the transformation moves outward into the far reaches of the organization. All the key players, informal and formal, at all places in the organization must embrace the charter, take ownership of it, and move it to the next levels of application. No formal mechanism of generation is required. Those who "get it" are brought on board when they are ready, and then they do their part to find and lead others who can get it as well. As might be guessed, the various organizational committees, from medical staff committees to management councils, are great vehicles for publicizing the vision and expanding the conspiracy.

This kind of revolution must be fully transparent. Everyone eventually must be on board to help in the creation of a preferred future. The work of the conspiracy is merely to stimulate this journey for all members of the organization, from those at the point-of-service to those in the boardroom. Joining the conspiracy to operational processes already under way is a good mechanism for getting the charter on the table of those who most need to engage with it.

Be Strategic and Patient

There are no enemies in this revolution—only those not yet part of it. The conspirators must understand which stakeholders they need to bring on board to give the charter both life and legs. They must also understand when to approach these individuals and groups or include the charter in their work.

Further, they should know the local politics of communication and action and identify which strategies are best for addressing specific challenges and circumstances. Getting specific individuals to perform certain required actions (because of their relationships, positions, or skills) is a part of the strategic process of managing the charter and guiding it through the political landscape. Indeed, one-on-one interactions with key players are as important as group meetings. In approaching key players, the conspirators need to translate the charter into their language to obtain their acceptance and advocacy. Key players have to be able to see how the process benefits them and advances their own opportunities and circumstances—that is part of the political process.

Seek Out Significant Champions

As the conspiracy grows, it must incorporate champions able to take the charter farther on its journey. The transformation process is like a relay race: different runners with different skills are required at different points in the process. The organizational leader must anticipate the new focus, person, or skill necessary for getting to the next stage and must ensure that each is applied in the right format and at the right time to move the process along.

As in most conspiracies, movement toward the goal is not along a straight line. Backward or horizontal steps are occasionally required to refresh or expand the process. In addition, as progress occurs, the kind of champions needed often can be found at new locations. That is as it should be. The conspirators must celebrate any support that moves the transformation along to the next stage and increases its chance of success.

Ensure Small Successes Occur Early and Often

Successes must take place along the way to maintain momentum. Creating a plan for substantive change and getting the whole organization to embrace it are long, gradual processes, and people will remain unmotivated if they perceive their efforts as unlikely to make a difference. Even small accomplishments show that movement has occurred, and without some deliverables the organization is sure to lose interest before it gets very far. The accomplishments give the transformation process "legs" and ensure that the process's champions can overcome objections and opposition in a manner that allows them to incorporate new ideas into the process and convert possible opponents into supporters.

Make the Transformation the Mainstream Activity

The goal is to enable the whole organization to thrive well into the future. The conspiracy is simply a means of ensuring the organization's survival at a time when the organization appears to be missing an opportunity to prosper. Thus, the conspirators must always keep in mind that the purpose of their efforts is to benefit the organization, not themselves. They also must avoid becoming so committed to the conspiracy that their attention is diverted from the real end and their energies wind up misdirected. Once the conspirators have attained their objective—to make the transformation the central activity of the organization—the nature of their endeavors shifts toward initiating work processes related to the new reality. The conspirators must now fully embrace the character, context, and content of the new reality, which means redefining the work, retooling the workplace, and focusing on the conditions that allow the organization to thrive. In a sense, the conspiracy has now become the new reality.

Of course, the metaphor in this section of a conspiracy is merely a way of highlighting the focused commitment to fundamental change that leaders in an organization must have when options are limited or opportunities are being missed. It pinpoints the sense of urgency the leaders must impart to the entire organization to get everyone to make the kind of effort needed to ensure the organization's ability to thrive in a highly charged and changing set of circumstances. It also emphasizes the understanding that engagement and response to the demand for major change is a process with specific stages and points at which different stakeholders engage and accelerate their involvement in the journey of change. The leaders, acting as change agents, must stimulate the staff and other stakeholders to raise their own levels of energy and refocus their efforts. The conspiracy enlists them in an effort that is greater than they are as individuals, giving them a sense of meaning and purpose and generating the energy, emotion, insight, spirit, and commitment they need to adapt and grow. Focused commitment and strong motivation, along with appropriate processes, methodologies, and techniques, round out the requisites of revolutionary yet sustainable transformation.

Innovation Coaching

A team leader has the responsibility to create the right conditions for the team and its members to learn and grow. In fact, the main purpose of team leadership is to ensure that the team members can develop and become what they must to thrive in shifting circumstances. The achievement of this goal, of course, requires the team leader to overcome existing obstacles to effective coaching (**Exhibit 12-4**).

To become successful in the new age, leaders and staff members must relate to the processes of transformation so that they see them as the essence of their work and not as mere responses to a demand to do things differently. Adaptability is as much an attitude as it is a way of doing business, and the goal of leaders should be to help everyone be different, not just perform new job activities. After all, in this era of revolution, it is not just the work that is changing, it is the very workplace itself—the conditions, elements, and technologies of work.

Because the working conditions are being substantially altered, leaders must ensure that the differences do not escape the attention of those who do the work. They need to help the workers revise their mental model of work and turn every worker into a revolutionary. In other words, they need to publicize the fact that innovation is now a way of life and help the workers develop the skills and attributes they require to live that way of life and become part of the transformation of the workplace (**Figure 12-3**).

To convert work into innovative effort, leaders need to follow several rules, discussed subsequently. They should also keep in mind that workers must figure out the emerging context for their work and relationships and create the structures and content for the journey itself.

Exhibit 12-4 Impediments to Effective Coaching

Use of power
- Inadequate power
- Autocratic application of power
- Lack of empowerment
- Nonstrategic use of power

Self-image
- Poor self-esteem
- Unclear role
- Psychological flaws

Knowledge
- Undeveloped knowledge
- Learning needs
- Inexperience
- Lack of personal technique

Problem solving
- Inadequate worldview
- Intolerance of diversity
- No clear process
- Situational solutions

Figure 12-3 Innovative as a Way of Life. The leader focuses on the central components of personal transformation to ensure that each person can embrace change.

Set the Bar High

Leaders need to convince workers that expectations for their performance are high, but not so high they cannot be met. The challenge is to set expectations that prevent workers from falling back on old behaviors and practices but that also do not discourage them. The expectations should stimulate the workers to engage in different thinking and to change the very nature of the work.

Another way of saying this is that the transformation of work requires new models for thinking, a new context for work, and goals that demand new ways of working. The goals should not be so easily attainable that the workers can retain their old ways of doing things.

Be Clear About Who You Are

In the new world of work, people need to redefine who they are and their definition of success. For example, hospitals, which were originally defined as places where sick people were cared for, have been redefined as places where healthcare services are delivered. The range of services that falls under the rubric *health care* differs from the range that falls under the rubric *caring for the sick*.

Because the health services landscape is moving toward more accountable care models, healthcare leaders must highlight the changes in the context of work and the implications for its performance, including the new demands that have arisen. They must then revise the structures and processes of work to meet the new demands and to assist staff in adjusting their insights, attitudes, and behaviors appropriately. Staff members must live the image of the organization in all they are and do. Making sure that staff members see the shift and can live the new perspective in their work and relationships is a critical element in the journey into the future.

Treat Transformation as a Mission, Not a Job

The staff of an organization must not simply change the way they do their work but also change the way they live their work. Therefore, the organizational leader, acting as a coach, must be able to explain how to live and work differently using the broadest and clearest language possible. Transcending simple notions of labor, the leader creates an image of healthcare delivery as having a purpose beyond its immediate effects. By showing how work efforts can influence the world of health care, the leader transforms the performance of work by an individual into the pursuit of a mission. People want to support good and noble causes that take them outside of themselves and also want to view their efforts as having a profound value. The leader can help them take this leap from the mundane to the honorable and incorporate a sense of mission into the very fabric of their work activities.

Expose Staff to Different Messages and Different Messengers

To motivate staff members, the leader must give them encouraging messages that differ from those they have often heard in the past. The leader must also communicate new expectations and provide opportunities for staff members to learn what they need to know to meet these expectations. The encouragement and the expectations communicated must be consistent with the transformation on which the organization has embarked. The goal is to stimulate staff members to think about how to do their work more effectively.

New voices should also be heard. Young workers, workers who are quiet and reserved, and workers from outside the particular work group should be included in the collective dialogue. The leader should do as much as possible to "push the walls" to move people out of their comfort zones to stretch into new ways of thinking and doing.

> **Key Point**
> The leader must be so consumed by the organization's mission that transformation becomes second nature. In addition, by being committed to this mission, the leader presents a visible example of transformation in action that has the power to inspire others to transform themselves and their job activities.

Create an Egalitarian Organizational Structure

Hierarchy should be minimized in times of great change. In fact, in the new age hierarchy has limited value. Horizontal relationships, defined not by position but by role, are the cornerstone of accountability. The leader of an organization must therefore facilitate relationships with those he or she depends on for planning and performing the organization's work.

In other words, the leader must value the work and the worker equally. Each worker has a contribution to make. Because the workers know best what produces results, the leader's job is to get each to offer innovative ideas on how to improve methods and processes. The leader therefore needs to make it safe and easy for workers to become part of the collective dialogue and put forth suggestions. Barriers to interaction, sharing, and challenging simply cannot exist if the spontaneous communication of ideas is to become the organization's modus operandi. Ideas are an important form of capital for any enterprise and can come from any place. For them to be released, the organization's culture must make it not only possible but routine.

Put Money Where the Ideas Are

For an idea to be implemented, some level of resource support is required. Although not every idea is worth supporting, funding for good ideas must be available because staff members need to know that their ideas have the potential to go somewhere and make a difference. If their ideas are ignored for lack of funding, they will eventually go back to old routines and refuse to contribute. If their ideas, on the other hand, are taken seriously and investigated, they will continue to make suggestions.

The funding or budgeting process must make it possible to explore ideas and innovations to an extent commensurate with their likely utility. Out of 1,000 ideas perhaps only 10 will ever be used, but those 10 could not have emerged unaccompanied by the rest. In short, the exploration of all ideas is critical to the discovery and application of the few that do become part of the organization's practice.

Let the Talented Experiment

It is impossible to apply new thinking by rote or through using a "straight line" approach. Talented people must be gathered together and supported. This means, among other things, allowing them to take risks. The outcomes of ideas are often unpredictable, and thus a certain amount of trial and error is necessary. Ideas must be tried and possibly modified before their worth can be known. If an idea is not shown to be beneficial after a trial period, it should be discarded.

Nothing should be set in cement. Strategies should be implemented and then modified as necessary. Structures and permanent processes should be avoided because they create barriers to necessary revisions. In addition, enough creative people must be included in the organization to ensure that innovative thinking occurs. Constant attention to bringing in and keeping such people is critical for sustaining the transformation. The leader must be comfortable with those who are bright and creative and come up with ideas that challenge the leader to think and act differently.

> **Point to Ponder**
>
> Experimentation is critical to innovation and adaptability. An organization not willing to experiment is doomed to failure.

Allow People to Share in the Fruits of Their Creativity

This is perhaps the most challenging notion for healthcare leaders. For some unfathomable reason, the practice of rewarding people for their contribution has not become common practice within the healthcare arena. However, people own their creativity and ideas and lose interest and move on if their ownership is not honored. Keeping creative people means investing in them, and investing in them means rewarding them for their innovations.

Creative people often do not seek to be compensated financially. For them, seeing their originality have an impact can be reward enough. Nonetheless, the leader should acknowledge contributions in a meaningful way. Although a bonus is the most recognized and established kind of reward and should be seriously considered, there are a host of other kinds of recognition, including public acknowledgment (celebrations and events), publishing the work inside or outside the institution, gain sharing (sharing the rewards), and shared ownership. Whatever rewards are defined by the organization, the reward granted to an individual for a given contribution should fit the needs of the person and the kind of contribution. Remember, highly creative people are looking not for long-term, permanent positions but for opportunities to express their gifts and talents. Keeping them on as employees depends on whether the organization's culture provides them with an ability to create, grow, and advance.

The leader is always attentive to the need to keep the organization moving and to respond to current demands (**Figure 12-4**). Creating the environment, structure, and processes necessary to ensure the organization's adaptability is the leader's single most important task. Because inventive people are essential to the organization's ability to respond to new demands, the leader is forever looking for, challenging, and rewarding such people in an effort to maintain a pool of creative talent (**Figure 12-5**).

Innovation Coaching

Figure 12-4 The Dynamics of Continuous Adaptation. The leader ensures that each element of adaptation is addressed by those whose work must be transformed.

Figure 12-5 The Elements of Personal Transformation. Change is not complete until the cycle of transformation is complete. The leader brings personal passion to moving people to a new level of performance.

Making Integration Work

Because of the systems-oriented dynamics of health care and the effort to create a seamless and population-based approach to ensuring health, making things fit together is very important. The leader of a healthcare organization must evaluate the fit between elements and improve it wherever possible (**Exhibit 12-5**). When a merger or alliance occurs, however, creating proper fit can be a great problem. People bring to the new entity their past ideas, commitments, cultures, and notions of how the work is to be done, and they resist or find it difficult to create the level of integration that is required. Much of the energy of the leader is devoted to making the new arrangements not just workable but productive.

> ### Group Discussion
>
> A common topic of discussion today in accountable care is the nature of true integration. As a group, brainstorm the basic elements of integration. Identify areas where group members disagree. Break into two debating teams of two or three members each and have each team take a position and argue for it. The remainder of the group will critique the debate and evaluate the arguments. After the debate, the group members should discuss how their view of integration has been altered or reinforced. Finally, identify three or four common elements of integration that can be used as criteria to determine whether integration has been achieved.

Perhaps the greatest concern is the speed with which things seem to happen today. Although time itself has not accelerated, the extra complexity of work has made it difficult to accomplish tasks at the pace once expected. The sheer complexity of the transformation processes currently under way in the American healthcare system challenges both pace and intensity. Because staff members find they no longer have enough time to do what they used to do, the leader must help them replace their focus on doing lots of activities with a focus on doing the right things.

In the old days, healthcare clinicians did a lot for patients. In fact, this reality drove the definition of caring. Today, although caring is still central to health care, it is expressed differently. The independence and accountability of the users of health services are now as important as the services delivered by care clinicians. People must acknowledge their responsibility for their own health and be empowered to act in the right way at the right time to ensure their own

Exhibit 12-5 Elements of Integration

- Accountability
- Alignment
- Focus on the whole
- Goodness-of-fit
- Integrity
- Interdependence
- Orientation toward outcomes
- Role congruence

well-being. Clinicians consequently are faced with a different mix of activities and priorities and must recognize that doing everything for patients is not the best way to render needed assistance.

To many health professionals, the idea that patients are unilaterally responsible for their health borders on heresy. At the very least, it goes against a long tradition of provider-owned "doing for." Nonetheless, in this age of consumer control and accountability, the complexity of health care and the added demands on the providers' time require many of the tasks to be placed in the hands of patients. This transfer of responsibility, of course, changes the character of the patient–provider relationship.

The leader must ensure not only that the transfer of responsibility is carried out but also that clinicians and patients change their attitudes, beliefs, and practices accordingly. Replacing the expectation of "doing for" with the expectation of "doing with" is an arduous task, not just for staff but for patients as well. Patients, too, have grown up with a certain image of health care and certain expectations of what they should obtain from the healthcare system. They can feel disappointed when these expectations are not fully met. They, too, operate with a dependency model under which they surrender responsibility, accountability, and control to healthcare clinicians in return for being tended. In fact, their surrender sometimes facilitates their descent into conditions and lifestyles that contribute to the illnesses for which they seek treatment.

Today, part of the healthcare clinician's role is to alter patient expectations of "being taken care of." Part of the healthcare leader's role is to work with clinicians in creating a new model of health care and revising the patient–provider relationship. The ultimate goal is to help clinicians use their time more effectively and appropriately in delivering care and providing services to those in need.

In particular, clinicians must focus on teaching and otherwise empowering patients to see more and do more in their own interest. They must also involve family members and significant others in the delivery of services and in counseling, supporting, and caring for loved ones in need of assistance. For these changes to occur, healthcare leaders need to focus on four important responsibilities, described subsequently.

Speeding Up Processes

Time is of the essence. Clinicians have less and less time to talk with patients about their healthcare needs and provide appropriate services, and therefore clinicians and patients must make better use of their time together. For example, follow-up now means making sure patients can gain access to the resources they need (i.e., connecting them to a network of resources, including sources of information that can guide their actions when they are no longer within the healthcare system).

As noted, the locus of control is with patients (where it really belongs). Clinicians must make sure that it never shifts away from there and that patients have what they need to take care of their health. Healthcare leaders have the task of helping staff become comfortable with this reality and

> **Key Point**
> The healthcare system is changing in fundamental ways, so clinicians and patients need to act differently and "expect differently." The clinicians, in particular, need to change their behaviors and expectations and educate the patients to change theirs.

guiding them into practices that allow patients to make the best decisions and carry out those decisions. For the transition to the new patient–provider relationship to occur, both clinicians and patients must develop new skills and skill sets.

Orchestrating the Dynamics of Change

Making the shift to new ways and new roles is difficult for everyone. Complicating the situation is the fact that new rituals and routines must replace those that reinforce behaviors suitable to the older model of service. Staff members, having lived for so long with the more traditional dependent practices, now need approaches, tools, and skills to help them initiate and sustain new behaviors. Leaders must ensure that they develop and use these in ways that fit their culture and experience with change. By exchanging best practices, staff members can connect with others who are busy creating and constructing methods and models for improving services and changing their relationships with those they serve.

Building Relationships

Everything is built on good and sustainable relationships. The most important leadership task is to ensure that everyone is "singing off the same song sheet." Keeping an organization's staff on target and focused on its mission is difficult yet critical work. The leader continually tests, challenges, and extends personal and collective relationships with stakeholders throughout the process of changing behavior. When things get tough or stuck, the leader's only resource may be the personal relationships and the accompanying trust he or she has developed during this process. Identifying with the difficulties that staff members are experiencing and supporting them through the changes they encounter are critical to sustaining their efforts. Testing, stretching, evaluating, renewing, supporting, and challenging are steps in the normal cycle of action, relationship, and response that every leader needs to know how to do (**Figure 12-6**).

Putting Necessary Structure in Place

New behaviors are not sustainable without accompanying structural supports. Care providers for those with chemical dependency issues know that addressing an addict's behavior is not enough—the environment also must be changed. Creating a context for change means building an environment that leads to desired behaviors. When workers fully participate in creating their environment, chances increase that they will own the appropriate behaviors and achieve the desired outcomes.

Leaders often fail to pay close attention to the structural realities, allowing staff to fall back into old patterns of behavior. Creating structures that limit old patterns and foster preferred patterns, along with rewarding the performance of desired behaviors, can make the difference between an effective workplace and one that is unproductive and problematic. As an impetus for positive change, structure is at least the equal of behavior itself.

Addressing Problems Head On

People who do not approach problems proactively acquire a "firefighting" mindset. Unfortunately, because of the large number of problems and issues that confront leaders daily, they often end up spending more time on daily skirmishes than on substantive issues. A focus on firefighting, by leaving their real responsibilities unattended, simply begets more fires to fight.

Unlearning/learning
Perceiving
Modeling
Acting out
Affirming new behavior

Sustaining
Externalized
Evidenced
Reaffirmed
Taught
Normalized

Maintaining
Coding
Entrenching
Replaying
Exemplifying

Figure 12-6 Cycle of Transformational Learning.

Group Discussion

Tracy Polus, the head of the respiratory department, had a difficult time confronting behavior problems. She habitually used the third person when discussing such problems and could often be heard saying, "When a person does . . ." or "If someone would . . ." or "If people could . . ." The staff never really knew if she meant to refer to their behavior in particular or to the behavior of people in general. Eventually, they began to discount her comments, and because no one else was dealing with problematic behaviors, relationships in the department suffered. What recommendation would you give Tracy? How could she change her own behavior to make her a more effective manager? Is there a type of developmental program that she should undergo? Is it too late for her to establish new ground rules for her staff? What would some of the ground rules be?

Some ways of dealing with problems allow leaders to do their transformational work. Indeed, problem solving can be a source of growth and can support a leader's transformational work. The trick is not to look at problems situationally and attempt to resolve them within the context of the situation but instead to investigate the circumstances in which they occur.

> **Point to Ponder**
>
> Behavior changes cannot be sustained without structural supports in place, and leaders must pay as much attention to these as to the changes themselves.

Rather than filling holes in the staffing schedule on the spur of the moment, for example, a leader should identify and address the underlying causes; otherwise, the problem will occur again, often in a form more difficult to resolve.

A patchwork approach to solving problems creates more problems than it solves. It also creates problems in related but remote parts of the system. When a process is broken, other processes that interact with it pay the price. For instance, a delay in laboratory testing results in a delay in treating patients. In a complex system, problems can cascade through the system, causing difficulties for everyone.

Leaders, in dealing with problems, should follow a few basic rules. Although simple, they are often forgotten, to the detriment of the problem-solving process.

> **Key Point**
>
> Not all problems can be solved quickly, so the leader of an organization must prioritize problems to make sure the critical ones are dealt with immediately. People problems always come first, relationship problems second, and external problems last. Structure and process problems are ongoing, as are the procedures for handling them.

Solve Problems Selectively

It is unbelievable how many leaders take on, all at once, the full range of problems affecting their organization. Not all problems can be or need to be solved immediately. Leaders must approach problem solving like any other deliberative process. In particular, they must develop strategies for prioritizing problems and bringing order and focus to the effort of addressing problems critically.

Because problems are omnipresent and affect everything that people do, leaders must look at the relationships among problems, explore the way in which they interact, and then decide the order in which the problems are addressed. Not every problem has the same weight or the same ability to obstruct work and the achievement of desired outcomes. Setting up a list of problems to be dealt with first is a necessary step in the problem-solving process.

Work on the Fundamental Problems First

Many leaders believe they should work on the most urgent problems of the day. Yet problems that seem small can be the source of these seemingly more critical problems. If the root problems are not resolved, all others caused by them also do not get resolved. In addition, problems that appear to be critical to people in the midst of a crisis usually turn out to be mere symptoms of more fundamental problems. Thus, an important goal in problem solving is to determine which problem is a root cause and which is an effect.

Include People with the Necessary Skills and Power in the Resolution of Problems

Although it is best for people to assert ownership of the problems that concern them, it is not always possible for everyone affected by a problem to be part of the problem-solving effort. What is more important is that the right people be involved—those who have the skills to resolve the problem and the power to make the resolution permanent. In most cases, finding and implementing a solution to a problem requires the engagement of a broad range of players and stakeholders.

Be Accountable for Ensuring Problems Are Solved

Although leaders are obligated to see that problems are solved, they are not obligated to solve problems they do not own. The important consideration in determining who should deal with a problem is who owns it and who is best placed to resolve it (i.e., usually one and the same person or group). The role of the leader, in most cases, is merely to provide the proper people with everything they need. As a result, the leader's focus is not so much on the problem as on the process.

If the owners of a problem turf it outside of their locus of control, the problem is unlikely to remain fixed for long. Therefore, leaders must make sure that problem-solving skills and processes are embedded in the organizational culture and that those who are attempting to deal with a problem have the wherewithal to take care of it.

Counterproductive beliefs and practices are significant barriers to the permanent resolution of problems. For example, despite what many leaders believe, being committed to resolving problems is not nearly as important as being committed to using good problem-solving techniques and processes. These techniques and processes create the insights and skills necessary to deal with problems effectively and quickly enough to avoid long-term trauma.

Eliminating Firefighting Altogether

The best thing the leader of an organization can do is replace firefighting activities with much more productive behaviors. The research and work of Roger Bohm have been important in codifying what is wrong with most problem solving and in publicizing better methods (Savitch, 2008). To make problem solving truly effective, the leader needs to use analytic and tactical methods and strategic approaches and to alter the organization's culture (Schabracq, 2007; Zedeck & American Psychological Association, 2011).

Tactical Methods

The advantage of tactical methods of problem solving is that they can be put into place quickly to deal with problems in the short term while the infrastructure for the more lasting approaches is constructed. *Tactics* simply means making a change applicable and practical so that it can be successfully implemented. Tactics provide a means that is useful and can be replicated, evaluated, and changed when required. They are not cast in stone and can be readily adapted to new realities or necessary changes. The dynamic nature of tactics allows the leader to bring flexibility to bear on issues or problems and to introduce adaptability in the work process.

> **Point to Ponder**
>
> Firefighting is not a good problem-solving approach because it keeps the focus off the root issues and on the symptoms. In fact, the more firefighting a leader does, the more firefighting the leader has to do.

Getting Help from Outside the Circle

It is often wise to have someone from outside the service or unit help with the response to problems inside. A person from outside has a fresh view of the issues and is not invested in the issues or the solutions under consideration. Leaders often refrain from using outside resources because they are uncomfortable with others knowing their problems or simply because they have not attempted this maneuver in the past. Yet the more insight that can be obtained from those who do not own the issues, the more objective and effective the solutions are likely to be. In the new age, one of the expectations should be that leaders will call on each other as outside consultants in dealing with the deeper and more complex problems and issues that undoubtedly arise.

Trying Something New

People have a tendency to do the same things while expecting different outcomes. They become attached to rituals and routines that are inherently problematic and refuse to face the challenge of learning new practices. Most problems in organizations occur because the members hold on to old practices that have become barriers to smooth functioning and effective performance. The leader of an organization, acting as a change agent, must begin at the fundamental level—by creating a good fit between form and function and establishing a culture that supports changes in behavior. Here again, it is by creating the right context for change and creativity to occur that leaders can most help reduce the impact of habit and make it possible for people to let go of past practices.

Triaging Problems

Problems are always occurring. The goal is to solve them as soon as possible so that they do not incubate greater problems. It therefore makes sense to sort through current problems quickly to determine which are normal or trivial and which are pivotal and likely to cause other problems. A conflict between two practitioners, for example, might create a bottleneck in the flow of work, especially if they sabotage each other's efforts. Resolving their conflict would therefore prevent a range of difficulties down the road, and so the conflict would appear high on the list of problems to be tackled immediately.

Strategic Approaches

Strategic approaches, because they are embedded in an organization's way of working and doing business, take longer to plan and implement than do tactical methods.

Prioritizing Problems

Problems should be viewed as a normal part of organizational operations and their solution as a normal part of the leader's work. As much as possible, the leader should help the staff see problems as normal and develop categories for classifying problems according to their potential impact. Problems that affect staffing and the availability of clinical support resources, for example, would be treated as more urgent than office supply problems, and conflicts between departments would rank higher than conflicts between individuals on a given unit. Prioritizing problems is not intended to diminish the importance of any problem; it simply ranks them so that more critical issues are not left hanging.

Using Learning Scenarios

The leader of an organization is crippled if she or he is the only one to take on the responsibility of solving problems. The "mama" syndrome, in which problems are seen as exclusively within the leader's jurisdiction, prevents problem-solving processes from being built into the system. Everyone needs to develop problem assessment and problem-solving skills and the independence to take care of problems at the right time.

There is no way to avoid or eliminate all problems, and indeed problems are a sign of life in the universe. Once staff members understand this, the leader can use present or past problems as vehicles for teaching problem-solving skills. Through this kind of scenario learning, the leader can help staff members alter their attitudes toward problems and can change the locus of control for solving them. The staff can embrace problems as tools and develop the skills necessary to manage them to the organization's benefit.

Building a Problem-Solving Tool Chest
The solution of each problem should build the skill sets necessary to solve subsequent problems more quickly and easily. In a sense, each solution serves as a database for future problems. Codifying and recording approaches to specific kinds of problems increases the likelihood that recurrences will be solved in a similar fashion. Better still, it increases the likelihood that recurrences can be dealt with early enough to prevent a negative impact. In addition, banding together the strategies for dealing with particular types of problems creates a good framework for handling problems effectively.

Cultural Changes
An organization's attitude toward its own problems is as critical to their permanent resolution as any other single factor. If the organization refuses to see its own problems, nothing it does will ensure its ability to thrive in the long term.

Rejecting Patching as a Problem-Solving Approach
Focusing on situations instead of issues—or being sucked into situations and seeing the issues only from the inside—is sure to lead to failure. The best policy is to help the staff develop problem-solving skills so that they see clearly the problems that arise as part of their work and act as independent troubleshooters. Everyone who faces a problem wants the associated pain taken away. However, the pain is merely a symptom, and focusing solely on it ensures that the underlying issues never hit the table. In other words, the patching approach to problems must be challenged and eliminated from the set of permissible approaches.

Making Problem-Solving Deadlines Irrelevant
It is true that problems cannot be allowed to go on forever. Rather than set deadlines for solving problems, however, the leader should embed a problem-solving methodology into the work itself. If the methodology is effective and problem solving is fostered by the organization's culture, deadlines become moot. The problems that arise are not avoided or treated as belonging to "the other guy," but instead are viewed as opportunities for growth.

Refusing to Reward Firefighting
In health care, a premium tends to be placed on those who can make critical decisions quickly and correctly. Health professionals with this ability are treated as heroes by every medical soap opera and documentary. Heroes make poor citizens, however, and require a great deal of ego feeding. In fact, they are not necessarily good models except in war and can cause more problems than they are credited with solving.

It is better to implement good problem-solving methods and mechanisms than to have staff use individualistic approaches. It is better to build an organization committed to problem solving than to reward good firefighters. Waiting for problems to manifest means being a day late and a dollar short—by the time the problems are addressed, most of the damage has been done. The preferred strategy is to anticipate problems and incorporate their resolution into the life and work of every member of the organization.

TABLE 12-1 Personal and Group Stages on the Journey of Transformation

Stage	Personal	Group
Stage 1	Unlearning Letting go Reacting	Seeing change Acknowledging Resisting Mourning
Stage 2	Naming new skills Learning new skills Applying new skills	Discerning impact Finding meaning Experimenting Giving form
Stage 3	Reinforcing the new Evaluating behavior Teaching the new Extinguishing the old	Shifting expectations Relating in new ways Celebrating Taking ownership

Conclusion

For a leader, transformation can be a way of life. It is a journey consisting of logical stages made up of specific actions and processes. At its best, the journey is rational, progressive, and purposeful (**Table 12-1**).

Leaders who accept the role of transformational coach must embrace and cope with the vagaries of these changing times. Through role modeling and commitment to self-direction and growth, they create a context for new expectations and new behaviors. Through living the reality of change, they ensure that others can embrace their own changes and respond appropriately. In all their actions, they fulfill the aims of transformational coaching by remaining fully engaged with the staff and guiding them on the way to a productive future.

Chapter Takeaways

1. It is important for professionals to both comprehend and successfully translate the real meaning and value of accountability, distinguishing it from responsibility and emphasizing its critical role in the process and production of value-based clinical service outcomes.
2. The learner and learning organization are part of the same complex adaptive environment that continuously and dynamically responds to changes in its environment and to the demand for innovation in the work it facilitates. In this scenario, worker and workplace are identified as one in this "membership community," and the collective behaves in ways that enhances its value and assures its sustainability.
3. The revolutionary leader and the innovative coach are simply two elements of the same dynamic. Each skill recognizes the need of individuals and teams to develop their mutual understanding of the demand for growth and change, calibrate their collective response, charter a set of communal actions, undertake a plan of action, and evaluate effective movements within a positive team dynamic.

4. Integration is the medium through which all systems work. The current effort of health systems is to create a seamless population-based approach to ensuring health along the life continuum in a way that broadens the quality and impact of the service and effectively manages the relationship between cost and value.
5. Leaders do not avoid problems; indeed, they embrace and engage them. Leaders develop a strategic and structured process for problem identification, engagement, and resolution. By investing in problems as a normative part of the business of management of human systems, the leader avoids late stage reaction, the failure of timely engagement, and the erroneous perspective that problems are an unwelcome contradiction to the happiness and effectiveness of the work and workplace.

Case Study 12-1

Coaching for Growth

Casey is recognized in her organization as one of its most innovative and progressive leaders. The directors who report to her also seem to be more progressive than many of the other department directors, and they are frequently the leaders or chairs of various hospital councils. Casey's department is always on the leading edge of change, and they have the highest nurse, patient, and physician satisfaction scores when compared to other hospital departments. The entire department seems to run like a well-oiled machine.

Sandra is in her second year of a PhD program in executive leadership for nursing, and she has been assigned to Casey for her practicum experience. She is required to spend 100 hours with Casey for a semester as a participant-observer to all that Casey does in her role as chief nursing officer (CNO) and vice president (VP) of Patient Services. Sandra's professor has told her about Casey's reputation for being a transformational leader not only in her hospital but also in the entire community. The professor suggests that Sandra interview Casey to gain insight into how Casey has developed her own leadership skills, as well as the leadership skills of those who report to her. Sandra develops a list of questions that she wishes to discuss with Casey and her learning objectives for the practicum experience. Sandra will work with Casey and her directors over the semester and will accompany them to the group/council meetings and individual meetings with their direct reports. She plans to observe how the directors interact with one another as well as how they interact with Casey and other executives in the hospital.

It does not take Sandra long to recognize the differences between Casey and her colleagues at the VP level. In the nurse executive meetings, Casey is engaged and involved in the discussions and constantly looks for opportunities to expand her scope of responsibility and to demonstrate the accomplishments of her department. She frequently shares some of the innovations that have been developed by her directors to improve patient care outcomes, develop the clinical nurses, improve relationships with physicians, or ensure the best experience for patients and families. The other VPs do not seem nearly as engaged in the discussion and rarely come to the meetings as prepared as Casey is.

In a meeting with Casey, Sandra asks Casey, "What attributes do you desire in your directors as leaders of their units?" and "How have you developed the directors to be successful in their roles?" Casey explains that she looks for individuals who could develop their staff to reach their fullest potential. She looks for individuals who are risk takers and who are open to new ideas for innovation.

When observing Casey with the directors who report to her, Sandra observes a very dynamic and active team who obviously enjoy working together and who support each other as they present their challenges and successes.

During Casey's individual meetings with her directors, Sandra observes Casey constantly teaching and coaching each director and giving support and advice as needed. Casey often shares articles with the directors to expand their knowledge on leadership topics. She encourages the directors to assess the strengths of their direct reports and to seek out individuals who could be groomed for future leadership positions. They discuss specific clinical nurses who could champion various changes and innovations on the clinical units. Casey also encourages each director to develop a succession plan with developmental goals for individuals who demonstrate leadership potential.

When possible, Casey invites one or more of her directors to accompany her to meetings. She is transparent about issues that she deals with in her role, and she explains to Sandra that it is her philosophy to ensure that each of her directors is prepared to step into her role at a moment's notice if needed. Sandra marvels at Casey's personal commitment to mentoring her directors because some VPs might be threatened by strong direct reports, fearing that they might usurp authority or try to position themselves for the VP role. In contrast, Casey states, "If I stepped out of this role, I hope to be missed personally, but any one of my direct reports should be able to step into the role without even a ripple felt by the organization."

While accompanying Casey to her hospital-wide meetings, Sandra notices Casey is also very encouraging to her colleagues and frequently observes Casey "managing them up" to the chief operating officer. Casey spends time building her relationships with the VPs of other departments, which, she explains, is critically important as a foundation for times when challenges or problems might arise. She states, "Building positive relationships with others makes problem resolution much easier, and potential problems can be avoided with early discussions rather than waiting for the problems to escalate." Casey not only lives these principles, she also holds her own direct reports accountable for developing relationships with their peers as well.

Questions

1. What attributes of a transformational leader do you think that Casey exhibits in her role as CNO and VP of the nursing department?
2. How does Casey hold herself and her direct reports accountable for the department's outcomes and outputs?
3. How does Casey demonstrate the coaching aspect of her role as a leader?
4. If you were Casey, what might you do to develop your own team of directors?
5. In the Institute of Medicine's *Future of Nursing Report* (2011), there is a recommendation that every nurse be groomed to become a leader. With this in mind, what might you do, if you were Casey, to ensure that every clinical nurse is developed to become a leader?

Case Study 12-2

Mentoring Frontline Leaders

Andy has been the chief nursing officer (CNO) of Whitefish Community Hospital for the past 5 years. He has done an excellent job of advancing the knowledge, skills, and self-confidence of his directors, and the hospital was recently awarded Magnet designation with special commendation for research and innovation. Andy considers this to be a major accomplishment because when he first came to Whitefish Community the nursing department was led by a very authoritative leader in a hierarchical organizational structure. Andy has made many changes to the nursing organization and has won the respect of the executive team for all that has been accomplished. Physicians in the hospital have also commented on how nursing has improved dramatically over the past 5 years. Although Andy has every right to feel proud of nursing leadership and the clinical staff, he feels uneasy about the level of preparedness of the frontline leaders at the point-of-service.

The nursing organizational structure consists of directors who report to Andy, managers who report to the directors, and assistant managers who are shift leaders with responsibility for the day-to-day direction of staffing and the interface with the clinical nurses for their schedules and performance appraisals. In addition to the assistant managers, the more advanced clinical nurses are also designated as charge nurses, who are responsible for leading the clinical activities of the unit, including the patient assignments for each shift.

What concerns Andy is that the least experienced "manager" has the greatest interface with the clinical nurses, other professional partners, and the patients and families. He recognizes a need to improve the knowledge and competencies of the frontline leaders to improve patient outcomes, increase nurse and physician satisfaction levels, and ensure that there are adequate numbers of prepared individuals for a viable succession plan should the need occur. Andy realizes that the frontline leaders who are unprepared for their roles could significantly affect the hospital's reputation for excellence.

Andy often states, "A good reputation is hard won, easily lost, and sometimes never regained." He encourages his direct reports to focus on the issues that define quality from the perspective of the patient, physician, and employees. "It matters significantly that our nursing-sensitive indicators and all other quality metrics meet and exceed our targeted goals, but it's also critical that we address issues that are perceived by our customers as quality indicators. A clean environment, meal trays delivered on time, medications given when requested, and a comfortable space for the families are all issues of quality for the patients. Having information and resources available, the presence of the nurse during rounds, and an efficient hospital visit are all issues of quality for physicians. Having needed resources, adequate staffing, and a healthy work environment are all issues of quality for the nursing staff. We as leaders need to ensure that our nurses have the resources that they need to do what they do best, and then we need to get out of their way and let them do it! We need to assure our physicians that we have the best, the brightest, and the most competent nurses in the world who can provide excellent care for their patients and their families. We need to provide a calm, pleasant, healing environment for patients and their families. The only way that we can accomplish these goals is to be authentic leaders who are physically and emotionally present in our support for our nursing staff and particularly for the frontline leaders who are the least prepared for their critically important role."

Andy shares his concerns with his directors and the other executives on the healthcare team. He gathers their ideas, and they develop a mind map of all possible ways that the frontline leaders can be developed in the most cost-efficient way. They decide to develop a Leadership Institute with an array of courses and classes offered online and in quarterly presentations. They design a leadership development program that includes lectures online and in class, reading materials, video presentations, and group discussions of actual case presentations. It is decided that after the participants earn 25 units of education, they will be given a leadership certificate and pin presented at a graduation ceremony. The graduation will include a national speaker and recognition of the new graduate in the Whitefish Community Hospital publication that is distributed to all employees, physicians, patients, friends of the hospital (financial donors), and the board of directors.

Andy is pleased that this plan provides an educational foundation for the frontline leaders who may not have had the opportunity for leadership education beyond their basic nursing education; however, he still feels that something is missing in advancing the leadership skills and competencies of the frontline leaders. During the budget season, Andy had the opportunity to review all of the programs and services offered by the nursing division and other hospital divisions to ensure their "worthiness" of being financially supported in the upcoming year. During this analysis of all programs, Andy reviewed the annual report for the New Graduate Residency Program, and the data clearly indicated the positive outcomes and cost-efficiency of the program. Nested in the program was a strong and viable mentor program for the new graduate residents. Feedback from the new graduates indicated that the mentor program provided the social support that they needed to be acculturated on their units and provided a "safe resource" for them when they had questions, concerns, or frustrations they did not feel comfortable sharing with their direct supervisors. When Andy read the annual report and the anecdotal comments, he had an "aha!" moment. "Of course! This is the support that is missing for frontline leaders. We need to pair them with more prepared and experienced managers or directors who have clearly demonstrated success in their roles and who are willing and able to mentor the frontline leaders beyond the planned educational courses and sessions." Andy is excited about developing a leadership mentoring program not only for new leaders in the organization but also for the existing less-experienced frontline leaders. He strongly believes that a mentor from another department would provide the social and experiential support that is often missing in formal education.

When Andy shared his vision with the directors and executive colleagues, they are also interested, particularly when he shares the positive outcomes of the mentor program for the new graduate residents. He mentions that he would be using that program as a pattern for the development of the leadership mentor program. He also shares how he would be evaluating the program's effectiveness with outcome metrics that he would report back to the executive team. He indicates that the program would be provided within existing budgeted educational funds, and the return on the investment would not only be measured in financial terms but also in terms of patient, physician, and provider outcomes because the frontline leaders strongly influence these outcomes. Andy's next steps are to engage some of the directors, managers, selected frontline leaders, and the research nurses in the design, development, and measures of the leadership mentor program.

Questions

1. What is your opinion of Andy's plan to advance the knowledge and competencies of the frontline leaders?

2. What additional benefits, if any, do you see resulting from the development of a leadership mentor program?
3. What attributes of a transformational leader and coach does Andy demonstrate in his role with his direct reports, executive colleagues, and the nursing division as a whole?
4. Compare and contrast the similarities and differences between an authentic leader and a transformational leader.
5. In reviewing the attributes of quantum leaders, how do these attributes intersect with the attributes of authentic and transformational leaders?
6. If you were in Andy's role, what would you do to advance the knowledge, skills, and competencies of frontline leaders, and how would you measure whether you were successful in this endeavor?

References

Argote, L. (2013). *Organizational learning: Creating, retaining, and transferring knowledge.* Springer.

Argyris, C. (2006). *Reason and rationalizations: Capital limits to organizational knowledge.* Oxford University Press.

Bleich, M. R., & Hessler, C. (2016). Appreciative inquiry and implementation science in leadership development. *Journal of Continuing Education in Nursing, 47*(5), 207–209.

Brewer, G., & Sanford, B. (2011). *Decade of change: Managing in times of uncertainty.* Gallup Press.

Butani, L., & Plant, J. (2016). Building connections with role models using an appreciative inquiry approach. *Academic Pediatrics, 16*(4), 411–412.

Clavelle, J., Porter-O'Grady, T., Weston, M., & Veran, J. (2016). Evolution of structural empowerment: Moving from shared to professional governance. *Journal of Nursing Administration, 46*(6), 308–312.

D'Alfonso, J., Zuniga, A., Weberg, D., & Orders, A. (2016). Leading the future we envision nurturing a culture of innovation across the continuum of care. *Nursing Administration Quarterly, 40*(1), 68–75.

Guzman, G., Fitzgerald, J. A., Fulop, L., Hayes, K., Poropat, A., Avery, M., Campbell, S., Fisher, R., Gapp, R., Herington, C., McPhail, R., & Vecchio, N. (2015). How best practices are copied, transferred, or translated between health care facilities: A conceptual framework. *Health Care Management Review, 40*(3), 193–202.

Hickey, M., & Kritek, P. B. (2012). *Change leadership in nursing: How change occurs in a complex hospital system.* Springer.

Hu, A., Shewokis, P. A., Ting, K., & Fung, K. (2016). Motivation in computer-assisted instruction. *Laryngoscope, 126*(Suppl. 6), S5–S13.

Institute of Medicine. (2011). *The future of nursing: Leading change, advancing health.* National Academies Press.

Lencioni, P. (2008). *The five dysfunctions of a team.* Wiley.

McCarthy, B. (2016). Appreciative inquiry: An alternative to behaviour management. *Dementia* (London), *16*(2), 259–253.

Naylor, M., & Kurtzman, E. (2010). The role of nurse practitioners in reinventing primary care. *Health Affairs, 29*(5), 893–895.

Pesut, D., & Thompson, S. A. (2018). Nursing leadership in academic nursing: The wisdom of development and the development of wisdom. *Journal of Professional Nursing, 34*(2), 122–127.

Porter-O'Grady, T. (2007). *Implementing shared governance.* Tim Porter-O'Grady Associates.

Porter-O'Grady, T. (2009). *Interdisciplinary shared governance: Integrating practice, transforming health care.* Jones & Bartlett Learning.

Porter-O'Grady, T. (2013). From tradition to transformation: A revolutionary moment for nursing in the age of reform. *Nurse Leader, 12*(1), 32–37.

Porter-O'Grady, T. (2020). The structural framework for nursing professional governance: Foundation for empowerment. *Nurse Leader, 18*(2), 181–189.

Rowland, C., & Hall, R. (2014). Management learning, performance and reward theory and practice revisited. *Journal of Management Development, 33*(4), 342–356.

Savitch, W. (2008). *Problem solving with C++.* Addison-Wesley.

Schabracq, M. (2007). *Changing organizational culture: The change agent's guidebook.* Wiley.

Schein, E. H. (2013). *Humble inquiry.* Berrett-Koehler.

Shomaker, T. S. (2011). Commentary: Preparing for health care reform: Ten recommendations for academic health centers. *Academic Medicine, 86*(5), 555–558.

Stanford, J. R., & Wilkins, D. S. (2016). Changing physician behavior by integrating a risk-adjusted database into a quality improvement program. *American Journal of Medical Quality, 31*(6), 596–597.

Watkins, S., Dewar, B., & Kennedy, C. (2016). Appreciative inquiry as an intervention to change nursing practice in in-patient settings: An integrative review. *International Journal of Nursing Studies, 60*, 179–190.

Westerwick, A., Johnson, B. K., & Knobloch-Westerwick, S. (2016). Change your ways: Fostering health attitudes toward change through selective exposure to online health messages. *Health Communication, 1*, 1–11.

Wilensky, G. (2016). Changing physician behavior is harder than we thought. *Journal of the American Medical Association, 316*(1), 21–22.

Zedeck, S., & American Psychological Association. (2011). *APA handbook of industrial and organizational psychology.* American Psychological Association.

Suggested Readings

Heibing, D. (2012). *Social self organization: Understanding complex systems.* Springer.

Northouse, P. (2012). *Leadership: Theory and practice.* Sage.

Sandberg, S. (2013). *Lean in: Women, work and the will to lead.* Knopf.

Quiz Questions

Select the best answer for each of the following questions.

1. Which of the following is always true of accountability?
   a. It is generated externally.
   b. It is delegated from above.
   c. It is generated internally.
   d. It moves from the bottom upward.

2. How do accountability and responsibility differ from one another?
   a. They measure different kinds of processes.
   b. Responsibility is more results oriented.
   c. Accountability is measurable and responsibility is not.
   d. Accountability is defined in terms of outcomes.

3. In confronting change, what do most people find is their first response?
   a. To personalize it
   b. To feel excitement
   c. To challenge the necessity for change
   d. To refuse to change

4. In transformative learning, how can theory-in-use be described?
   a. It consists of the conceptual foundations for an action.
   b. It is an automatic thought process related to an action.
   c. It is the theoretical validation of an action.
   d. It is a research-based response to a need.

5. What is the first step in gathering staff together for the purpose of learning and adapting?
   a. Identify a good methodology to use.
   b. Enumerate the rules of engagement.
   c. Understand the stages of the change process.
   d. Get to work on the problems immediately.

6. The issue of resources plays a critical role in all problem solving. In dealing with this issue, leaders should keep in mind which of the following rules of thumb?
   a. It is always possible to find more money if you look for it.
   b. Providing additional resources is not the way to reach a sustainable solution.
   c. Allocating more resources is necessary for solving problems.
   d. Budgeting adequate resources is part of all planning.

7. In problem solving, leaders must remember that which of the following is the one absolute unforgivable?
   a. To leave problems unresolved too long
   b. To create inadequate processes for resolving problems
   c. To lack a methodology for change
   d. To solve other people's problems for them

8. The coach is the chief:
   a. facilitator.
   b. problem solver.
   c. learner.
   d. agent of change.

9. When a coach is acting as a revolutionary, which of the following is the most important task?
   a. Get action underway quickly.
   b. Bring down existing structures as quickly as possible.
   c. Expand the circle of conspirators.
   d. Construct an individual plan of action.

CHAPTER TWELVE   Coaching for Unending Change: Transforming the Membership Community

10. In innovation coaching, risk is critical for success. What else is critical?
    a. Experimentation
    b. Planning
    c. Creating ideas
    d. Brainstorming

11. In undertaking tactical changes, which of the following is the first thing the leader does?
    a. Get out of the way.
    b. Outline a process for change.
    c. Direct the participants in their work.
    d. Create a set of priorities.

12. In managing strategic changes, what does the leader focus on?
    a. Processes, elements, and tasks
    b. Priorities, learning scenarios, and problem-solving tools
    c. Context, functions, and solutions
    d. Vision, solutions, and outcomes

13. In facilitating cultural change, what does the leader avoid?
    a. Fighting, opposition, and conflict
    b. Directing, controlling, and disciplining
    c. Patching, setting deadlines, and firefighting
    d. Narrowing, limiting, and refining

14. With the growing demand for value-based accountable care, _____ is no longer the key element of work performance.
    a. accountability
    b. responsibility
    c. ownership
    d. faithfulness

15. The change from responsibility to accountability suggests which of the following?
    a. Shifting from a narrow focus on process to a broader perspective that encompasses the impact and results of the process
    b. Leaving a focus on process behind in emphasizing the achievement of outcomes
    c. Continuing to emphasize process but focusing more on skill development
    d. Emphasizing sustainability instead of maintaining a linear goal focus

16. In the 20th century the emphasis was on functions and work processes. In the 21st century, the focus is on:
    a. outcomes.
    b. processes.
    c. value.
    d. work.

17. Structure, relationships, and process should be directed toward:
    a. facilitating ownership so the organization's work can be sustained and advanced.
    b. advancing processes and structures to support the fulfillment of work obligations.
    c. advancing complexity in order to ensure that all the components of work are addressed.
    d. sharing work obligations in order to make sure that mutuality is valued.

18. Accountability has three major elements: the right to decide and to act, the power to decide and to act, and:
    a. the skills to act and undertake work.
    b. the insight to understand and to act.
    c. the leadership necessary to facilitate action.
    d. the competence to decide and to act.

19. All persons have specific and unique "mental maps." These maps form the contextual framework out of which:
    a. learning flows.
    b. behavior flows.
    c. action flows.
    d. outcomes flow.

20. The fourth element/characteristic of appreciative inquiry is:
    a. discovery.
    b. delivery.
    c. dream.
    d. design.

21. What is the fifth principle of appreciative leadership?
    a. Integrity/inclusion, the way of leading
    b. Accountability, the ownership for outcomes
    c. Collaboration, building relationships
    d. Ownership, investment and partnership

22. As much as possible, the leader should help the staff see problems as normal and:
    a. define the elements of problems so they can be seen clearly.
    b. identify responsibility for resolving problems.
    c. develop categories for classifying and prioritizing problems according to their potential impact.
    d. identify urgent problems and begin to work on them immediately.

23. _____ approaches to specific kinds of problems increase the likelihood the recurrences will be solved in a similar or related fashion to the originating problems.
    a. Sorting and naming
    b. Prioritizing and identifying
    c. Locating and isolating
    d. Codifying and recording

CHAPTER TWELVE   Coaching for Unending Change: Transforming the Membership Community

24. In appreciative principle 4, one of the important performance metrics in demonstrating impact is:
    a. ownership.
    b. communication.
    c. timeline.
    d. clarity.

25. Which of the following is one of the critical elements of appreciative leadership principle 1, emphasizing relational capacity and accountability?
    a. Sense of self
    b. Strategically crafted questioning
    c. Inclusive language
    d. Adult-to-adult interaction

CHAPTER THIRTEEN

The Leader's Courage to Be Willing: Building a Context for Hope

> Something unforeseen and magnificent is happening. Health care, having in our time entered its dark night of the soul, shows signs of emerging, transformed.
> —Barbara Dossey and Larry Dossey

Chapter Objectives

At the completion of this chapter, the reader will be able to:

- Review the sources of healthcare professional disenfranchisement.
- Describe the behavioral concept of willingness as it relates to the role of the leader.
- Describe a process for identifying and evaluating dogma in the healthcare system.
- Define the five essential qualities of will.
- Identify specific situations in which leaders can positively affect practice using the five essential qualities of will.

This chapter explores the concept of willingness and related concepts (e.g., will, the will, and willpower), the personal and organizational context in which willingness unfolds, and the factors that may erode its expression. It explains how the will of a person generally operates, how leaders can maximize their will, the evolutionary stages that a person's will goes through, and the purposes toward which a person's will can be directed. It also describes the five essential qualities of will (or willpower): courage, passion, energy, discipline, and trust. Finally, it presents nine strategies for facilitating willingness and associated assessment questions for leaders.

Why do healthcare workers, especially nurses, become discouraged? Where does the hope go? Job-related stress, emotional exhaustion, moral distress, and feelings of depression, helplessness, hopelessness, and entrapment are some of the reasons for dissatisfaction and discouragement among all clinicians, including physicians and healthcare administrators. The combined assault of staffing shortages and heavy workload, excessive regulations, and reduced reimbursement has left a pall of apathy over the healthcare profession. The human and social interactions that once were part of patient care have been replaced with technologies such as the electronic medical records that eliminate human interdependency and support independent work. This separates clinicians from the human connection they once received from working with each other.

First, staffing shortages are challenging leaders to find quick solutions—a nearly impossible task. Second, state and federal regulations require healthcare leaders and workers to perform numerous procedural tasks to document compliance, with associated high costs in time and money. A recent article identified more than 30 regulatory bodies at the national level and 8 or more licensing agencies per state that have jurisdiction over healthcare organizations (American Hospital Association [AHA], 2017). The complex laws and regulations generated by these agencies are often conflicting, and their benefits to the public are generally unknown.

How care is provided, documented, and reimbursed are all part of the changing landscape of the U.S. healthcare system. These issues have profound effects on clinical practice and on the professionals who provide patient care—the clinicians—and patients and their families. Yet, despite the problems in the nursing profession, the public has more regard for nurses than for any other type of health professional. Nurses have a powerful voice in their communities—perhaps even more powerful than they know and actualize. Consumers and politicians want to know what nurses think about prescription issues, ensuring access to care, and changing the health system to meet the needs of patients and their families.

Why are some leaders more successful than others in leading an organization through the transformational change necessary to address staff shortages, reimbursement, consumer needs, and regulations? Why do some leaders fail to sustain their commitment to a change, letting it slowly subside or disappear altogether? Why can some people create an environment of hope and calm despite desperate or difficult circumstances? One answer can be found in the notions of will and personal willingness. Willing leaders are the cocreators of change. They recognize that no one person or situation can take away their personal peace, joy, and sense of competence, and they transmit these feelings to others.

Because of feelings of desperation, personal investment in the status quo, or a need for psychological preservation, some very knowledgeable leaders lose their willingness to take the initiative in making changes. Instead, they replace their willingness with an organizational mask, becoming what they believe the organization or a powerful other wants them to be. Such leaders may be incapable of seeing the whole and acting on their vision of it because they have lost their calling to nursing and health care. The dark side of the calling takes over and our calling becomes a job, economics drives our decisions rather than quality and safety, and passion for the profession abates, along with our willingness to embrace healthcare challenges to the fullest. Willing leaders not only see the whole but also claim responsibility for creating their personal experience of transformational change. Willing leaders also work to move from the middle-of-the-road positions to clarify and strengthen their positions on important issues. Paralysis and mediocrity are replaced with passion and engagement.

A Context for Hope

Leaders of quantum organizations can move only in one direction—toward building and sustaining the context for healthcare services and reinforcing expectations for a better future. These leaders behave in new and bold ways and see things from an optimistic and futurist perspective. Further, they are willing to do the work that needs to be done to meet patient needs, adhere to professional standards, and stay within the limits of available reimbursement. By their commitment to creating a hopeful context, they ensure that healthcare workers are better able to do the work of healing and health promotion.

The degree of a leader's willingness to lead can be explained by the extent to which he or she possesses courage, passion, energy, discipline, and trust. By possessing these qualities in abundance, the leader can engender in others not only hopefulness but a greater willingness to provide service.

> **Point to Ponder**
>
> Hope springs not from trying to remodel the past but rather from being willing to continually create the future with our colleagues to meet the changing needs of the community.

Will

Will (or willpower) has been defined as an inner power—a power over nature and over the self (i.e., self-control). Only the development of this inner power can offset the risk of our losing control of the tremendous forces at our disposal and becoming victims of our own achievements.

The terms *will* and *willpower* are typically used to refer to this inner power in the abstract, apart from the consideration of any individual person. The phrase *the will* is used when discussing willpower as evidenced by an individual person. In this usage, a person is said to have a will, and this will, typically viewed as the center of the person's self, is what exhibits willpower (or lack of willpower). Because the development of each person's will depends on the person's culture and the current circumstances, including political and economic factors, a person's will can be very powerful, very weak, or some degree in between these two extremes.

In coaching others, leaders should recognize that developed willpower has an enormous potential for creating and adapting to change. Once leaders gain an appreciation for how the qualities of willpower are expressed, they can comprehend the dynamics of those whose will is less strong and understand their rationale for pulling away. Reframing the work of leadership in terms of willpower can serve to create or rebuild hope and to redirect others toward greater achievement and satisfaction.

Discovery of Will

This section explores the view that a quantum leader's will is critical to his or her leadership success. The leader needs to discover the essence of his or her will and create the conditions for others in the organization to discover and honor their own will.

For each person, the discovery of his or her will encompasses the following five phases:

1. Recognizing that willpower exists
2. Realizing that one has a will
3. Living one's personal will
4. Recognizing one's soulfulness (an awakening of the self resulting from insight and self-exploration)
5. Recognizing that awakening the will can be risky and can even threaten paralysis

> **Key Point**
>
> Will is the self-directing capacity of human beings—the internal body of personal power. The simplest and most frequent way in which a person discovers his or her will is through determined action and struggle. When a person makes a physical or mental effort or actively wrestles with some obstacle or opposing force, the person feels a power, or energy, rise up inside.

Self-exploration, particularly investigation of one's will, does not appear to be widely embraced by those in leadership positions. Overworked and sometimes taken for granted, leaders must struggle with a number of issues before they can embark on an examination of their will. These issues include the following:

- Leaders often have a Victorian conception of will, according to which it is associated with stern control over others.
- Most people are reluctant to change, particularly if it involves personal examination. Also, change requires time and patience—two commodities that are in short supply. It is easier to sit back and let others carry the ball.
- Leaders often do not want to pay the price for becoming more involved in change (or becoming less involved).
- Leaders are hesitant to discuss willpower and its characteristics with the executive team for fear of job loss.

Not surprisingly, the organization's culture strongly influences whether an exploration of willpower does in fact occur. The values, practices, and longevity of employees can facilitate or obstruct meaningful changes that foster a readiness to investigate the nature of willpower.

Initially, a person's will has a regulatory and directive function. Take the case of a rehabilitation patient. He knows what his legs are supposed to do and in which direction he is supposed to move, but in addition to the normal power he uses to propel his legs, he needs the encouragement of the physical therapist, giving him the willpower to act. Without this encouragement, the patient's willpower would be weak or sporadic and might disappear altogether.

When individuals discover that willpower exists within themselves and realize that the will and the self are intimately connected, they become more oriented toward the self and concomitantly less oriented toward others and the world. Recognizing that the power to make changes is located primarily in the self and not in others, they are now free to use their willpower to choose, relate, and bring about changes in themselves and others. They feel a new sense of unlimited potential for action, whether this involves altering themselves or acting on the outside world.

Consider the prevalence of noise in patient care areas. It is well known that noise prevents patients from resting and sleeping. Care providers know they should be less noisy and also remind others of the importance of quiet, but only rarely does an individual with a high degree of courage speak up about the need for a restful environment. In other words, the will to act is usually missing or is not sufficient for action. Although solving the problem of noise would seem to be simple, the fact is that noise in patient care areas continues to be one of the most common causes of patient complaints.

Another example concerns the resistance of workers to changes in their work routines. They may believe that the current work routines are the best way to achieve the desired goals, but often they are merely fearful of what will happen to them after the changes are implemented. Thus, their fear, rather than their will, drives their behavior. Overcoming resistance to change is a consistent theme in management literature, and efforts to guide leaders in developing the skills needed to foster change and innovation are well documented.

Given that any complex adaptive system exhibits self-organization, unpredictable interactions, and interdependencies, leaders can learn to work with the natural energy of the system. They can learn this and overcome resistance to change more effectively by developing an understanding of will and willingness. It is helpful to note that will, despite the Victorian conception of it, is not about sternness but rather about the multidimensional directive and regulatory balances used by an individual.

It is not difficult to let the easygoing side of one's nature take control and to allow internal or external influences to dominate change when negative pressures exist. Such behaviors reinforce apathy and discouragement. Leaders can oppose negative behaviors. They should not expect training of the will to be accomplished without the expenditure of energy and persistence required for the successful development of any other quality, physical or mental. Effort lies at the base of any worthwhile leadership activity and is a requisite for success.

> ## Group Discussion
>
> Identify at least two situations in which you thought about reacting to a problem situation but did not. Was your reluctance related to patient care, the behaviors of coworkers, organizational policy, or something else? Now that you have identified a situation that should be managed, how can each member of the group support you in summoning the courage to react in the future?

Nature of Will

Because will is embedded in the self, self-exploration and the astute observation of colleagues are starting points for gaining an appreciation of the significance of will for leadership. Self-exploration can help a leader:

- Control his or her own will.
- Identify areas that need to be developed.
- Assess the application of willpower by others.
- Intervene in cases of inappropriate use.

Awakening of the self requires insight, self-absorption, and struggle. In the journey through transformational change, leaders discover the power to make choices, relate to others, and bring about changes in themselves and others. As a result of the new insights they gain during this journey, leaders could withdraw their support for certain projects or change priorities. Both positive and negative actions can be conscious or unconscious, depending on the degree of self-examination. When self-examination is a conscious process, the effect on the individual can be profound because the self shifts its orientation inward.

Unfortunately, there are obstacles to and dangers in self-exploration of the will. All too often, leaders work to become who they believe the organization wants them to be, preventing themselves from becoming who they really are. When this happens, they struggle and perceive themselves stuck in a persona that is not authentic, with the result that they feel impotent, apathetic, and insincere and do not draw from their natural strengths.

> **Key Point**
>
> Are you willing to want what you get when it comes or to force yourself to get what you want? How strong is your will?

The questions that leaders, not to mention other individuals, need to ask themselves are these: Are you willing to say yes—to act, think, and feel as you really are? Can you picture what this would be like? Would it not be joyful to do things because they reflect your will and are authentic rather than solely because the organization expects such behaviors?

By developing their will, leaders are better able to make decisions intuitively and rationally. By integrating their personal heart and objective mind, they become more authentic individuals and increase their willingness to act. Alternatively, if they act solely for reasons and values outside of themselves, they will continue to suffer and be disinclined to participate in the changing environment.

Further, denying one's personal will is a way of avoiding personal accountability. Assuming accountability, on the other hand, means never experiencing anything that is not a product of one's vision, mental model, or emotions. The self, not the external world, is the source of experiences. It follows that nothing can take away one's peace, joy, or sense of adequacy—each of these must be given up voluntarily.

Types of Will

Characterizing the types of will that people have can help clarify what will is. For example, it is relatively common to hear people described as having a strong will, a skillful will, or a good will. A brief account of each type follows.

To say that someone has a *strong will* is to say that that person has significant power or determination. A typical mistake is to believe that strength of will is the essence of the whole will—that having a will means always attempting to get one's own way.

Someone who possesses a *skillful will* is able to achieve desired results with the least amount of energy. People who have this type of will must understand their own habits, goals, and desires, and the relationships among these, to use them skillfully.

A person with a *good will* is benevolent, has a high degree of integrity, and does not use his or her will to overpower or corrupt the will of others.

Essential Qualities

The notion that a person's will consists only of strength or weakness, or goodness or badness, is incorrect and can lead someone engaged in self-exploration in the wrong direction. Instead, for individuals to exhibit will or willpower, they must possess a certain set of qualities; namely, courage, passion, energy, self-discipline, and trust (**Figure 13-1**). Leaders who are interested in increasing their expertise should use this set of qualities as a paradigm of will during periods of self-examination or when evaluating the behavior of others.

Courage

Courage is that quality of mind or spirit that enables individuals to face difficulty, danger, and pain without fear and to act in accordance with their beliefs. Courage is required to stay the course during the shaking and shuddering of the chaotic stage of change and to manage resistance to change to reach new levels of knowledge and performance. It is also required to tolerate paradox—to function while holding two competing forces inside. Courageous individuals also tend to be creative, daring, and trusting of their intuition, whereas individuals who lack courage are cautious, to put it politely (**Exhibit 13-1**).

Courage often does not emerge until the pain of not doing something exceeds the fear of doing it. The fear that we feel when we encounter an unfamiliar pathway and must enlarge our

Figure 13-1 The Five Essential Qualities of Will Lead to Hope for the Future.

Exhibit 13-1 Qualities Associated with Willingness and Reluctance

Willingness	Reluctance
• Courage	• Fear
• Passion	• Apathy
• Energy	• Lethargy
• Self-discipline	• Self-indulgence
• Trust	• Skepticism

---

thinking is a signal that we are on the brink of learning. It is like traveling in a foreign country and being seized by a vague fear and the instinctive desire to go back home. Similarly, during periods of change we experience an instinctive desire for the protection of old habits. At that moment, we are tense but also porous to learning.

Numerous explanations for the lack of courage exist. Most point to fear of the unknown or discomfort with what is happening. Fear is paralyzing and brings out the worst in people—their most basic instincts, those for self-protection and survival. Yet healthy fear—the kind of fear that enhances the acquisition of new knowledge—needs to be valued, reinforced, and fostered.

To create a more hopeful culture, leaders need to assist others in finding the courage to deal with the type of fear that causes imperviousness to learning and shuts down the

> **Points to Ponder**
>
> To know what is right and not to do it is the worst cowardice.
>
> —Confucius
>
> There is nothing more difficult to take in hand, more perilous to conduct, or more uncertain in the success, than to take the lead in the introduction of a new order of things.
>
> —Machiavelli
>
> Ships in port are safe, but that is not what ships were built for.
>
> — Antoine de Saint-Exupéry, *The Little Prince* (1943)

capacity for connectedness. Believing in others and remaining patient while they endure and experience the process further support their personal growth and accountability.

The Nike slogan "Just do it" calls individuals to jump out of the comfort zone and into the fringe of the unknown. Leaders need the same "just do it" attitude. This does not mean acting impulsively and without a plan, but instead doing the best that one can in light of what one knows and expects at that particular time.

As an example, although the perceived conflict between financial viability and professional standards will probably continue forever, decisions still need to be made. Leaders must often "just do it"—make a decision that balances standards and reimbursement. To develop the courage to make such decisions, you must let go of what others believe you should be and boldly show the world who you are. Courageous leaders:

- Face their fears.
- Explore their vulnerability.
- Lean toward risk.
- Celebrate failures.
- Never give up.

Passion

A sense of passion and willingness in individuals happens when we work from our purpose, which for clinicians is usually about caring for patients, improving health, and providing hope. Leaders who create a culture that ignites purpose and focuses on doing what is right for the patients engage employees by fulfilling their calling of caring for patients. The goal is to create an organizational culture that turns employees and patients into thunderous evangelists for the organization. This type of culture is very different from the traditional organizational culture, in which the following occur:

- Employees are expected to encourage patients to use a select group of providers in a specific geographic region.
- Employee productivity is closely monitored.
- Policies are strictly enforced.

Successful organizations carefully and intentionally balance passion and performance.

Energy

Energetic individuals are vigorous and active, with a capacity for serious effort. Such individuals also have an intensity of will capable of overcoming opposing forces, like an athlete in competition. This intensity of will is a form of power and needs to be recognized and used

Group Discussion

After reading the following summary of an event, identify the presence (or absence) of courage, energy, trust, passion, and discipline in the behavior of the nurse.

A clinical nurse admitted a terminally ill patient and reported to her manager that she believed she really had made a difference in the care of the patient and in the final outcome. She also stated that she had required a total of 2 hours for the admission process—an hour in excess of the allocated time. The manager, in response, showed concern about the extra time used in the admission process and the additional expense for this type of care.

The clinical nurse then explained the situation more fully. A female patient with terminal cancer, accompanied by her husband, was admitted for pain management and relief of abdominal ascites. She was scheduled for a fluoroscopy-guided paracentesis to relieve the fluid and to receive IV pain medication. The patient was exhausted and wanted relief from her discomfort. Also, in the course of the admission, the patient informed the nurse that she was ready to die, that she had fought hard and long enough and knew nothing could be done to extend her life. Her husband agreed.

The nurse asked the patient if she knew that draining the fluids from her abdomen would relieve the pressure temporarily but would leave more space for the fluids to collect again. The patient was told that she could be kept comfortable without the paracentesis and could be assisted to die as comfortably as possible. This approach was discussed with the physician, who gave it his approval. The patient and husband chose to have pain management only. The patient died peacefully 2 days later.

In discussing the case with her manager, the nurse argued that use of 2 hours for the admission process resulted not only in a desirable outcome but in an economic savings. True, the admission cost the organization an additional hour of RN time, but eliminating a fluoroscopy-guided paracentesis avoided the addition of approximately $2,500 in charges to a DRG bill. The organization was saved this entire amount because the reimbursement for the patient was fixed. Thus, the nurse maximized the quality of the care while minimizing the organization's costs.

Group Discussion

Reflect on a situation in which you were at your wits' end and finally reacted. At what moment and for what reason were you inspired or forced to respond? In the future, will you react more quickly? Why or why not?

positively. The energy required for optimal willingness is never limitless; rather, energetic individuals learn to temper and manage their energy expenditure, balancing high-energy times with quiet times.

In contrast, low-energy individuals are apathetic, uninterested, or burned out. Some are fearful of getting involved or becoming too hopeful because of past disappointments. For these individuals, the lack of a clear, defined sense of self is often at the root of their inaction. If they see themselves as disempowered, which many of them do, their stagnation is reinforced. What low-energy individuals need is assistance in reentering the unfolding processes of life. In particular, they need to assess their goals, focus on the future and on what is positive and working, and accept that human beings are inherently imperfect.

Self-Discipline

Self-discipline is the personal willingness to adhere to standards and meet responsibilities. It is the ability to check impulsive actions while persisting in selected activities. Self-discipline is regulation of one's own behavior, not that of others. Without self-discipline, a leader with a strong will acts impulsively and unpredictably, negating the positive spirit of leadership willingness.

When leaders develop self-discipline, they are better able to focus their attention and minimize impulsive and scattered activities. Their inner concentration grows, allowing them the steady control and clarity of action and thought they need to gain the support of colleagues.

Trust

Developing trust between colleagues requires congruence of values, nonpossessive warmth, effective communication, and empathy (i.e., the ability to understand the perceptions and feelings of others). Trust and purpose also yield happiness (Zak, 2017). It requires knowledge that the shared values are ethically sound and that the work of the care providers is truly intended to further the public's interest. The trust that has been built up between colleagues is reinforced when everyone consistently behaves in accordance with accepted patient care standards and uses resources wisely, shares information appropriately, and discusses new ideas openly.

Paul Zak (2017) identifies eight leadership behaviors that foster trust and can improve performance:

- Recognize excellence.
- Induce challenge—assign a difficult but achievable job.
- Give autonomy.
- Enable creativity.
- Share information broadly.
- Intentionally build relationships.
- Facilitate growth of people in skills and as human beings.
- Show vulnerability as a leader—ask employees for their help.

A leader with a fully developed will, characterized by courage, passion, energy, self-discipline, and trust, creates a positive and encouraging context in which employees are expected to practice within professional standards and values. This type of leader also instills a sense of hopefulness in all members of the organization, increasing the chance that together they will bring about a better and more meaningful healthcare future (**Exhibit 13-2**).

> **Exhibit 13-2** Attributes of a Willing Leader
>
> - *Openness to change*: Willingness to approach changes in staffing, organizational structure, and roles with a positive attitude while maintaining a focus on patient care; willingness to be a cocreator of change rather than a defender of the past
> - *Acceptance of diverse perspectives*: Willingness to look at multiple reasonable alternatives while giving up the role of patient advocate; willingness to acknowledge that some situations may not be acceptable but are a major part of one's work life and must be handled patiently
> - *Focus on value*: Willingness to educate others to understand evidence-based approaches as the new context for providing healthcare services
> - *Awareness of the larger system*: Willingness to move between micro and macro views of issues—from the patient to the team to the department to the organization to the community to the state to the world and back

Hope

Hope is the feeling that what is wanted can be had or that events will turn out well. People find it difficult to be hopeful if they do not believe things are going satisfactorily. They become less inclined to get involved and less willing to do the right thing because it does not seem to matter. When the qualities of will—courage, passion, energy, self-discipline, and trust—are present, a beacon of hope emerges to begin a positive cycle of behaviors. Discouraged and disenfranchised workers start to see new opportunities and develop a new willingness to focus on the present and future, leaving the past behind.

Strategies to Facilitate Willingness

Once leaders understand the nature of will, they are in a position to facilitate willingness as a means of achieving their goals. Following is a discussion of strategies that incorporate the qualities of courage, passion, energy, discipline, and trust. Note that these do not exhaust the strategies for increasing the willingness of individuals on the team, but constitute a beginning on which to build.

Removing the Dogma Brick Wall

So much health care is done routinely and automatically, with little thought to its rationale. As science advances, new technologies and practices emerge and become popular. These and the older technologies and practices should be examined to ensure that the evidence-based care that results in value to the patient is provided at the lowest cost. Examining technologies and practices demands significant courage, because it can involve challenging the system and its players. It also requires openness to new ideas and the recognition that change is (i.e., change is inevitable and should not be avoided). The ongoing complexity in the healthcare environment can be a source of burnout. To moderate this risk, a shift from bureaucracies to adaptive individuals and environments is essential. Nurse leaders' roles are not just to keep the system running but to help it run better (Uhl-Bien et al., 2020).

In surveying health care for the purpose of making improvements, leaders should not look first to see what additional products, services, and providers are needed in the future, but rather review the current situation to identify nonvalue-adding services for elimination. Or, at

Group Discussion

The following questions are posed for reflection. Examine behaviors related to all five categories: courage, passion, energy, self-discipline, and trust. Are some behaviors more prevalent than others? How can you improve behaviors in each category? Finally, develop a plan to incorporate the desired behaviors into the interview process for new employees and in the annual performance review competency set.

Courage
- Is there evidence that members of the organization are able to share their values and ideas in a nonthreatening manner?
- Is there evidence that members are able to stand their ground in defending their values and ideas?
- Are the members brave enough to ask the right questions?

Passion
- Is there evidence in the organization of a strong and vocalized commitment to ideas? To projects?
- Is there evidence that all employees take great pride in their work?
- Are there groups or projects in which enthusiasm is lacking? If so, which are they?

Energy
- Does the organization's leader exhibit vigor and vitality when managing projects?
- Does the leader's opinion dominate the ideas or actions of others?
- Are employees willing to participate in organizational group activities, social events, and/or committees?

Self-Discipline
- Does the organization's leader regulate his or her activities appropriately?
- In managing projects, does the leader act impulsively?
- Are meetings or programs well thought out and implemented with little chaos?

Trust
- Is the organization's leader honest, forthright, and candid with others, or does the leader tell half-truths, damaging the trusting bond between leader and colleague?
- Are team members open and honest with each other?
- Does the leader rely on team members, and do team members rely on each other?
- Is information shared broadly?
- Do team members have discretion in how they do their work?

best, they should review both the current and the proposed improvement simultaneously. This approach, besides helping to create excess capacity for future needs, revalidates what is important in health care. All too often, practices become integrated into the system and continue to be used long after their rationale is lost or forgotten. "We have always done it this way" is not a good reason to keep on using a nonbeneficial practice.

For one thing, we have not always done it this way. At one time, only physicians were allowed to take blood pressures, insert nasogastric tubes, administer IV bolus medications, and write prescriptions. Now aides, technicians, and nurses perform these same tasks. The fact is that health professionals, especially physicians, often hesitate to relinquish technical tasks that the state practice act does not really require them to perform. New research and evidence examining the value of the nursing history has challenged one of nursing's sacred cows (Ackman et al., 2012). The authors report in a performance improvement project that the nursing history was a one-time, nonvalue-added process. There are many patient care processes that don't add value or are duplicative of what other clinicians do.

Unquestioning adherence to authority and tradition is a well-known barrier to the development of knowledge. Although authority and tradition provide a seemingly stable foundation, blind faith is problematic and can be detrimental to survival. Continuing progress in nursing and other areas of health care thus warrants an examination of all dogmas and a release from those that are without foundation.

Dogmas pertain to professional roles as well as procedures and practices. Patients deserve the best of every discipline, and efforts to delineate the boundaries of each discipline and profession need to be ongoing. Those responsible for delineating the domains of the various health professions must look at the received wisdom (conventional beliefs) within each profession, the profession's knowledge base (science), and the profession's application of that knowledge (art). The practices of any professional healthcare worker go beyond science as traditionally conceived to include, for instance, the use of intuition and the therapeutic use of the self. Likewise, the emerging principles that pertain to building relationships and partnerships beg for inclusion into the healthcare disciplines.

The real work of quantum leaders is to deconstruct the dogmas of traditional Newtonian science and transform current organizational underpinnings to reflect the essence of complexity science. The realities of current organizations—the great number of connections and

Group Discussion

Questioning practices requires courage and evidence. The following practice has been identified as questionable given the lack of evidence:

Using Trendelenburg position to treat hypotensive episodes. Evidence indicates that the Trendelenburg position has little, if any, positive effect on cardiac output and blood pressure. It impairs pulmonary gas exchange and increases the aspiration risk.

As the organizational leader, how would you go about changing the use of Trendelenburg positioning? Consider code situations, use in the surgical suites, emergency areas, and the functioning of hospital beds. Who are the key stakeholders? Who will support this change? Who will resist this change?

Flynn, M. B. (2013). Questioning common nursing practices: What does the evidence show? *American Nurse Today, 8*(3), 6–7; Makic, M. B. F., Rauen, C., Jones, K., & Fisk, A. C. (2015). Continuing to challenge practice to be evidence based. *Critical Care Nurse, 35*(2), 39–50.

relationships among the many elements and the inherent capacity for change or adaptation—demand a better explanation than can be delivered by the linear thinking characteristic of Newtonian science. Once the nonvalue-added work is identified, the processes to engage nurses to actually change practice may in fact be more challenging than identifying the outdated work.

Unlike the mechanistic Newtonian paradigm, complexity science affirms that no leader is an island. In other words, the achievement of desired outcomes in a system is beyond the talents of any one individual or discipline. Instead, outcomes result from the relationships between individuals and disciplines. Although the abilities of a single individual are important, they are not completely useful until the individual establishes relationships and works together with other individuals. Thus, the attention of leaders shifts from individual performance to appropriate patterns of interrelationship. A context that frees individuals from the traditional role of implementer of decisions from others to one of collaborators who work together to enhance the overall adaptability of the healthcare system (Uhl-Bien et al., 2020) is essential. The following are strategies for minimizing dogma:

- Examine and assess the value of at least three current practices each month. Retain or eliminate each practice depending on its value.
- Believe in the value of process so strongly that at least three employees gain the same appreciation each month.
- Approach difficult situations in which there is personal impact with the same enthusiasm as situations that do not affect you personally.
- No matter how long current practices have been used, be willing to examine them and consider other evidence-based practices.
- Review prevalent dogmas in a patterned way. Commit to making no change impulsively. Instead, first talk with colleagues to ensure that every proposed change makes good sense or if employees have a better idea.
- Know that colleagues share concerns about long-held practices and believe there are better ways as well but may not be quite ready to address the issues. Patience is needed.

Continuous Learning

High-quality healthcare services can be delivered only by educated, compassionate, and skilled clinicians. Further, such clinicians need to maintain or increase their competence levels through professional development and advancement. Following through on a commitment to professional growth, however, can be incredibly difficult in an organization steeped in reorganization. Everyone's energy is channeled into the redesign and maintenance of the new context, making continuing education hard to pursue. The quantum leader must therefore support the acquisition of new knowledge and skills by employees, while at the same time sustaining the reorganization efforts. According to Schein (Contu, 2002), learning and change that inevitably accompany new knowledge are part of a complex process that includes both the achievement of increased knowledge and the frustrations of the change dynamic. Following are some ways for a leader to ensure that continuous learning becomes part of the organization:

- Create and maintain a culture that fosters continuous learning.
- Recognize that new knowledge is essential for all to survive.

- Participate enthusiastically in professional development, and share the knowledge you gain with colleagues.
- Support continuous learning consistently—through every budget cycle and challenge throughout the year.
- Identify and trend performance measures that support the value of professional development.

Minimizing Professional Antagonism

In hierarchical departmental organizations, the work groups can become competitive and adversarial. In healthcare organizations, for example, departments battle for resources and position.

In addition, nurses have been reported to "eat their young." A recent panel of student nurses working in a particular healthcare organization identified the nurses who coached and mentored them in a positive way and those who reinforced their novice status in the presence of others. One student freely shared why she would not select that organization for employment: she had been assigned a preceptor who was a nationally recognized nurse expert but who was avoided by students because of her intimidating behaviors and perceived intolerance.

Antagonism exists among new employees often because of poor interpersonal skills of managers, preceptors, and colleagues. In nursing, the nurses (the staff and the nurse manager), not nonnurse coworkers, have the greatest impact on nurse stress. Thus, in this regard, nurses truly can be their own worst enemies—and consequently the solution may lie within nursing rather than outside the healthcare system. Millennials are the largest proportion of the nursing workforce, and their greatest need is to connect with their team and patients and feel like they belong. Nurses need to care for each other—just as they do for their patients. They need to be their brothers' and sisters' keepers. The leader's role in reducing professional antagonism is to do the following:

- Bring issues into the open for discussion and minimize behind-the-scenes dialogue.
- Realize that relationships truly can be therapeutic. Expecting collaboration is the only way to develop the culture and context for high-quality, low-cost patient care services.
- Incorporate interpersonal development into clinical professional development.
- Address issues as they arise.
- Stay focused and remain objective.

Group Discussion

The assumption that people working in health care are shallow, single-minded, materialistic, and socially unfettered is consistent with Newtonian science. These beliefs support the practice of attracting new employees by giving them sign-on bonuses. Do you agree or disagree with this rationale? What are the effects, positive and negative, of this approach to recruitment on quality, productivity, and cost? What types of reward and recognition practices would be consistent with complexity theory? What are the effects of these reward and recognition practices on quality, productivity, and cost?

Meeting the Needs of Employees

There are two categories of employees: those who have jobs and those who have careers. Those with jobs report to work, perform their duties as well as possible, and go home at the end of their tour of duty to get on with their lives. In contrast, those with careers not only do the necessary work, but plan where they are going in their chosen profession and participate in professional activities outside of the workplace.

Not every person is seeking a career. Some individuals are satisfied with a job that is meaningful and fairly compensated. Expecting to motivate all employees to commit to a career is unrealistic. It is especially ill-advised to dangle cash before professionals as a way of inducing desired behaviors and changes. This strategy is based on the assumption that people are motivated only by material gain, and is likely to lead to a healthcare workforce that is indeed petty and greedy. It is also based on the assumption that individuals act independently of their social institutions and that social systems are nothing more than the sum of individual actions. This is a shallow notion of human decision making and ignores the way our values and actions are conditioned and constrained by social relations.

The world of work today is very different from what it was in the past. Workers stayed with one company or organization for a lifetime, whereas now workers may have several career pathways, and mobility rather than promotion is the symbol of advancement. The notion of loyalty needs to be redefined to reflect the marketplace of the 21st century. Loyalty to an organization may have been appropriate at one time, but now loyalty to one's core values is more suited to the way work is organized.

Leaders need the courage to recognize this phenomenon and ensure that both types of employees—job holders and career seekers—are valued and treated fairly. The organization must meet not only the needs of the customers but also those of the individuals it employs. The presence of employees from different generations and with different values requires leaders to use multiple strategies:

- Create a compensation system that recognizes the multiplicity of employee values and needs. In addition, the system should support retention and guide employees to new opportunities when the organization's needs change, the required job skills change, or the employees' desires change. Become a partner with employees in managing their work and planning for the next position and coaching them for success.
- Be vigilant and persistent when implementing and maintaining an appropriate compensation system and recognition and reward program.
- Stay focused and committed despite resistance from those who would like the current compensation system and recognition and reward program to remain unchanged.

Providing Value-Based Services

What one does and what difference it makes are the key issues for all providers. If an organization provides 1,000 services and only 25 make a difference, then the other 975 services must be considered for elimination—even if the 975 services have billing codes that render them reimbursable.

Provider and clinician accountability for contributions to patient care outcomes is a missing piece of health care. All clinicians must focus their actions on achieving desired outcomes and implement only interventions that have a basis in science or a realistic chance of benefiting patients.

The measurement of healthcare outcomes is becoming more meaningful and reflective of patient needs (Pappas, 2013). Nursing care can now be documented and linked quantitatively to healthcare value (Pappas & Welton, 2015). Unfortunately, some key indicators are often evaluated as if there is no relationship between these indicators, which fails to take into account the basic goal of health care—health improvement. For example, staffing productivity measures are typically examined separately from patient outcome measures and the cost of an episode (hospital stay or clinic visit) of patient care. If productivity targets reflect there is too many staff for a unit of work, there is pressure to decrease staff to improve productivity; however, in addition, nurses must evaluate changes in staffing in the context of a potential impact of decreased staff on patient outcomes and the cost of an episode of care. If staffing costs are reduced and the episode cost increases because the patient acquired an infection, cost reduction has not been accomplished and quality erodes. Achieving positive clinical and cost outcomes is how healthcare value is defined.

Consumers of healthcare services expect that the services received are based on logic and scientific knowledge and that the intended outcomes are likely to occur. Further, they view the primary goal of healthcare organizations as providing effective clinical services, not making a profit. The problem for these organizations is how to provide value-based, high-quality care that is affordable and at the same time receive reimbursement that covers operating costs and generates capital (this is different from making as much money as possible).

The call for healthcare value in the Affordable Care Act further challenges leaders of the system to determine the optimal mix of value-based care with available resources. Unfortunately, many leaders are caught in the cost–quality balancing act and are not always sure how to achieve value-based care. This raises the question whether we can afford to spend money on quality initiatives. Ethically, the answer is a resounding yes! And that is the public's expectation as well.

Perhaps it would be helpful to reframe the quality question as a value question. Value is determined by the three elements of cost, quality, and service (Malloch & Porter-O'Grady, 1999). Cost is the amount of resources used to provide direct care. Quality is described by the outcomes of care. Service is a matter of the time and type of care provided. Thus, the following question becomes relevant: Are healthcare leaders obligated to provide value-based services to patients and family members? The issue of spending money on quality is now linked to both cost and service, and many organizations invest in quality and service because good performance can lower the cost of care.

Achieving value-based health care faces an additional challenge: drawing conclusions about quality initiatives and return on investment when there are multiple factors involved. A further complication is the extensive use of a type of cost–benefit analysis that is not sensitive to healthcare objectives. If the benefits of a program can be priced in dollars, then a cost–benefit analysis can identify the alternative with the largest benefit-to-cost ratio. However, many decisions involve benefits that are not easily quantifiable in monetary terms or otherwise, such as psychological benefits and environmental benefits (clean air and water).

Healthcare leaders and clinicians are now required to examine services using the value equation and to make decisions accordingly. If resources are limited, leaders must ask whether every patient sign and symptom requires intervention, particularly if minimal or no improvement in the patient's clinical condition is the likely outcome. Paying close attention to the health improvement value of healthcare services is an incredibly difficult challenge for providers and leaders schooled in the doctrine that increasing access to health care and growth in the healthcare system were absolute goods. Unfortunately, accountability and control were absent

---

Exhibit 13-3 Myths and Truths About Employee Productivity

Accepted Notions
- If employees work more hours, they will be more productive.
- If employees work faster, they will be more productive.
- If employees are paid more, they will be motivated to work harder and produce more.

The Reality
- Employees perform optimally for 6 to 7 hours and may be able to work longer in a burst of energy or inspiration, but then they must rest.
- Employees need balance; they need a life outside of work.
- Slower, intuitive thinking is often more effective in solving problems than mental agility.
- Studies show that in Germany, where individual performance is not rewarded with pay increases, productivity is often higher than in the United States.
- Employees are most productive when their employers pay them equitably and then do everything possible to help the employees put money out of their minds.

Data from Johnson, C. B. (2000). When working harder is not smarter. *Inner Edge, 3*(2), 18–21.

from the cost-based payment system, and the results are well known—exhaustion of resources. Health professionals are currently challenged to move from "use all the healthcare resources needed" care to "use only resources that outcomes show the benefit" care.

Another value-related issue of interest is productivity. Because business still operates under questionable assumptions regarding productivity—that the more hours employees work, the more productive they are; that the faster employees work, the more they accomplish; and that the more employees are paid, the more motivated they are to be productive—leaders are challenged to better understand the reality of employee productivity (**Exhibit 13-3**). Health professionals in this country are working more hours than ever before and getting less done. In fact, Americans have the dubious distinction of being first in the number of hours worked each year. The U.S. Department of Labor, Bureau of Labor Statistics, noted only a slight increase in productivity from the first quarter of 2019 to the first quarter of 2020, and the productivity increase in the last 10 years is attributed to technological advances, particularly the development of the internet. The Coronavirus impact on productivity was significant, with a 2.5% decrease that will require significant industry response in health care and manufacturing (Bureau of Labor Statistics [BLS], 2020).

High rates of burnout are reported among healthcare clinicians, with physicians and nurses reporting substantial symptoms of burnout (The National Academies, 2019). Burnout is a work-related phenomenon associated with the workplace and not an individual mental health diagnosis. Society depends on a healthcare workforce that functions at its highest level. Time for reflection and contemplation of ideas and issues on how to improve the work system to support clinician well-being is sorely missing in health care. The never-ending task list is always present and demanding attention. Further, technology, such as the electronic medical record, has caused clinicians to work independently instead of in human interaction. In general, clinicians desire to do meaningful work most of all, next they desire opportunities for collaboration through group decision making and collegiality.

What drives people to work at their best? Experts report that pay is not the chief motivator. How can healthcare leaders revitalize the lost passion of employees? What retention strategies support the rebuilding of a hopeful culture? Interestingly, the answer is simple. When

> **Exhibit 13-4** Optimizing Performance: Productivity or Fruitfulness?
>
> **Productivity**
> - Productivity is mechanistic.
> - In a productivity-driven organization, employees are treated like machines and judged on the quantity of their output.
> - The predominant concern is getting more "bang for the buck."
> - Efforts to increase employee motivation are dependent on external sources, pay, benefits, and so forth.
>
> **Fruitfulness**
> - Fruitfulness is humanistic.
> - Fruitfulness involves a respectful, holistic view of each person that recognizes values, beliefs, and expectations.
> - Fruitfulness honors the inner need of each person to express his or her uniqueness and talents and to develop and expand.
> - Fruitfulness engages the inner selves of employees and causes them to grow and be sustained naturally and enduringly.
>
> Data from Johnson, C. B. (2000). When working harder is not smarter. *Inner Edge, 3*(2), 18–21.

employees believe their work is meaningful—productive in the sense of producing beneficial results—they are motivated to work harder and experience a renewal of passion and hopefulness derived from their work. Productivity is not only about quantity; it is also about quality.

Optimizing employee performance takes on a whole new meaning in this context. All human beings have a need to express their uniqueness and their talents in the work they do and be recognized for their contributions (**Exhibit 13-4**). Therefore, employees are typically motivated by jobs that develop their skills and expand their minds, demand individual initiative, involve working on teams, benefit others, and spark a desire to make a difference in the world.

Jobs that have these characteristics possess what Cedric Johnson (2000) called *fruitfulness*—work flows from one person to another in a way that is both respectful and valued. To ensure that healthcare work possesses fruitfulness, leaders need to do the following:

- Continually examine services, measures, and systems to assess their impact on patient outcomes. Retain those that improve patient outcomes, and eliminate those that have no effect or a negative effect.
- Believe that hope can be restored to care providers through restoring value to the work they do.
- Believe intensely that individuals give their best when treated like adults and professionals.
- Be committed to doing what is best for patients.
- Consistently expect only value-adding services to be delivered to patients. Publicly recognize individuals who focus on value, and guide those who require assistance in eliminating unnecessary and nonvalue-adding work.
- Believe that all healthcare clinicians and providers intuitively know that restoring value to work is the right path but have not been able to translate their perceptions into practice. Believe that most, but not all, will eventually make the transition.
- Believe that the healthcare system will not only support but also require increases in the value of healthcare services. Know that colleagues support caring, healing work that makes a difference.

Becoming Mentally Fit

Some care providers appear to be tougher than others. In fact, their "toughness" might be a kind of mental fitness resulting from their sense of commitment, perception of control, and ability to view change as a challenge. Mental fitness involves taking responsibility for one's reactions to adversity. Through this kind of fitness, individuals can prevent emotional exhaustion and turn stressful events into meaningful challenges. Often, the expectations of altruism as a basic nurse value and behavior are different from societal values in which altruism is sometimes seen as not in the best interest of the patient (Guiffra, 2013).

Mental fitness is helpful for handling role modifications and reductions in the workforce. Employees who lack mental fitness often develop an attitude of learned helplessness. For example, if they are laid off, they react with anger, believe getting laid off is beyond their control, blame themselves, and generally feel helpless. Their helplessness triggers a downward spiral of self-defeat in which they see themselves as increasingly unable to get ahead.

Goal setting, mental imagery, emotional mastery, and positive thinking are all part of the mental conditioning that is necessary to overcome this helplessness and survive substantial changes. The mentally fit alter the perception of stress and mobilize effective coping techniques, lessening the trauma of stressful events. In fact, they transform these events into opportunities for increased meaning in life. Leaders who are mentally fit learn to manage the context of the work as well as the specific content of their discipline.

Mental fitness among leaders is associated with leadership resilience and leadership agility. As leaders become more mentally fit, they also become more resilient, decreasing the probability that they will experience burnout. Many leaders, particularly those at the vice-presidential level, work persistently to support and guide the chief executive in clinical matters in addition to meeting their own responsibilities. The relationship between the nurse executive, for example, and the chief executive is not only critical for organizational success but typically requires more from the nurse, who is continually providing feedback about the impact of decisions on patient outcomes and clinician engagement in addition to the executive accountabilities of strategic financial management. Not surprisingly, the nurse leader, if lacking in mental fitness, will be prone to burnout.

Leaders who are downsized experience a much greater emotional and psychological impact than typically has been acknowledged, and their ability to deal with such trauma is minimal at best. For one thing, the skills needed to handle disappointment are seldom taught in educational programs. Therefore, downsized leaders spend considerable time second-guessing past decisions and become reluctant to make decisions for fear of further emotional insult. If they get follow-up counseling, it is directed toward helping them cope with their behaviors, rather than preparing them for future disappointments. Becoming mentally fit, on the other hand, is a matter of learning to expect, anticipate, and plan for job-related disappointments and defeats and taking a proactive approach to managing one's personal destiny (**Exhibit 13-5**).

Leadership agility is the ability to respond quickly and appropriately to input from employees and colleagues, the actions of competitors, and developing crises. Leaders with this ability are better able to manage the stress of situations and to calculate the odds of success or failure. Once they acquire agility, along with resilience and mental fitness, leaders are in a good position to handle their responsibilities without becoming exhausted and incapable of experiencing the pleasures of their work. They are also in a good position to appreciate the

Exhibit 13-5 Planning for Position Elimination

- Recognize that no position is forever, nor should it be if the work of the organization is changing to meet the needs of the marketplace.
- Consider other roles that might be of interest in the future and begin to develop skills in the relevant areas.
- Discuss your interests with your immediate supervisor, request assistance in continuing to meet current expectations, but also be prepared for changes. (Note: Although it may be difficult to discuss role changes, open and honest communication is always the best approach.)
- Retain control of your career—avoid letting other factors control you.

---

virtues of mental fitness and to understand its importance for the organization as a whole. To ensure that the organization's entire workforce is mentally fit, leaders should do the following:

- Create a culture that recognizes that good and not-so-good events occur, understand that employees need support when things do not go well, and provide the necessary support to those who require it.
- Develop a personal commitment to help others acquire mental fitness, resilience, and agility.
- Continually strive to increase their own mental fitness and create a culture that requires others to do the same.
- Extract hope and energy from the mission of health care.
- Establish a program of self-examination and self-renewal.
- Recognize that no individual is an island and that each person needs relationships, support, and feedback.

Balancing the Use of Time

The transition into the Information Age has left many people with far too many activities on the to-do list and too little time to accomplish them. Constant attention to digital communication distracts individuals from any significant attention to tasks at hand. Each beep of the device breaks what little concentration there might have been. Leaders must therefore guide employees toward looking at time use in a different way. No individual ever has enough time for all the things he or she would like to do. Time management strategies may assist employees in eliminating nonproductive or nonessential tasks, but the employees still need to find a good balance between the things that are truly important to them. More specifically, they need to achieve an equilibrium between the activities of work and personal activities so that they can find joy and pleasure in both.

Some progress has been made in creating more balance between work and personal life, but more needs to be done to minimize the burnout and keep employees from feeling discouraged and disenfranchised. When organizations identify balancing work and personal life as a goal, they tend to focus on the time at work. An organization might develop initiatives to help employees have flexibility in work hours, for example, but at the same time it might leave vacancies unfilled and ask employees to do more with less. It does not matter that the employees have flexible hours if they also have to work 5 or 10 more hours each week. Because they are not much better off as a result of the initiative, the employees view the message as ambiguous.

In addition, leaders might then perceive the employees as ungrateful, causing the employees to feel that the executives just do not get it.

Leaders must build a culture of respect for employees and their accomplishments. When people feel successful, leaving the workplace at the end of the day is easier both physically and mentally because the shadow of work is not hanging over their heads. Leaders also should help employees feel successful in other aspects of their lives. Sometimes the support needed might seem like it falls outside the leader's jurisdiction. However, quantum leaders recognize that no individual ever enters the door of the organization and leaves his or her personal life behind. They understand that personal issues have an impact on any employee's ability to work effectively and that assisting the employee might be critical to the team's success. Employees have a wide variety of needs that change as their lives change. Few have the personal skills to achieve and maintain balance. A strong mentoring program not only produces better employees but also can teach the skills needed to balance work and personal life.

> **Point to Ponder**
>
> What are the characteristics of the best companies for work-life balance? Glassdoor.com, a social jobs and careers community where people share information and opinions about the places they work, identified popular perspectives for work–life balance: a flexible work schedule, the option to telecommute, paid time off, compressed work weeks, family-friendly work environments, ease of access to food and fitness amenities, and support from supervisor for work–life balance.
> https://www.glassdoor.com/index.htm

Once employees feel supported and successful in the workplace, they are better able to direct energy to the goals of the team.

Selflessness, not selfishness, can be a time-waster as well. Saying yes to every request is not realistic. Learning to say no on occasion lets the individual take back some of the time he or she has been losing. The hardest part of saying no is doing so guilt-free.

The following strategies should be used by leaders to help themselves and employees balance their work and their personal lives and avoid activities, behaviors, and emotions that consume time to no good purpose:

- Recognize that everyone has the capacity to balance his or her use of time better.
- Focus on balancing time use as an opportunity for increasing meaningfulness and not as an opportunity for increasing control and regimentation.
- Share the reality that time is short, desires are many, and every person engages in a never-ending struggle to close the gap.
- Be persistent in examining personal activities for balance and avoid the tendency to shift back to being task focused.
- Be intentional in coaching others in how to balance work and personal life, deal with incivility, and hold conversations that uphold a culture of respect.
- Believe that colleagues know that a good balance between work and personal life results in higher productivity and greater job satisfaction.
- Consider the addition of work–life balance goals to the annual performance review.

Increasing the Focus on Patients

It is no secret that the locus of control for healthcare services should be the patient, not the provider. Yet in spite of all the efforts to create patient-focused care delivery systems, few patients would agree that they are in fact the focus of services or in control of anything. In explanation, they could cite facts such as these:

- Clinicians continue to prescribe and perform treatments without discussion with the patients.
- Visiting hours are still in effect.
- Appointment times for services are based on Monday-through-Friday, 8AM–5PM schedules.
- Patient procedures and their scheduled times are determined by providers with minimal input from patients or families.

Leaders have plenty left to do to transform the healthcare system into one that is truly based on the will of the patient. A good place to begin is the internet, which should be pushed as a proactive means of assisting consumers in interpreting healthcare information. Other strategies leaders should use to increase the patient focus of health care include these:

- Find the courage to continue the journey to creating a better system. Avoid the tendency to believe that the system is as consumer focused as it can be.
- Recognize that personal experiences as a patient can be invaluable for learning the truth about healthcare service delivery.
- Remain committed and focused when complaints override positive feedback. Resist the temptation to retire from health care.
- Never stop asking patients to share their experience of the healthcare system. Learn from them and share the information gained with other health professionals to improve the system.
- Believe that every clinician possesses courage, passion, energy, and self-discipline but may need reassurance and encouragement to exhibit them fully.

Becoming Politically Competent

Political competence encompasses the ability to accurately assess the impact of public policies on one's domain of responsibility and the ability to influence public policy making at both the state and the federal levels. Politically competent leaders are aware of relevant regulations, laws, proposed acts, and certification procedures and are able to remove or mitigate outside barriers to the delivery of services. They also work within the organization to define issues affecting the delivery of patient care services and identify internal policies or procedures that should be altered. Nurse leaders can become involved in health policy development, study the processes of policy making with a mentor and create internal strategies to engage all nurses in understanding the relevance of meaningful participation in health policy creation and modifications (Shariff, 2014).

However, these are only the first steps. The leaders need to ensure that all members of the organization have a degree of political competence, can address concerns in a timely manner, and can suggest possible solutions both internal to the organization and externally to legislative bodies. The point-of-service staff members experience the real concerns and successes that occur at the delivery of services, know when things do not go well, and can offer recommendations for change. Their input is needed not only in the executive suite but, in many cases, in the legislative arena as well. Strategies for increasing the political competence of the organization as a whole include the following:

- Develop the ability of all employees to share information about system effectiveness. Be aware that the empowerment of employees, if not guided, can result in chaos.

- Recognize that empowerment can light a fire throughout the organization. When a person's personal contributions are valued, the fire in that person's heart is fueled.
- Patiently guide employees to communicate and share information. Never give up trying to ensure that the information necessary for identifying and implementing improvements is available to the members of the organization.

Pay close attention to the desired outcomes of care as well as to the processes used to achieve them. On the other hand, never circumvent necessary processes for the sake of efficiency.

Relighting the Lamp

Nursing and health care have always been hard work. But today's healthcare environment has additional challenges of complexity, declining revenues, difficult government regulations, and shortages of qualified workers. All these add up to the need to work more effectively than ever and to achieve job satisfaction in an atmosphere of tremendous pressure and shrinking support. Cost-saving measures may be crucial to an organization's survival, but to healthcare providers they mean stress, frustration, and attrition if not coupled with the elimination of nonvalue-added work and improved patient care.

With job stress high and morale at an all-time low, interdepartmental tensions have grown to epidemic proportions. Patient needs are complex, and there is simply not an adequate supply of some types of clinicians, straining the existing workforce. Clinicians are expected to provide care with great sensitivity, patience, and empathy. It is ironic that the emphasis on patient satisfaction in health care comes at a time when the pressures make high-quality care challenging. Nurses have a clear line of sight to outcomes that associate directly with nursing practice—nurse-sensitive outcomes. To meet the social mandates, to learn from the past, and to continue to create new and better methods to integrate technology, information, and the wisdom of providers and leaders is a path forward. Leaders must realize that the key to moving forward rests with the clinicians, and the leaders' role is to facilitate actions from a work context where the voices of the clinicians are evident and valued.

Some days the work of leadership seems like more than a person can handle, yet dedicated leaders continue on through seemingly insurmountable challenges. Most likely, the work of leadership has become an internal calling. The calling to leadership or the urge to give away one's gifts and make distinct contributions to the world not only uncovers the joy that everyone seeks but also affirms one's life work and contributions to a better world. It is the calling to leadership that energizes, affirms, and sustains leaders in times of great challenge.

According to Leider (2004), engaged leaders not only know who they are and what they stand for but also are able to assist others to heed their own life callings. They are able to guide others to uncover their embedded destiny and to see beyond today to what they can become tomorrow. This is the ultimate coaching and mentoring process! Thus, the engaged leader with emotional competence can both identify personal destiny and assist others in the journey of discovery and commitment to their calling as a part of the larger design of the world. Not surprising, engaged leaders recognize their calling not as a destiny or goal, but as a wellness issue; leading is doing what needs to be done, and not doing the work of leadership would be frustrating and stress producing. The calling of leadership guides the leader in integrating the internal personal self with the outer world—a struggle that is continuously present in many leaders. Knowing from the internal self what needs to be done and living those beliefs and values in the real world marks the leader's journey. The leader must role-model the integration of the personal, authentic self with the real, external world. The journey starts with the self and moves toward others and the needs of the world. The fully engaged leader emulates a high level of consciousness or spiritual connection with those in the world. The leader is fully present in each situation, listens carefully with an open mind, and, on the basis of core values, interacts assertively and honestly.

The words of Florence Nightingale offer hope and gentle reminders for all clinicians. Her perceptions are consistent with the public and political consciousness of today, namely, that public health and human caring are supremely important. Further, as in her time, many are now calling for reform of basic social and healthcare practices. In our era, for example, there are many critics of our society's response to the needs of the homeless, the medically indigent, those who are HIV positive, those who are living with AIDS or another incurable or chronic illness, and those who are relatively powerless or neglected, including pregnant women, children, and older adults.

Consider these themes from Nightingale's writings:

- Basic caring and healing practices must be restored.
- The moral, the spiritual, and the metaphysical must be reintegrated.
- The knowledge and values of women—the sacred feminine healing spirit—must be allowed to play an essential role in health care.
- Healing professionals must recapture their sense of "calling."
- The public's requirement of personal and professional caring competencies and commitments must be honored.
- The wisdom of connected oneness and wholeness—the interrelationship among person, nature, environment, and health—must also be honored.

Group Discussion

In our rush to reform education, we have forgotten a simple truth: Reform will never be achieved by renewing appropriations, restructuring schools, rewriting curricula, and revising texts if we continue to demean and dishearten the human resource called the teacher on whom so much depends. Teachers must be better compensated, freed from bureaucratic harassment, given a role in academic governance, and provided with the best possible methods and materials. But none of that will transform education if we fail to cherish—and challenge—the human heart that is the source of good teaching.

The preceding comments by noted educator Parker Palmer (1998) were about the education system, and these words still resonate today. With these words in mind, answer the following questions: In what way is the state of health care similar to the state of education? Is it possible that health care already has enough financial resources and that the solution to the problems in the healthcare system is to rearrange funding, reduce bureaucracy, and increase involvement? Are there other important strategies that need to be part of the solution? How do the concepts of will and willingness apply to the current situation in health care?

Aren't these same themes relevant today? Is there any doubt that the transformative journey we are on dates back at least to the 19th century? As Watson (1999) noted, our work should be about relighting the lamp and helping our colleagues to reintegrate and reconnect to restore the professional wholeness that was wounded during the recent modern era.

Conclusion

The Age of Complexity encompasses exponential increases in information, technology, and interaction between diverse people and cultures, confirming that our world is truly global. In addition, despite the fear that many people feel today, the complexity of this new age can be a source of hope. The speed of change, the blurring of work and home life, and the new global relationships enrich each one of us directly or indirectly.

Leadership thinking must be more humanistic and more sensitive to the complex interrelationships in the world. Hope in the future and willingness to transform bureaucracies into self-renewing organizations are other aspects of the journey of leaders into and beyond the millennium. To accomplish their goals, leaders require courage to do the right thing, passion for the work of healing, energy to stay the course, self-discipline to remain focused, and trust that others are partners in the process. Finally, they must be steeped in the belief that the future will indeed be better because they have designed it.

Chapter Takeaways

1. Developing one's will and willingness strengthens commitment and capacity as a professional and leader.
2. Being hopeful about the future provides a positive focus and reinforces expectations for a better future for all employees.
3. Eliminating dogma and nonvalue-added work reinforces the importance of evidence-based practice.
4. Employee productivity metrics do not reflect the quality of outcomes; examination of quality metrics focused on outcomes provides a more accurate representation, such as the absence of adverse outcomes, satisfaction of patients and employees, and achievement of clinical outcomes.
5. When discouraged, refocusing on the calling of nursing can revitalize professional practice and personal satisfaction.

Case Study 13-1

Managing Pressure to Decide

Al has noticed that two of his directors are exact polar opposites of each other in their leadership style, skills, and competencies. He often thought to himself that they are classic textbook pictures of leadership skills on a continuum. Pete is a strong thinker and is full of innovative ideas to improve his department and the hospital as a whole. He doesn't perceive traditional lines of authority or regulations as a barrier to his innovative ideas, but views them as a potential challenge, as a chess master would regarding his opponent. Pete is full of ideas and energy and is constantly changing, fixing, and moving things forward in his departments. Al had personally witnessed Pete discussing his ideas with the president of the organization with such confidence and courage that even Al did not possess. It seemed that Pete was fearless and disregarded the commonly understood rules of organizational hierarchy. He spoke to the president as if they were best friends or individuals who worked together frequently. Al secretly coveted Pete's ability to be "out there" or "in your face" on issues that Pete was passionate about.

In contrast, Caroline is a very quiet but effective leader. She has been in her role for more than 25 years and has 35 years of seniority in the organization. She is highly regarded as an expert in her clinical area and as a soft, compassionate leader with her staff. Caroline is nearing retirement and probably would have retired a few years ago had it not been for the sudden death of her husband. Caroline had shared with Al that she is not retiring now because of her fears and concerns about her financial stability in the present economy. Al noticed that Caroline rarely brought forth any new or innovative ideas, but her departments seemed to hum along without much controversy, crisis, or change. Although Caroline is open to new ideas, she certainly put forth no effort to promote innovation or change in her departments. She seems quite content with the status quo.

When reflecting on these two individuals and their strengths and areas needing development, Al would have characterized Pete as a strong-willed and engaged individual who was like a "dog with a bone" when he felt strongly about a proposal or situation. In contrast, Caroline simply and quietly got the job done and changed things when necessary. Caroline could be characterized as a person with a soft, good will who exuded caring and compassion for others but had little energy or will to change the status quo. Al's boss, the chief operating officer (COO), once mentioned to Al that they needed to develop a strategy to deal with the "walking retired," and Al silently wondered if he was referring to Caroline along with some of the others whom they both knew were no longer effective in their roles. Al felt protective of Caroline because of her long years of service and because her performance was essentially good. She met all of the performance goals required of her, her staff seem to be satisfied with her as a leader, and the patient satisfaction scores were also within expected limits. It was just her quiet and unengaging demeanor that caused others to perceive her as low energy and ineffective. In some ways Al thought she was a good balance to Pete's constant whirlwind of energy, excitement, passion, and eagerness to put forth his agenda and to please others. Caroline, on the other hand, had shared with Al that she no longer felt the need to impress others and that she had no desire to move up in the organization to promote herself for other positions. She stated that "my performance speaks for itself, so why do I need to behave differently just to impress others."

Al was under constant pressure from the COO to do "something" with Caroline—reassignment to a less visible position or encouragement to retire. Al was a bit concerned about his boss's perception of his own skill incompetency in his role if he didn't do something with Caroline. He was saddened that she was perceived as "burned out" when she met all of the performance requirements and was positively perceived by her staff and physicians. He realized that the organization valued high-energy, quick-thinking, innovative individuals who not only got the job done but also were constantly moving the organization forward into new service lines, care delivery methods, and strategies to improve the workplace environment for staff and physicians. What a quandary! Al was absolutely conflicted about what he should do with Caroline. He knew with certainty that there would be chaos among the clinical nurses and physicians if he should encourage her to move to a new position or to retire. He knew that Caroline did not want to retire, and therefore he could expect a backlash from his actions to encourage her to do so. In his mind he questioned the COO's intentions and the congruency with the organization's values. Looking at it differently, however, Al realized the potential benefits of having an individual in the role who was more energetic and innovative. Such a person might propose new programs and services that would accelerate the department's success and make changes to improve patient care, physician satisfaction, and employee engagement (although these metrics were already within expected ranges). It was more of a "decision of potentiality" than "necessity," which made Al all the more unsettled about pressure to make a change in Caroline's role.

Questions

1. What is your perception of Al's personal conflict in this case?
2. How would you describe Al's level of courage in facing the COO's pressure for Al to make a change in Caroline's role when Al clearly feels conflicted about the fairness and appropriateness of the change given that she meets expectations in assigned organizational goals?
3. What do you think Al's best strategy should be in meeting the COO's agenda, being fair to Caroline, and making the best decision for the overall good of his departments and hospital?
4. If you were Al, how would you perceive the political correctness of Pete's informal interactions with the president of the organization given the circumstances described in this case?
5. What qualities does Al demonstrate that may characterize him as being a willing leader, and which attributes might he continually develop to improve his own authenticity as a leader?
6. If Al determines that Caroline should stay in her role, what methods might he consider to "relight her lamp" as described earlier in this chapter?

Case Study 13-2

Courageous, Tenacious, and Resilient

Susan has been in her role as executive director of Women's Services at Community Memorial Hospital for nearly 7 years. During this time, she has witnessed tremendous growth in the annual volume of deliveries, women surgeries, and neonatal intensive care admissions. The phenomenal success of the department has led to her managing issues related to the tremendous growth in volume and a lack of an adequate number of beds to place newly delivered mothers, neonatal admits to the ICU, and even surgical admits for pre- and postoperative services. It's clear that Community Memorial Hospital needs to expand its building for maternal–newborn services and women's surgery services or build a new building on an adjacent site. Susan has been to a number of national conferences and talked with other leaders of freestanding women's hospitals who have shared stories of how the new hospital has positioned them well as market leaders and provided opportunities to expand services for patients. When sharing her observations with her physician colleagues, they agree that a proposal for a freestanding women's and newborn's hospital should be developed for the executive team to consider. Susan meets with the market research department to acquire data about the patient catchment areas and projections for potential growth in the women's service line. She also meets with the director of finance to review the current financial data and requests assistance in developing the projected pro forma with growth assumptions built into the financial scenarios.

The executive team at Community Memorial Hospital is well aware of the burgeoning growth of the women's service line. The planning committee reviewed options for expanding the existing building on campus but quickly determined that an expansion would not be a viable option because the current building had many deficiencies that would also need replacement or repair. The building no longer meets current patients' requests for private rooms and space for mother–baby couplet care, and the normal newborn nursery and neonatal intensive care unit are completely undersized for the obstetrical volume. Although most of the gynecological surgeries are performed in the department, the patients have to be moved to a different building for postoperative care because all available beds are used for maternity patients. Not building new space soon would result in loss of market share.

Susan and the medical directors for Perinatal Services and Neonatal Services worked with the financial department to develop a feasibility analysis proposing a new freestanding women's hospital with a new birthing center, private postpartum rooms, private rooms for high-risk maternity patients, a large neonatal intensive care unit, a 10-room surgical center, and a women's postoperative unit. Once the feasibility analysis was prepared, Susan and the medical directors presented the concept proposal to the executive team at Community Memorial Hospital. They asked for resources and financial support to hire a hospital planning company to do a preliminary space program outlining the departmental needs and overall space requirements so that the project costs could be correctly estimated and entered into the pro forma equations to determine the return on investment and internal rate of return.

Susan could never have anticipated the initial pushback that she received from some of the members on the executive team who previously acknowledged that the women's and newborn service line had outgrown the current facility. Discussion ensued about the need to build a new facility for the cardiovascular service line, which was also growing exponentially and had a greater revenue base than that of the women's and newborn service line. The proposal was sent forward to the board of directors, who were also split in their support for either the new women's hospital or the cardiovascular pavilion. When Susan attended the meetings, she was often the brunt of jokes by some board members who scoffed at the need for a women's hospital. Some of them asked, "Why don't we just build a men's hospital as well?" Susan had carefully scripted responses to such questions and reiterated the importance of appealing to women because the evidence supported that women were often the healthcare decision makers for families. Susan explained that market research information validated that the women in the family often guided decisions related to choosing healthcare plans during open enrollment periods and in choosing physicians. By providing a women's hospital, Community Memorial Hospital could position itself well as a market leader in women's health for both inpatient and outpatient services.

The executive director of the cardiovascular service line also had a compelling rationale for building a new cardiovascular pavilion instead of a women's hospital. Many advances in technology, interventional radiology, and the medical and surgical care of cardiovascular patients supported the need for more space for these patients. Because there were only enough resources for one new facility or expansion, the executive team and the board of directors had to decide which of the two options would provide the greatest value and position the hospital for future growth, financial stability, and recognition for excellence.

Susan was passionate about the vision for a new women's hospital, and she spent many hours discussing the vision with potential donors, community organizational leaders, hospital executives, and the board of directors. She believed so strongly in the vision that she was willing to meet with anyone who could assist in moving the vision to reality. Susan also realized that the executive director for cardiovascular services was equally passionate about his vision for a new cardiovascular service line and was aligning supporters for his vision as well. Both were articulate in expressing how patient outcomes could be positively influenced with the new buildings and that the hospital would be viewed positively in the community with the new facility. Susan presented the story of her vision over and over and was courageous in "the line of fire" when people challenged the need for a new women's hospital. In the end her persistence was fruitful, and she successfully persuaded the executive team and board of directors to allocate resources for the planning of a new women's hospital. Although Susan was triumphant with this news, she was also sensitive to her colleague's dismay that his vision for a cardiovascular pavilion would be put on hold for a few years.

Questions

1. How did Susan show courage when proposing the new women's hospital?
2. In what ways did Susan demonstrate her tenacity and resilience in proposing the women's hospital?
3. How would you strategize to propose your vision of a new building in the face of a competing proposal that also has great value to the success of the organization?
4. Healthcare executives rarely have the resources to fund all the needs for capital equipment, operational expenses, and facility improvement, so resources must be carefully allocated based on the merits of the proposal in adding value to patients and to the organization. With this in mind, how would you weigh the merits of the two proposals in this case study for a new women's hospital or the cardiovascular pavilion?

References

Ackman, M., Perry, L. A., Wolfard, E., Steckel, C., & Hill, C. (2012). Changing nursing practice: Letting go of the nursing history on admission. *Journal of Nursing Administration, 42*(9), 435–441.

American Hospital Association (AHA). (2017). *Regulatory overload: Assessing the regulatory burden on health systems, hospitals, and post-acute care providers.* American Hospital Association Publishing.

Bureau of Labor Statistics (BLS), U.S. Department of Labor. (2020). *Productivity and costs: First quarter 2020, revised.* https://www.bls.gov/news.release/pdf/prod2.pdf

Contu, D. L. (2002, March). The anxiety of learning: An interview with Edgar Schein. *Harvard Business Review, 79,* 100–106.

de Saint-Exupéry, Antoine. (1943). *The Little Prince.* HMH Books.

Flynn, M. B. (2013). Questioning common nursing practices: What does the evidence show? *American Nurse Today, 8*(3), 6–7.

Guiffra, M. J. (2013). Letter to the editor: Altruism is the heart of our story. *Nursing Outlook, 61,* 67–69.

Johnson, C. B. (2000). When working harder is not smarter. *Inner Edge, 3*(2), 18–21.

Leider, R. (2004). Is leading your calling? *Leader to Leader, 31,* 36–40.

Makic, M. B. F., Rauen, C., Jones, K., & Fisk, A. C. (2015). Continuing to challenge practice to be evidence based. *Critical Care Nurse, 35*(2), 39–50.

Malloch, K., & Porter-O'Grady, T. (1999). Partnership economics: Nursing's challenge in the quantum age. *Nursing Economics, 17,* 299–307.

National Academies of Sciences, Engineering, and Medicine. (2019). *Taking action against clinician burnout: A systems approach to professional well-being.* The National Academies Press.

Palmer, P. J. (1998). *The courage to teach: Exploring the inner landscape of a teacher's life.* Jossey-Bass.

Pappas, S. H. (2013). Value, a nursing outcome. *Nursing Administration Quarterly, 37*(2), 122–128.

Pappas, S., & Welton, J. (2015). Nursing: Essential to healthcare value. *Nurse Leader, 13*(3), 26–29, 38.

Shariff, N. (2014). Factors that act as facilitators and barriers to nurse leaders' participation in health policy development. *BMC Nursing, 13*(20). doi:10.1186/1472-6955-13-20

Uhl-Bien, M., Meyer, D., & Smith, J. (2020). Complexity leadership in the nursing context. *Nursing Administration Quarterly, 44*(2), 109–116.

Watson, J. (1999). *Postmodern nursing and beyond.* Churchill Livingstone.

Zak, P. (2017, January–February). The neuroscience of trust. *Harvard Business Review.* https://hbr.org/2017/01/the-neuroscience-of-trust

Suggested Readings

Berenson, R. A., & Docteur, E. (2013). *Doing better by doing less: Approaches to tackle overuse of services.* Robert Wood Johnson Foundation/The Urban Institute. https://www.rwjf.org/en/library/research/2013/01/doing-better-by-doing-less--approaches-to-tackle-overuse-of-serv.html

Buerhaus, P. (1998). Milton Weinstein's insights on the development, use, and methodologic problems in cost-effectiveness analysis. *Image: Journal of Nursing Scholarship, 30,* 223–227.

Drucker, P. F. (2006). What executives should remember. *Harvard Business Review, 84*(2), 145–152.

Gifford, W. A., & Davis, B. (2008, Fourth Quarter). Doing the right things to do things right: A commentary on leadership and the use of evidence in practice. *Worldviews on Evidence-Based Nursing,* 170–171.

Gordon, S. (2005). *Nursing against the odds: How health care cost-cutting, media stereotypes and medical hubris undermine nurses and patient care.* Cornell University Press.

Hamel, G. (2009). Moon shots for management. *Harvard Business Review, 87*(2), 91–98.

Huber, C. (1998). *The key: And the name of the key is willingness.* Keep It Simple Books.

Mankins, M. C., & Garton, E. (2017). *Time, talent, energy: Overcome organizational drag and unleash your team's productive power.* Harvard Business Review Press.

O'Malley, M. N. (2000). *Creating commitment: How to attract and retain talented employees by building relationships that last.* Wiley.

Rauen, C. A, Vollman, K., Arbour, R. B., & Chulay, M. (2008). Challenging nursing's sacred cows. *American Nurse Today, 3*(4), 23–25.

Williams, L. L. (2006). The fair factor in matters of trust. *Nursing Administration Quarterly, 30*(1), 30–37.

Zimmerman, B., Lindberg, C., & Plsek, P. (1998). *Edgeware: Insights from complexity science for health care leaders.* VHA.

Chapter Thirteen   The Leader's Courage to Be Willing: Building a Context for Hope

Quiz Questions

Select the best answer for each of the following questions.

1. Which of the following is *not* among the reasons that healthcare workers report disenfranchisement?
   a. Staff shortages
   b. Excessive regulations
   c. Loss of patient respect
   d. Job stress

2. Which of the following characterizes the fully developed will?
   a. The fully developed will creates an enormous potential for change.
   b. The fully developed will requires significant coaching and mentoring.
   c. The fully developed will is inherent in all leaders.
   d. The fully developed will avoids expressing authentic feelings.

3. From the perspective of a leader, the will emerges through several phases of discovery. In the most important of these phases, what does the leader do?
   a. Evaluates colleagues' perceptions of the leader's degree of willingness
   b. Informs his or her supervisor of the intention to explore the concept of will
   c. Makes an attempt to identify areas in which personal growth is needed
   d. Recognizes the will as a unique and describable phenomenon

4. Among the obstacles to a leader's exploration of his or her will, which of the following is the most common?
   a. Peer pressure to avoid additional work
   b. Organizational pressure to conform to established practices and norms
   c. Lack of time
   d. Lack of knowledge about exploration of the will on the part of the leader's supervisor

5. Passion as an essential quality of will is expressed in which of the following ways?
   a. Employees share their values and ideas in a nonthreatening manner.
   b. People in the organization take pride in their work.
   c. In decision making, the leader's opinion dominates the opinions of others.
   d. Power is distributed equally among all leaders.

6. Dogmas obstruct the transformation of the healthcare system for which of the following reasons?
   a. Policies require too much time to review.
   b. Employees are allowed to retain jobs that no longer are needed.
   c. The boundaries between professions continue to remain unclear.
   d. The use of resources is not always related to patient outcomes.

7. Regaining balance between work and personal life requires courage to do which of the following?
   a. Create new compensation systems to recognize the differing values of employees.
   b. Pursue change with zeal until satisfactory human resources policies are created.
   c. Accept that employees are interested in the recommendations of the leader.
   d. Remain focused on creating change.

8. Value-based services differ in several ways from the kind of services most commonly delivered. Which of the following would *not* be affected by the transformation to value-based services?
   a. Quality of the services
   b. Research base of the services
   c. License of the provider
   d. Available reimbursement for the services provided

9. Leaders who are mentally fit are better able to manage the complexity of the healthcare system. Which of the following is *not* a benefit that mental fitness bestows on leaders?
   a. Ability to handle the disappointment of not being selected for a position
   b. Ability to take responsibility for one's actions and one's reactions to adversity
   c. Increased sensitivity to the situation of employees who have been laid off
   d. Ability to avoid confrontations and the discussion of pertinent issues

10. Maintaining the status quo or leadership mediocrity is not reflective of willing leaders. Which of the following is not reflective of a willing leadership?
    a. New ideas are implemented in a strategic manner.
    b. Patient safety risks are avoided.
    c. Clinical conflicts are readily addressed.
    d. Provider personal practice preferences are supported.

11. The relationship between willpower and creating change:
    a. allows for more collaboration in the process.
    b. allows leaders to better understand resistance to change.
    c. is positive and results in positive outcomes.
    d. is required for strategic planning and implementation of new ideas.

12. Developing one's will is strongly influenced by organizational culture and is supported by:
    a. establishing policies.
    b. educational programs.
    c. determined action and struggle.
    d. performance reviews.

13. How does courage differ from willpower?
    a. Courage is about the absence of fear; willpower is about the abstract inner strength of an individual.
    b. Courage is about giving up ground when pressured; willpower is about standing one's ground.
    c. Courage is about withholding opinions when there is conflict present; willpower is about addressing conflicts quickly.
    d. Courage is about holding true to controversial beliefs; willpower is about letting go of controversial beliefs at the appropriate time.

14. A willing leader develops attributes that embrace future opportunities wholeheartedly. Acceptance of diverse perspectives is one of these attitudes and includes:
    a. examining the perspectives of each member of the team.
    b. engaging in dialogue to inform others how to fit into the team.
    c. ensuring that there is value in the differing perspectives before integrating them into the team's work.
    d. accepting the perspectives of each team member.

15. Hopeful leaders provide value to an organization through:
    a. belief in the value of current performances.
    b. focus on the future to advance personal goals.
    c. focus on the future to envision opportunities.
    d. encouraging others to consider the need to be prepared for layoffs.

16. Dogmatic practices are often difficult to identify. Sources of these practices can originate from all of the following, *except*:
    a. evidence-based practice implementation.
    b. physician-dominated cultures.
    c. perceived beliefs of effectiveness.
    d. respect for traditions.

17. The Evidence-Based Practice team identified the Trendelenburg position as ineffective. All of the following are obstacles to eliminating this practice, *except*:
    a. organizational culture influences.
    b. multiple random clinical trials.
    c. provider personal preferences.
    d. positive clinical experiences from the use of the Trendelenburg position.

18. Moving from dogma to value-based care requires:
    a. engagement of stakeholders.
    b. access to evidence-based practice and research resources.
    c. approval of providers.
    d. access to a list of nonvalue-added interventions.

19. The difference between evidence-based practice and value-based care can be described as:
    a. the cost-effectiveness for a desirable change in patient condition.
    b. the number of randomized clinical trials performed.
    c. the degree of satisfaction of patients and providers.
    d. the level of research/evidence-based practice rigor.

20. Acquiring new knowledge is a professional role expectation. Learning while working is inadequate for the professional because:
    a. employee productivity is negatively impacted.
    b. employee productivity is positively impacted.
    c. willingness to attend workshops is not consistent among employees.
    d. it is not wholly adequate to demonstrate competence in using the new knowledge.

21. Political competence is important for healthcare leaders to achieve which of the following?
    a. To identify the source of resistance to new ideas
    b. To engage in meaningful dialogue with elected officials
    c. To provide input specific to healthcare policies
    d. To impact the cost of health care

22. Relighting the lamp of Florence Nightingale is important to achieve:
    a. recommitment to the calling of nursing.
    b. reduction in job stress.
    c. increased engagement with policy makers.
    d. public health.

23. Mental fitness in leadership is best described as:
    a. the same as transactional leadership.
    b. readiness for external disasters.
    c. the ability to respond quickly to multiple inputs appropriately.
    d. the ability to address employee expectations appropriately.

24. Monitoring work–life balance requires time, focus, and commitment. Which statement best reflects the optimal approach for emotionally competent leaders to support work–life balance?
    a. Paying attention to daily schedules to ensure promptness with start and stop times
    b. Engaging in regular reflection on meeting desired expectations for work time and personal time
    c. Obtaining family feedback
    d. Eliminating time-wasting activities and gossiping

25. Hope or the state of being hopeful includes all of the following, *except*:
    a. a feeling of accomplishment and being appreciated.
    b. a willingness to do the necessary work to be successful.
    c. a necessity for an organizational culture.
    d. anticipating a positive future.

CHAPTER FOURTEEN

Engaging the Spirit of Leadership: Becoming a Living Leader

I am being driven forward into an unknown land. The pass grows steeper, the air colder and sharper. A wind from my unknown goal stirs the strings of expectation. Still the question: shall I ever get there? There where life resounds, a clear pure note in the silence.

—Dag Hammarskjöld, "Markings"[1]

Chapter Objectives

At the completion of this chapter, the reader will be able to:

- Describe the personal needs that relate to self-care and development as a leader and as a person.
- Construct a personal plan for self-direction and self-development that addresses professional, personal, and spiritual needs.
- Distinguish between the various competing aspects of life as a leader and understand the creative skills necessary to manage the leadership role and make a difference.
- Understand how to set time aside in a format that permits deepening of the spiritual journey.
- Enumerate 10 spiritual rules for personal growth that incorporate the principles of chaos and complexity.

In the concentrated chaos and complexity of multiple systems conflict and change, it is hard for the leader to find and to take moments for self-reflection and development. The intensity of focus and attention of the leader's role draws a great deal from the spirit and energy of the leader. Without a sense of spiritual centering and integrity, leaders do not have adequate sustenance because much of the needed support must come from within. Leaders must have self-discipline, resolve, insight, and a sense of direction to prepare for the tough experience

---

[1] "Thus it was" from MARKINGS by Dag Hammarskjold, translated by Leif Sjöberg and W. H. Auden, translation copyright © 1964, copyright renewed 1992 by Penguin Random House LLC and Faber & Faber Ltd. Used by permission of Alfred A. Knopf, an imprint of the Knopf Doubleday Publishing Group, a division of Penguin Random House LLC. All rights reserved.

of engaging others to manage their own lives. Leaders must also focus on their own resources and enter into a process of self-reflection, centering, and nourishing the spirit. This chapter describes the elements and processes associated with leadership self-care and support, including spiritual and personal routines.

Leadership is more than a set of learned skills. Effective leaders possess a deep comfort with themselves and an engagement with life that is appreciative, generative, and harmonizing. They exhibit an excitement and a way of embracing life that are encouraging and hopeful to those they lead. They have a depth of commitment and a reservoir of spirit and energy that are inspiring, along with a sense of being fully in touch with who they are and what moves them. At the same time, effective leaders appear never fully content, having a sort of personal restlessness, as though on a journey or in search of something still just out of their reach that continues to drive them on.

Leaders who are more than just effective—who qualify as great leaders—have an understanding or acceptance that some deep force runs through all existence, giving it form and life and direction, yet at every level of consciousness this force remains mysterious. This force comes in many forms and goes by an unlimited number of names, but it operates regardless of what it is called. Great leaders sense, indeed, feel, this force and at some point are driven by an awareness of its movement within. In the lives of most great leaders, a question arises about what they would do in response to the call deep within, and they respond by moving in concert with this inner force and by making out of it whatever they can. In short, they commit to the great "yes" of their lives and as a result are driven to do great and meaningful things.

This "call" is not just reserved for the great of the world; it is actually part of the greatness that is in each of us. Regardless of the place we occupy in society, moments of opportunity, risk, and commitment surround us. We all experience the sense that a call is being made to our own greatness. We all possess gifts and strengths that determine our uniqueness and that, when fully expressed, can have a valuable impact on our lives and, at least by reflection, on the lives of others. We each simply need to be aware of the stirrings of the force within and to act in concert with it. Our awareness of the force does not simply happen, however; it comes out of the insight born of a spiritual discipline (**Figure 14-1**). Spiritually grounded leaders undergo a cycle of interactions that demonstrates their ongoing commitment to personal growth and development.

> **Point to Ponder**
>
> The spiritual and consciousness-centered leader focuses each eye separately: one eye focuses on the close-up realities and vagaries that must be addressed now, and the other focuses on the farthest horizon of the future.

Chaos and the Call to Leadership

In these times, it is difficult to find enough moments of peace to think reflectively about anything. Days seem filled with activity, change, and movement, responses to ever-increasing demands for the new and different. As we more fully move into the Postdigital Age, we can sense the significance of the changes in understanding, work, relationships, and life itself. All the science fiction we have read appears to be coming to life before our very eyes.

The pace of change has in fact picked up during the past 20 years, leaving the 20th century and the Industrial Age forever behind us. Our movement through this Postdigital Age tempts us with the loss of all the beliefs and practices that characterized the Industrial Age, especially

Figure 14-1 The Cycle of Spiritual Discipline.

the linearity and vertical orientation of our thinking, which had a defining influence on all our traditional social institutions and practices, from science to government and religion.

The unidirectional and linear notions associated with the Newtonian view of the universe have now been significantly eclipsed. The quantum theorists, for example, proved that life cannot be understood in terms of unilateral and vertical mental models. The chaos of the universe has a rhythm and flow that moves multidirectionally, and through the cloud of chaos a discrete and elegant simplicity (hidden order) can be seen that defies the chaos that created it.

These realities often confound and confuse us. They disrupt our sensibilities and our rituals and routines. They create incongruities in our beliefs and understanding. The uncertainty they cause makes us disquieted and anxious. The confidence we garnered from settling on a set of practices and beliefs that brought order to our lives has been undermined. Yet we are not sure with what to replace those practices and beliefs. We hunger for some certitude and some sense of the absolute that can guide our thinking and acting, but finding these tools of life is turning out to be extremely difficult.

> ## Group Discussion
>
> Recall a serious tragedy or overwhelmingly painful experience you thought you would never recover from. Then, discuss with the other participants what it was that moved you on, got you past the pain, and enabled you to reengage with life and make a difference once again.

There is a tremendous backlash associated with the loss of certainty. Groups on the political extreme express a high level of anger and anxiety and call for a return to fundamental beliefs and historical practices as a solution to the loss of certainty. However, this approach does not engage with the facts recently revealed by science and research—facts that will not disappear because they are disconcerting and incongruous with what we believe should be true (O'Rourke et al., 2016).

Change is always a challenge to human beings. It presents us with the task of confronting ourselves and everything that defines our lives. It reminds us that life is forever in movement and is more journey than event. Truth is also more journey than event. We want truth to be immutable to avoid the discomfort, uncertainty, and ambiguity associated with change and to keep from questioning the premises of our actions (Shin et al., 2016). Absolutism removes control over our lives from our hands and puts it someplace outside of us. It frees us from the obligation to own what we know and how we must change, and it limits the experience of "noise" that accompanies all aspects of life. The surrender of control to an external absolute eliminates the pain, challenge, risk, and suffering that arise out of the struggle to cope with the vagaries of existence.

It is into this fray that the leader enters, attempting to engage with the vagaries of life and to incorporate the uncertainties of the experience into the work of adaptation and growth (Nilsen et al., 2016). The leader finds comfort not in the safe haven of an unchanging external reality, but in staying the course and deepening his or her personal journey (Black et al., 2016). The spiritually aware leader recognizes that being available to the challenges and opportunities embedded in the endless process of change is critical to personal growth. By connecting to the experience of change and demonstrating growth within his or her life, the leader encourages others to continue on their own journey of discernment and development (Pradarelli et al., 2016).

Chaos is pervasive throughout the universe. Yet, to understand the chaos, it is important to visualize the simplicity that lies at its center. Touching that center brings confidence and order to an individual's life and encourages experimentation and engagement. It is hard work, however, to move through the clouds and shrouds of the chaotic experience to land at the center—the place where the elements of chaos converge and create the mosaic that represents—at the same time—mystery and order. Endeavors to get to that place make up much of the work of personal leadership (Menaker, 2016).

> **Key Point**
>
> Chaos and the loss of certainty provide an opportunity to let go of those things that are inherently changing and passing. Chaos is a fundamental element of the spiritual discipline, severing us from our false certainty about what can never be certain, refocusing us on the journey, and allowing us to hear the journey's call to adapt and grow.

Certain principles can illuminate the conditions of participation in change and help to explain the proper role of leadership in a world defined by chaos and complexity:

- The universe is a work in progress, still unfolding, yet in creation, moving everything in it forward in a web of energy and understanding.
- Chaos and complexity are the essential characteristics of the universe. The universe cannot be understood independent of its own complex reality.
- Everything in the universe is self-organizing. The patterns, webs, and intersections of life create a mosaic of intense goodness-of-fit that reveals the ultimate connection among all the elements of the universe.
- People, too, are part of the universal network of relationships and are cocreators in the ever constant unfolding and self-organizing activity.

- Organizations (systems), as smaller reflections of the universe, are self-organizing, complex, and adaptive entities in which people purposefully express their creativity, energy, and meaning together.

Quantum science revealed many of these principles in its attempt to understand the physics of the universe. From the moment of the Big Bang (itself a complex uncertainty) to the present, all aspects of the universe, including those that involve life, operate within the context of the principles of chaos and complexity (Bains & Schulze-Makuch, 2016).

The leader's role is to apply these principles to the organization. This includes showing a willingness to act in concert with quantum design—that is, to engage with chaos and harness its implications. The traditional institutional and vertical views of work and relationship are inadequate for understanding how to lead and implement changes. Instead, a "whole systems" view must underpin the work of the leader and inform the actions and priorities of the organization's members.

Leaders of organizational units, such as services, departments, and divisions, must recognize that, rather than merely leading their units, they lead the whole organization from the perspective of their units. Most leaders see their primary responsibility as making their units operate as effectively as possible. Although this is a laudable goal, no unit can thrive if the other units do not. Thriving requires an intersection of actions, each advancing the others and together ensuring the health of the whole. All the leaders of units are working to harmonize the efforts of everyone in the organization in an array of connections that together advance the organization's mission. Chaos and complexity are simply the normal context for all work and relationships, and therefore leaders must use their understanding of chaos and complexity in every element of their work.

Self-Management and Creativity

There are those who suggest that the universe is a cold, mechanical process and that life is harsh, hierarchical, accidental, and beyond the ability of human beings to affect. This view of the universe as mechanistic and indifferent or even hostile is inaccurate (Wheatley, 2009). Work by quantum scientists reveals that the universe is an exploring, experimenting, adapting process that is continuously and endlessly in the act of creation. Potential, change, adjustment, and becoming represent the character of existence, indicating that life is more challenging and dangerous than previously imagined. Because all things are essentially related, no action

Group Discussion

Reflect on three words that describe your fundamental beliefs about life. Then, present your words to the group, spending no more than 2 minutes to explain what they mean. Write all the words from all participants randomly on a flip chart. At the end of the session, look at the composite of words, and on a second flip chart write the one word that best describes what each participant sees or feels about all the words on the first flip chart. When all the participants have finished, that page represents the prevailing spiritual culture of the group.

CHAPTER FOURTEEN   Engaging the Spirit of Leadership: Becoming a Living Leader

Creative universe
Exploring
Unfolding
Experimenting

Creative processes
Changing
Adjusting
Becoming

Creative self
Passionate
Open
Searching
Responsive

Figure 14-2 The Creative Spirit.

is without a wide-ranging influence. In particular, each person's behavior has an effect on the processes of life everywhere. The well-known fact that small events can have large effects far away—encapsulated in the notion that the gentle flapping of a butterfly's wings in China can influence the unfolding of a hurricane in the Atlantic—is a reminder of the interconnectedness of everything.

For leaders, the implications of these newer notions are profound. Leaders, by the smallest of their actions, can have a significant impact on others at every level in the organization. By their behavior, which is under constant scrutiny, they create the organization's culture and build the framework for responding to the challenges and uncertainties of a world forever in flux. They exemplify the normalcy of change by embracing and engaging with it and responding with acceptance and adaptation.

It is important for leaders to fully live up to the expectations of their role. If a leader is not personally disposed to live in the potential, he or she cannot ask others to live there either. Leaders must demonstrate in their leadership practices a personal pattern of response to life's calls. For example, the universe delights in exploration and transformation, and leaders must exhibit in their behavior the enthusiasm of experimentation, challenge, and engagement (**Figure 14-2**). Indeed, they must be the living representatives of this dynamic. In this section, we discuss some issues that leaders need to consider to live and lead in accordance with the realities of life.

> **Point to Ponder**
>
> Rather than being harsh and unforgiving, life is full of opportunity. All it asks is that you desire it enough, work at it the right way, patiently build your personal resources, and then grab it when it calls. Whether good things happen to you depends more on you than on the good things.

Life is joyful. If the leader of an organization is not excited, neither are the other members. The leader creates the context for work and relationships. If the mental model of the leader implies that life is hard and treacherous, it will be hard and treacherous in that organization.

Self-Management and Creativity

The leader must believe that life is exciting and full of adventure so that everyone feels they are being invited on a journey of discovery and transformation. Otherwise, the environment is rife with the fallout of what the leader does believe about work and relationships.

Time must be allowed for reflection. Leaders need to spend time thinking about their role and the context of their role. No leader can be in touch with what is influencing his or her work if there is no room in the day for personal reflection. Call this activity what you will—meditation, deliberation, or some other term—it leads to renewal, insight, engagement, and reenergizing response. Both the external and internal elements of life's changes are considered in a way that has meaning for the leader. The focus is on the person of the leader and that individual's own life issues, priorities, challenges, and growth.

Leaders are cocreators. Leaders know that things do not simply happen by accident or without meaning. They are always seeking to discern the relationship between specific actions and their significance (Cullen & Donahue, 2016). Sorting through the vagaries of change to find its prime movers and intersections is a part of the work of transformation. People do not make change. Change is. People give change the form it takes and link it to all the elements that either constrain it or facilitate it. By "seeing" the inner life of change and identifying what it is trying to reveal, leaders attach to it the factors that give it form and meaning for those it affects. Knowing this, leaders act as cocreators, operating in concert with the change, digging for its meaning and impact, and working with others to determine the most appropriate response.

Chaos is always the route to order. Leaders know that chaos is a constant. They also know that order is generated out of chaos. Looking at the simplicity that lies at the center of complexity, leaders search for the connections that the chaos is breaking up or reformatting on a way to the very next stage of the change journey. They tie the forces at work to the mission, purposes, and direction of the organization to fit the pieces together to converge around the change. Leaders recognize that chaos is a requisite of order and are thus better able to accept chaos as an element in their own lives. They also recognize that chaos is normal and to be welcomed as a part of life. Further, they embrace chaos before expecting others to engage with their own experience of chaos.

Leadership is a contract with possibility and opportunity. Leaders understand that experience is simply the application of potential to present circumstances and that their role is to give substance to the changes occurring by making them real for those they lead. In other words, they translate the potential reality into language that has meaning for staff members in their present situation. In addition, they put staff members' current experience into a much broader context by treating it as a stage, a milepost, on a longer journey. By operating with this frame of reference, they can help staff members understand the context of their work and actions. Here again, leaders must live in the embrace of the potential, always seeing it ahead and translating its implications into language staff members can understand. As has been repeatedly noted, leading is a way of life, not just a skill set.

Life gets messy before order shows up. Living with mess is hard for many people. We desire logical, rational, and visual order and usually manage our lives to obtain such order. The problem is that while we are busy establishing and maintaining order, life is getting ready to put sand in its gears. In our desire for order, we sometimes treat the journey of life as a stationary condition that can somehow be fenced off by an unchanging set of self-created parameters. The journey, however, soon reasserts itself, sometimes dramatically, as when it brings down our neatly constructed world of supposed impervious order. This type of disruption reminds us of the impermanence of order and the essential character of the journey that is life, which is to move from where we currently are through a process of change, challenge, and, hopefully, growth. The movement does not occur in a straight line, however, and messiness is one of the reminders that we need to continuously adapt.

Leaders must preserve their identity. All living things seek to preserve their identity and sustain themselves. Leaders are no different. Yet leading is demanding work and can lead to depletion and burnout and damage to one's personal integrity. Living in the world means finding a place in the world. For leaders, it means recognizing that they occupy a space that is influencing all the surrounding spaces. How well they live in their own space, respond to the demand for movement, address personal issues, and confront the challenges to growth determine their ability to affect others through their personal leadership. Leaders cannot help others adapt to that which they cannot adapt. The paradox of identity is that persons must change to maintain their identity. Leaders must adapt to assist others in becoming reconciled to their own changes.

> **Point to Ponder**
>
> If leaders have no idea what drives them, how can they expect anyone else to know? Self-knowledge is the beginning point of self-direction.

We all participate in each other's evolution. We all have an impact on others—there are no foreigners on life's journey. Everything everywhere ultimately connects to facilitate change at every level. The rules, processes, and conditions of growth are ever-changing and cannot be counted on to act in the same way at different times and places in the change cycle. The leader knows this, understanding that synthesis rather than analysis, fluidity rather than solidity, principle rather than law, and focus rather than function are the real operating conditions of life. Discernment is a more valuable gift than definition. Direction is more important than location. These truths merely indicate how different the workings of change are from our linear expectations. We confront the patterns and movements of change in our responses to life, but change continues regardless of our responses. Our success in the journey of life depends mostly on the congruence of our responses and our recognition that we are fundamentally interdependent (Bakker, 2013).

Leadership work is important and influential, and thus requires care and concerted effort. The personal engagement of leaders in their own journey, for example, is a means of demonstrating that they have an obligation to confront the challenges presented by change and also a means of guiding them in their attempts to adapt to change (Bodaken & Fritz, 2006; Hickey & Kritek, 2012). On the other hand, leaders who have not attended to the personal issues of adaptation and have failed to sustain their insights, courage, and creativity probably will be unable to help others gain the self-understanding and discernment they need to meet their own challenges successfully.

Creativity and Innovation

We are born creative. No matter what else or who else we perceive the spiritual force in our lives to be, this spirit is the source of creativity. Artists, musicians, writers, creators of every type all make reference to some deep source of power from which flows the energy of creativity. Yet, although creativity is inextricably linked to the life force in each of us, many of us talk of creativity as something we can own or control and manipulate. We treat it as external to ourselves and profess to believe we could do so much more if we only could get hold of it.

We fail to realize that we all have it—it is a part of who we are. We do need, however, self-awareness and discipline to access it and to give it form and direction.

There is a direct relationship between creativity and discipline. Creativity needs its own time. We need to allow it the space to take form and to have expression. Although accidents of creativity and innovation regularly occur, rarely are they accidentally refined and developed. If it is visible, it is because it was made visible, disciplined by the action that brought it forward and molded it into a format that could be experienced and then shared with the world, for all to marvel at and enjoy (**Figure 14-3**). For its expression, creativity demands a format and also a context. By setting a specified time and place for its expression, we provide the discipline necessary for the elements of creativity to converge and produce something of value. The products of creativity could not exist without the work of creativity, requiring that we appreciate the latter as much as the former.

> **Key Point**
> We are all creative. We are, however, naturally creative in different ways. Although creativity is deeply hardwired within each of us, it is malleable enough to be expressed in almost any way we choose. The only requirement is that we do decide to do something with it because it can wither and die if left unattended.

At the same time, creativity demands release from the slavishness of routine and the straitjacket of habit, rote, and ritual. Only within the chaos of experience can the elements of creativity converge. Further, the format for its expression must be allowed time and space to emerge. Forcing creativity into prescribed structures of expression limits its ability to take shape. This does not mean that no format is required. There is no pottery without the potter's wheel, no painting without a canvas.

It is difficult to live creatively. There is always some reason not to. We have all made comments about creative people who seem eccentric, even weird. Because they appear to live fully in their own world or to walk their own way, they make us feel uncertain or uncomfortable. In general, we experience uncertainty and unease if people fall outside our definition of what is appropriate, and because creative people tend to operate outside the parameters of normal behavior, we wonder whether getting in touch with the creative in ourselves will make us become like them. The answer, of course, is that creativity does not have a look and a walk and that we can connect with our creativity without changing in every way possible.

Ideas / Notions / Thoughts / Fragments / Dreams / Knowledge / Concepts	→	Frames / Images / Forms / Parameters / Formats	→	Structures / Substance / Processes / Products

Figure 14-3 Requisites of Creativity.

It is important to recognize that leaders cannot get the best out of those they lead if they cannot touch the best in themselves. This means they need to develop an awareness of who they are and how their essential self is expressed in the normal course of living each day. Leaders must understand that their spiritual part is frequently expressed in their most creative moments. Getting in touch with one's own creative center means discerning the spiritual values that lie within as well. For creativity to find expression, of course, requires discipline and habit and the meeting of certain conditions.

Mindfulness and Personal Creativity

There is a strong relationship between mindful centeredness and creativity. Personal self-awareness and reflection is an important part of the preparation for availability to the process of creativity both in one's self and in working with others. Centering oneself and team members in the beginning of any creative exercise helps open the mental junctures and pathways to be able to "flow" freely in ways that enable creativity. Through centering, and opening awareness in the mindful process of managed breathing and intentional listening to the sounds of quiet, allowing them to simply move through the mind and body freely and openly, a sense of inner freedom emerges. Noticing the character, resonance, and uniqueness of each surrounding sound in becoming aware of their individual contribution to the symphony of sound allows an availability to emerge within that sets the individual and team up to listen, hear, and be available to the sounds of each other. End the process with either a personal reflection of one thing you feel the sounds you've heard are saying to you, or in the team process, have team members share one thought with each other about the sound's meaning to them as a way of generating collective awareness and appreciation for the breadth and diversity of insights gained from this shared mindful experience. Using mindful and centered exercises such as this provides a vehicle for the leader to focus and concentrate thoughtful energy and the personal capacity for creativity and individual and team in a way that allows them to both engage the potential of their own contribution and to be receptive to the insights and contributions of others. Good leaders are intentional with regard to the individual and collective work they do. Out of this intentionality comes the need to fully engage in the use of tools, such as mindfulness, in ways that are proven valid and valuable to specific activities, such as stimulating creativity, that are proven to be beneficiaries of mindfully focused activities (Raney, 2014) (**Figure 14-4**).

Finding the Source of Creativity

A person's creativity does not simply appear on demand. The person has to search for it and then develop ways to give it expression. The best way of getting in touch with it is to set aside a regular time during the day to focus on nothing but the inner self. Journaling is a helpful tool in this endeavor because regularly writing down one's thoughts establishes the habit of focusing on the creative and bringing it out into the open. The process need not be complicated or demanding. The goal is to write from one to three pages about whatever comes to mind at the moment. No one need see what was written because the purpose is merely to make sure that something has been done. In time, the act of writing begins to touch a deep part of the self, and expressing what lies within becomes easier. How long it takes to achieve fluency depends on how many blocks are standing in the way.

Creativity and Innovation

Circles labeled (top to bottom): Curiosity, Forgiving, Grateful, Compassionate, Peaceful, Vulnerable, Appreciative acceptance

Annotations: ...Reflective, ...Intentional, ...Discipline, ...In the moment

Figure 14-4 Personal Attributes of Mindfulness.

Group Discussion

Getting in touch with the unrestrained child within is critical to touching our own creativity. Take a moment to reflect on a childhood episode in which you did something that was different or even unique (at the time)—in a word, creative. Those who wish to can tell their story to the rest of the participants. During each story, the listeners write down what each perceives as the key elements of the story. The group then discusses these elements and considers whether they are present in creativity regardless of age or time. Finally, the participants identify ways in which they can incorporate these elements into their own efforts at touching their individual creativity.

Everyone possesses an internal auditor who judges what is written or spoken or thought as appropriate or not. Often the auditor appears just as an individual is about to get in touch with his or her creativity and prevents the expression of ideas on the grounds that they are, for example, inappropriate, not right, not good, or not normal. This review and approval function is the person's own creation. A good way to bypass it is to commit to the process of daily writing and go wherever it leads. In time, the auditor will disappear and be replaced by a sense of freedom and openness, which is the groundwork for creative expression.

Journaling is a way of meditating that is often easier than the more defined forms of meditation. What often happens is that the wisdom that lies deep within emerges through the process and finds expression in a language that can inform, inspire, and guide. It is a chance for the inner voice to assume an outward form, deepening the meaning of our lives and perhaps moving us in a new direction.

Spending Time with the Child Within

As Jung and many contemporary psychotherapists revealed, we each have a child embedded deep within us that resides there throughout our lives. This child is the enthusiastic, joyful, excited part of ourselves that embraces life fully and without reservation. It is only when we are wounded by the behavior of others or by negative experiences that our inner child loses touch with the primordial joy that typifies the experience of the spirit. And even when the child loses touch with the joy of life, it continues to seek it until it finds joy again, renewing itself in the process.

The creative process often, if not always, meets up with this inner child. Many say it is impossible to get in touch with one's creativity without confronting this inner child and giving it a voice. Indeed, it is this voice that is the expression of creativity. Further, because the inner child, by its very nature, is not bound by the rules and parameters of adulthood, these are rendered powerless to limit the expression of creativity. However, whatever the child is feeling, whether pain or joy or some other emotion, will emerge as a part of the journey to the place of creativity, and until these feelings are expressed and dealt with in a meaningful way, the creative expression will remain blocked at the very place where it resides. That is why we must take up our unfinished business with this child (the pains and hurts of our life experiences and journey to adulthood) to free the creativity within.

Through the process of journaling, a person typically arrives at the door of creativity but is prevented from entering by the remnants of past pain. In verbalizing these on the daily pages of the journal, the person can get them out of the way and open the route to creative expression. In some circumstances, working on the issues with a professional or other trusted person may be a necessary step in the journey to freeing the inner child and releasing the creativity residing within.

Opening the Gates of Creativity

When we complete the journey to the center of our being, we find a deep well of creativity—a place filled with things that can be used as vehicles for creative expression (Leonard-Barton, 2011). We are all artists of one kind or another. Some of us are creative with our hands, some with our heads, some with our hearts—all of us with something. By using our regularly set aside time to explore different avenues, we can find that form of creative expression that most resonates with our inner self. Some people, of course, may discover more than one form. In any case, to give shape to our creativity we need to release the energy that lies within the urge to create. Creativity always seeks a way out into the world, and once touched and released it cannot be contained and must find expression, enriching the lives of everyone it touches and connecting all of us in ways we cannot even imagine.

Creativity is expressed in symbols and images. Even the wordsmith has a vision before forming that vision into words. Leaders also express their creativity through the construction of a vision. They then present this vision to others as evidence of their commitment to make some difference, to cause something to happen that enhances the life experience of everyone.

In this dynamic, leaders recognize that the critical ability is to be available to the creative force without attempting to master it. Creativity is very much a mystery and requires awareness instead of readiness. The creative force must first be seen before it can be expressed. Further, to give it form the creative mind must be attentive to what it might be saying. Form comes as a product of good discernment and the discipline of translating the creative force into words or substance (Breland et al., 2016).

> **Point to Ponder**
>
> The creative leader recognizes that what is critical is being available to the creative force, not mastering it.

Creativity leads each of us inward and then onward. We must spend time in the "inward place." As Georgia O'Keeffe and Brenda Ueland caution us, we must spend time watching the flowers, puttering around in the imagining, idling, seeing, forming stuff that lives within. Leaders must identify the activities that guide them to the creative place within. Each of us can recall where we got our best ideas. For some it is in the shower; others, the car; still others, hiking mountain trails. From wherever the ideas come, the creative force is always seeking expression; we need only be aware of where and how it operates.

Overcoming the Fear of Being Wrong and Not Being Perfect

Many artists and psychologists have noted that the opposite of love is not hate but fear. Fear closes off access to the creative—indeed, to most of life. Fear is a mental door that keeps the spirit imprisoned and unaware. How much faith is an expression of fear and as a result narrow, ritualistic, and rigid? How many people neurotically seek the spiritless road, comfortable in their own rightness but devoid of life and joy?

Fear, like a trap from which there is no escape, imprisons the heart and keeps it from experiencing the fullness of life. It closes the mind and shuts the door on life. It is the ultimate indicator of nonengagement. It keeps people from reaching out toward those very things that advance their experience and reduce the chance that fear will rule them. It is all too common to see people failing to confront fears that affect their expression of life—or to see someone struggling to avoid something infinitely less painful than the life of fear the person is living.

There is virtually nothing redeeming about fear. Yet much of the relationship that so many people have with life is tinged by their accommodation of their own fears. In addition, the structures of 20th-century organizations were largely grounded in the concept of fear. In hierarchical organizations pervaded by the culture of "bossism," the negative power of the boss is what keeps people in line, and the power that managers wield is often articulated in the language of control and punishment. It is no wonder that changing the way the leadership role is perceived and expressed is so difficult. To make the necessary changes and remove fear from organizational life, leaders must therefore confront the history of the role and people's perception and experience of it.

Being wrong is an essential constituent of creativity. In fact, creative people spend more time being wrong than being right. The road to rightness is paved with experimentation, innovation, mistakes, and redoes. In fact, in systems language success of any kind is simply the culmination of sufficient error. When the right amount of error has occurred and a sufficient amount of learning in relationship to the error has been obtained, then success emerges. Mistakes are the signposts of the journey toward achievement. The only error that is untenable is the same error repeated. An error repeated indicates that no learning occurred, and the error's lesson was missed.

Mistakes are to be embraced by the organization as the tools of growth. The more fully an error is incorporated into the expectations of work, the fewer errors are present and the more certain the leader is that the right errors will emerge. By celebrating error, the leader takes the fear out of it and puts it into the right category—the category of devices for determining where people are on the journey toward their goals.

> **Key Point**
> Being wrong is not a defect. We learn as much from our errors (Stewart et al., 2006) as we do from our successes. The critical issue is to learn the specific point from any error so that we do not repeat it or stay imprisoned in a never-ending cycle of repetition and decline.

Failure is a normative element in the journey toward any sustainable value (Porter-O'Grady & Malloch, 2019). Without it, there is simply no measure against which any success can be compared. The leader must see failure as an evaluative mechanism, a tool set, that helps develop insight, mechanisms for evaluation, and enable methodologies for corrective action and alternative approaches. The role of the leader is to free negative emotional content from the value of failure so that he can be used in a way that is truly positive and value-grounded, helping the leader and participants identify opportunities for growth and change and build toward meaningful success.

Confronting personal fear and fear in the workplace is a challenging process (**Exhibit 14-1**). So much of human experience is defined by fear that it becomes nearly impossible to push it out of people's lives. From regulation to accreditation, there are plenty of opportunities to be afraid of something or someone in a way that limits creativity and engagement with life. So many folks worry about whether they will "get in trouble" because of projects or activities with which they might be associated. For example, instead of thinking about how their behavior enables the organization to deliver high-quality services, individuals waste their time worrying about whether they will offend someone, or do the wrong thing, or even cause a patient's death.

Of course, the probability of any one person doing sustainable damage is very low. People in an organization are generally incapable of permanently jeopardizing its integrity and functioning unless they have that goal as their evil intent. Of late, much work has been written on fear in the workplace and how unnecessary it is, not to mention detrimental to performance and even dangerous. One of the main goals of leadership should be to drive fear-based behavior

---

Exhibit 14-1 Overcoming Fear

Sources of Fear	**Means of Identifying Fear**	**Ways of Overcoming Fear**
• Parents	• Self-awareness	• Meditation
• Teachers	• Therapy	• Risk-taking
• Peers	• Reflection	• Therapy
• Self	• Input from others	• Focused action
• Authorities	• Trauma	• Confrontation
• Religion		• Surrender–embrace
• Events		

out of the workplace and replace it with the commitment to relationship and creativity and the importance of taking risks in order to improve.

So many people in the professional workplace spend much of their time concentrating on the "floor" of their practice. Establishing standards, maintaining standards, benchmarking, developing protocols, and establishing routines are all names for the mechanism of focusing on the foundation, or the floor, of work and practice. Although it is essential to establish and use evidence-based standards, the leader must keep in mind that these standards represent the ground upon which practice builds. Excellence is never achieved simply by maintaining standards. Excellence is achieved after standards have been established and as people climb from these foundations toward the "ceiling" of their work and practice. Excellence occurs when people and organizations aim for the ceiling, moving beyond the floor of their practice in a way that advances and transforms it into higher levels of value, meaning, and impact on others. This pattern of behavior eclipses fear, which limits perspectives and keeps people focused merely on avoiding error instead of advancing excellence.

How much of the fear present in the workplace is there because of the fear within the leaders? If leaders have not resolved their own fear issues, do these issues affect their relationships with others and affect the organization as a whole? If their language is laced with fear-based terminology, are they helping to create an atmosphere of anxiety and suspicion?

Fear-based behaviors—judging, blaming, pointing fingers, complaining, and so on—kill innovation. In the new age, there is simply no place for them. The job of the leader is to eliminate fear-based behaviors by giving them no room. Leaders begin this process by making sure that their own fear issues have not negatively influenced the environment. By focusing on fear issues and grappling with their presence in each individual's life journey, leaders have a good chance to create a workplace of trust and joy and creativity.

> **Point to Ponder**
> Fear kills all creativity.

In addition, leaders need to be aware of the importance and vitality of transparency in the expression of their own humanity and challenges in their leadership journey. Perhaps one of the most significant personal characteristics of excellent leadership is the capacity to demonstrate personal vulnerability and openness regarding the individual journey of development and change. This vulnerability demonstrates the capacity of the leader to engage and embrace openly in the vagaries of risk, error, experimentation, and adaptation and serves as a visible template for staff to emulate, model, and replicate in their own journey of transformation and change. This vulnerability gives others a window into the authentic and legitimate self which shows the leader as an individual who is unique and special. The leader's vulnerability gives individual staff members permission to demonstrate and express their own experiences and challenges of growth and adaptation in a way that provides advantages to each organizational member, the service unit or department, and, ultimately, those they serve.

Confronting the Core Negativity Within

As we move through life, we collect flawed mental models, negative stereotypes, and unsupported generalizations. These become deeply embedded in our consciousness and are reflected in our attitudes and behaviors. They often surface in our self-talk and our conversation with those closest to us. Although the generalities we use are typically inaccurate, even groundless,

CHAPTER FOURTEEN   Engaging the Spirit of Leadership: Becoming a Living Leader

we still fall back on them in the midst of stress or during periods of difficulty. Following are a list of examples (to which each of us could add):

- I always do this.
- No one likes me.
- I'm going to die of . . .
- I'll always be poor.
- I cannot study.
- I've never been able to . . .
- I'm just not good at . . .
- It's too late for me to do . . .

How many of these phrases have we caught ourselves saying at some time or other? Most people are surprised that this type of language is so pervasive. Think about how limiting and just plain incorrect these statements are. The challenge for every leader is to look carefully at his or her own language and assess the extent to which it is laced with negativity. The fact is that most leaders use (and hear) more negative language in a day than any other type.

Most of our negative ideas and images are untrue, including those that pertain to our own abilities. If we really could not do most of what we imagine cannot be done, we could not do what we have already done. Most of our core negatives come from outside ourselves—from parents, friends, religion, society, and so on. On top of these we add other negatives based on our experience. Eventually we have so many that they cannot help but impair our relationships and degrade other aspects of our lives.

What is important to remember is that negative beliefs are just that—beliefs. They are also obstacles blocking the enriched experience and the creative endeavors everyone is capable of. They shut the door on awareness and limit the places where talent or opportunity can make a positive change in our lives. Further, they give us all an excuse not to address challenges: no matter what we do, we will not succeed anyway. Keep in mind, they are simply beliefs, often, actions of the mind, reinforced by brief experiences. Individuals often "talk themselves" into these negative beliefs in ways that give them a reality and legitimacy they simply do not have.

Sitting on the sidelines of life, we can join others in spreading negativity. When we see others struggling to be creative, we can assure them that they will not succeed and thus need not strain themselves. The most threatening person to a negativist is the person who has agreed to engage with his or her negatives, take on a creative task, and follow wherever it leads. This person creates a risk that the negativist will see someone achieve all that the negativist has failed to do and thereby make the role of negativist very uncomfortable.

Leaders struggling to fight their own negatives should remember that affirmation is the enemy of negativity, that affirmative beliefs are just as viable and powerful as negative beliefs, only they have more mileage. They also need to replace the negative terminology they have used in the past with affirmative language, demonstrating their commitment to a different set of images and mental models, raising the level of the dialogue in the organization and creating a healthier organizational culture. Here are some examples of affirming language:

- I am very good at . . .
- I've always been able to . . .
- You're an excellent . . .

- I am a brilliant . . .
- I am challenged by . . .
- It's great fun to . . .
- What a great idea . . .

> ## Group Discussion
>
> Discuss the content of your self-talk with the group—the things you say to yourself when you are alone. What are the words used? What are the themes? Are the comments primarily positive or negative? Then, share your self-talk words with each other. Taken as a whole, is the group's self-talk supportive and encouraging or negative and punishing?

If leaders fight the urge to blurt out a negative comment and substitute an affirming statement, they will notice the different results. Language and behavior are themselves strong change agents. Contemporary research shows that positive statements, even when untrue, can become true through changing behavior over time (de Bono, 2007).

The transition to a more positive culture does not happen overnight. The bombardment of negative images and generalizations that most of us have undergone eventually turns negativity into our second nature. Leaders therefore have to make the overcoming of negativity a focused part of their leadership work. To not get sucked into the drama of constant negativity, they must have a way of exploring the sources of their own negativity and lack of creativity, past and present (Simons & Havert, 2012).

For leaders, getting in touch with their own journey means looking squarely at themselves and at how their nature affects their relationship with and leadership of others. How much do they understand about negativity and what causes it? What overwhelms their creativity? What affects their ability to embrace innovation? What personality characteristics keep them from relating to the elements of life that challenge or frighten them? How can they help others reflect on their attitudes and behaviors if, as leaders, they have no mechanism for doing that in their own lives?

Leaders cannot ask others to go to places they themselves are not willing or able to go. They thus need to routinely engage in reflection to gain essential insights about themselves, including whatever internal obstacles block their own creativity, engagement, and courage and decrease their ability to guide others and help them overcome the many challenges they face on their individual journeys. Leaders can ask themselves: Why would anyone I lead be willing to be creative or courageous if I don't practice those behaviors?

Equally important to the leader is the willingness to demonstrate vulnerability and openness to what the personal journey teaches and reveals to each of us. Good leadership and mentorship require that leaders share the personal reflections that come with the struggle to growth. No secrets or mystical unmentionables are imbedded in the leadership journey. Every leader's story is food for another's journey and can be a stimulus for new learning and advancing others' experiences of leadership.

CHAPTER FOURTEEN   Engaging the Spirit of Leadership: Becoming a Living Leader

Exercising the Spirit

We all know how important it is to exercise the body. Almost all medical literature about longevity tells us that exercise is an essential part of our lives. Regular exercise leads to good health and lifelong productivity, and failure to exercise is one of the major causes of untimely death.

Stretching the Spirit Within

Each person's spirit of consciousness—the source of creativity, energy, and engagement and seat of the self—has precisely the same need for exercise (**Exhibit 14-2**). When the spirit of consciousness is not exercised, it becomes weak and flabby and fails to grow. A weak spirit cannot provide the meaning that people need and look for in their lives. In the case of leaders, a weak spirit limits their effectiveness and causes them to lose direction. When that happens, their enthusiasm is diminished, and they cannot motivate others to embrace the challenges of change. They then become disengaged or depersonalized and subject to all and any of the diseases of the spirit. Without exercise, both the muscle (spiritual strength and creativity) and the immune system (moral courage and focus) of the spirit cease to operate effectively. They become susceptible to spiritual infections, such as evil intent, lack of direction, poor decision making, depression, and lack of focus.

Many leaders who want to pursue self-development read to learn and gain meaning of who they are as a leader. Self-clarity and self-knowledge enables them to discuss similar topics with others. Reading alone never calls people to do the deeper task of stretching their spirits in a way that actually changes their lives. The personal journey of touching the spiritual energy within requires regular discipline—and focus!

Developing an Exercise Routine

Every leader needs regular spiritual workouts every day. The stress caused by confronting so much change requires a regular recess for recentering and refocusing on the meaning that drives the work of leading. This daily period of reflection and connection to one's spiritual energy should last at least 15 minutes. Of course, each leader must adjust the routine and time based on his or her individual needs and circumstances. The length of the period can be extended as the leader develops more skill and as the spirit increases its tone and strength. It is recommended that the leader gradually work up to spending 30 minutes on spiritual exercises each day.

Exhibit 14-2   Exercising the Spirit Within

Requisites	**Obstacles**
• Setting aside time daily	• Fear
• Exercising regularly	• Tiredness
• Being self-disciplined	• Distractions
• Using a specific format or method	• Laziness
	• Excuses
	• Other commitments
	• Family responsibilities

> **Exhibit 14-3** A Spiritual Exercise Routine
>
> *Deep breathing.* Transitioning from a high energy level to a lower one.
> *Spiritual warm-up.* Reading a selection from a source that has special relevance.
> *Stretching the spirit.* Reflecting on an incident or theme.
> *Strengthening the spirit.* Applying knowledge and experience to gain wisdom.
> *Spiritual cooldown.* Breathing, letting go, and choosing a thought to keep for the day.

A large body of research indicates that a spiritual/psychodynamic-conscious and intentional workout should encompass five specific steps: deep breathing, a spiritual warm-up, spiritual stretching, spiritual strengthening, and a spiritual cooldown (Gotink et al., 2016; Tarrasch et al., 2016; Vago & Zeidan, 2016). The following paragraphs demonstrate one of many different suggested approaches to establishing a regular routine of reflection and spiritual centering (**Exhibit 14-3**). Leaders are advised to find the discipline to allow the approach to be unique to their own personal needs and capacity for reflection and discernment. The method they choose is not nearly as important as is the regular, consistent discipline of time spent in self-reflection.

Deep Breathing

At the beginning of every exercise routine, you need to transition from one level of energy to another lower level. You also need to move from a primarily external focus to looking inward. Deep breathing is a technique that helps you make the necessary journey.

Deep breathing facilitates the transition from a high level of energy to a lower level. In a relaxed position, slowly but continuously breathe deeply through your nose. After each inhale, hold your breath for a second and then let it go fully out through your mouth all at once. You need to do 10 to 20 of these before you begin to feel the relaxation unfold. The routine should be slow and continuous, completely unrushed, allowing you to peacefully and quietly relax yourself and refocus your attention on yourself and the reflective work you are about to undertake. Every time you sit down to do your reflective work, you should begin with deep breathing because it sets you up for the steps to follow.

This is where the heavy exercise occurs. Your response to your insights has an important impact on your choices, approach, method, and focus for the day. The insights you obtain during this strengthening exercise may accumulate over a number of days and eventually come together to clarify what course you should take in dealing with a challenge, problem, or issue. You should spend 5 to 10 minutes (and no more than 10 minutes) on this part of the workout.

Spiritual Warm-Up

The next step is to read a brief selection from a source that has relevance to your own life or experience. The reading is meant to move your spirit and mind into a reflective mode. By making the transition to a quieter, more peaceful perspective, you become ready to begin the journey to an intensive internal experience. This exercise should last anywhere from 3 to 5 minutes.

Stretching Your Spiritual Energy

You can use a real-life event or situation to center your attention on a particular theme or aspect of life. For example, you might choose an event that exemplifies the theme of the selection read during the warm-up. Using an actual incident or circumstance as a focal point is designed to narrow the reflective work so that it fits within the workout period but is still illuminating. This exercise, like the warm-up, should last 3 to 5 minutes.

Strengthening and Focusing the Mindful Spirit Within

During reflection, a question or series of questions arises. These might concern an aspect of your life or experience or a component of your role, relationships, or work. At this point you apply your knowledge and experience to learn about yourself—about your issues, relationships, problems, and concerns—and gain wisdom.

> **Key Point**
> Spending time with ourselves is the most valuable and most difficult thing we can do in life.

Cooling Down

The spiritual workout is concluded with a brief period of breathing and letting go. This exercise brings the workout to a close and transitions you back into your daily activities. You should choose an important thought or moment in the reflection to remember and keep with you for the rest of the day. You might even write it on a small card. Writing down important thoughts or memorable moments allows you to recollect them at any time during the day and to apply them whenever and in whatever way appears right. This finishing exercise should take between 2 and 3 minutes. Please keep in mind that the effort here is to provide an opportunity for quiet reflection as a vehicle for providing the kind of directed discernment related to your person as a leader and to deepen your capacity for insight, self-reflection, purposefulness, and intentional personal transformation.

Quiet, Please

A quiet place is necessary for proper exercise of the mind and spirit. Unlike the body, which can be toned by exercising to vigorous music and enthusiastic encouragement, the spirit needs quiet to be stretched and strengthened. The quieter it is during spiritual exercises, the better the results.

Finding and maintaining quiet can be difficult. Some people even feel initial anxiety in a quiet place. Today, distraction is the name of the game, and we have become conditioned to continuous assaults on our consciousness. For leaders, the very work of leading forces them into a host of relationships, conversations, processes, and problems that leaves no time for consideration and reflection.

> **Key Point**
> In developing self-awareness, the discipline of regular reflection can make an important difference. Progress is always variable, but no progress will be achieved if the process is not a regular habit.

Focusing on our spiritual resources is inner exercising. The better we get at it, the deeper we go, and the more we desire the joy and peace that come from going deeper. Regular spiritual reflection leads to a surprising yet extremely satisfying calm, accompanied by a deep sense of peace and contentment. The secret to discovering this place is the quiet and calm that surrounds us when we undertake our exercise routines. Each workout should be done in a quiet place and at an available time (i.e., a time free of other commitments), and preferably the same time and place should be used for all the workouts.

A wide variety of mental and spiritual resources has emerged over the history of humankind. The warm-up exercises, for example, can be drawn from a broad selection of spiritual or reflective works. The goal of reflective exercising is to stretch the spirit through a variety of growth experiences and challenges that fall inside and outside of the person's usual life context. These experiences and challenges instigate growth by pushing the person to use a diverse set of learning resources as a tool kit.

The notes written during the spiritual cooldown act as "memory joggers" to help connect our experiences to the wisdom gained through the exercises. In the midst of daily activities, our consciousness periodically generates windows or moments of perception that affirm the insights that arose from that day's reflection. The notes from a particular exercise session can also serve as a doorway back to the work done during that session, allowing the wisdom gained to continue to play a role in meeting life's challenges.

> **Key Point**
> A leader is never off duty while in the leadership role. Leaders are under constant observation of others while they try to turn every moment, every interchange, every experience into an opportunity to make a difference in the lives of those they lead.

Importance of Mindful Exercise Every Day

Regularity is the key to good spiritual work. It is recommended that these exercises be done first thing in the morning or as early as possible in the day. Although morning is best, exercising the spirit is valuable any time it is done. As mentioned, exercising for 15 to 30 minutes a day is enough for the benefits to accrue.

If a leader does the exercise routine daily, he or she will begin to see a difference in the areas of feeling, acting, and thinking. The leader will have more energy, experience more enthusiasm, exhibit more creativity, and feel more centered. As a result, the leader's work relationships will improve, among other positive consequences. As the spirit uses better strategies to handle stress, anger and tension will ease and then dissipate, sleep will come more easily, and worry will begin to lessen. After faithfully completing a full 100 days of regular workouts, the leader will almost certainly see dramatic changes in his or her life.

There are also opportunities to bring mindfulness to the daily activities of a clinician in a less structured way. Consider the simple mindfulness practice of paying attention to what is before you in the process of caring for a patient—using your stethoscope. With a calm body and clear mind as you are performing auscultation, warm the stethoscope in your hands and take several mindful breaths. On the last exhale, remember why you are a nurse. Place the stethoscope on the patient's chest and give your full attention to listening—reconnecting to your calling as a nurse. Listen with intention for a full minute, considering every aspect of what you hear—heart rate, rhythm, and others. Thank your patient and internalize the benefit to your patient that your effort brought—peace (Rushton & Turner, 2016).

The First 100 Days

The leader commits to a set of daily exercises for 100 days. This commitment is meant to help the individual continue the workouts long enough to experience some of the benefits of mindful reflection and seek out other sources and methods of spiritual strengthening. The spiritual energy of every person matures in its own fashion, and by the time the mindful workout routine is well established the leader's spirit will thirst for further spiritual experiences. Indeed, the leader will come to find that he or she cannot live without them.

CHAPTER FOURTEEN   Engaging the Spirit of Leadership: Becoming a Living Leader

Spiritual Intelligence: 10 Mindful Rules of the Road

Leadership is not simply a set of skills but a whole discipline. As such, it requires a commitment to constant growth, self-development, and reinforcement by the work of being a leader. Leaders, in living the role, not only direct the process of change and adaptation but also exemplify adaptability, modeling it for others. This means that personal change, maturation, and development make up a fundamental part of the life of any leader. Consequently, leaders are always involved in reaching for the potential within the self.

Following is a discussion of 10 basic themes that thread through the life of a leader. These themes underscore the fact that leaders, in virtue of their role, are on a journey of exploration and growth (**Exhibits 14-4** and **14-5** and **Figure 14-5**).

1. *The leadership role demands courage.* For leaders, risk is a pervasive fact of life. Leaders live in the potential, by definition a place of great risk and vulnerability. Leaders who avoid and reject vulnerability eliminate the chance of joy from a potential outcome that is positive. The leaders' willingness to engage with their own vulnerability determines the depth of their courage. When leaders don't face their vulnerability because they wait until they are perfect or have the perfect answer to a problem, time is wasted because their unique gifts are withheld (Brown, 2012). They have a responsibility to translate the potential into real experiences in a way that helps others see how the journey requires their engagement. Leaders are often required to live on the cutting edge, pushing against the walls of reality, forcing team members to confront their own perceptions and behaviors, and challenging them

---

Exhibit 14-4   Ten Spiritual Rules of the Road

1. The leadership role demands courage.
2. Caring for the self is the first priority.
3. Setting a few focused goals and achieving them are preferable to setting and failing to achieve a broad range of goals.
4. Mindful reflection and/or prayer can be a powerful tool of leadership.
5. Challenge and change are normal features of the universe.
6. The universe is full of creative and transforming energy as well as mystery.
7. Leaders can seek out others who are committed to change and growth.
8. The goal of leadership is to connect to the journey of transformation.
9. Judgment is an enemy of the spirit within.
10. You cannot love your creation if you do not love the creator.

Exhibit 14-5   Requisites of the Spiritual Journey

- A desire for truth
- Self-love
- Creativity
- The support of others
- A disciplined process
- Ability to see life itself as a journey

Figure 14-5 The Journey of Spirit.

to create their own futures. Leaders frequently appear to be running counter to the prevailing sensibilities and must confront the noise that their actions create, holding strongly to what is right and necessary in a way that advocates for these things in the face of the noise—certainly a challenging reality but a requisite of the role.

2. *Caring for the self is the first priority.* Leaders are not self-sacrificing, long-suffering, passive personalities who mindlessly implement the organization's directives. Instead, they have a strong sense of self and are fully in touch with their own motives and intentions. They are clear where they are in relationship to what motivates action and response, and they always act on the basis of their understanding of this. They also recognize that they cannot address the needs of others if their own neediness is greater. Therefore, they realize that they require time for reflection, opportunities for self-development, and the skills necessary for dealing with critical growth issues. It is only through self-understanding that leaders can help meet the needs of others.

3. *Setting a few focused goals and achieving them are preferable to setting and failing to achieve a broad range of goals.* There is nothing more debilitating than setting a host of goals and not meeting them. Thus, it is wise to set a small number of goals and commit to achieving them. Being less ambitious ensures that the focus does not get lost and that significant progress can be made. Personal development is a work in progress and requires a lifetime commitment.

Focusing only on key issues of self-development makes it possible to resolve them and move on. Not every behavior or habit can be altered at the same time. Leaders need to be kind to themselves, express gratitude for small successes, and not expect progress on every front. Small successes can serve as the foundation for significant change and as the means for attaining ultimate goals.

Leaders need to be similarly kind to those they are helping to change. They should assist them in setting priorities so that they can better succeed in revising their behaviors and practices. By being realistic and not expecting too much, leaders can turn success into a way of being. Success does much to alter attitudes and reenergize performance, changing both the milieu and the spirit of the work.

4. *Mindful reflection and/or prayer can be a powerful tool of leadership.* Although there are as many religious traditions as there are leaders, mindful reflection and prayer is central to all of them. Whatever their convictions, leaders should know that mindful reflection and prayer has been determined to have a great impact on the quality of decisions and the comfort with which challenges are faced. Prayer is simply a reflection of a reality beyond one's own. When used with mindfulness and intentionality, it harnesses the spiritual forces within and without to help create the stamina required to carry on. It centers the mind and calls it to focus in a way that leads to new insights and deep, strong relationships. This reflective capacity has value for the secular mind as well. Time set aside in deeply reflective activity has demonstrated psychobiological benefits that affect positive well-being.

   Prayer and mindful reflection ensure the constancy necessary to any meaningful effort and link the effort to the forces needed for something to happen. They encourage and strengthen the individual, realigning the individual's energy to fit the requirements of the task. They help keep things in perspective and pull the mind and heart back to the journey, putting the work into a life framework rather than an event model. In reflection and prayer, the issue or situation takes on broader and deeper implications and gets connected to a whole range of intersections that give it meaning and call people back to the larger picture. Prayer and/or reflection renews, strengthens, encourages, and connects people in a way that ensures their faithfulness to the effort and to each other. Prayer and reflection are also vehicles for gratitude.

5. *Challenge and change are normal features of the universe.* Stability is equivalent to death. Change is the normal state of existence. The role of leaders is to walk the tightrope between stability and chaos, with a tendency to favor the latter. Chaos is a sign of life in the universe and pervades human experience. Realizing this, leaders do not expect stability to last for long. Any stability they find is simply a resting point on the journey to the next place.

   > **Key Point**
   >
   > Sometimes all that is possible is to embrace the mystery, the unknown, of a situation and allow it to be beyond reach or understanding for a while. Going with the flow of an experience helps position the leader to discern something different or new and advances the leader's insight and experience in a way that simply cannot be controlled or managed.

   Opposition, including the clash between differing interests, is part of change. Thus, leaders are always prepared for opposition and contrary arguments, practices, and behaviors. Indeed, the techniques of managing relationships encompass ways of challenging people's mental models. Leaders begin by clarifying their own perceptions, roles, and commitments and then challenge others to make their own commitment to fostering change and meeting the challenges that arise on the journey.

6. *The universe is full of creative and transforming energy as well as mystery.* Regardless of their personal belief traditions and perceptions, leaders need to understand what this means at the individual level because they must harness the internal energy of

the staff and the external energy embedded in all transformation. This combined energy reflects a resonance with change that itself can keep people focused and directed. Leaders can appreciate that influence and the wisdom that is often evident in the demand for change.

Because everything is always in motion, everything that the leader does and creates somehow reflects change and adaptation. A particular change does not happen for its own sake. It is a reflection of a grand concert of changes that, when connected together, cocreate the next stage of the universe. Leaders, along with everyone else, are participants in this universal dance or exchange of energy, and by understanding this fact they can deepen the meaning of their work and change efforts. Becoming aware of the wisdom deeply embedded in the action of the universe is the first step in discerning a deepening level of meaning and value in the individual efforts of all who are contributing to the transformation.

7. *Leaders can seek out others who are committed to change and growth.* Companionship on the journey of leadership is a great gift—but only if the companions are of the right kind. There are those who, for some reason, are committed to making the journey of life difficult and rocky. They want others to be in their condition. They obstruct the processes of transformation and suck the life out of the experience of leadership.

   These people should be carefully managed in the leader's life. Leaders need as much support as they can get in doing the work of leadership. They should expect colleagues and friends to be as committed to personal and organizational transformation as they are. The work of leadership takes a lot of energy and demands the support of good people who can clarify the work and stimulate the person doing it. Leaders must seek out those who are themselves well motivated and can act to advance, rather than limit, the leadership role. Likewise, they must break their relationships with people who are somehow driven to try to discourage them or deflate their energy. The work is tough enough as it is.

8. *The goal of leadership is to connect to the journey of transformation.* When surrounded by the challenges of leadership, leaders can lose sight of the fact that change is normal and that people cannot keep from changing. The issue, thus, is not whether they will transform but how they will change and what condition they will be in at the end of the change cycle.

   People can change by design or by default, and it is part of the leadership role to help them change by design—to guide them on the journey of transformation rather than letting them be carried down the rapids. Working with people through their own tough times, however, can skew a leader's perceptions and obscure the fact that change is unavoidable. Therefore, leaders need to get away from their work occasionally or talk to colleagues to reaffirm their commitment to leading change and reestablish their connection with the journey and their vision of the future. Indeed, this is an essential part of leadership—staying grounded in transformation.

9. *Judgment is an enemy of the spirit within.* How many people have been sacrificed on the altar of judgment? Other than in courts of law, judgment is usually destructive. The appraisals that people make of their own activities are usually negative and have the effect of suppressing their creativity. The appraisals of others can be just as negative and just as counterproductive.

People's judgments reflect their feelings about what they are judging, and their judgments obviously are formed by their values and prejudices, fears, and uncertainties. People rarely see things as they really are but instead make what they observe into shadows of their own biases. In addition, judgments about actions are often more concerned

> **Point to Ponder**
>
> Judgment is always finally destructive. It puts up a barrier in our consciousness that prevents leaders from seeing the potential at their disposal. It keeps them stuck in the present and the superficial, unable to dig to a deeper place where meaning resides and truth can be found.

with the agents than with the actions themselves. An action or performance, for example, might be condemned just because the person who did it was assumed to be unskilled or inept or lacked the right to do it. Everything has value when seen in a valuable way. Even negative behavior can have meaning if it is understood.

> ## Group Discussion
>
> As a group, brainstorm the ways in which judgment obstructs progress. Then, brainstorm impeding judgments and place these on a flip chart. Next, discuss possible approaches to use to prevent the various mechanisms of judgment from taking control of a leader's consciousness. Finally, enumerate the characteristics of the judgment process, identify clues that someone is habitually making judgments and acting on them, and discuss ways in which the tendency to make judgments might be managed or avoided.

When judgments are made, they usually reflect some weakness in the individual making the judgment. The ability to see things within their actual context and from a perspective generated from within that context (Hosmer, 2006; Massaro et al., 2012). Judgments are generally loaded with fear content, and fear disables and limits human responses and kills the creative urge. Leaders who develop the ability to seek and understand the source of judgment will disable the impact of judgment and set a course for change.

10. *You cannot love your creation if you do not love the creator.* No person can love another in a healthy way if the person feels unloved or even without the right to be loved. This is as true for leaders as for anyone else. How many people have aspired to hold formal leadership positions because they are seeking recognition? How many actual leaders have a greater neediness than those they lead? How many are looking for satisfaction in the adulation and dependencies that can accompany the leadership role? How many leaders keep a tight rein out of the fear they will lose control and no one will love them because they failed to do their job or cannot own the glory?

Many seek the leadership role not solely out of a desire to make a difference. Instead, they seek it because of their own need to shine, to be noticed, and to get from their position what they could not get elsewhere: recognition, reward, and love. They do not realize that if they cannot find satisfaction within themselves, they will not find it in the leadership role either. Also, they do not understand that they must first love themselves before they can expect to get from the role what it truly has to offer. Unfortunately, others are held back and organizational success is elusive.

> **Point to Ponder**
>
> You simply cannot love another for long if you cannot love yourself first.

These 10 themes are simply suggested "givens" around which the leadership role is built. Consequently, they can serve as a personal template for leaders as they learn to make sense of their role and find the center within that informs each of them about their own growth. In addition, leaders who embark on a mindful spiritual exercise regimen of the sort described previously can incorporate a personal assessment of the individual implications of these themes into their initial workouts (or periods of mindful reflection).

Becoming Self

All creation is good. There is simply no other way to evaluate it. Life appears because it wants to. Life wants life. Life seeks fullness, expression, identity, emergence, and flowering. In every aspect of creation, it appears as though life wants to live. The evidence is to be found in all of its acts of self-creation, change, adaptation, and growth.

Life's drive toward self-organization is a fundamental feature of the universe, and it has operated from the beginning of existence as we know it. We simply needed the right science, the right moment, and the right perceptions to grasp these facts.

> **Key Point**
>
> Life wants life. Life seeks fullness, expression, identity, emergence, and flowering. In every aspect of creation, it appears as though life wants to live. The evidence is to be found in all of its acts of self-creation, change, adaptation, and growth.

Francisco Varela, a famous biologist, coined a term for life's creation of more life out of itself. He named this process *autopoiesis*, which means "self-formation." He affirmed that life is unique in having the ability to create itself—to continue to generate more life.

The process of autopoiesis is continuous and cyclical. And it is generative in that life enlarges itself, growing the options and the potential and the fullness that make it what it has become at any moment in time. Life cannot stay the same. It complicates and diversifies itself, constantly becoming something more than it was.

The journey of life is an experience without boundaries. It moves in all directions and offers choice without limit. Once a selection has been made, however, boundaries emerge, forcing the selection to take form, to be lived fully in the form that it takes, expressing the reality that the selection now represents. Yet, paradoxically again, the boundaries themselves, while disciplining the selection into form and action, allow choice to move in a new direction and seek options that could not have arisen without the discipline imposed by the boundaries.

Each person must find the way into this mosaic of simplicity and complexity that best exemplifies the person's own journey. This self-referencing process, in which the discipline of choice requires living consistently with any selection made, operates at every level of the universe. For instance, the patterns or "habits" of role can appear anywhere, from the operation of scientific laws to the simplest routines of human behavior. This self-referencing also influences how we see the world because it affects what our eyes see and what form our seeing takes in our lives. Our self-perception informs our world, not usually the other way around. We begin to create what makes sense to us, and the limits and permissibles embedded in our personal worldview create boundaries around whatever it is that supports our worldview.

Self-referencing tells us a lot about how we change, grow, and adapt at every level, from the personal to the societal to the systematic to the universal. As Teilhard de Chardin (2015), the famous Jesuit paleontologist, eloquently pointed out, we are cocreators of the universe, working in concert with the energies and forces of creation to engage with the requirement to keep creating. Each component of life is working within its parameters, intersecting with others, and interacting with the components it most directly touches. Together, all the components operate in a way that ultimately changes everything in an endless cycle of creativity and growth.

This paradox of boundary and intersection is critical to the role of the leader. Nothing in life operates outside of this paradox. Each boundary intersects and interacts in a dynamic way with every other boundary in a dance that ultimately causes each of them to change. The energy of life comes out of this complex interaction of intersecting boundaries moving in a constant flux of relationship that transforms each of them singly and collectively. Such are the physical laws of the universe and conditions under which leaders must act out their role.

Life evolves in a context of cocreation. No one acts independently of anyone else. Indeed, there is no real independence but only interdependence, and this fact gives both form and direction to the role of the leader. Leaders are always working to understand the interdependence of situations, circumstances, and people. They know that in the workplace everything has an impact on everything else. Yet every person is acting out of his or her own space, doing the work that is expected. It is the aggregation of all the elements of the work and the efforts of the workers that, when brought together, makes something sustainable happen.

Leaders live life in the white spaces—the boundary land—between people, places, and processes. They do their work in the context of the potential future to which the confluence of their efforts ultimately leads. They read the signposts of the journey by identifying the elements of the journey and the forces that, when aggregated, tell the story of direction and process. At the same time, they are working to evolve, to respond to the demand for personal change. In short, they are managing both the journey and their personal experience of it.

Each member of the organization must do the same thing. The main leadership task is to make it possible for all members to have an awareness of this work, know its implications for their personal journey and the collective journey, and respond to the demand for change by applying their creativity.

The leaders of an organization must also see the undercurrent of linkage that exists in every place in the organization. To achieve this goal, they need to be highly receptive and hear the sounds of the universe in the language of persons, movement, and self.

Listening for the Sounds of Change

Perhaps the most important and, at the same time, difficult skills for a leader to obtain are listening skills, including those needed to hear the sounds of direction and change. We are always getting ready to speak or respond even as we listen to someone else talk. In short, much of the time we are not really listening. Listening intently is an important belonging cue to build psychological safety into culture (Coyle, 2018).

To exercise good leadership, leaders must listen from the very core of their being. They must listen to the sounds of change and to the more spiritual sounds of life, hearing themes as well as words, seeing intent as well as message, determining direction as well as impression. Listening intently is essential to hearing themes and undercurrents, leaders can anticipate events and take the right action at the right time. Building safety in groups can signal bonds of belonging and connection.

No one can listen deeply without preparation and development of listening skills. Leaders must assess their level of attention to the words and actions of others, as well as their focus on the ebbs and flows of the work. They must ask themselves about their readiness to respond to the issues affecting health care and their ability to detect the trends, including economic trends, that will affect its future.

Deep listening comprises contextual listening and content listening (**Exhibit 14-6**). Both are critical. The purpose of contextual listening is to become aware of the surrounding circumstances—the external events that affect what work people do and what resources are available to them. The purpose of content listening is to hear what people are saying, understand what it means, and grasp its implications. The deep listener listens to content while maintaining an awareness of the context, at the same time recognizing that what people say is always influenced by their beliefs, experience, perspectives, and prejudices. Listening with a broad frame of reference provides the listeners with an accuracy gauge—a way of placing what they see and hear within a context that validates, challenges, or alters its meaning.

Leaders develop an inner ear through mindful reflection and self-awareness. They must understand their own perspectives and perceptions—those things that might skew their ability to hear with openness and acuity—to hear the voices of others accurately. If leaders cannot hear their own notions, values, fears, and prejudices and give them a language and a place in the journey, they will be unable to incorporate incoming information into their knowledge base, undermining their ability to lead effectively.

Leaders who have not yet done deep spiritual and personal work still have filters in place that adjust messages from the outside to their comfort level or even block messages that are not congruent with their beliefs and values. By modifying what is heard, these filters reduce the leaders' ability—and the ability of the entire organization—to respond appropriately and effectively to the messages.

By using their inner ear to access their beliefs and attitudes, leaders can become alert to the same dynamic going on in others. They can then perceive more completely the struggles,

Exhibit 14-6   Contextual and Content Listening

Contextual Listening	**Content Listening**
• Circumstances	• The message
• Conditions	• Components
• Framework	• Players
• Environment	• Truth
• External factors	• Perception
	• Issues

uncertainty, barriers, and challenges embedded in the utterances they hear and also understand better how information is received and used by the staff as they attempt to deal with the realities affecting their own work and relationships.

Spending time in quiet and mindful self-reflection is a proven way of enhancing one's ability to listen deeply. If leaders can get past their self-constructed barriers to self-knowledge, they can see behind the words, read into the language, and look beyond the present, all gifts that, among other things, help them create a more accurate profile of the issues they face.

Finding Spirit in the Chaos

Art and nature have always had an impact on the human spirit. The culminating beauty of a mountain vista or a symphony orchestra has the power to move the spirit and bring great contentment. Yet each of those is the fractal image of smaller units of what would otherwise be seen as chaos. Imagine looking at the tangle of infrastructure of a forest or listening to each individual instrument play its own music. Clearly, only when the elements of the forest or the symphony aggregate can the beauty of the collective intersections be revealed and fully enjoyed.

It is the ability to see the whole and recognize its beauty that inspires the spirit and deepens the character. Further, although the art of Mandelbrot sets (mosaics created when aggregated chaos reveals the order within) can be enjoyed to a degree, the addition of human consciousness, as occurs in the art of the human spirit, intensifies the experience and raises the level of appreciation.

The human story and the art and spirit of life are filled with metaphors, contradictions, challenges, myths, and created scenarios. Using patterns of self-similarity and self-discord, artists and mystics create in ways that stimulate, challenge, and resonate with our humanity. By experiencing these convergent and divergent realities, we can fathom our connection to each other and to the universe and can grow in ways that intensify and enrich our lives.

The art of chaos can also have an impact on the way in which leaders address uncertainty, diversity, and variability. Leaders must come to prize divergent and convergent realities at the same time. Suspending the expectation to see order right away is the first step toward appreciating what complexity has to offer. By looking broadly at problems and opportunities, leaders can understand what they are and what they entail, whereas examining them too closely would obscure their meaning. Standing on the balcony of experience gives leaders the chance to observe both actions and their context and to perceive a reality that might otherwise make no sense.

> **Key Point**
>
> It is important not only to listen to the words of the message but also to listen for the intent, value, passion, focus of the message, and the speaker's relationship to what he or she is communicating. By listening deeply, the listener gets the message and the meaning as well.

The ability to see things broadly, one of the foundations of wisdom, takes time to acquire. Only after observing enough from the balcony can leaders develop the depth of insight and understanding needed to put everything into its proper context. Leaders, like other people, frequently get stuck in their own experience and are co-opted by their attachment to it, making it impossible for them to place it in a broader frame. By keeping unattached to any particular position, leaders can see every event, situation, or issue from outside and also can link it to other elements

Figure 14-6 The Realms of Spirit Within the Chaos.

of the system invisible from inside. There is no indictment intended here of the perspective of those inside an issue, for example. The point is to celebrate the distance and wisdom of the leader coming from the outside and thus the leader's ability to place the issue into a context that gives it meaning.

The ability of leaders to operate in this manner of appreciative inquiry and leadership is enhanced by personal work directed toward putting life in perspective—that is, seeing it as part of a chaotic and complex world (**Figure 14-6**). Spending time reflecting on the mystery of life and integrating this fact into their lives gives leaders a firm center and inspires confidence and composure.

We have, all of us, seen leaders of this type and observed with interest and not a little awe how balanced they appear, even in the midst of a notable crisis. Their ability to see around, through, or beyond the crisis inspires us, especially when their insight stands the test of time. Having gained a deeper perspective (really, a broader one), these leaders show how everything, even a crisis, fits into the multiplicity that is life and experience.

The Compensations of Ignorance

Paradoxes are forever there to challenge each of us in our certainty. There is clearly more we do not understand than there is that we know. Much of what is written in this text, although true at our current level of understanding, soon enough will no longer be true. The authors can recall the commitment they brought to previous books and the energy with which they articulated the truth of the time, only to note how much has changed and how little of what was written 30 years ago is as true today.

> **Point to Ponder**
>
> Truth is a journey, not an event. Honor those who are seeking truth; avoid those who have found it.

Still, every generation, through its work, builds the foundation for the next. No work is an end in itself; no process or experience simply comes to a dead halt. Each piece is part of the mosaic of revelation that got us to today and will get us to tomorrow. This longer-term perspective must inform the leadership role. Even in the midst of a vital crisis or critical life event, leaders must use the fabric of complexity to put the circumstances in a larger frame of reference because this frame of reference better reflects the reality of the time than do the experiences and stresses of the event itself. It is so easy for leaders to get sucked into an event and allow it to become the center of their reality, losing all sense of its place in the course of events.

Koans, in the form of a riddle, are used by Buddhists to focus the mind in a way that heightens understanding and intuition, keep us from putting temporal and spatial boundaries around our lives and experience. They invalidate our parameters. The minute something makes sense to us or becomes clear, the intersections of our clarity take us back into the chaos to the next level of intellectual or perceptual challenge. Rather than a negative, this feature of reality keeps us always on the edge of creativity and discovery. It also reminds us that there is no place to rest (at least for very long) and that nothing is an end in itself. For the leader, the journey of discernment is always deepening and broadening understanding and informing its translation into practice and application in the role of leadership and in the lives of others.

The challenge for leaders and others lies in the engagement with the flow of life. If religious or intellectual beliefs become strongly entrenched, they can serve as the barriers to subsequent discoveries, insights, or revelations. As has been said, truth is a journey, not an event. It is a lived dynamic, not simply a fact of life.

None of us can know everything. Even those of us who are well educated come to understand how little we know of all that is knowable. Further, our quest for knowledge is a delusion if we think of knowledge as a thing. Knowledge is not a thing but rather a dynamic—a revelation bound up in the time and circumstances that make it available. Although it is valuable, knowledge is not an end in itself. Nor is it ever complete. In mathematics, when equations are carried out to the third decimal, they reveal a particular product. When carried out to the sixth decimal, they reveal a different product. This process can continue ad infinitum.

> **Key Point**
>
> For leaders, the issue is not how much information they have but how much they need in order to act. No amount of information eliminates all risk, and beyond a certain point gathering more information does not reduce the risk but the timeliness of any action taken.

In decision making, the issue is not the total quantity of information possessed but whether there is enough information to make a decision. In no case will more information eliminate all the risk associated with choosing. Indeed, the collection of information can be pursued for so long that any action that would have been effective becomes untimely. Leaders must recognize that the leadership role is rife with risk, just like every other aspect of life. The demands of the time are part of a broader canvas that resists comprehension, and every decision sends into motion effects that can never fully be known.

In considering a particular decision, leaders need to be concerned about three things: Am I the correct individual to make this decision, is it the right decision for the time, and does it set a direction that fits the circumstances of the journey? In short, do the signposts appear to validate the decision? If they do, that is the best indicator that the decision is the correct one. After all, the overarching goal is to make decisions that, over time, take the organization and everyone in it to a better place where knowledge and the quality of life are advanced. Thomas Edison made more than 1,000 attempts before the light bulb went on. After which failed attempt should he have stopped? All 999 were necessary for the journey to light, and we can be thankful for every one of them.

Mystery

Perhaps the most notable need of leaders today is to be reenchanted by a sense of mystery. In every area of life, the more questions get answered, the more questions get raised. Indeed, the explicit lesson of chaos and complexity is the profound inscrutability of it all.

Despite the advances of science and the discoveries of medicine, we still are largely in the dark about the nature of the universe and the things that it contains. The billion-dollar effort to decipher the human genetic code was a seminal event in the course of human history. Of course, besides finally revealing the code, what it did was open the door to a whole new project: identifying the billion or so proteomes that do the work of the genes and discovering how the genes perform their myriad tasks through these proteomes. Collating and codifying the proteomes are tremendous undertakings, yet it is the work demanded by the revelations of the genome project. One level of complexity leads to an even deeper and broader level of complexity.

Wherever there is progress, there is a temptation to become arrogant and controlling. We are easily lured into believing that what we are doing is magnificent and grand—that we are creating the future of humanity. Because we know so much, we become deluded by our knowledge, giving it more credence and more importance than it merits. If history has taught us anything, it is that we are forever learning. That is to say, what is unknown is infinitely greater than the combined knowledge we humans have garnered on our short journey through time.

In the United States, our enthusiasm and egotism often insulate us from the depths of our ignorance. Being so busy making discoveries and applying them in different and exciting ways, we have little time to set aside for contemplating the fathomless mysteries that remain and feeling awe at the very small part we play in the unfolding of the universe. It is this awe for the unknown, this respect for the mystery of life, that is so important to leaders in the midst of the chaos of transformation. Leaders can put their efforts into perspective as the Industrial Age gives way to our current age—one filled with promise but, as of yet, lacking much substance.

Leaders today, besides regaining a sense of mystery themselves, face the additional challenge of deepening the appreciation of staff for the chaos and complexity that pervade the universe. They can do this by engaging with change directly and exemplifying in their behavior an awareness of the mystery in all movement. By not knowing, by not having all the answers, by being uncertain and exploring alternatives, leaders demonstrate their vulnerability to the effects of complexity. They also create a safe space for staff members to express their own uncertainty, discomfort, anxiety, and excitement. A further consequence is that leaders and staff

> **Point to Ponder**
>
> The wonderful thing about mystery is that it relieves us of the obligation to know everything. It allows us to appreciate the uncertain, the unformed, indeed, the journey of life. Mystery opens us up to discernment and discovery and moves us away from definition and control. It deepens our appreciation for the experience of life rather than the management of life.

together, through their appreciation for the mystery of their journey, will come to realize that they are about important things—that they are all participating in a larger project as cocreators and that what they do makes a difference, sometimes apparent, at other times unknown, but an inexorable difference nonetheless. And this is the centerpiece of the mystery.

Synthesis and Synergy

Finally, leaders are reminded that the work of leadership itself is filled with mystery. We have all done apparently inconsequential things that, we later discovered, had a profound impact on someone else. In some secret way, quietly and steadily, our words or actions thoroughly changed that person's life. Caught up in the moment, a leader might see an act as unimportant—and as a single act it might be. When connected to some other reality, it can take on a new form and new dimensions and have a significant impact on another's life.

Unseen forces are embedded in all reality, and mystery is present in all aspects of life. Everywhere, unknown influences, relationships, and intersections exist just beneath the surface of the actual and operate synergistically to continue the movement of change. Because some of these have no form or are not yet perceived, their effects can sometimes be traumatic. As part of their role, leaders are always looking for the unseen, the intersections, the goodness-of-fit among the elements of chaos and change. By looking for the linkages and connections, reading the signposts of the journey, looking within or behind motives, they are able to give language to the experience and the journey. Being disciplined to see the whole and to distinguish the contribution that the whole makes to the parts, and vice versa, they are in a position to appreciate the greater mystery to which everything relates, to be awed by its implications and moved by its inscrutability.

> **Point to Ponder**
>
> The imagery of complexity pervades the world, from artwork to zebras. The order embedded in complexity—an order made visible as a mosaic of intersections and interactions—reflects the synthesis and seamlessness of creation and the connections within and among all things.

There are always missing pieces. We may be tempted to believe that by discovering those pieces we can unravel the ultimate secrets of the universe and know everything we need to know. Of course, this is just plain foolishness. Every secret unlocked reveals a host of new secrets not yet addressed—meaning that the process of discovery is endless. Understanding this, leaders see and experience their role as the journey it really is. All parts of the journey intersect in visible and invisible ways, and the array of interactions and intersections necessary to the experience of life is also the work of life and the raw material for the work of leadership.

> **Key Point**
>
> Any knowledge that we gain forms the foundation for the next mystery. Inscrutability outruns understanding as long as there is life.

Operating within the context of their own journey, facilitating the experiences of others, and finding and defining the relationships among the elements and forces of movement and change, leaders are faced with the challenge of seeking and seeing the synergies that allow them to pursue their work and support the collective work of the organization. In harnessing these synergies, they represent for everyone in the organization the action of creation, complete engagement with life, and the full embrace of the mystery of complexity.

Chapter Takeaways

1. In the leadership experience in a time of great intensity and change, it is difficult to find sufficient time or moments where intentional mindfulness and reflection can be practiced. Yet such spiritual centeredness and the capacity for purposeful reflection is a critical characteristic of sustainable leadership and an important part of leadership self-management.
2. Creativity demands leadership availability to the creative "urge." Mindful and creative leaders recognize themselves as cocreators in partnership with the human community in the act of becoming, exploring, discovering, and innovating. In the midst of the chaos of change and transformation, the leader's sense of the creative spirit within recognizes the convergence of the universe yet unfolding, with the leader's connection to the creative dynamic, and of the elements of the creative process necessary to ensure sustainable change.
3. Intentional mindfulness is critical to the effectiveness of good leadership in that it advances in the leader a recognition and practice of maintaining a nonjudgmental state of awareness and presence through conscious sensitivity to thoughts, feelings, and processes in-the-moment within a heightened state of consciousness. This available and intentional level of awareness and the acceptance of insights gained from it help inform the leader in his or her own self-development and availability to the needs and growth of others. Mindfulness as a discipline is embedded in a regular routine of personal and spiritual self-exploration and the manifestation of self-discovery in every aspect of leadership practice.
4. Continuous mindfulness and spiritual awareness is not self-sustaining; it is, in fact, a discipline. There are processes associated with the internal (spiritual) journey and specific processes and activities through which it is refined and developed. Through use of the discipline, and approach or routine, the leader begins to deepen perceptions of self-awareness, development, growth, and maturation. Through the use of a methodology, the leader develops the capacity to utilize insights gained and to inform leadership practice in ways that improves and advances it.
5. Leaders demonstrate the capacity and skills to lead through relationship, interaction, and self-expression. Through the openness of personal vulnerability demonstrated through intentional mindfulness, transparency and self-truth influence all interaction and reveal congruence between the leader's thoughts, words, and deeds. By example, the leader engages the learning and working community in their own vulnerability and exploration of their role and work in cocreating and transforming the human experience, advancing learning and discovery, innovation, and quality of life for the whole human community.

Case Study 14-1

What Should I Do for an Encore?

Sarah just celebrated her 60th birthday, and this milestone in her life has caused significant self-reflection. Sarah has been a nurse consultant for the past 15 years and the president of her own consulting firm, Nursing Leaders Consulting Group (NLCG). NLCG has 10 employees, including Sarah, an executive assistant, a part-time chief financial officer (CFO), a part-time data analyst, a part-time writer/editor, and a part-time marketing/promotions person. The

CHAPTER FOURTEEN Engaging the Spirit of Leadership: Becoming a Living Leader

rest of the employees are all master's-prepared or PhD nurse consultants with various clinical backgrounds. NLCG provides strategic planning, operational improvement, professional development, and organizational culture transformational services to hospitals and healthcare organizations throughout the United States and internationally.

Reflecting on the last 15 years, Sarah is proud of the tremendous growth and reputation of the organization that she has built with her expertise and that of her colleagues. The consultants for NLCG not only have conducted numerous on-site consultations but also have made presentations at national and international conferences, written articles for professional journals, prepared their own booklets, and presented webinar conferences for various audiences for continuing education units (CEUs). Although Sarah has truly enjoyed the consulting experience, the rigorous travel schedule and on-site consulting demands have made her physically and emotionally weary. It has been difficult to schedule time away from her work because, as a principal member of the firm, she typically fields all of the calls inquiring about their consultation services. Once she speaks to the prospective client and determines the client's specific needs, she either delegates the consultation to one of the nursing specialists or takes the lead herself on the project. Lately, there has been a tremendous demand for the services of the nurse consultants at NLCG, and the consultants have been spread thin trying to meet the needs of numerous clients, maintaining contact with existing clients, and marketing their services to prospective clients through speaking engagements and writing for publications.

Sarah and the other consultants have enjoyed the independence and autonomy that consulting affords them as contrasted to being employees for a major organization. Sarah often comments that she is "engaged in many of the nation's leading healthcare organizations," which gives her a very unique perspective in contrast with an individual who has worked for the same organization for most of his or her career. Sarah states, "I have truly seen the good, the bad, and the ugly in healthcare organizations." Overall, she is extremely satisfied and fulfilled with the work and feels that she and her colleagues have made a tremendous difference in the growth and development of leaders nationally and internationally. The consulting role has allowed her to be extremely creative and innovative in the work that she does and in mentoring and coaching nursing leaders to manage the complexity of their organizations.

Although Sarah feels great pride with her work and career accomplishments, she also feels that she will be unable to keep the current pace for much longer. She feels that few understand how difficult it is to be a consultant. Considering all of the complexity of travel, trying to rest or sleep in different hotels night after night, and managing the long consulting hours with few breaks during the day have taken their toll. Sarah recalls many examples of starting the consulting day at 7 o'clock in the morning over a breakfast meeting, consulting with groups all morning, making a presentation over lunch, meeting with groups again in the afternoon, and attending dinner meetings or even evening meetings before the day ends and she can return to the hotel or catch a flight home. On many such days, she hardly has time allotted for a bathroom break. Being a consultant means being "on stage" all during the engagement. Sarah also realizes that although she has developed many professional relationships with her clients and colleagues, these relationships are very different from personal friendships, and it would be inappropriate to share her feelings with her clients.

Reflecting on her career and the options for the future, Sarah feels perplexed and wonders, "What shall I do for an encore?" She is at the top of her game, and she wants to end her consulting career at her peak, instead of becoming resentful of all of the hours it took to be a successful consultant. She thinks about selling the firm to one of the other nurse consultants or to an outside interest, but she fears leaving her consulting life and her own firm. She still needs a steady income, benefits, interaction with colleagues, and outlet for her sense of creativity. At times her head is filled with negative self-talk because she feels that it would be a mistake to do anything other than consulting. On the other hand, she has visions that there must be a way that she could give back to the nursing profession, to her community, and to emerging and developing leaders in the sunset years of her career. She just needs to take that first step of faith and explore the possible opportunities for a career change despite her overwhelming success as a nurse consultant and business owner.

Sarah explores many options available to her. She could apply for a chief nursing officer (CNO) role at a local hospital, interview for a tenure-track faculty position at the university near her home, or relocate to another city for a position in professional development in a large multihospital healthcare system. All of these alternatives have merit and would provide a steady income, benefits, and an opportunity to "make a difference." Not entirely sure of the direction she should take in designing her future, Sarah decides to sell her firm to her colleagues. She offers her assistance to ensure the smooth and successful transition to the new ownership and to continue to market and promote the expertise of her colleagues.

Realizing that she is completely exhausted mentally, emotionally, and physically, Sarah gives herself permission to "not make a decision" immediately. She decides to take some time off and take care of herself. She takes a trip to a sunny location to sit on the beach, to read some fun books instead of professional material, and to share experiences with a close, long-time friend who has been always accepting of Sarah and honest in her assessment of situations and recommendations when asked. Upon returning home, Sarah takes time to meditate, take long walks, and enroll in a yoga class. She does many of the things that she did not have time for when she was working as a consultant. She buys season tickets to the symphony, attends several plays, and joins a literary group that reads and discusses literature.

After a few months of getting in touch with herself again, Sarah applies for the tenure-track faculty position at the local university. She feels that she wants to "give back to the community" and teach and mentor emerging leaders in the graduate nursing program. Although the transition from complete independence and autonomy to a more structured position is challenging, Sarah finds that she really enjoys the intellectual stimulation that she receives from the inquisitive students who are eager to learn. She has lots to share, not only about nursing theories but also about practical applications and case studies that she experienced as a nurse consultant in many different types of healthcare organizations. At first her new life seems very chaotic with trying to keep up with the readings to make her courses current and practical, preparing innovative methods for teaching and delivering course content, and reading, editing, and advising students in their written work. It does not take long for Sarah to say, "I love this new life that I have planned for myself, and it is a healthy transition for me in the last chapters of my fantastic nursing career!"

Questions

1. Sarah had a very satisfying career and successful business enterprise. How do you feel about her decision to leave that behind and pursue other career opportunities? What other changes could she have made to continue as a consultant?
2. We are often confronted with a personal "fork in the road," with both opportunities and challenges in either direction that we might choose. Describe the forks in the road that Sarah faced and the potential opportunities and challenges of each.

3. What are your thoughts about Sarah's personal journey to renew herself spiritually and physically?
4. What might you do if you were making such a large decision and feeling the internal conflict and the physical and emotional exhaustion that Sarah was feeling?
5. Describe how innovation and creativity are affected by emotional and physical exhaustion and possible solutions to energize the creative spirit again.
6. How did Sarah manage the negative self-talk that she experienced? How do you manage both negative and positive self-talk?

Case Study 14-2
Lifelong Learning and Striving for What Is Around the Corner

Brook has had quite a nursing career! As he reflects on the past 15 years, Brook is surprised at himself for having accomplished so much in such a short period of time and at such a young age. He graduated at 21 with a bachelor's of science in biological sciences, and then decided that he had wasted the last 4 years of his life earning a degree in an area that he did not want to work. Considering all of his possible career options and dabbling for a year in pharmaceutical sales, Brook decided to apply to a second degree nursing program to become a nurse. He had always been interested in the healthcare field and assumed that after he received his BS he might return to graduate school in pharmacy, public health, or healthcare administration. He had not really considered nursing before, but the idea became more and more intriguing to Brook. Perhaps he was influenced by the recent illness and death of his mother, and observing the compassionate care that she had received sparked an interest in his soul. He watched the nurses and admired their knowledge and competence coupled with sincere compassion when caring for his mother and other patients. He had not realized before how much science that nurses are exposed to in their education, but in talking with them he realized that his own background in biological sciences would be a great platform for a new career in nursing. It was a great choice for Brook, and he not only obtained a master's degree in nursing in the second degree program, but he also made a firm decision that he would continue on in his education.

His first job as a nurse was not only stimulating but also absolutely invigorating to his spirit. He loved every minute working with the patients, his colleagues, and the physicians. He worked as a clinical nurse in the surgical intensive care unit initially, but after a year, he asked to be transferred to the emergency department (ED). He loved the pace and the constant challenge of the ED, and he recognized and appreciated the physical and emotional challenges that his patients faced as they came into this unknown and often threatening environment. Every day he left work feeling that he'd made a positive difference for his patients, and he felt good about himself. Yes, life was good . . . but he yearned for something more. He asked himself, "Am I crazy, or what?"

Brook enrolled in a doctor of nursing practice (DNP) program, and although he thoroughly enjoyed exposure to the class content, he also found it challenging to be a full-time student and a full-time clinical nurse. The hours were long, and he had to make every minute count to keep up with the volumes of reading material, long practicum hours, and his work in the ED. At times he was completely and utterly exhausted and spent emotionally and physically.

Brook took every opportunity during the semester breaks to take paid leave from the hospital and to travel. He went hiking in the Grand Canyon, spent a week on the beach in Hawaii, and took a fun trip with friends backpacking around Europe. After these excursions he felt refreshed and renewed, eager for school to start, and ready return to work. He asked himself, "Am I crazy, or what?"

It did not seem long until Brook graduated with his DNP. The degree opened several new career opportunities, and Brook landed a phenomenal position in the San Francisco Bay area as the director of research and professional development for the emergency services of a large healthcare system with hospitals throughout northern California. It was a great position with many challenges but strong leadership and resources to ensure his success in such a role. Brook had the opportunity to work with other directors to lead one hospital on its Magnet journey and to facilitate meaningful evidence-based practice projects and research studies to improve patient outcomes in the emergency service experience. It was an exciting time in Brook's personal and professional life for a few years, but it was not long until he felt restless again. He could not believe that he felt motivated to go back to school to earn his PhD in nursing. He asked himself, "Am I crazy, or what?"

Brook admired several of his PhD-prepared colleagues and their depth of knowledge about research. Although the DNP prepared him to use research evidence in practice, he yearned for a greater depth of understanding about research, statistics, and the entire qualitative and quantitative research processes and theory development. So, Brook applied and was accepted into the PhD program, and he continued his career while earning his PhD. Reflecting back, he never would have guessed that this would be the path his nursing career followed, yet he appreciates all that he has learned about himself in his formal educational experiences and in his real-life experiences caring for patients and their families in his nursing role. Brook realizes that he arrived at this point in his life and career by living in the potential as well as the reality of his life. It has not been an easy path, but he feels that he is a better person for having taken the journey. He can honestly say that he feels inner peace with the decisions that he made and the path that he chose.

Questions

1. What are some examples of self-talk that you could find in this story about Brook and his career path?
2. Going to school while working full time is not easy for anyone. What did Brook do that rejuvenated his spirit and refreshed him physically? What do you do to refresh yourself and rejuvenate your spirit?
3. What were some of the challenges that Brook faced in his journey, and what inner strength did he employ to meet these challenges?
4. What might have been the consequences if Brook had taken a different course when he realized that he was unfulfilled with his BS degree in biological sciences?
5. How do our life's experiences shape and influence our personal and professional decisions?
6. How can we know when we have made the right decision for ourselves and our career?

References

Bains, W., & Schulze-Makuch, D. (2016). The cosmic zoo: The (near) inevitability of the evolution of complex. *Macroscopic Life. Life (Basel), 6*(3), 25.

Bakker, A. B. (2013). *Advances in positive organizational psychology* (1st ed.). Emerald.

CHAPTER FOURTEEN   Engaging the Spirit of Leadership: Becoming a Living Leader

Black, H., Soto, L., & Spurlin, S. (2016). Thinking about leadership: Metacognitive ability and leader developmental readiness. *New Directions for Student Leadership, 149*, 85–95.

Bodaken, B., & Fritz, R. (2006). *The managerial moment of truth*. Free Press.

Breland, J. Y., Asch, S. M., Slightam, C., Wong, A., & Zulman, D. M. (2016). Key ingredients for implementing intensive outpatient programs within patient-centered medical homes: A literature review and qualitative analysis. *Healthcare (Amsterdam, Netherlands), 4*(1), 22–29.

Brown, B. (2012). *Daring greatly*. Avery.

Coyle, D. (2018). *The culture code*. Bantam Books.

Cullen, M., & Donahue, M. (2016). Partnership negotiations: Innovation for nurse contract negotiations during turbulent times. *Nursing Administration Quarterly, 40*(1), 33–38.

de Bono, E. (2007). *Tactics*. HarperCollins.

de Chardin, T. (2015). *The phenomenon of man*. R. P. Pryne.

Gotink, R. A., Meijboom, R., Vernooij, M. W., Smits, M., & Hunink, M. G. (2016). 8-week mindfulness based stress reduction induces brain changes similar to traditional long-term meditation practice—A systematic review. *Brain and Cognition, 108*, 32–41.

Hickey, M., & Kritek, P. B. (2012). *Change leadership in nursing: How change occurs in a complex hospital system*. Springer.

Hosmer, L. T. (2006). *The ethics of management* (5th ed.). McGraw-Hill/Irwin.

Leonard-Barton, D. (2011). *Managing knowledge assets, creativity and innovation*. World Scientific.

Massaro, M., Bardy, R., & Pitts, M. (2012). Supporting creativity through knowledge integration during the creative processes: A management control system perspective. *Electronic Journal of Knowledge Management, 10*(3), 258–267.

Menaker, R. (2016). Leadership strategies: Achieving personal and professional success. *The Journal of Medical Practice Management, 31*(6), 336–339.

Nilsen, E. R., Olafsen, A. H., Steinsvag, A. G., Halvari, H., & Grov, E. K. (2016). Stuck between a rock and a hard place: The work situation for nurses as leaders in municipal health care. *Journal of Multidisciplinary Healthcare, 9*, 153–161.

O'Rourke, N., Canham, S., Wertman, A., Chaudhury, H., Carmel, S., Bachner, Y. G., & Peres, H. (2016). Holocaust survivors' memories of past trauma and the functions of reminiscence. *The Gerontologist, 56*(4), 743–752.

Porter-O'Grady, T., & Malloch, K. (2019). Failure and resilience: Driving sustainable innovation. In D. Weberg & S. Davidson (Eds.), *Leadership for evidence-based innovation in nursing and health professions* (2nd ed., pp. 207–233). Jones & Bartlett Learning.

Pradarelli, J. C., Jaffe, G. A., Lemak, C. H., Mulholland, M. W., & Dimick, J. B. (2016). A leadership development program for surgeons: First-year participant evaluation. *Surgery, 160*(2), 255–263.

Raney, A. (2014). Agility in adversity: Integrating mindfulness and principles of adaptive leadership in the administration of the community mental health center. *Clinical Social Work Journal, 42*(3), 312–320.

Rushton, C. H., & Turner, K. (2016). Ethics in everyday practice: Pick up your stethoscope. *Ethics in Critical Care, 27*(4), 462–464.

Shin, R. Q., Ezeofor, I., Smith, L. C., Welch, J. C., & Goodrich, K. M. (2016). The development and validation of the contemporary critical consciousness measure. *Journal of Counseling Psychology, 63*(2), 210–223.

Simons, M., & Havert, M. L. (2012). Using appreciative inquiry to support a culture shift in transition. *Technical Services Quarterly, 29*(3), 207–216.

Stewart, R., Corneille, M., & Johnson, J. (2006). Transparent and open discussion of errors does not increase malpractice risk in trauma patients. *Annals of Surgery, 243*(5), 645–651.

Tarrasch, R., Berman, Z., & Friedmann, N. (2016). Mindful reading: Mindfulness meditation helps keep readers with dyslexia and ADHD on the lexical track. *Frontiers in Psychology, 7,* 578.

Vago, D. R., & Zeidan, F. (2016). The brain on silent: Mind wandering, mindful awareness, and states of mental tranquility. *Annals of the New York Academy of Sciences, 1373*(1), 96–113.

Wheatley, M. (2009). *Turning to one another: Simple conversations to restore hope to the future.* Berrett-Koehler.

Suggested Readings

Brown, J. (2012). *The art and spirit of leadership.* Trafford.

Cordeiro, W. (2009). *Leading on empty: Refilling your tank and renewing your passion.* Baker Publishing, Bethany House.

McKee, A., Boyatzis, R., & Johnston, F. (2008). *Becoming a resonant leader: Develop your emotional intelligence, renew your relationships, sustain your effectiveness.* Harvard Business School Press.

Palmer, S. (2012). *Digital wisdom: Thought leadership for a connected world.* York House Press.

Rothwell, W. (2012). *Becoming an effective mentoring leader: Proven strategies for building excellence in your organization.* McGraw-Hill.

Wheatley, M. (2006). *Leadership and the new science: Discovering order in a chaotic world.* Berrett-Koehler.

Quiz Questions

Select the best answer for each of the following questions.

1. Most great leaders can recall a time when:
    a. situations made them what they became.
    b. all greatness was simply chance and mystery.
    c. they felt a deep call within to leadership.
    d. they thought that leadership was simply learned.

2. The spiritually focused leader emphasizes the importance of:
    a. the here and now.
    b. the longer and more distant road.
    c. keeping focused on the emerging issues.
    d. only focusing on the future.

3. Chaos is always the route to:
    a. order.
    b. complexity.
    c. uncertainty.
    d. mystery.

4. We all participate in each other's evolution because:
    a. all things are ultimately interconnected.
    b. the universe acts independently on all other creation.
    c. we have been made masters of creation.
    d. genomics shows that we are essentially the same.

5. Creativity is expressed in which of the following ways?
   a. Art and music only
   b. The scientific process
   c. Symbols and images
   d. All of these are correct.

6. There is virtually nothing about fear that is:
   a. unnecessary.
   b. redeeming.
   c. invalid.
   d. just.

7. Exercising the spirit requires which of the following?
   a. Prayer
   b. A fixed approach
   c. A regular routine
   d. A guru

8. According to the 10 spiritual themes of leadership, leaders must have the ability to:
   a. point in the proper direction.
   b. see all issues with clarity.
   c. embrace the needs of others.
   d. take risks.

9. Which of the following is a major enemy of the spirit within?
   a. Anger with others
   b. The tendency to make judgments
   c. Lack of regular reflection
   d. Lack of strong relationships

10. Which of the following is a fundamental tenet of the universe?
    a. All life is self-organizing.
    b. All things can ultimately be understood.
    c. All action is rational.
    d. All change is impermanent.

11. There is no more important ability for leaders to develop than the ability to:
    a. direct.
    b. act.
    c. listen.
    d. take risks.

12. To those they lead, what do leaders represent?
    a. The respect for the mystery that is present in all aspects of life
    b. The hardships that attend every action
    c. The challenges that arise out of all action
    d. The internal logic that guides all creation

13. Quantum theorists proved that life cannot be understood in terms of:
    a. structure and function.
    b. beliefs and perceptions.
    c. unilateral and vertical action.
    d. sensibilities and rituals.

14. As disquiet arises and we all shift further into the complexities of our contemporary times, people yearn for:
    a. confidence.
    b. calm.
    c. routine.
    d. certitude.

15. With the loss of the certainty of past beliefs and practices, there is a tremendous _____ expressed in high levels of anger, anxiety, and reaction and a call for a return to the fundamental beliefs and historical practices of yesterday.
    a. backlash
    b. threat
    c. pain
    d. rejection

16. The leader's role is to apply quantum principles to the organization, including showing a willingness to:
    a. embrace and accept tradition.
    b. engage with chaos and harness its implications.
    c. reject historical values.
    d. celebrate the chance to change everything.

17. If a leader is not willing to live in and fully experience the _____, he or she cannot ask others to embrace change in their own lives.
    a. future
    b. challenge
    c. potential
    d. present

18. Leaders cannot touch the best in those they lead if they are unable to:
    a. touch and express the best in themselves.
    b. empower others to do what they need them to do.
    c. direct others to change.
    d. guide others to change themselves.

19. One of the significant values of journaling is:
    a. finding out what's wrong that needs work.
    b. allowing hidden wisdom to find expression.
    c. expose errors one might not want to confront.
    d. share your personal challenges with others.

CHAPTER FOURTEEN   Engaging the Spirit of Leadership: Becoming a Living Leader

20. Vulnerability is an important personal value for the leader because it:
    a. shows others that the leader has the same challenges/failings as they do.
    b. helps eliminate others' expectations of the leader that may be inappropriate.
    c. identifies the leader's self-challenges before others do.
    d. allows the leader to expose his or her true self and live with transparency.

21. In leadership, failure is definitively seen as:
    a. an error, which once identified, can always be corrected.
    b. an essential element used to evaluate progress toward success.
    c. the problem in the system that calls for recalibrating system priorities.
    d. an unacceptable occurrence that should be permanently eliminated from good work process.

22. Mistakes, errors, and failures are the signposts of the journey toward:
    a. disaster.
    b. increased challenges.
    c. achievement.
    d. dysfunction.

23. Which of the following principles is exemplified in the statement "the leader is a cocreator"?
    a. In creation, everything acts interdependently.
    b. The leader seeks others to share in her or his vision.
    c. Interdependence is not as important as independence.
    d. The leader is responsible for creating direction that others can embrace.

24. The grounded leader embraces the mystery of existence because:
    a. all answers about creation and existence will reveal themselves with persistence.
    b. mystery helps keep us from confronting unanswered questions and irresolvable problems.
    c. issues are irresolvable, and leaders can demonstrate how embracing mystery keeps us from being afraid.
    d. it deepens the appreciation of the complexity of life's journey and encourages continuing curiosity.

25. Leaders should avoid:
    a. making judgments about themselves or others, and should not seek out or pay attention to the judgments of others.
    b. self-evaluation and self-criticism leading to self-doubt and role uncertainty.
    c. negative people who can create an environment of failure and uncertainty.
    d. too much engagement of others, which leads to familiarity and disrespect of the leader role and role ambiguity with the staff.

APPENDIX

Quiz Answers

Chapter 1
1 (d), 2 (b), 3 (a), 4 (b), 5 (a), 6 (b), 7 (c), 8 (c), 9 (a), 10 (b), 11 (c), 12 (b), 13 (d), 14 (c), 15 (a), 16 (a), 17 (a), 18 (c), 19 (b), 20 (c), 21 (d), 22 (c), 23 (d), 24 (c), 25 (b)

Chapter 2
1 (d), 2 (b), 3 (a), 4 (a), 5 (c), 6 (d), 7 (b), 8 (c), 9 (c), 10 (a), 11 (b), 12 (d), 13 (c), 14 (b), 15 (a), 16 (d), 17 (c), 18 (a), 19 (d), 20 (c), 21 (b), 22 (a), 23 (d), 24 (b), 25 (b)

Chapter 3
1 (a), 2 (b), 3 (a), 4 (c), 5 (a), 6 (b), 7 (b), 8 (d), 9 (a), 10 (c), 11 (c), 12 (a), 13 (d), 14 (d), 15 (c), 16 (c), 17 (b), 18 (a), 19 (b), 20 (d), 21 (a), 22 (b), 23 (d), 24 (a), 25 (c)

Chapter 4
1 (c), 2 (d), 3 (a), 4 (b), 5 (c), 6 (b), 7 (a), 8 (d), 9 (b), 10 (c), 11 (a), 12 (c), 13 (d), 14 (b), 15 (c), 16 (d), 17 (a), 18 (d), 19 (b), 20 (a), 21 (b), 22 (c), 23 (a), 24 (a), 25 (b)

Chapter 5
1 (d), 2 (c), 3 (b), 4 (c), 5 (a), 6 (c), 7 (d), 8 (d), 9 (b), 10 (c), 11 (c), 12 (a), 13 (d), 14 (a), 15 (b), 16 (d), 17 (c), 18 (c), 19 (c), 20 (a), 21 (d), 22 (b), 23 (a), 24 (b), 25 (b)

Chapter 6
1 (c), 2 (b), 3 (a), 4 (d), 5 (a), 6 (b), 7 (b), 8 (d), 9 (b), 10 (b), 11 (c), 12 (b), 13 (a), 14 (d), 15 (b), 16 (d), 17 (b), 18 (a), 19 (c), 20 (b), 21 (d), 22 (a), 23 (c), 24 (c), 25 (c)

Chapter 7
1 (a), 2 (c), 3 (b), 4 (d), 5 (a), 6 (d), 7 (b), 8 (c), 9 (a), 10 (d), 11 (b), 12 (c), 13 (a), 14 (c), 15 (b), 16 (d), 17 (d), 18 (b), 19 (b), 20 (a), 21 (c), 22 (a), 23 (b), 24 (b), 25 (d)

Chapter 8
1 (d), 2 (a), 3 (d), 4 (b), 5 (b), 6 (c), 7 (c), 8 (a), 9 (b), 10 (c), 11 (b), 12 (b), 13 (a), 14 (d), 15 (c), 16 (d), 17 (c), 18 (b), 19 (a), 20 (c), 21 (b), 22 (d), 23 (d), 24 (a), 25 (d)

Chapter 9
1 (c), 2 (c), 3 (d), 4 (c), 5 (a), 6 (d), 7 (b), 8 (d), 9 (a), 10 (a), 11 (c), 12 (d), 13 (c), 14 (a), 15 (c), 16 (d), 17 (a), 18 (b), 19 (d), 20 (a), 21 (b), 22 (c), 23 (d), 24 (d), 25 (a)

Chapter 10
1 (b), 2 (a), 3 (d), 4 (b), 5 (c), 6 (a), 7 (d), 8 (a), 9 (d), 10 (a), 11 (c), 12 (c), 13 (b), 14 (c), 15 (d), 16 (a), 17 (c), 18 (a), 19 (b), 20 (c), 21 (d), 22 (b), 23 (d), 24 (a), 25 (c)

Chapter 11
1 (a), 2 (a), 3 (b), 4 (d), 5 (b), 6 (c), 7 (a), 8 (d), 9 (d), 10 (a), 11 (a), 12 (b), 13 (d), 14 (b), 15 (c), 16 (c), 17 (c), 18 (a), 19 (a), 20 (d), 21 (d), 22 (d), 23 (c), 24 (b), 25 (d)

Chapter 12

1 (c), 2 (d), 3 (a), 4 (b), 5 (b), 6 (b), 7 (d), 8 (c), 9 (c), 10 (a), 11 (a), 12 (b), 13 (c), 14 (b), 15 (a), 16 (c), 17 (a), 18 (d), 19 (b), 20 (d), 21 (a), 22 (c), 23 (d), 24 (c), 25 (d)

Chapter 13

1 (c), 2 (a), 3 (d), 4 (b), 5 (b), 6 (d), 7 (a), 8 (c), 9 (d), 10 (d), 11 (c), 12 (c), 13 (a), 14 (d), 15 (c), 16 (a), 17 (b), 18 (b), 19 (a), 20 (d), 21 (c), 22 (c), 23 (c), 24 (b), 25 (a)

Chapter 14

1 (c), 2 (b), 3 (a), 4 (a), 5 (d), 6 (b), 7 (c), 8 (d), 9 (b), 10 (a), 11 (c), 12 (a), 13 (c), 14 (d), 15 (a), 16 (a), 17 (c), 18 (a), 19 (b), 20 (d), 21 (b), 22 (c), 23 (a), 24 (d), 25 (a)

INDEX

Note: Page numbers followed by exhibit, *f*, and *t* indicate material in exhibits, figures, and tables, respectively.

A

absolutism, 590
abuse of power, 469–470
   intolerance toward diversity, 470
   mandatory overtime, 470
accident, defined, 374 (exhibit 9–1)
accountability, 505, 506
   based organizations, 505
   conflict resolution and, 244
   for error management, 382
   expect, 488
   fiscal, 387
   in healthcare system, 189
   horizontal relationships and, 529
   individual *vs.* system, 374 (exhibit 9–2)
   internal, moving from external oversight to, 391
   living, 392
   personal will and, 556
   relational capacity to mobilizing, 519
   from responsibility to, 504–507, 505 (exhibit 12–1)
   shared, for learning, 402
   systems evaluation and, 314
acting as agent of transformation principle, 486–487
acting out, conflict and, 228
action
   identity-based conflicts, 243–245
   learning tools, 515 (exhibit 12–3)
   risk and, 30
active listening, 258, 483
active members, conflict resolution and, 228
actual reality, 7, 57
   potential reality *vs.*, 57 (exhibit 2–1)
acuity, 211, 318, 396, 402
adaptation, 34, 76, 79. *See also* flexibility
   borderland of chaos and, 282
   dynamic, 515
   effective, 513
   error and, 72
   leaders and requirements for, 516–517
   as more important than anticipation, 291
adaptive capacity, 57
   change and, 277–279
   in human organizations, 280–282
adaptive effectiveness
   crisis preparedness and, 312–315
   DCTM details of components for assessing, 309*f*
additional intelligences, valuing of, 118
advanced beginner stage
   in emotional competence development, 440 (exhibit 10–3), 441
   team emotional competence, 443–444 (exhibit 10–4), 444
advancing organization, rational risks and, 336

adverse event, defined, 374 (exhibit 9–1)
advocacy leadership, 479
Affordable Care Act, 386, 417, 567
Agency for Healthcare Research and Quality (AHRQ), 381
agenda, for action, 244
Age of Accountability, 505
Age of Enlightenment, 8
Age of Health Reform, 5
Age of Technology, 8*f*
aggregation, across systems, 70*f*
agility, leadership, 570
agreement, interest-based conflict resolution and
   formalizing of, 256
alignment, innovation and, 149–154, 169*f*
Alzheimer's disease, 17
ambiguity, 424
   conflicts and, 233
   evidence in healthcare system, 189–192
   messages, 476
anger, unresolved, 465
anomaly, value of, 119–120
antagonism
   identity-based conflict and, 237–239
   professional, minimizing, 565
anticipation
   ability to, 58
   adaptation more important than, 291
antisocial behavior, tolerance of, 473–474
apparent cause analysis (ACA), 375
appreciation of knowledge, 425–426
appreciative inquiry, 518
appreciative leadership
   critical value of, 517–519
   principles
      integrity/inclusion, 520
      language expectations and obligations, 519
      performance and demonstration of impact, 519–520
      relational capacity to mobilize accountability, 519
      self-awareness/self-confidence, 519
apprenticeship model, of training, 3
Argyris, Chris, 511
ARIA conflict engagement theory, 236
art, of chaos, 616
artifact, change and, 87
artificial intelligence (AI), 121
authentic leader, 331
authority
   effects from unquestioning adherence to, 563
   systems evaluation and, 314
autocatalysis, 14
autocratic leadership behavior, 477
automatic reflex, identity-based conflict and, 240
autopoiesis, 14, 613

B

baby boomers, 447, 473
bad attitude, displaying, 442
balance
- passion through, 429–430
- use of time and, 571–572

Barrett, R., 480
behavior. *See also* people and behavior; toxic behaviors in organizations
- antisocial, 473–474
- disciplinary line, errors and, 384
- dysfunctional, 481 (exhibit 11-5)
- fear-based, 600–601
- inspirational, 335
- learning organizations and focus on, 511
- patient and provider, engagement of, 202–203
- team members and patterns of, 438, 445
- toxic, 466–479

beliefs, unquestioned, 563
Benner, P., 484
biological metaphors, 77
biological research, organizational survival and, 510
biotechnology, 109
biotherapeutics, 11, 17, 18
blame
- assigning, 375, 375 (exhibit 9-2)
- conflict and, 237
- identity-based conflict and, 237
- punishment and, 373

blogs, 122
bodily intelligences, 118 (exhibit 3-4)
Bohm, Roger, 537
boredom, 473
"bossism" culture, 599
boundary
- setting, 343
- wireless technologies and loosening of, 55–56

brainstorming, 118
breakdown, defined, 374 (exhibit 9-1)
breathing deeply, 605
Buber, Martin, 63
Buddha, 459
Burden, Virginia, 217
bureaucracy, minimizing, 391
bureaucratic theory, 77
burnout, 472, 568, 571, 594
business
- case
  - healthcare story, 204–207
  - innovation, 204
- models, 111 (exhibit 3-1)
- in syndicated world, 356*t*

C

capitalism, competition and, 34
Capra, F., 338
career development programs, 487
career entrapment, 472
- behaviors, 472 (exhibit 11-2)

career entrenchment, 471, 485
- strategies to minimize, 487 (exhibit 11-6)

career seekers, job holders *vs.*, 566
caregivers, patients and, engagement of, 202–203
care providers
- mandatory error reporting and, 380

caring, for self, 608 (exhibit 14-4), 609
Carson, K. D., 471
Carson, P. P., 471
cash register, 335
caucusing, 256
CDO. *See* Chief Data Officer
cell phone technology, 66
CEO. *See* chief executive officer
certainty
- backlash associated with loss of, 589
- giving up quest for, 332
- longing for, 332

challenge
- around toxic situations faced by leader, 459
- with conflict, 217–218
- healthcare, 111 (exhibit 3-1)
- leading to toxic situations, 459
- as normal feature of the universe, 608 (exhibit 14-4), 610
- related to change, 590, 608 (exhibit 14-4)
- related to work-life balance for female leaders, 477–478

champions, seeking out, 526
change
- adaptive capacity and, 277–279
- avoiders/resisters, identifying, 13
- from center outward, 82–85
- challenges related to, 590, 608 (exhibit 14-4)
- courage and, 556
- crisis and, 271–272
- developed willpower and, 553
- dissipative leadership, 420–421
- and effectiveness, 38–40
- elements of personal transformation and, 531*f*
- endless, 10–14, 54
- error and, 72
- essential elements of, 87
- external forces and, 301–302
- failure and, 89
- internal forces and, 302–303
- leaders and constancy, 304
- listening for sounds of, 614–616
- management, 279
- as normal feature of universe, 608 (exhibit 14-4), 610
- orchestrating dynamics of, 534
- overcoming resistance to, 554
- results of, 87
- transformation and, 509
- willing leaders and, 551
- work routines, 554

chaordic organizations, 356
chaos, 24, 38
- call to leadership and, 588–591
- characteristics of, 56–59
- complexity, crisis and, 281–282

diversity and, 71
energy and, 81
finding spirit in, 616–617
language, 14 (exhibit 1–5)
paradox and, 29–30
practice within marketplace and, 387
realms of spirit within, 617*f*
route to order, 593
theory, 24, 33, 53, 281
character, 431, 432
leadership, quantum, 14–35
charisma, 328
chemotherapeutics, 11, 17, 18
cherishing new knowledge gained, 341
Chief Data Officer (CDO), 199
chief executive officer (CEO)
compassionate leadership and, 427
feedback given to, 439
knowledge base for, 393
child raising, workplace flexibility and male participation, 477
child within, spending time with, 597
chunking, 32, 68
"circle of innovation," 145, 146*f*
clarity
conflict management and, 227
goal setting and, 294
clients, organizations in crisis and partnerships with, 299
clinical decision making, financial resources and, 386
clinical teams
disciplinary isolation, 287
evidence-based practice, 290
strategic core and, 288
two-pronged focus on outcomes and, 292
closed components, in systems, 76
coaching, 419. *See also* innovation, coaching; transformational coaching
effective, impediments to, 527 (exhibit 12–4)
of employees, in vulnerable risk-taking behaviors, 342
through error recovery process, 378
upward, 439
cocreation, 593, 614
cognition, 423 (exhibit 10–1)
coherence, 89
collaboration, evidence of, 68
collateral thinking, linear thinking *vs.*, 75 (exhibit 2–4)
collective mindfulness, 352
complexity communication and, 348*f*
open communication and, 353–355
strategies for cultivation of leadership vulnerability, 353–357
syndication, 355–357
Collins, J., 425
command-and-control style, of leadership, 418
common orchards, outcome of, 338
communication, 258
complexity. *See* complexity, communication
innovations in, 122
interest-based conflict and, 255
open, 353–355

environment, 223
preventing unnecessary conflict and, 223
systems, adaptive capacity, change and, 278
technology, 2
vertical structure and restrictions on, 467
community
consciousness, 480 (exhibit 11–4)
identity-based conflicts and, 230
innovation, assessing, 112–113
compartmentalization, 19, 20
compassion, 426–427
higher productivity, 437
measuring emotional competence of teams and, 447
compensation systems
for both job holders and career seekers, 566
inequitable, 468–469
competence, 15, 423 (exhibit 10–1). *See also* emotional competence
political, 392–393
team process factor, 293*f*, 294–295, 295*f*
competency grids, 289
competent stage
in emotional competence development, 440 (exhibit 10–3), 441
team emotional competence, 443–444 (exhibit 10–4), 444
competition, 33–35
complexity, 38, 590
adaptation and, 25–26
adaptive systems, 21
chaos, crisis and, 281–282
characteristics of, 56–59
communication, 348–351, 348*f*
collective mindfulness and, 348*f*
critical listening, 348–349
critical questioning, 349–350
critical thinking, 351
dealing with lack of time and, 520
energy and, 81
harnessing of, 82
in health care, 459
imagery of, 620
knowledge and, 32
language, 14
leader's focus in times of, 518*f*
organizations and, 273
process, outcome and, 22
quantum science and, 14–15
science, 6, 276, 563–564
simplicity and, 31, 69
system, aggregation across, 70*f*
of teams, 288
technology and, 275–276
theory, 2, 281
complex systems
linking of simple systems in creation of, 31–33
simple systems and make up of, 68–70
component-centered behavior, traditional organizations and, 77

Index 635

component systems
  effectiveness of, 69
  within larger systems, 69
comprehensive system, 23
compromise, identity-based conflicts and, 241
computer chip, 6
computerized calendar, 123 (exhibit 3-6)
conceptual foundations, Newtonian vs. quantum, 6 (exhibit 1-3)
conflict
  avoidance, 430
  challenges with, 217-218
  growth, transformation and, 220-222
  in human community, 275-276
  human condition, as source of, 222-223
  identity-based, 229-245
  information, 225f
  interaction, 225f
  interest-based, 225f, 229, 245-257
  management, 218-219, 222
    productive handling of, 224-227
  people, behavior, and, 257-259
  resolution
    ARIA format for, 236
    stages in process of, 254f
    win-win, 243
  sources, 220 (exhibit 6-1)
  structural, 224f
  team-based, 228-229
  unnecessary, avoidance of, 222-227
  unresolved, 231, 235
  of value, 224f
Confucius, 558
congruence
  goals, and prevention of conflict, 223-224
  point of service and, 64
connectivity, 22
  healthcare systems, 190t
connectography, 22
conscious error, 72
"constructive voice" approach, 487
contemplation, 477
  healthcare and need for, 568
contemporary leader, work of, 109
contemporary research, 603
contextual listening, 615 (exhibit 14-6)
contingency approach, 77
contingency staffing plans, 297
continuing education, 295, 394, 402
continuing learning, 564-565
continuous adaptation, dynamics of, 531f
continuum-based teams, in healthcare, 259
continuum-driven approaches, to conflict resolution, 245
contradictory messages, 476
control
  identity-based conflicts and need for, 230
  point of service and locus of, 83
corporate culture, levels of, 480 (exhibit 11-4)
cost, 387
  effectiveness analysis, 388
  shifting, 188-189
cost-to-benefit ratio, 388
counterproductive beliefs and practices, 537
courage, 556-558, 557f, 573
  examining behaviors related to, 562
  leaders, 556-558
  leadership role and, 608, 608 (exhibit 14-4)
course corrections, 124, 341
creative spirit, 592f
creative thinking, 118
creativity
  borderland of chaos and, 282
  crisis and, 90
  defined, 107
  error essential to, 72
  innovation and, 594-603
  inspiring, 335
  intrinsic motivation and, 419-420
  requisites of, 595f
  self-management and, 591-594
  sharing in fruits of, 530
  transformation and, 509
crisis
  adaptive capacity in human organizations, 280-282
  change and adaptive capacity, 277-279
  chaos, complexity and, 281-282
  complexity
    and organizations, 276-277
    and technology, 275-276
  conflict in human community, 275-276
  creativity and, 90
  critical planning process, 280
  cybernetic and interacting environmental scanning process, 300-301, 300f
  defining, 271-272
  developmental freeze and, 396
  early warning, 272-273
  ensuring a strong service core, 303-304, 303f
  environmental scanning and, 304-308
    signals and, 306-308, 306f
    triggers, 307-308, 307f
  human resource focus, 280-282
  impact on outcomes, 299-301
  internalization and externalization
    external forces, 301-302, 302f
    internal forces, 302-303, 302f
  leader's perception of, 273-274
  management, 273
    dynamic cybernetic team model, 284-285
    strategic, 282-285
  normative crisis, 272-273
  plan group, 309
  preparedness, 308, 309f
    adaptive effectiveness and, 312-315
    environmental scanning system and, 310f
    issues addressed for, 309-310
    planning and, 308-310, 310f
    recovery/salvage stage and, 310-311, 311f
    systems evaluation and, 312-315, 313f
  strategic core, 288, 289f

synthesizing external and internal factors, 287–288
team outcomes, 290–291, 291f
team performance, 289–290, 290f
team process factors, 293–299, 293f
    competence, 293f, 294–295, 295f
    goals, 294, 294f
    resources, 296–297, 296f
    results, 298–299, 299f
    work demands, 297–298, 297f
understanding, 274
user expectations, 292–293
critical events, impact on outcomes, 299
critical listening, 348–349
critical questioning, 349–350, 350 (exhibit 8-5)
critical thinking, 351
C-suite leaders, 158–159, 159 (exhibit 4-7), 160f
CT scanners, 81
cultural changes in problem solving, 539
    making problem-solving deadlines irrelevant, 539
    refusing to reward firefighting, 539
    rejecting patching as problem-solving approach, 539
culture
    historic focus of work, 141 (exhibit 4-2)
    hopeful, 557
    identity-based conflicts and, 230
    and innovation, 140–141
    leadership and, 463–464
    negative side effects, 140
    point of service and, 64
    positive, transition to, 603
    toxicity and, 461–462
customer expectations, teams and, 292–293
cybernetic (s), 276, 279
    and interacting environmental scanning process, 300–301, 300f
    interface of evidence and innovation, 117f
cycle of vulnerability, 331–343, 332f
    becoming vulnerable, 332–333
    beginning the cycle again, 342–343
    cherishing the new knowledge gained, 341
    course corrections, 341
    evaluating the results, 339–341
    living the new reality, 338–339
    rational risks and negative fantasies, 335–337
    stages of, 331 (exhibit 8-2)
    stretching one's capacity, 338
    taking risks, 333–335
cynicism, 465

D

damage assessment, 311
Darwin, Charles, 85
data-based conflicts, 250–251
DCTM. *See* dynamic cybernetic team model
deadlines, for problem-solving, 539
de Chardin, T., 614
decision, and structures, 143–147
decisional control, innovation and, 144 (exhibit 4-5)
decision making, 618
    information and, 26

innovative organization, 143
mosaic of, in system, 83, 83 (exhibit 2-5)
open communication and, 353
point of service and, 147–149
style, team members and, 438
vertical structures and, 467
decision tree, process design, 5f
deep breathing, 605, 605 (exhibit 11-3)
deep listening, 615
deliberation, 27, 593
demeanor, of mediators, 258
department leaders, crisis, environmental scanning and, 304
dependency model, 533
developing skills, rational risks and, 336
developmental freeze, 396
devil's advocate, acting as, 442
dialogue
    conflict resolution and personal ownership of, 222
    differences and, 231
    open communication and, 353
differences
    dialogue and, 231
    finding, identity-based conflict and, 235–236
differentiation between parties, identity-based conflicts and, 243
Digital Age. *See* Industrial Age
digital world, 120
dignity, identity-based conflicts and need for, 230
directed creativity, 118
direction, 594
disaster, 274
    planning, 308
discernment, 27, 594
discipline, 557f, 560
    creativity and, 594
    and leader's willingness, 553
    remediation *vs.*, 384–385
disclosure, 380–381
discontinuance, 124
disenchantment discontinuance, 124
disenfranchisement, workers, hope for, 561
disequilibrium, equilibrium and, 79–82
dishonesty, inconsistency and, 476–477
disruptive innovation, 107, 115
disruptive technologies, 139, 140 (exhibit 4-1)
dissipative leadership, 420–421
dissipative structures, 14
distributors, syndication and, 356
diversity
    intolerance toward, 470
    as necessity of life, 71–72
    valuing, 343–344
dogma
    brick wall, removing, 561–564
    strategies for minimizing of, 564
Dossey, Barbara, 551
Dossey, Larry, 551
double-loop learning, 514

Index   637

downsizing, 477, 483
  of leaders, 570
Dreyfus, H. L., 439
Dreyfus, S. E., 439
Drucker, Peter, 5, 30
Druskat, V. U., 437
dyadic model of leadership, emergent model of leadership *vs.*, 420
dynamic adaptation, learning and, 515
dynamic cybernetic team model (DCTM), 284–285, 284*f*, 309*f*
dynamic systems, 88
dysfunctional behaviors, principles for minimizing, 481 (exhibit 11–5)

E

Edison, Thomas, 619
education programs, 114
effective adaptability, 513
efficacy, identity-based conflicts and need for, 230
egalitarian organizational structures, creating, 529
ego, quantum leadership and absence of, 328
Einstein, Albert, 74
electronic health record, 106, 108, 195
electronic medical record, 301–302, 305
Elizabeth I, 349
embarrassment, minimizing feelings of, 375
emergence, healthcare systems, 190*t*, 194–196
Emerson, Ralph Waldo, 53
emotion, 423 (exhibit 10–1)
emotional competence
  advanced beginner stage, 440 (exhibit 10–3), 441
  behavioral assessment categories, 424*t*
  competent stage, 440 (exhibit 10–3), 441
  developing, 439–442
  expert stage, 440 (exhibit 10–3), 441–442
  interviewing for, 436 (exhibit 10–2)
  measuring, 447–448
  nature of, 422–432
    compassion, 426–427
    impulse control, 430–431
    knowledge appreciation, 425–426
    mindfulness, 428
    nonverbal emotional competence, 428
    openness to new ideas, 425
    passionate optimism, 428–429
    passion through balance, 429–430
    presence, 427
    resilience, 429
    self-awareness, 424–425
  novice stage, 440 (exhibit 10–3), 441
  principles, 422
  proficient stage, 440 (exhibit 10–3), 441
  underpinnings of, 419–422
    dissipative leadership, 420–421
    holism, 419
    integrated leadership, 421–422
    intrinsic motivation, 419–420
emotional intelligence, 431–432
emotionally incompetent behaviors, 442–443

emotional mastery, 570
emotional risks of leadership, 433–434
  employment insecurity, 434
  inconsistent feedback, 433
  lack of feedback, 433
empathy, 431, 560. *See also* compassion
employees. *See also* workers
  meeting needs of, 566
  productivity, myths and truths about, 568 (exhibit 13–3)
  revitalizing lost passion of, 568
  satisfaction surveys, 448
  workgroup, 141, 145
employment insecurity, 434
empowering employees principle, 484–485
empowerment, issues of, 15
endless change, 10–14
energy, 481, 557*f*, 558, 560
  complexity, chaos and, 81
  examining behaviors related to, 562
engagement, in health care, 417
environmental scanning, 305*f*
  crisis and, 304–308
  recovery/salvage and, 311*f*
  signals and, 306–308, 306*f*
  systems evaluation and, 313*f*
  triggers, 307–308, 307*f*
equilibrium, disequilibrium and, 79–82
equity
  conflict management and, 221, 227
  and partnership, 142–143
errors and failures. *See also* medical errors; mistakes
  context creation for safety, 372–373
  defined, 374 (exhibit 9–1)
  essential to creation, 72–74
  evidence-based practice, 382
  failure to rescue, 395, 396
  in healthcare leadership
    dehumanization of healthcare providers, 394
    demanding the impossible, 402–403
    developmental freeze, 396
    failure to own healthcare products, 391
    failure to shift to value-based healthcare services, 386–387
    fragmented leadership, 393
    hiring bonuses, 396–397
    living accountability, 392
    revaluing healthcare providers, 397–401
    staffing by ratios, 395–396
    work force reductions, 394–395
  in healthcare service, 379–383
  just culture, 373–375
  leadership, 383–385
  learning, 375–376
  management, summary on, 404–405
  marketplace, 387
  mistakes *vs.*, 73 (exhibit 2–3)
  as opportunity approach, 385
  patient-centered care, 383
  recognizing and recovering from, 378–379, 378 (exhibit 9–5)

staffing levels and, 395
system *vs.* individual, 373–374
teamwork, 376–381
   communication, 379–380
   disclosure, 380–381
   expecting perfection, 377, 377 (exhibit 9–4)
   healthcare providers, failures and error, 378–379
   honoring excellence, 377–378
   mandatory error reporting, 380
tolerating, 442
two strategies for handling of, 377 (exhibit 9–4)
ethical issues, disclosure, 381
ethnicity, identity-based conflicts and, 240
evaluating results, 339–341
evidence, inconsistent use of, 189–192
evidence-based practice, 67
   errors and failures and, 382
   team outcomes and, 290–291
evidence-based processes, 117–118
evidence-based staffing, 397–401
evidentiary leadership, 187–207
evolution
   of each other, 594
   and revolution, 510–511
   revolution *vs.*, 84
evolutionary change, 90
excellence
   honoring, 377–378
   outcomes and, 291
executive leaders, 159
   challenging for, 62
   change dynamic and, 277
exercising the spirit, 604–607, 604 (exhibit 14–2)
experimentation
   change and, 87
   by talented people, 530
experts
   conflict resolution and use of, 259
   stages
      in emotional competence development, 440 (exhibit 10–3), 441–442
      team emotional competence, 443–444 (exhibit 10–4), 445
exploitation, leaders and, 88
exploration, 592
   change and, 87
   leaders and, 88
external communication, 380
external forces
   change and, 301–302
   strategic core and, 288
externalization/internalization, 301–303, 302f
external oversight, moving from, to internal accountability, 391

F
facilitating, 419
facilitators
   knowing what people want, 236
   leaders as, 223

trust building and, 236
failure
   common causes of, 125 (exhibit 3–8)
   and errors. *See* errors and failures
   to manage unmotivated employees, 471–473
   strategies to increase success and avoid, 125 (exhibit 3–8)
   to thrive, 513
fallibility, 332
False Claims Act, 337
family, identity-based conflicts and, 230
faulty situations, correcting, 418
fear, 556–558
   of being wrong, overcoming, 599–601
   and failure, 600
   overcoming, 600 (exhibit 14–1)
federal regulations, 552
feedback
   giving to CEO, 439
   inconsistent, 433
   lack of, 433
female leaders, challenges related to work-life balance for, 477–478
fiber optics, 8
financial resources, clinical decision making and, 386
financing, implementing ideas and, 529–530
"firefighting"
   eliminating, 537–539
   mindset, 534
   refusing to reward, 539
first-line leaders, 159–162
   defined, 159
   role of, 161
fiscal accountability, 387
fit, systems theory and, 59. *See also* goodness-of-fit
fixed payment systems, 391
flexibility
   borderland of chaos and, 282
   of internal environment, 302
   plan, 298
fluidity, 2
   compression of time and, 36
   contextual/strategic role of board, 155–158
   of internal environment, 302
focused goal setting, 608 (exhibit 14–4), 609–610
Follett, Mary Parker, 346
foolproof elasticity formula, 192
forethought, 485
fractals, 15
   organizations and, 15, 27
fragmented leadership, 393
framing issues, related to conflicts, 235
fraud, 391
fruitfulness, healthcare work and, 569 (exhibit 13–4)
fundamental problems, working on first, 536
funding, implementing ideas and, 529–530
future
   developing charter for, 525
   state mapping, 118

G

game playing, team-based conflict and, 228
GDP. *See* Gross Domestic Product
gender, identity-based conflicts and, 240
generations of workers, connecting with, 446–448
generation X worker, 447
generation Y worker, 447
genetic (s), 9
    profiling, 18
genomics, 9, 11, 17, 85
geographical information system (GIS) model, 201
George, B., 330
germ theory, 17
globalization, 9
global/unity consciousness, 480 (exhibit 11-4)
goals
    congruence between, 223–224
    team process factor, 293*f*, 294
goal setting, 570
    focused, 608 (exhibit 14-4), 609–610
Goleman, D., 431
goodness-of-fit, 16, 78, 505, 521
    internal forces and, 302
    issues, opportunities, and, 385
    leaders and, 59
    living the new reality and, 338–339
    organizations and achievement, 300
    results and, 298
    systems evaluation and, 312
    team performance and, 288
    thriving and, 277
good will, 556
governance level in health systems, 64
government regulations, 574
grasping, 484
great leaders, 588
Gross Domestic Product (GDP), 188
group identity and efficacy, 437
groupthink, minimizing, 484
growth
    conflict and, 220–222
    mistakes as tools of, 600
guilt, shame and, 385

H

Hammarskjöld, Dag, 587
handheld digital device, 81
handwritten calendar, 123 (exhibit 3-6)
happiness, 516
harnessing complexity, process of, 82
Harvard Business Review, 328
Hawking, Stephen, 38, 54
HCAHPS survey, 191 (exhibit 5-1)
healing, 461, 479
healthcare, 17
    benefits of emotional competence in, 434–439
        coaching upward and, 439
        focused hiring, 435–436
        higher productivity, 437–438
        improved succession planning, 436–437
    as both risk adverse and conflict adverse, 222
    challenges, 111 (exhibit 3-1)
    collective mindfulness in, 352
    conflict resolution and effectiveness of, 259
    early-engagement, 18–19
    example of disruptive innovation, 115
    external forces and, 301–302
    identity-based conflicts and, 229
    innovation, rationale for, 108–115
    leaders, 11, 12, 17
        compression of time and, 36
        conflict resolution and, 259
        dialoguing about failures with, 379
        finding value of healthcare services and, 387–388
        mandatory reporting and, 380
        revitalizing lost passion of employees and, 568
        revolutionary changes and, 86
    leadership, 344–345
        issues and opportunities, 385–403
    local nature of, 63–66
    methods of delivery, 109
    organizations, increasing political competence within, 573
    outcomes, measurement of, 567
    potential for conflict in, 243
    products, failure to own, 391
    professions
        fluid boundaries and, 62
        goals of, 19
        productivity issues and, 568
    value-driven, leader, 20 (exhibit 1-7)
    virtual, services, 120
healthcare providers, 6
    dehumanization of, 394
    demanding impossible from, 402–403
    finding value of healthcare services and, 387–388
    revaluing, 397–401
healthcare services
    decisional structures, positional control, 144 (exhibit 4-5)
    determining value of, 387–388
    historical culture of, 141
    rewarding value-adding behaviors in, 488–489
    values in, 166
healthcare systems
    Chief Data Officer, 199
    complex system
        connectivity, 194
        emergence, 194–196
        interdependence, 194
    current valuation model, issues in
        cost, 188
        cost shifting, 188–189
        demand without accountability, 189
        evidence, inconsistent use of, 189–192
        partial measurement, 189–192
    errors and, 371–372
    funding, 189
    qualitative information in, 190
    transformed valuation model for. *See* valuation model

health services, deconstruction of, 37
health structure, functional components of, 35f
health systems
    adaptive effectiveness and, 312
    complex, view of, 82f
    disaster planning by, 308
    recovery/salvage stage of crisis preparedness and, 310
    strong service core and, 303
    systems evaluation and, 313
healthy organizations, characteristics of, 460–461
heritage, identity-based conflicts and, 230
hidden agendas, team-based conflicts and, 228
hidden information, interest-based conflict resolution and looking for, 256
hierarchical control, 20
high-reliability organization (HRO), 333
high-reliability processes, 114
hiring
    bonuses, 396–397
    focused, 435–436
Hock, Dee, 355
holism, 419
Holmes, Oliver Wendell, 105
hologram, 15, 78
holographic leadership, 393–394
holography, 15
homogeneity, 71
honest feedback, 433
hope, 461, 471, 552–553, 561
    for future, five essential qualities of will leading to, 557f
hopelessness, 473
horizontal linkage, 76
horizontal relationships, accountability and, 529
horizontal thinking, 61
hospitals
    adaptive effectiveness and, 312
    disaster planning by, 308
    mandatory overtime in, 395
    patient safety tips for, 382 (exhibit 9-6)
    radical transformation of, 86
    recovery/salvage stage of crisis preparedness and, 310
    strong service core and, 303–304
    systems evaluation and, 313
hours per patient day (HPPD), 191
HRO. *See* high-reliability organization
Huang, C. A., 478
human error, 384
human organizations, adaptive capacity in, 280–282
human relations school, 77
human resource focus, 280–282
human systems, 170
humility, 424

I
"I" approaches, conflict resolution and, 226
idea
    financing and implementation of, 529–530
    new, openness to, 425
identifying what-ifs, 118
identity, characteristics of, 232 (exhibit 6-2)
identity-based conflicts, 218, 222, 226, 229–245
    action, 243–245
    antagonism, 237–239
    ARIA, 236
    finding differences, 235–236
    giving parties voice, 231–233
    interest-based conflicts *vs.*, 231
    invention, 241–243
    knowing what people want, 236
    resonance, 239–241
    time and patience, 233
    trust building, 233–234
ignorance, compensations of, 617–619
imagery, of complexity, 620
imbalance, between work and personal life, 477–478
implanted defibrillators, 118
impulse control, 430–431
    higher productivity and, 437
    measuring emotional competence of teams and, 447
incompetence, 442
inconsistency
    and dishonesty, 476–477
    feedback, 433
incremental innovations, 115
individual emotional competence skill levels, behaviors and, 440 (exhibit 10-3)
individuals, characteristic behaviors in, 119
Industrial Age, 8f, 9, 22, 24, 588
    assessments of value in, 66
    in-control leaders during, 326
    leadership, 3, 22, 78
    and orientation towards, 66
    perception of vulnerability in leaders during, 327
    work in, 3
inequitable reward and recognition practices, 468–469
informal network, pay attention to, 30–31
information, 9
    conflicts, 225f
    decision making and, 26
    exchange, conflict resolution and, 258–259
    importance of, 55
    overload, dealing with, 349
    team-based conflict and role of, 228
    technology, 109
Information Age, 8, 55
    balancing use of time during, 571
    critical questioning in, 349
    relationships in, 344f
inner child, spending time with, 598
inner power. *See* will
innovation
    alignment, 149–154
    balancing with value, 166–167
    board, contextual role of, 155–158, 162 (exhibit 4-8)
    borderland of chaos and, 282
    business case, essential components of, 204–205
    capacity for rational risk taking, 120–121
    "circle of innovation," 145, 146f
    coaching, 527–531

innovation (*Continued*)
    allowing people to share in fruits of their creativity, 530
    be clear about who you are, 528
    creating egalitarian organizational structure, 529
    exposing staff to different messages and messengers, 529
    letting the talented experiment, 530
    put money where the ideas are, 529–530
    treating transformation as a mission, not a job, 528–529
  course corrections, 124
  creativity and, 594–603
  cross-fertilization of, 112
  C-suite leaders, 158–159, 159 (exhibit 4–7)
  cultural context, 140
  decisional control, 144 (exhibit 4–5)
  decision and structures, 143–147
  descriptions of, 167
  differentiating roles in, 167–170
  disruptive, 139
  equity and partnerships, 142–143
  evidence-based processes, 117–118
  first-line leader, 159–162
  forum for priority management, 168 (exhibit 4–10)
  infrastructure, 145
  label *vs.* role, 115–125
  leadership, 170–171. *See also* leadership
  locus of control, 144
  management-driven control, 144
  measurement, barriers to effective, 124 (exhibit 3–7)
  and membership community, 164–166
  metrics and evaluation strategies, 122–124
  motivation and, 149
  operationalizing, 116
  organizational network
    contextual role of, 155–158
    leaders and, 148
    nodes and links, 148–149*f*
  point of service, 147–149
  quantum leader, 110–111
  safety in, 163
  senior team, 159
  stakeholder value, creating, 154–155, 155*f*
  supporting, 116
  time for reflection and idea generation, 118–119
  uncommon partnerships, formation of, 121
  value of anomaly, 119–120
  valuing multiple intelligences, 118
  as way of life, 527
  in workplace, 152–153
innovators, 119
  organizational support, 162–164
insight, 587
inspiration, work of, 111
Institute for Healthcare Improvement, 383
Institute of Medicine (IOM), 188, 380, 385
  To Err Is Human goals, 380
institutional model, 77
institutions, systems *vs.*, 60 (exhibit 2–2)

insulin pumps, 118
integrated leadership, 421–422
  components of, 435
integration, 66
  elements of, 532 (exhibit 12–5)
  evidence of, 66
  making it work, 532–534
integrity, 89, 331, 431, 432, 520, 587
  of systems, 78
intellectual capital, 343
intelligence (s), 118
  defined, 423 (exhibit 10–1)
  emotional, 431–432
intentionality, 596, 610
intentional rule violations, 384
interaction
  conflicts, 225*f*
  issues of, 15
interconnected Internet accessed calendar, 123 (exhibit 3–6)
interconnectedness, 14, 592
interdepartmental tension, 574
interdependence, 23 (exhibit 1–10), 75 (exhibit 2–4), 241, 532 (exhibit 12–5)
  healthcare system, 190*t*, 194
interdisciplinary forum, development of, 168
interest-based conflicts, 218, 225*f*, 245–257
  beginning resolution process, 254*f*, 255–256
  building trust and communication, 254*f*, 255
  constructing initial database, 254*f*, 255
  data-based conflicts, 250–251
  defining concerns and setting priorities, 254*f*, 256
  developing strategies to guide process, 254*f*, 255
  establishing initial relationship, 254*f*, 255
  finding potential solutions and presenting to parties involved, 254*f*, 256
  formalizing agreement, 254*f*, 256
  identity-based conflicts *vs.*, 231
  isolating interest-based conflicts, 251–253
  keeping process on track, 256–257
  looking for hidden information, agendas, and interest, 254*f*, 256
  organizing plan for mediation, 254*f*, 255
  relationship-based conflicts, 246–247
  resolution process, 252*f*
  structure-driven conflicts, 249–250
  ten steps for resolution of, 253, 254*f*
  types of, 246
  values-based conflicts, 247–249
interests, identity-based conflicts and, 242
internal accountability, moving from external oversight to, 391
internal forces
  change and, 302
  strategic core and, 288
internalization and externalization, 301–303, 302*f*
internal stakeholders, 121
Internet, 17, 80, 108, 109, 573
  healthcare and, 86

interaction, 2
syndication and, 357
interoperable systems, 66
interpersonal intelligences, 118 (exhibit 3-4)
intersections, systems thinking and, 32
interviewing, focused hiring and, 435–436
intolerance toward diversity, abuse of power, 470
intrinsic motivation, 419–420
intuitive, rational integrated with, 25
invention, identity-based conflicts, 241–243
IOM. *See* Institute of Medicine
irrational risk, 121
isolating interest-based conflicts, 251–253
"I" statements, identity-based conflict resolution and, 240

J
James, William, 139
job candidates, for dysfunction principle, screening, 487
job holders, career seekers *vs.*, 566
Jobs, Steve, 271
Johnson, Cedric, 569
The Joint Commission, 380
journaling, 598
"journeying," leaders and, 40
journey of spirit, 609*f*
judgment, 27, 611–612
  leadership, 332

K
Kellner-Rogers, M., 187, 338
Keynes, John Maynard, 1
kindness, 464
kinesthetic intelligences. *See* bodily intelligences
knowledge, 619
  appreciation, 425–426
  cherishing, 341
  complexity and, 32
  management of, 55
  nursing profession and, 141
  as power, 329
  as utility, 55
  workers, 164
knowledge-based digital world, transformation to, 108
knowledge workers, 3
  emergence of, 75
know thyself principle, 481–482
koans, 618
Kouzes, J. M., 343
Kurtsman, J., 330

L
label innovation *vs.* role innovation, 115–125
lack of respect, for workforce, 470–471
language
  conflict resolution and use of, 226
  expectations/obligations, appreciative leader and, 519
  identity-based conflicts and, 230
lasers, 17
LASIK surgery, 35
layoffs, 397

leadership presence and, 427
mental fitness and, 570–571
leaders, 139, 503–504, 505. *See also* quantum leaders
  accountability of, 116
  in advancing work of innovation, 112
  agents of change, 87
  assess functional proficiency of individual workers, 16
  authenticity, 329–331
  aware of professionals, 23
  behavior, 10
  building strong service core and, 303–304
  challenges around toxic situations faced by, 459
  change and effectiveness, 38–40
  cocreators, 593
  companionship for growth and, 611
  complexity harnessed by, 81
  compression of time and, 35
  conflict management skills for, 222
  confronting the core negativity within, 601–603
  courageous, 558
  cycle of vulnerability and, 332–343
  decision-making styles of, 120
  development of will by, 554
  downsizing of, 570
  driving concerns of, 68
  energy, flow of change and, 81
  error and, 73
  experimentation and, 30, 87
  as facilitators, 223–224
  failure as evaluative mechanism, 600
  focused hiring of, 435–436
  goodness-of-fit, 59
  great, 588
  healthcare, 11, 12, 17
  innovation skills, 161
    alignment, 149–154
    C-suite roles, 158–159, 159 (exhibit 4-7), 160*f*
    equity, 142 (exhibit 4-3)
    equity and partnerships, 142–143
    first-line manager, 159–162
    locus of control, 144
    management, role in, 164
    motivation, 149–154
    point of service, 147–149
    stakeholder value, 154–155
    value, 166
  innovative, titles, 115 (exhibit 3-3)
  "journeying" and, 40
  mental fitness among, 570–571
  mindfulness, 596
  mission and purpose, 167, 168*f*
  motivated *vs.* unmotivated, 39 (exhibit 1-12)
  new models of, 21–23
  open communication and, 223
  perception of crisis, 273–274
  planning and, 24–25
  politically competent, 573
  productive conflict management by, 224–227
  professional antagonism and role of, 565
  resiliency in, 335

leaders (*Continued*)
  responsibility, 37
  as revolutionaries, 524–527
    be strategic and patient, 525–526
    building the conspiracy, 525
    creating argument for revolution, 524–525
    developing a charter for the future, 525
    ensuring that small successes occur early and often, 526
    seeking out significant champions, 526
  risk-disposed, 335
  role, 10–11, 27
  self-awareness/self-confidence, 519
  self-exploration, 554
  of service systems, 84
  as signpost readers, 57
  spiritual workouts, 604–605
  strategic crisis management and, 282
  team construction and, 290
  team performance and, 289–290
  as transformational agents, 511
  of vertically structured organizations, 467
  vulnerability in, 327–328
  whole system orientation and, 69
  willing, 551
    attributes of, 561 (exhibit 13-2)
  work-personal life balancing strategies and, 571–572
leadership, 504. *See also* opportunities in healthcare leadership
  in accountability-based organizations, 511–516
  adaptive capacity, change and, 38, 277–279
  agility, 570
  appreciative, 517–519
  and balance, 26–28
  change in, 7
  chaos and call to, 588–591
  compassionate, 426–427
  compression of time, 35–38
  context of, 19–21
  culture and, 463–464
  definitions and concepts update, 107–108
  dissipative, 420–421
  effectiveness, 38–40, 421*f*
  emergent, 420
  emotional competence, 419–434
  emotional risks of, 433–434
  endless change, 10–14
  errors and failures, 383–385
  fitness, in new millennium, 326–327
  fragmented, 393
  healthcare, 344–345
  healthcare innovation, rationale for, 108–115
  holographic, 393–394
  in Industrial Age, 3, 22
  and innovation, 170–171
  innovation label *vs.* innovation role, 115–125
  journey of transformation and, 611
  judgment, 332, 334
  leading in post-digital age, 5–7
  mystery and, 619–620
  Newton and organizational design, 4–5
  organization, goal of, 27
  postdigital, 8–10
  potential reality and, 7
  and professional governance, 105–108
  quantum character of, 14–35
  quantum leader and innovation, 110–111
  risk and, 618
  role, complexity and impact on, 53
  spiritually aware, 590
  transformational, 479
  vulnerability, 327 (exhibit 8-1)
    strategies for cultivation of, 353
  in world of constant movement, 2–4
learning, 33
  continuing, 564–565
  double-loop, 514
  error's role in, 73
  fostering, 513
  leaders and requirements for, 516–517
  organization, 511–516
  shared accountability for, 402
  single-loop, 514
  transformational, cycle of, 535*f*
  triple-loop, 514
leisure, 478
Lencioni, P., 331
life spans, increasing, 63
life-threatening errors, 73
Lincoln, Abraham, 503
"line and box" approach, to workplace configuration, 5*f*
linear thinking, 14
  vs. collateral thinking, 75 (exhibit 2-4)
linguistic intelligence, valuing of, 118 (exhibit 3-4)
listening
  active, 258
  content, 615 (exhibit 14-6)
  contextual, 615 (exhibit 14-6)
  for sounds of change, 614–616
  suffering silence and, 425
living the new reality, 338–339
local changes, revolution and aggregation of, 85–90
locus of control, 144
Longest, Beaufort, 392
longevity, exercise and, 604
lower levels of innovations, 115
loyalty, redefining notion of, 566
Lundin, K., 466, 480
Lundin, W., 466, 480
Lynch, J., 478

M

Machiavelli, N., 558
malpractice suits, disclosure and, 381
"mama" syndrome, 538
mandatory overtime, 395
  abuse of power, 470
mandatory reporting
  error, 380
  rational risks and, 336–337

Mandelbrot sets, art of, 616
Marion, R., 59
Marx, D., 384
Maslow's hierarchy, team-based conflict and, 228
mathematical intelligence, valuing of, 118 (exhibit 3–4)
mature workers, 447
measurement, of health care outcomes, 567
measures of success, change and, 79
mediation, organizing plan for, 255
mediators
  demeanor of, 258
  interest-based conflict resolution and, 255
medical errors
  disclosure and, 380–381
  external communication, 380
  patient safety and, 373
  staffing levels and, 395
medical therapies, old therapies *vs.* new therapies, 12 (exhibit 1–4)
meditation, 593, 598
meeting places, conflict resolution process and, 258
membership communities, 164–166
  rights and obligations, 165
  role in innovation, 164–166
  systems as, 89
  transforming, 503–504
    evolution and revolution, 510–511
    lack of time, dealing with, 520–524
    leaders as revolutionaries, 524–527
    learning organization, 511–516
    from responsibility to accountability, 504–507
    transformation, organizing for, 516–520
    work and worker, transforming, 508–510
mental boundaries, 346
mental imagery, 570
mentoring, 419
  emotional competence and, 437
  of employees in vulnerable risk-taking behaviors, 342
  toxic, 475–476
mentorship of new members, 165 (exhibit 4–9)
metrics, 405
  and evaluation strategies, 122–124
    guidelines for selection of, 122 (exhibit 3–5)
  of value-based health care, 388–389
micromanipulation, 9
micronization, 11
Middle Ages, 8
millennial nurses, 464–466
mindfulness, 428, 596, 597*f*, 610
mind mapping, 118, 200–201
miniaturization, 9
mission
  innovation-based, 112 (exhibit 3–2)
  strong focus on, 303–304
mistakes
  defined, 374 (exhibit 9–1)
  errors *vs.*, 73 (exhibit 2–3)
  as tools of growth, 600
model building, 118
modesty, union of willfulness and, 425

momentum, conflict resolution and maintenance of, 243
motivated leaders, unmotivated *vs.*, 39 (exhibit 1–12)
motivation, 149–154, 431, 569
  elements of, 151 (exhibit 4–6)
  intrinsic, 419–420
  team members and, 438
multiple perspectives, 484
musical intelligences, 118 (exhibit 3–4)
mutuality, 464
mystery, 619–620

N

nanotechnology, 109
national differences, identity-based conflicts and, 239, 240
National Quality Forum (NQF), 381
natural tensions, recognition of, 113–115
needs, identity-based conflicts and, 242
needs-resources gap as a team, management of, 403
negative emotions, tempering, 430
negative fantasies, rational risks and, 335–337
negative outcomes, recommendations related to, 340
negativity, confronting core of, 601–603
negligence, 384
net income margin, 388
net present value, 388
new age
  characteristics, organizational levels and, 87*f*
  new rules for, 17–18
New Age imperatives, 17 (exhibit 1–6)
new millennium, leadership fitness in, 326–327
new relationships, 343–347
  healthcare leadership inclusivity, 344–345
  opportunities for change, 345
  privacy, 345–346
  relationship skills, 347
  self-disclosure, 347
  valuing diversity, 343–344
Newton, Isaac, 19, 74
Newtonian characteristics, 20 (exhibit 1–8)
Newtonian mechanics and organizational design, 4–5
Newtonian principles, 3
Newtonian science, deconstructing dogmas of, 563–564
Newtonian thinking, 21
Newtonian worldview, quantum leader's worldview *vs.*, 419
Nightingale, Florence, themes from writings of, 575
nimbleness, 303
noise, 280
  in patient care areas, 554
  therapeutic shifts and, 306
nonvalue-added services, eliminating, 389–390
nonverbal emotional competence, 428
normative crisis, 272–273
  early warning, 272–273
novice stage
  in emotional competence development, 440 (exhibit 10–3), 441
  team emotional competence, 443–444 (exhibit 10–4), 444

nurses
  adaptability an, 512
  conflict management skills for, 222
  leaders, burnout and, 570
  millennial, 464–466
  professional antagonism and, 565
  staffing, selected references on, 398–400 (exhibit 9-8)
  surveillance role played by, 395
nurse-to-patient ratios, patient needs and, 401
nursing
  and knowledge, 141
  public's view of, 551
  relighting the lamp and, 574–576
  shortages, 574

O

O'Keeffe, Georgia, 599
O'Leary-Kelly, A. M., 474
open communication
  collective mindfulness and, 353–355
  environment, 223
  preventing unnecessary conflict and, 223
open components, in systems, 76
open meeting laws
  basic principles of, 353 (exhibit 8-6)
  open communication model and, 353–355
openness, 337, 351, 597, 603
  to new ideas, 425
operationalizing innovation, 116
opportunities in healthcare leadership
  eliminating nonvalue-added services, 389–390
  holographic leadership, 393–394
  managing the needs-resources gap as a team, 403
  moving from external oversight to internal accountability
    living accountability, 391
    political competence, 392–393
  practice within the marketplace
    metrics of value-based health care, 388–389
    value description, 387–388
  revaluing healthcare providers as vital capital
    evidence-based staffing, 397, 401
    shared accountability for learning, 402
    staffing for patient needs, 401–402
  team-based health care, 390–391
opportunity
  for change, 345
  leadership as contract with, 593
optimism, passionate, 428–429, 435, 441, 447
order, chaos as route to, 593
organizational chart, 61
organizational learning theory, 281
organizational levels, new age characteristics and, 87f
organizational metrics, 122
organizational models, changing, 5f
organizational network
  contextual role of, 155–158
  leaders and, 148
  nodes and links, 148–149f
organizational syndication, 355

organizational toxicity, 465
  sources of, 467 (exhibit 11-1)
organizations, 383. *See also* toxic behaviors in organizations
  adaptive capacity in, 280–282
  commitment to innovation, 112
  complexity and, 276–277
  consciousness, 480 (exhibit 11-4)
  formal structure in, 30
  fractals and, 15, 27
  healthcare, reducing risk from errors, 74
  innovation behaviors into, 116
  leadership, goal of, 27
  learning, 511–516
  mechanisms in, 165 (exhibit 4-9)
  Newtonian thinking and, 19
  operationalizing innovation, 116
  orientation to outside information, team members and, 438
  patterns of relationships in, 21
  structure of, 27, 113
  of 21st century, 109
  view errors and negative outcomes, 120
organ printing, 9
Orsburn, J. D., 437
outcomes
  impact on, 299–301
  moving from responsibility to accountability and, 504–505
  team, 290–291, 291f
overtime
  family boundaries and, 346
  mandatory, 395
ownership, 520
  accountability and, 505
  issues of, 15

P

paradigmatic moment, 85
paradox, 29 (exhibit 1-11), 614, 617
  chaos and, 29–30
  courage and, 556
partnerships
  process factors, 293–299, 293f
  uncommon, formation of, 121
parts, within wholes, 59–63
passion, 481, 557f, 558
  examining behaviors related to, 562
  hope and, 553
  sustaining, 430
  through balance, 429–430
passionate feelings, conflict and expression of, 236
passionate optimism, 428–429, 435, 447
  higher productivity and, 437
  measuring emotional competence of teams and, 447
  proficient stage of emotional competence and, 441
patching, rejecting as a problem-solving approach, 539
patient care
  areas, "noise" in, 554
  compassionate, 427

delivery, 111 (exhibit 3–1)
    outcomes, provider accountability for contributions to, 566–567
    services, 117
patient-centered care
    and errors and failures, 383
patient needs, staffing for, 401–402
patient outcomes, selected references on, 398–400 (exhibit 9–8)
Patient Protection and Affordable Care Act, 386, 417, 567
patient-provider relationship, 18
patients
    and caregivers, engagement of, 202–203
    disclosure to, 380–381
    increasing focus on, 572–573
    locus of control shift, 18
    satisfaction surveys, 448
    support healing and healthy behaviors, 202
patient safety, 188
    medical errors and, 373
people and behavior, 257–259
    communication technique, 258
    demeanor, 258
    information exchange, 258–259
    meeting setting and schedule, 258
    use of experts, 259
perfection, expecting, 377, 377 (exhibit 9–4)
performance
    of appreciative leaders, 519–520
    feedback, lack of, 433–434
    optimizing, 569 (exhibit 13–4)
Performance Measurement Matrix, 340 (exhibit 8–4)
personal assessment, 482
personal boundaries, 346
personal calendar, creating and managing, 123, 123 (exhibit 3–6)
personal creativity, 596
personality, of teams, 289
personal journeys, 604
personal life
    balance between work and, 571–572
    imbalance between work and, 477–478
personal transformation, elements of, 531*f*
personal willingness, 552
pessimism, 429
pharmaceuticals, 86
pharmacotherapeutics, 17, 18
physical boundaries, 346
physicians
    adaptability and, 513
    disclosure by, 380–381
    role of, 140
place, conflict management and role of, 226–227
planning
    crisis preparedness and, 308–310, 310*f*
    for trajectory, 24–25
planning, organizing, leading, implementing, controlling, and evaluating (POLICE), 3
podcasting, 122
point of service

culture and, 64
decisions, in systems, 84–85
innovation and, 147–149, 148*f*
sustainability of service systems and, 83
systems design, 33, 34*f*
POLICE. *See* planning, organizing, leading, implementing, controlling, and evaluating
policymakers, healthcare leaders and, 110
political competence, 392–393
    achieving, 573–574
Polus, Tracy, 535
population model, 77
position elimination, planning for, 571 (exhibit 13–5)
positioning, identity-based conflict and, 234, 238
positive statements, 603
positive thinking, 570
possibility, leadership as contract with, 593
Postdigital Age, 588
    leading in, 5–7
postdigital leadership, 8–10
Post-it notes, 376
posturing, identity-based conflict and, 234, 238
potential reality, 7, 57
    actual reality *vs.*, 57 (exhibit 2–1)
power, 328–331
    knowledge as, 329
    quantum leaders and, 329
power issues, source of conflict, 229
    mutual appreciation, team integrity and lack of, 229
prayer, as leadership tool, 608 (exhibit 14–4), 610
predictive capacity, 57
presence, 427
priorities, interest-based conflict resolution and setting of, 256
privacy, 345–346
problem solving, 257, 536
    accountability and, 537
    cultural changes and, 539
    deadlines, irrelevancy of, 539
    selective, 536
    strategic approaches to, 538
    tactical methods in, 537
    tool chest, building, 539
process
    design, 5*f*
    factors for team, 293–299, 293*f*
productive accountability, 507
productivity
    fruitfulness *vs.*, 569 (exhibit 13–4)
    higher, 437–438
    value-based services and, 567
professional antagonism, minimizing, 565
professional governance, leadership and, 105–108
professional mandate, 143 (exhibit 4–4)
proficient stage
    in emotional competence development, 440 (exhibit 10–3), 441
    team emotional competence, 443–444 (exhibit 10–4), 445
projection, identity-based conflict and, 238–239

project management, 112
prospective payment systems, 460
proximity, 464
psychoneuroimmunology, 465
punishment, blame and, 373
punitive culture, transforming, 383
purpose
    identity-based conflicts and need for, 230
    person, and performance, triadic relationship between, 67
    strong focus on, 303–304

Q

quality, 388
    question as value question, reframing of, 567
quantum character, of leadership, 14–35
quantum characteristics, 21 (exhibit 1-9)
quantum leaders, 474, 486
    collective mindfulness and, 352
    continuing learning fostered by, 564
    cycle of vulnerability. *See* cycle of vulnerability
    deconstruction of dogmas and, 563–564
    emotional competence and, 419
    engagement and, 417
    honoring excellence and, 377–378
    and innovation, 110–111
    integrated leadership and, 421–422
    intrinsic motivation and, 419–420
    issues and opportunities, 385
    living accountability and, 392
    in new millennium, 327
    power and, 329
    relationship skills and, 347
    team-based health care and, 390
    time management and, 572
quantum leadership
    absence of ego and, 328
    theory, emergent leadership and, 420
quantum mechanics, interpretation of, 56
quantum science, 591
    complexity, chaos and, 15
quantum theorists, 589
quantum theory, 2, 5, 21, 53
    directing change and, 7
questions, asking better, 376 (exhibit 9-3)
quiet place, spiritual exercise and, 606–607

R

random error, 72
rapport, building, 422
rational, intuitive integrated with, 25
rational risks, negative fantasies and, 336–337
rational risk taking, capacity for, 120–121
rationing of healthcare services, 388
ratios, staffing by, 395–396
reaction, to identity-based conflicts, 240
reactive advocacy, gone awry, 478–479
read, ability to, 58
Reason, James T., 371
reckless conduct, 384

recognition, identity-based conflicts and need for, 230
recovery/salvage, crisis preparedness and, 310–311, 311*f*
redeployment programs, 487
redundancy approach, 74
reflective members, conflict resolution and, 228
reflective response, identity-based conflict and, 240
reflexes, identity-based conflict and, 240
reflexive reframing, 240, 244
regular spiritual reflection, 604
regulations, 573
reimbursement, 388
    dramatic changes in, 386
    policies, toxic situations and, 460
relational algorithms, 14
relational design, 5*f*
relationship-based conflicts, 246–247
relationships
    building, 534
    built on respect principle, 485–486
    complexity science and, 56
    consciousness, 480 (exhibit 11-4)
    in Information Age, 344*f*
    issues of, 15
    skills, 347
    sustainable, 534
relaxation, failing to balance work and, 442–443
relevance of change, concept of, 80
religion, identity-based conflicts and, 230, 240
reluctance, qualities associated with, 557 (exhibit 13-1)
remediation
    discipline *vs.*, 384–385
    guidelines, 384 (exhibit 9-7)
    techniques, 384
replacement discontinuance, 124
reputation assessment and management survey, 447 (exhibit 10-5)
resilience, 429, 464
    in leaders, 335
    measuring emotional competence of teams and, 447
resolution of problems, including people with necessary skills and power in, 536
resolve, 587
resonance, 239–241
resources
    dependent approach, 77
    team process factor, 296–297, 296*f*
responsibility
    moving from, to accountability, 504–507
    vs. accountability, 505 (exhibit 12-1)
retrospective payment systems, 387, 391
return on assets, 388
return on equity, 388
return on investment, 388
    value-based health care and, 567
revaluing healthcare providers, 397–401
revolution
    aggregation of local changes and, 85–90
    creating argument for, 524–525
    evolution and, 510–511
revolutionary change, 90

reward value-adding behaviors principle, 488–489
rigidity, human systems, 170
risk, 608, 618
risk-intensive errors, 73
risk taking, 326, 333–335, 335 (exhibit 8-3)
Robinson, S. L., 474
robotics, health care and, 86
root cause analysis (RCA), 375
Rothman, J., 229, 236
Russell, Peter, 430

S

safety
   defined, 374 (exhibit 9-1)
   identity-based conflicts and need for, 230
   in innovation, 163
scenario learning, 539
scenario planning, 201
schedule, conflict resolution process and, 258
Schrödinger, Erwin, 7
Schrödinger's box, 7
Schrödinger's cat, 56
scientific thinking, shifts in, 21
screening job candidates for dysfunction principle, 487
Secretan, Lance, 325, 342
selective problem solving, 536
self-actualization, 276
self-awareness, 424–425, 431, 595, 596
   higher productivity and, 437
   of leaders, 519
   measuring emotional competence of teams and, 447
self-confidence
   of leaders, 519
self-control, 431
self-discipline, 560, 587
   examining behaviors related to, 562
self-disclosure, 347
self-esteem consciousness, 480 (exhibit 11-4)
self-examination, 555
self-exploration, 418
   leader, 554
   will and, 554
self-knowledge, 594
self-management, creativity and, 591–594
self-perception, 614
self-referencing, 614
self-regulation, 431
   measuring emotional competence of teams and, 447
senior executives, 158
senior management, change dynamic and, 277
service, 389
   core, strong, 303–304
   decisions, in systems, 83
service systems
   function of structure in, 63
   value of, 83
sexual differences, identity-based conflicts and, 240
shame
   guilt and, 385
   minimizing feelings of, 375

shared leadership model, 484
signals, 306–308, 306f
sign-on bonuses, 396, 397
signpost readers, leaders as, 57
signpost reading, 24, 58
simple systems
   complex systems and make up of, 68–70
   linking to create complex systems, 31–33
simplicity
   complexity and, 31
   system, aggregation across, 70f
single-loop learning, 514
single-metric evaluation, disadvantage to, 122
skill development, rational risks and, 336
skillful will, 556
skill sets, new vs. old, 2 (exhibit 1-1)
slow-knowing, 477
social capital, importance of, 343
social cues, 474
socialization/internalization/combination, 288
social media, 8
social networking, 122
social skill, 431
social systems management, complexity science and, 276
spatial intelligences, 118 (exhibit 3-4)
specialization, increase in, 522
specificity, goal setting and, 294
spirit
   exercising, 604–607, 604 (exhibit 14-2)
   finding in chaos, 616–617
   journey of, 609f
   realms of, within chaos, 617f
spiritual boundaries, 346
spiritual centering, 587
spiritual cool-down, 605 (exhibit 11-3), 606–607
spiritual discipline, 588, 590
   cycle of, 589f
spiritual exercise
   developing an exercise routine, 604–605
   first 100 days, 607
   quiet place, 606–607
   routine for, 605 (exhibit 11-3)
   stretching the spirit within, 604
spiritual intelligence: ten rules of the road, 608–613, 608 (exhibit 14-4)
spiritual journey, requisites of, 608 (exhibit 14-5)
spiritual traditions, 378
spiritual warm-up, 605, 605 (exhibit 11-3)
stability, 89
   dynamic interaction, 79
   human systems, 170
   and innovation, 114
staff
   communicating new expectations to, 529
   reductions in, 395
staffing, 350
   evidence-based, 397, 401
   for patient needs, 401–402
   by ratios, 395–396
   shortages in, 552

stakeholders
    creating value, 154–155, 155*f*
    healthcare leaders and, 11
    networks of, 121
standardization, clinical professions and fear of, 291
state regulations, 552
statistics, 568
status quo, challenging, 334, 335, 390, 425
steady-state career prototype, 472
stereotypes, 601
    toxic, 475 (exhibit 11–3)
"straight line" approach, 530
strange attractors, 14, 57 (exhibit 2–1)
strategic approaches to problem solving
    building a problem-solving tool chest, 539
    prioritizing problems, 538
    using learning scenarios, 538–539
strategic core, 288, 289*f*
strategic crisis management, 282–285
strategic imperative, team outcomes and, 290
strategic model, 77
strategic partnerships, 121
strengthening the spirit, 605 (exhibit 11–3), 606
stress, 574
    conflict and, 257
stretching, 326
stretching one's capacity, 338
stretching the spirit, 604, 605–606, 605 (exhibit 11–3)
strong will, 556
structural conflicts, 224*f*
structure
    meaningful and motivating work environment and, 517
    necessary, putting in place, 534
    organizational, evaluation of, 112
    wholes and, 14–16
structure-driven conflicts, 249–250
subjective meanings into leadership data set, integration of, 425
success
    change and measures of, 79
    ensuring, 526
succession planning, improved, 436–437
suffering silence, 425
superior attitude, displaying, 442
suppression, 418
survival consciousness, 480 (exhibit 11–4)
survival of the fittest, 34
sustainability, 21, 32
sustainable relationships, 534
Sutcliffe, Kathleen, 429
syndication, collective mindfulness and, 355–357, 356*t*
syndicators, 357
synergy, synthesis and, 620
systemization, evidence of, 68
systemness, leaders and, 89
systems
    aggregation across, 70*f*
    change generated from center outward in, 82–85
    complexity, 111
    context of, 89*f*
    decisions, 83
    evaluation
        crisis preparedness and, 312–315, 313*f*
        strong, elements of, 314
    institutions *vs.*, 60 (exhibit 2–2)
    intersecting/interacting functions of, 74–78
    leader's role and purposes of, 64
    mosaic of decision making in, 83
    policy and documentation of, 165 (exhibit 4–9)
    vs. individual errors, 373–374
        comparison of individual and system accountability, 374 (exhibit 9–2)
        key concepts, 374 (exhibit 9–1)
systems-oriented dynamics of health care, 532
systems science, 75
systems theory, 276
    fit and, 59
systems thinking, intersections and, 33

T

tactical methods of problem solving, 537
    getting help from outside the circle, 537–538
    triaging problems, 538
    trying something new, 538
taking risks, 326, 333–335, 335 (exhibit 8–3)
talented people, experimentation by, 530
task interdependence, 474
Taylor, Frederick, 3
team-based approaches, to conflict resolution, 245
team-based conflict issues, 228–229
team-based decisions, in systems, 83 (exhibit 2–5)
team-based health care, 390–391
team-based synthesis, 314
team emotional competence, 443–444 (exhibit 10–4), 443–446
    advanced beginner stage, 443–444 (exhibit 10–4), 444
    causes of team dysfunction, 445–446
    competent stage, 443–444 (exhibit 10–4), 444
    expert stage, 443–444 (exhibit 10–4), 445
    novice stage, 443–444 (exhibit 10–4), 444
    proficient stage, 443–444 (exhibit 10–4), 445
team process factors, 293–299, 293*f*
    competence, 293*f*, 294–295, 295*f*
    goals, 293*f*, 294
    resources, 296–297, 296*f*
    results/impact, 298–299, 298*f*
    work demands, 297–298, 297*f*
teams
    competence and, 294–295
    dysfunction, causes of, 445–446
    innovation skills, assessing, 113
    needs-resources gap management by, 403
    outcomes, 290–291, 291*f*
    performance, 289–290, 290*f*
    successful change and, 89
teamwork, measures of, 201, 202 (exhibit 5–3), 202 (exhibit 5–4), 376–381
technology, 9
    change in, 55
    communication, 2

complexity and, 275–276
compression of time and, 35
healthcare challenges, 111 (exhibit 3-1)
transformation and, 16–17
theory Y style of management, 419
therapeutic shifts, "noise" and, 306
thriving systems, 276
time
    balancing use of, 571–572
    conflict management and role of, 226
    dealing with lack of, 520
    with inner child, 598
    for reflection and idea generation, 118–119
    resolution of identity-based conflicts and, 233
    work and compression, 35–38
To Err Is Human (IOM), 380
Toffler, Alvin, 417
tolerance of antisocial behavior, 473–474
Torbert, W. R., 328
toxic behaviors in organizations, 466–467
    abuse of power, 470
        intolerance toward diversity, 470
        mandatory overtime, 470
    failure to manage unmotivated employees, 471–473
    imbalance between work and personal life, 477–478
    inconsistency and dishonesty, 476–477
    inequitable reward and recognition practices, 468–469
    lack of respect for the workforce, 470–471
    reactive advocacy gone awry, 478–479
    ten principles for minimizing of, 480–489
        accountability principle, 488
        acting as agent of transformation principle, 486–487
        empowering employees principle, 484–485
        know thyself principle, 481–482
        relationships built on respect principle, 485–486
        rewarding value-adding behaviors principle, 488–489
        screening job candidates for dysfunction principle, 487
        value truth of the whole principle, 484
        walk the talk principle, 482–483
        willingness to listen principle, 483–484
    tolerance of antisocial behavior, 473–474
    toxic mentoring, 475–476
    vertical authority structure, 467–468
toxicity
    culture and, 461–462
    development, 462
    level of, 461
    minimizing, 487 (exhibit 11-7)
toxic mentoring, 475–476
toxic situations, challenges leading to, 459
toxic stereotypes, 475 (exhibit 11-3)
tradition, unquestioning adherence to, 563
traditional culture, 116
traditionalists, 447
transdermal medications, 118
transformation, 480 (exhibit 11-4), 592, 593
    causes of, 509 (exhibit 12-2)
    conflict and, 220–222
    evaluating, 88*f*
    of healthcare system, 54

to knowledge-based digital world, 108
    as mainstream activity, 526–527
    as a mission, not as a job, 528–529
    organizing for, 516–520
        critical value of appreciative leadership, 517–519
        personal and group stages on journey of, 540*t*
    process of, 509
    sheer complexity, 532
    technology and, 16–17
    timelessness of, 1
    universal cycle of, 8*f*
    universal dynamics of, 10*f*
transformational coaching, 511
    dealing with lack of time and, 520–524
    eliminating firefighting altogether, 537–539
        cultural changes, 539
        strategic approaches, 538
        tactical methods, 537
    evolution and revolution, 510–511
    hitting problems head on, 534–537
        be accountable for ensuring problems are solved, 536
        including people with necessary skills and power in problem resolution, 536
        solve problems selectively, 536
        work on the fundamental problems first, 536
    innovation coaching, 527–531
    leaders as revolutionaries, 524–527
        be strategic and patient, 525–526
        building the conspiracy, 525
        creating argument for revolution, 524–525
        developing a charter for the future, 525
        ensuring that small successes occur early and often, 526
        seeking out significant champions, 526
    learning organization, 511–516
    making integration work
        orchestrating the dynamics of change, 534
        putting necessary structure in place, 534
        relationship building, 534
        speeding up processes, 533–534
    making it work, 532–534
    making transformation the mainstream activity, 526–527
    from responsibility to accountability, 504–507
    transformation, organizing for, 516–520
        critical value of appreciative leadership, 517–519
    transforming work and transforming the worker, 508–510
transformational leadership, 479
transformational learning, cycle of, 535*f*
triaging problems, 538
trial and error, living the new reality and, 338
triggers, 307–308, 307*f*
triple-loop learning, 514
trust, 342, 347, 557*f*, 560
    building, interest-based conflict and, 255
    examining behaviors related to, 562
    higher productivity and, 437
    hope and, 553
    identity-based conflict and building of, 233–234

truth, 590
turnover, cost of, 435

U

Ueland, Brenda, 599
Uhl-Bien, M., 59
uncertainty, 391, 424, 589
    emotional effects of, 434
    as norm, 326
    sharing, 338
uncommon partnerships, formation of, 121
unemployment, 472
unilateral decision makers, whole organizations held hostage to, 69
uniqueness
    identity-based conflict and, 233
    resolving team-based conflict and recognition of, 228
unit decisions, in systems, 83
unit leaders, crisis, environmental scanning and, 305
universe
    chaos pervasive throughout, 590
    Newtonian view of, 589
    as place full of creative and transforming energy and mystery, 608 (exhibit 14-4), 610–611
unmotivated employees, failure to manage, 471–473
unmotivated leaders, motivated *vs.*, 39 (exhibit 1-12)
unquestioned beliefs, 563
user expectations, 292–293

V

vagueness, conflict management and avoidance of, 227
valuation model
    business case, creation of, 204–207
    course correction work, 204
    healthcare story, documentation of, 196–199
    patients and caregivers, engagement of, 202–203
    teamwork, 201–202, 202 (exhibit 5-3)
    tools for, complex quality problems
        GIS model, 201
        mind mapping, 200–201
        scenario planning, 201
value-adding behaviors principle, rewarding, 488–489
value-based health care
    failure to shift to, 386–387
    metrics of, 388–389
value-based services, providing, 566–569
value-driven healthcare leader, 20 (exhibit 1-7)
values
    of anomaly, 119–120
    centerpiece of service delivery, 66–68
    conflicts, 224*f*
    description of, 387–388
    identity-based conflicts and, 230
    innovation and, 112 (exhibit 3-2), 166–167
    outcomes and, 291
    stakeholder, 154–155, 155*f*
    team members and, 437
    teamwork, quantify, 201–202, 202 (exhibit 5-3), 202 (exhibit 5-4)
values-based conflicts, 247–249

"value truth of the whole" principle, 484
valuing diversity, 343–344
Varela, Francisco, 613
vertical authority structure, 467–468
vertical control, 21
vertical thinking, 61
victim attitude, 430
virtual healthcare services, 120
VISA International, 355
vision, innovation-based, 112 (exhibit 3-2)
vital signs, 421
volition, defined, 423 (exhibit 10-1)
vulnerability, 327, 601, 603
    becoming, 332–333
    cycle of. *See* cycle of vulnerability
    in leaders, 327–328, 327 (exhibit 8-1)

W

walk the talk principle, 482–483
Warner Brothers, 335
Watson, J., 576
Weick, Karl, 429
Weiss, Karen, 31
Wheatley, M. J., 187
whistleblowing, rational risks and, 337
"white lies of leadership" syndrome, 476
wholes, parts within, 59–63
whole systems
    thinking, linear thinking replaced by, 14
    view, 591
will, 553–561
    defined, 553
    essential qualities related to, 556–561, 557*f*
        courage, 556–558
        energy, 558, 560
        hope, 561
        nature of, 555–556
        passion, 558
        phases in discovery of, 553
        self-discipline, 560
        self-exploration of, 554
        trust, 560
        types of, 556
willfulness, union of modesty and, 425
willingness
    to listen principle, 483–484
    qualities associated with, 557 (exhibit 13-1)
    strategies for facilitating
        balancing the use of time, 571–572
        becoming mentally fit, 570–571
        becoming politically competent, 573–574
        continuing learning fostered by, 564–565
        increasing focus on patients, 572–573
        meeting employee needs, 566
        minimizing professional antagonism, 565
        providing value-based services, 566–569
        removing dogma brick wall, 561–564
willpower. *See* will
win-win conflict resolution, 243
wireless communication, 17

wireless technologies, 55–56
Wolff, S. B., 437
women's movement, history of nursing and, 221
work
    balance between personal life and, 571–572
    compression of time and, 35–38
    demands, team process factors, 297–298, 297*f*
    failing to balance relaxation and, 442–443
    imbalance between personal life and, 477–478
    in Industrial Age, 3
    life reality shift, 4 (exhibit 1–2)
    routines, resistance to changes in, 554
    transforming, 508–510
    value of, as function of outcome not process, 16
workers
    connecting with generations of, 446–448
    new type of, 3
    point-of-service, congruency and, 65
    transforming, 508–510
workforce
    composition of, 446
    lack of respect for, 470–471
    leaders and mental fitness of, 570–571
    reductions, 394–395
workplace
    confronting fear in, 600
    innovation in, 152–153